THE IDEA OF EPILEPSY

THE IDEA OF EPILEPSY

A MEDICAL AND SOCIAL HISTORY OF EPILEPSY IN THE MODERN ERA (1860–2020)

SIMON D. SHORVON

UCL Queen Square Institute of Neurology

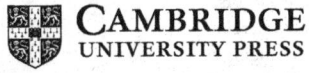

CAMBRIDGE
UNIVERSITY PRESS

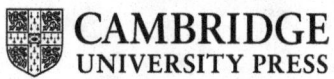

CAMBRIDGE
UNIVERSITY PRESS

Shaftesbury Road, Cambridge CB2 8EA, United Kingdom

One Liberty Plaza, 20th Floor, New York, NY 10006, USA

477 Williamstown Road, Port Melbourne, VIC 3207, Australia

314–321, 3rd Floor, Plot 3, Splendor Forum, Jasola District Centre, New Delhi – 110025, India

103 Penang Road, #05–06/07, Visioncrest Commercial, Singapore 238467

Cambridge University Press is part of Cambridge University Press & Assessment, a department of the University of Cambridge.

We share the University's mission to contribute to society through the pursuit of education, learning and research at the highest international levels of excellence.

www.cambridge.org
Information on this title: www.cambridge.org/9781108829519

DOI: 10.1017/9781108903684

First published 2023
First paperback edition 2024

A catalogue record for this publication is available from the British Library

Library of Congress Cataloging-in-Publication data
NAMES: Shorvon, S. D. (Simon D.), author.
TITLE: The idea of epilepsy : a medical and social history of epilepsy in the modern era (1860–2020) / Simon D. Shorvon.
DESCRIPTION: Cambridge, United Kingdom ; New York, NY : Cambridge University Press, 2023. | Includes bibliographical references and index.
IDENTIFIERS: LCCN 2022003648 (print) | LCCN 2022003649 (ebook) | ISBN 9781108842617 (hardback) | ISBN 9781108829519 (paperback) | ISBN 9781108903684 (ebook)
SUBJECTS: MESH: Epilepsy – history | History, 19th Century | History, 20th Century | History, 21st Century
CLASSIFICATION: LCC RC372.A1 (print) | LCC RC372.A1 (ebook) | NLM WL 11.1 | DDC 616.85/3–dc23/eng/20220323
LC record available at https://lccn.loc.gov/2022003648
LC ebook record available at https://lccn.loc.gov/2022003649

ISBN   978-1-108-84261-7   Hardback
ISBN   978-1-108-82951-9   Paperback

....

Every effort has been made in preparing this book to provide accurate and up-to-date information which is in accord with accepted standards and practice at the time of publication. Although case histories are drawn from actual cases, every effort has been made to disguise the identities of the individuals involved. Nevertheless, the authors, editors and publishers can make no warranties that the information contained herein is totally free from error, not least because clinical standards are constantly changing through research and regulation. The authors, editors and publishers therefore disclaim all liability for direct or consequential damages resulting from the use of material contained in this book. Readers are strongly advised to pay careful attention to information provided by the manufacturer of any drugs or equipment that they plan to use.

This book is dedicated to my wife Lynne and my son Matthew.

CONTENTS

PREFACE

This book has taken several years to research and write, and during this time I have been fortunate enough to have many friends and colleagues who have kindly commented on sections of the text and various drafts. I am especially grateful to Professor Walter van Emde Boas who read drafts of almost the entire work on more than two occasions and survived the process, made percipient and detailed suggestions and was exceptionally generous with his time; and also to Professor Matthew Walker, Professor Alastair Compston, Professor Reetta Kälviäinen, Professsor Eugen Trinka and Professor J. (Pete) Engel, all of whom were most helpful and insightful and corrected my grievous errors. My heartfelt thanks and deepest appreciation also go to my friend Ms Giselle Weiss, surely the best scientific editor in the world, who kindly read through the text in its various incarnations and made numerous suggestions with tact and grace, and with penetrating insight. I am also indebted to the truly exceptional UCL library services, which provided access to an extraordinary number of journals and books, archives and other material, without which the book could not have been written.

The artist David Cobley has had a long association with epilepsy, being first appointed artist in residence in the early 1990s at the Chalfont Centre for Epilepsy, where he provided paintings and drawings for the Epilepsy Research MRI unit. He kindly agreed to produce a series of illustrations for the text of this book, giving a layman's view of what it must have been like to have had epilepsy at various times in the century. His brilliant and well-crafted illustrations catch perfectly the emotional consequences of epilepsy.

Cambridge University Press is renowned for the quality of its publishing, and it is a reputation well deserved. I am especially grateful to Anna Whiting at the Press for facilitating the publication of this book and her encouragement, forbearance and patience with my obsessional and recondite requests. I am also grateful for the support and help from Katy Nardoni and Camille Lee-Owen during the whole of the production process. The copy editing was performed by Helen B. Cooper, who did a superb and thorough job in ironing out my many mistakes and rendering my manuscript suitable to see the light of day. Some of this book is based on, and borrowed freely from, other works of mine, and I freely acknowledge this debt; these works include Schmidt, D. and

Shorvon, S., *The End of Epilepsy? A History of the Modern Era of Epilepsy 1860–2010* (Oxford: Oxford University Press, 2016); Shorvon, S., Weiss, G. et al., *International League Against Epilepsy 1909–2009: A Centenary History* (Oxford: Wiley-Blackwell, 2009); Hodgson, H. and Shorvon, S., *Physicians and War* (London: Royal College of Physicians, 2019); Shorvon, S. and Compston, A., *Queen Square: A History of the National Hospital and Its Institute of Neurology* (Cambridge: Cambridge University Press 2019). Professor Dieter Schmidt, co-author of the first above-named book, is now deceased; I offer my gratitude for his friendship, wisdom and the stimulation of his discussion in the writing of that book – and his presence was missed in the preparation of the current text.

My professional life has been spent in epilepsy since 1973, when I was first appointed as a research registrar under the supervision of Dr E. H. Reynolds, and since 1978 at the National Hospital for Neurology and Neurosurgery and the UCL Queen Square Institute of Neurology in London. The study and the practice of epilepsy through these years have provided me with a privileged insight into this condition, with all its ramifications and complexities, and to Dr Reynolds, the Hospital and Institute at Queen Square, their staff, my close colleagues and, above all, their patients, I offer my deepest thanks for the understanding, opportunities and intuitions they have given me over the years.

Acknowledgements: I am grateful for permission to reproduce the following figures: David Cobley (Figures 1, 4, 13, 14, 22, 25, 32, 33, 35, 37, 38, 41, 42, 44, 45); Montreal Neurologic Institute (Figures 3,31,33); Queen Square archive (Figures 6, 7, 12); Royal Society London (Figure 8); *Punch* (Figure 9); Chalfont Centre for Epilepsy archive (Figure 10); New York Academy of Medicine (Figure 16); *Science* (Figure 18); Little Brown (Figure 26); Roche Medical (Figure 27); Penguin Random House (Figure 28); Professor A. W. Jones (Figure 36); Elsevier (Figure 39), International League Against Epilepsy (Figures 40, 43).

THE VOYAGE OF THE GOOD SHIP *EPILEPSY*

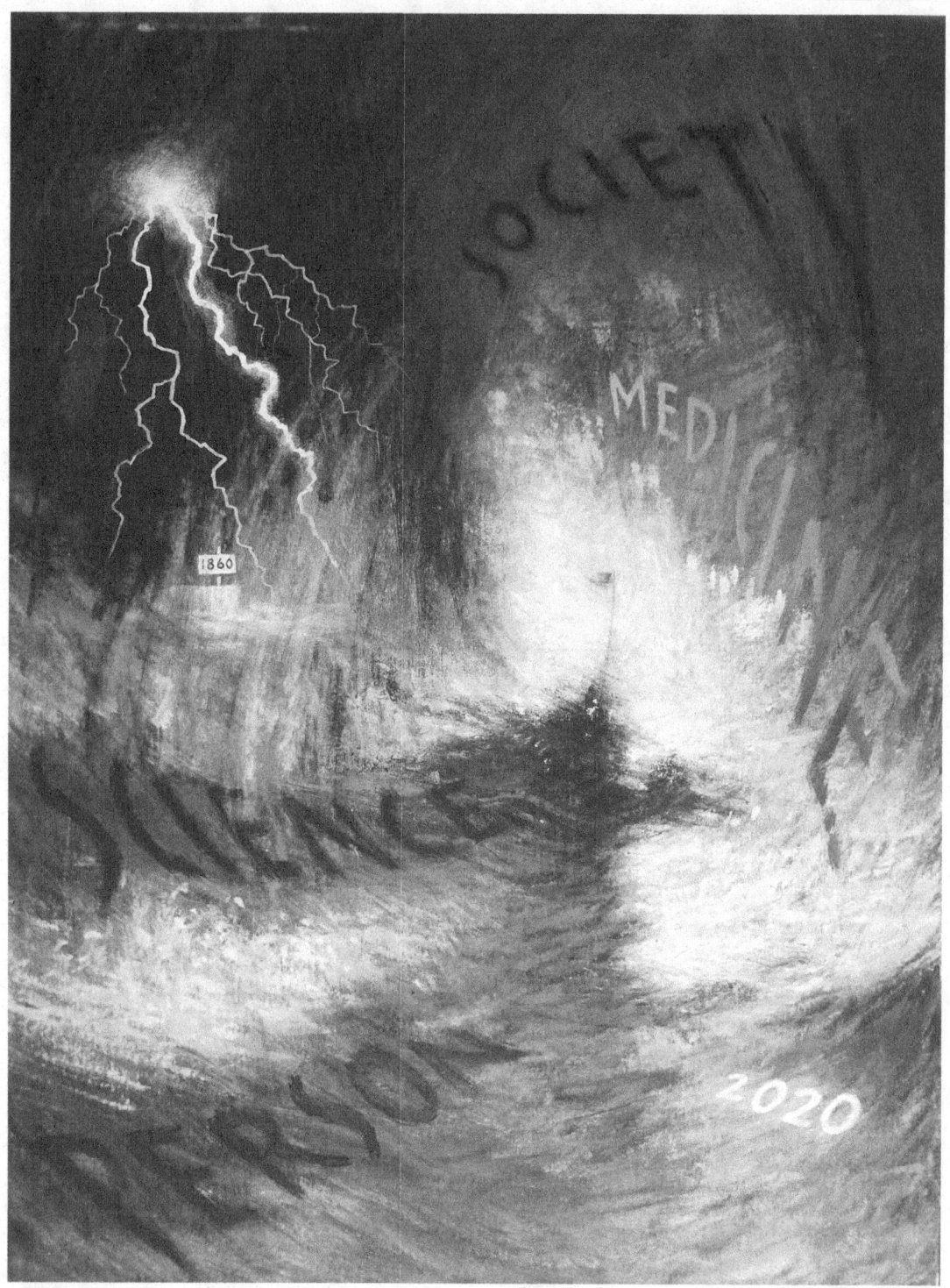

1. **The voyage of the good ship *Epilepsy***. On her journey from 1860 to 2020, rocked by the currents of science, medicine, society and the person with epilepsy (David Cobley, 2021).

INTRODUCTION

E PILEPSY OCCUPIES A UNIQUE POSITION AMONGST HUMAN AIL-
ments. In medicine, it is now, as it has always been, the unparalleled
hierophant of neurological disease. But at the same time, the notion of epilepsy
extends beyond that of a medical disorder. With its complex scientific, societal
and personal significations and meanings, it has attained a symbolism (an 'idea')
which has become deeply embedded in the culture of mankind. In consequence, although primarily a medical history, the topic of this book, the story
of *Epilepsy*'s voyage through the long twentieth century (1860–2020), has a
wider brief, to incorporate other themes in addition to those of medicine. To
ignore these would be to isolate epilepsy and deprive it of its deeper meanings.
Although similar considerations apply in many diseases, this is probably truer of
epilepsy than of most others. To Oswei Temkin, epilepsy was a 'paradigm of
the suffering of both body and soul in disease',[1] and with its broad and deep
connections, who can disagree?

Medicine occupies much of this book, but of the non-medical themes that I
have attempted to grapple with, three in particular stand out: the involvement of
science, the impact of societal trends on epilepsy and, not least, the often
harrowing personal experiences of individual sufferers. These themes are entangled one with another, but each is key to making sense of the meandering nature
of *Epilepsy*'s journey, the often illogical conceptions adopted and the sometimes
inefficient or harmful practices employed. The first theme is that of science – and
this grows in importance. Medicine could be defined as the art of transforming

---

[1] Oswei Temkin (1902–2002) was the leading historian of epilepsy. His book *The Falling Sickness: A History of Epilepsy from the Greeks to the Beginning of Modern Neurology*, first published 1945, is a brilliant and scholarly account of the history of epilepsy up to the end of the nineteenth century. This notable expression appears in the last sentence of the book (2nd ed., p. 388).

natural science into human experience; in making this transition, science becomes entwined in social, political, economic and psychological issues, and the result is an often messy business. As the extent of this interaction is at the heart of any epilepsy history, the second prominent non-medical theme is the exploration of the societal currents as they washed over *Epilepsy*'s decks. The most notable of these have been the impacts of capitalism, social democracy, legislation, public attitude, and, last but certainly not least, the social concepts of heredity. The third theme, the impact of epilepsy on the individual, is manifest most notably in prejudice and restriction of rights, on the individual's sense of identity, on stigma and on affect and confidence, which influence many facets of personal and public existence. Underpinning all this is the weight of the past. There is history in all men's endeavours; and it is the past which provides the context for the present. To ignore the past history of epilepsy is a form of illiteracy that condemns us not only to misunderstanding the present but also to bungling the future.

Why the long twentieth century ?. The year 1860 was chosen as the departure point for this journey as it was around then that the first modern conceptions of epilepsy appeared. It had been my initial intention to start the history in 1900, but the prior forty years proved so directly important for epilepsy that elongating the century made irrefragable historical, medical and scientific sense.

On launching into the process of writing, it also became immediately obvious that complexities had to be faced which were the consequences of the broad nature of epilepsy; some were unexpected and some indeed counter-intuitive – not least the proposition that epilepsy should perhaps not now even exist. I therefore decided – at a late stage – to include the following introductory section, outlining the aims and purposes of the book and surveying the complexities and the approaches taken to navigate around them. I was reminded of the words of Blaise Pascal, who himself died in status epilepticus, that 'The last thing we discover in writing a book is what to put in first',[2] and I found myself agreeing with him.

THE PURPOSE OF THE BOOK

Aims and Perspectives

As has been the case in medical histories of many conditions, the first aim of the book is to lay out a chronological story: to provide a ship's log of *Epilepsy*'s voyage, a gazetteer and a Pevsner's guide to her ports of call. In this sense, its primary purpose is to provide a straightforward narrative history. However, even this relatively modest goal is not without complications. Many 'facts' are far from absolute and, like the ocean wave, the appearance of a fact can change

---

[2] Translated from Pascal, *Pensées*, p. 265.

depending on scale, time and perspective; in a very real sense, many facts are thus at some level fake news – relative, subjective and dependent on context.[3] Nor, as sometimes assumed, are the facts of medical science immune to truth's elasticity – these too need to be viewed in a matrix that includes the influences of societal, economic and political trends, personal circumstance and contemporary intellectual fashion. In other words, medical facts, like all others, have meanings which are to a degree dependent on the cultural trends of the time.[4] Furthermore, not all is necessarily what it seems[5] in a world of spin and exaggeration, and neither truthfulness nor honesty in contemporary medicine and science can be taken for granted.[6] Despite such blurred edges, there is a still centre where objective evidence, if analysed impersonally, can guide a true understanding of the historical position and sequence of events, and I have proceeded on this basis

The level of detail is another consideration. I have put into this history considerable detail on the medical aspects with a medical readership in mind. Lay persons can skip the detail if they wish, and to facilitate this where possible I have endeavoured to bring out the salient points in summary. There is then the question of what items to include. In mapping the century-long journey, a navigator inevitably steers an arbitrary and intuitive course in choosing which tide to be swept along on and upon which star to point his sextant, as Temkin similarly noted.[7] It is also clear that the direction of travel is not one of seriate or unintermitted social or scientific progress, as of an ocean liner moving on the shortest trajectory between two points. Rather, it is a journey in which *Epilepsy* not infrequently travelled down blind fjords or tacked in aimless circles, routes which yet consumed much energy and time. This complicates the story, but to ignore the meanderings would be to sanitise the narrative.

If the first aim of the book is to be a chronicle of *Epilepsy*'s voyage, its second is of more than equal importance, and, one may feel, of more interest. This is to offer an explanation for the directions taken: to explain not only *what happened* but also *why it happened*. Exploring the 'why' of the story is a task more hazardous than defining the 'what', largely because of the fundamental problem

---

[3] As Orwell noted in 1943, 'The very concept of objective truth is fading out of the world' (*Looking Back at the Spanish War*, p.198). In 2022 it is difficult to disagree.

[4] See, for instance, the works of Roy Porter, Michel Foucault, Thomas Kuhn and Paul Feyerabend.

[5] As Sherlock Holmes observed, there is nothing more deceptive than an obvious fact (Doyle, *Adventures of Sherlock Holmes*, p. 91).

[6] A theme interestingly explored in a fictional way by Lauren Slater in her epilepsy biography (autobiography?) *Lying: A Metaphorical Memoir*, described in Chapter 5.

[7] 'But I have nowhere aimed at completeness; rather I have tried to obtain a picture of the thought of the different periods. That such a procedure is not without danger I am fully aware. The material used is only a fraction of the tremendous literature written on the subject and I may easily have overlooked material which would give a quite different aspect.' (Temkin, *Falling Sickness*, p. xi).

of perspective. The scientist, the physician, the everyman and the patient will each interpret the story of *Epilepsy*'s journey from their own vantage point, and their interpretations – their emphases and meaning – do strikingly differ one from the other. In this book, I have tried to represent the broad nature of the history by the inclusion of four particular perspectives:

The perspectives of science: As Peter Watson[8] has correctly pointed out, the influence of science on the history of the twentieth century is one often overlooked by historians. Indeed, science and its armies, officers and foot soldiers have played an overwhelming role in the history of modern epilepsy, both directly, and also indirectly by their impact on society and culture. Increasingly through this period, scientific thought and theory has infiltrated not only medicine, but also personal and social life. The influences, though, have been bidirectional. Political and economic issues have been powerful drivers of much of the scientific agenda, as have social influences on the direction of science. Science, at least as applied to epilepsy, has been frequently driven by the strong tides of the contemporary zeitgeist.

The perspectives of medicine: The primary concerns of medicine were (and are), as Francis Walshe – whose perspective was quintessentially that of the clinical neurologist – famously put it, 'the burning problems of . . . etiology, pathogenesis, and treatment';[9] and these have indeed remained at the centre of epilepsy medicine throughout the long twentieth century. The medicine of epilepsy is essentially an applied science, dependant on technological advances, for instance in neuroimaging, clinical chemistry and clinical genetics, and also on cultural fashion and societal trends. Because of their multiple and sometimes contradictory influences, many medical theories and practices, once hegemonic, are now viewed as bizarre aberrations, and once enthusiastically adopted were later completely rejected. No doubt the same fate will await many of our contemporary practices (and this is a point taken further in the Epilogue, and see also Appendix 2). The predominant attitude of doctors to epilepsy, and the style of medicine, have also varied greatly as have the medical facilities provided for epilepsy and these also have greatly influenced the social and personal course of epilepsy.

The perspectives of society: Often downplayed in scientific and medical treatises is the fundamental importance of contemporary culture and societal beliefs in setting the medical agenda. Throughout the long twentieth century, cultural attitudes defined how university and industry prosecuted science, and how doctors practised medicine. Capitalism dominated the century, and the impact of political and economic policy on epilepsy has been notably in the fields of pharmaceuticals,

[8] Watson, *A Terrible Beauty.*   [9] Walshe, 'The present and future of neurology'.

legislation and healthcare. Funding and societal norms to a large extent dictated how science and medicine were to progress. Pharmaceutical money, through sponsorship of professional organisations, bankrolled much of the epilepsy agenda. Social forces also exerted their influence through legislation, and laws and rules in relation to epilepsy were put in place in relation to consent, employment, education, driving institutionalisation and civil rights. Following the Second World War, centralised state-controlled healthcare systems were then put in place as part of the 'welfare state' and in this setting, healthcare for epilepsy (and most other conditions) has become to be perceived as a right not a privilege, with both positive and negative consequences. All these factors had a large impact not only on science and medicine but also the person with epilepsy.

The perspectives of the person with epilepsy: The final perspective is that of the sufferer – the insider's view of epilepsy. Although obviously vital to the history of epilepsy, this area has been the most difficult to unravel. No single answer exists to the question 'How does epilepsy feel?' as, of course, there are all sorts and conditions of man. Individual reactions differ and any attempt to provide definitive descriptions about what is a multi-layered and complex human experience is doomed to futility. Nevertheless, general statements are possible, and have some validity. A surrogate source of information about how epilepsy 'feels' and what it means is the depiction of epilepsy in biography, autobiography, literature and film – a mixture of first and third-person accounts, fiction and fantasy. These of course work on many levels, are open to different interpretations, and are sometimes deliberately ambiguous. However, within this corpus of work, the feelings, emotion and thoughts of those with epilepsy can be explored with the depth and subtlety that only the creative arts can convey. Graphic art can also assist – and the illustrations in this book by David Cobley are an example, designed as they are to indicate the emotional effects of epilepsy and its treatment in various guises.

Does Epilepsy Really Exist?

Epileptic seizures certainly do. But is epilepsy really a disease entity or a term worth preserving? It is argued in this book that by 2020 the condition may no longer exist, in part the result of the advances in epilepsy medicine which have brought into sharp focus the inherent vagaries of the concept of disease and the confusion between disease and symptom (this is a point expanded upon in the prologue and epilogue of this book). Throughout this text, I have used the word 'epilepsy' essentially as a reflection of contemporary convention. Often it would have been better and more precise to have rejected the word 'epilepsy' as a meaningful entity, but I have tried to maintain its historical context. At another level, epilepsy is a term of convenience and to some extent *a shorthand*, especially in the societal and personal context. Its existence is an issue which grates against linguistic precision – another under-rated virtue in the arena of science, wherein language is commonly mangled between the Scylla of unintelligibility and the Charybdis of blur. Perhaps now we have come to a point where the term 'epilepsy' should be recognised for what it is – a label, not an entity – and be dropped, not only in the interests of linguistic accuracy but for the benefit of medicine and its patients. This is an issue debated at the end of this book.

Complexities

Other difficulties and complexities have compounded the problems of writing this history and are briefly articulated here.

First, the story is divided, in the main, into chronological periods despite the obvious fact that the division is artificial. Currents ignore the boundaries of time and, for reasons of clarity in the telling of the narrative, chronology has been not infrequently breached; it is hoped this does not disrupt too much the tempo of the voyage.

Second is the bias of language. The choice of material has been made with a preference for documents written in English, a problem more troublesome at the beginning of this history than at the end, when much is published in English regardless of source. I also have tended to cite well- or interestingly-written works, a strong personal preference but one which does not necessarily have much relevance to historical importance.

Linked to language is geography, and the emphasis on the anglophone carries with it an inevitable tendency to overstate the Anglo-Saxon perspective. I have tried to avoid this as far as is possible, but realise that, particularly in relation to the social and personal aspects of this history, there is bias towards British and American material. It is these cultures and their history that I know best. In my defence is the fact that many trends in anglophone culture were shared in other countries, and the political and economic descriptions of such aspects as drug regulation and finances are to be read as *examples* of very similar trends elsewhere. Similarly, when referring to Europe, the text not infrequently confines its discussion to Western European countries, including Britain, at the expense of those of Eastern Europe. Where I have been able to, I have tried to temper this bias and maintain a broader perspective; and, at least in the second half of this history, the globalisation of epilepsy and its cultures has anyway diminished regional differences.

Third, in describing the progress of *Epilepsy*, the greatest emphasis has in general been placed on origins and foundations of trends and events, rather than on their subsequent course, and on the originators, not subsequent epigones. Elephants and butterflies are described, but not the worker ant. This emphasis seems justified but again leads to a bias of material with which all would not agree.

Fourth is the conundrum of where to include detail and where not to. Too much and the wood is obscured by the trees; too little and there is no wood at all. There is also a tension between providing a synoptical yet explanatory view of *Epilepsy*'s voyage, and so I decided to include great detail on those points in the journey in which the direction changed (examples are, for instance, the rise and fall of eugenics, the discovery of EEG and the changing funding structures of research in the post-war years) and to take a more abbreviated approach where progress was incremental and the trajectory more straight-forward – indeed, to the extent that mention of whole areas of work are severely truncated. Another bias is the fact that the developments in medicine are discussed in most detail, and science in the least, reflecting my own interests but also to rein in the length of the book. The last quarter-century provided particular problems in this regard, both because the amount of activity in all fields of epilepsy has massively increased, and also because the waters of history have hardly receded, leaving the ground too wet to know exactly what shape its landscape will take. The story of the last quarter-century is therefore described deliberately in a much more breviloquent and provisional form – particularly in relation to the science and clinical medicine of epilepsy.

Then there are the hurdles of intelligibility and jargon. The book is written in the hope that it will interest the informed public at large. But the language of science and medicine are inevitably technical, and the narration has not been dumbed down. A balance has to be drawn. Too technical and the conversation becomes closed to all but specialists; too loose and the science is rendered banal and tiresomely infantile. In this book, technical description is included, albeit modified with the intention where possible of making it comprehensible to the informed lay reader. A glossary of some of the technical terms is included to help bridge the gap of readability.

Another apology is needed regarding terminology. In parts of the text I have used terms which today are rightly considered prejudicial. For example, in the earlier chapters the word 'epileptic' is used in place of a 'person with epilepsy' and 'mental defective' in place of a 'person with learning disability'. Prejudicial wording has been retained where these were terms in contemporary usage, as in narrating the history it seemed to me more truthful to reflect the tone and nature of the historical voice as well as its content. I diverge from a 'cancelling' tendency, and believe that history should not be sanitised or rewritten by prohibiting terms which today are not appropriate. Similarly, I have in general described the science and medicine of epilepsy using contemporaneous terminologies, and not changes subsequently made (for instance, when referring to seizure types or treatments).

A final issue to be grappled with is determining the extent to which the course of *Epilepsy* has been due to the genius of individuals, as Thomas Carlyle put it to 'Great Men' (or, as Heinrich von Sybel pronounced, '[t]he masses do nothing') or conversely to the milieu in which they lived, the fertile soil in which genius could flourish.[10] There have been great men and women whose contribution to epilepsy has been epochal but whose work is embedded in a pre-existing clinical, scientific or societal framework, and on the shoulders of more minor work of others, and untangling how much this framework facilitated their contribution is not possible. In general, my preference has been to avoid hagiography (a constant danger in any medical history), and so the book is based more on factual action than on biography or people. But I have diverged from this rule for a small number of truly exceptional individuals whose accomplishments transcended the conventional to such an extent, and were so personal, that exemption seems justified; for those with more modest but nevertheless important contributions, a short biographical footnote is added.

An assessment of the value of any individual's contribution to any field can be made sensibly only after the passage of time, and indeed in some cases only over generations. It is for this reason that I have taken the decision *to avoid describing in any detail at all the personal contribution of any living individual*. This, I realise, is likely to be most contentious, and is bound to cause displeasure to the many still alive who are well worthy of inclusion. It is also a decision made in the full recognition that it weakens the focus of the most recent history, which, as mentioned, is abbreviated and more provisional. I hope those searching the index for the names of the living will understand the reasons for, and the logic of, this injunction and pardon the author for their omission.

This book was written by a clinician, one entranced by history but not a historian by trade or training. Incorporating the broader political, economic and historical trends, and their antecedents, has been the most difficult task – not least because, in describing the course of *Epilepsy*, efforts have been made to avoid value judgement, unifying theory or overarching political philosophy, or taking strong historiographical positions such as are often at the centre of other historical narration. In my view, key to describing history is the need to guard against one's own sympathies, but, however much one tries, an act of interpretation will always be a personal matter. The story thus has the inevitable biases of a Cambridge-educated, Caucasian, male, British, clinical neurologist, of the baby-boomer generation, and a university academic, with all the cultural baggage that this entails.

[10] Carlyle, *On Heroes*; H. von Sybel, cited in Thompson, *History of Historical Writing*, vol. 2, p. 214.

Whether the book succeeds in either satisfactorily documenting the narrative history or providing convincing explanations of it is for the reader to decide. For the author at any rate, its writing has been both a cathartic and an exciting voyage of discovery, as few subjects are as interesting or as complex as the story of this ancient disease.

THE STRUCTURE OF THE BOOK

One of the supreme works of medical history is Robert Burton's *Anatomy of Melancholy*.[11] The title of the current work is a deliberate homage to Burton's book in recognition of the many ways that it has set the standard against which all other disease histories should be matched.[12] Burton liked to paint a sprawling canvas, mixing up different themes and perspectives: as he put it, 'An Anatomy ... philosophically, medicinally and historically opened and cut up'; this I find attractive and have also attempted. For epilepsy (in Temkin's words, 'a paradigm of the suffering of both body and soul in disease', p.388) and melancholia (in Burton's words, 'this being a common infirmity of body and soul, and such a one that hath as much need of spiritual as a corporal cure', p. 27) share enough similarities to justify this approach.

He liked to draw in facts from many fields, in recognition of the fact that the effects on a disease are not limited 'to the confines of physic', and issued this warning: 'If any physician in the mean time shall infer, *ne sutor ultra crepidam*, and find himself grieved that I have intruded into his profession, I will tell him in brief, I do not otherwise by them, than they do by us' (p. 26). This is a sentiment shared in this book. Epilepsy, like melancholia, has both involvement in and implications for many areas of human endeavour.

The book is divided into three sections (similar to the 'partitions' in Burton's work), each of which has a specific purpose.

Section 1: The introduction and prologue adopt one of the purposes of Burton's *preface*, to briefly outline the aims of the book, its scope, structure and perspectives, and some of the complexities encountered in its writing. The prologue briefly reviews the changing concepts of epilepsy. Burton's preface was in part satirical, but here this story of epilepsy diverges and, in the wokish style of today, the condition is treated with more decorum.

Section 2: This is the heart of the book (and its fat) – a chronological narrative history (a log book) of the journey of *Epilepsy*. The five chapters cover

[11] The full title of the book is *The anatomy of melancholy, what it is, with all the kinds, causes, symptoms, prognostics, and several cures of it. In three partitions. With their several sections, members, and subsections, philosophically, medicinally, historically, opened and cut up. By Democritus Minor. With a satirical preface, conducing to the following discourse* (Oxford: printed by Henry Cripps, 1626 (second edition). Quotations are from the Preface.

[12] 'Idea' is substituted for 'Anatomy', as the latter word and page numbers from the Nonesuch edition now carries too strongly the imprimatur of science.

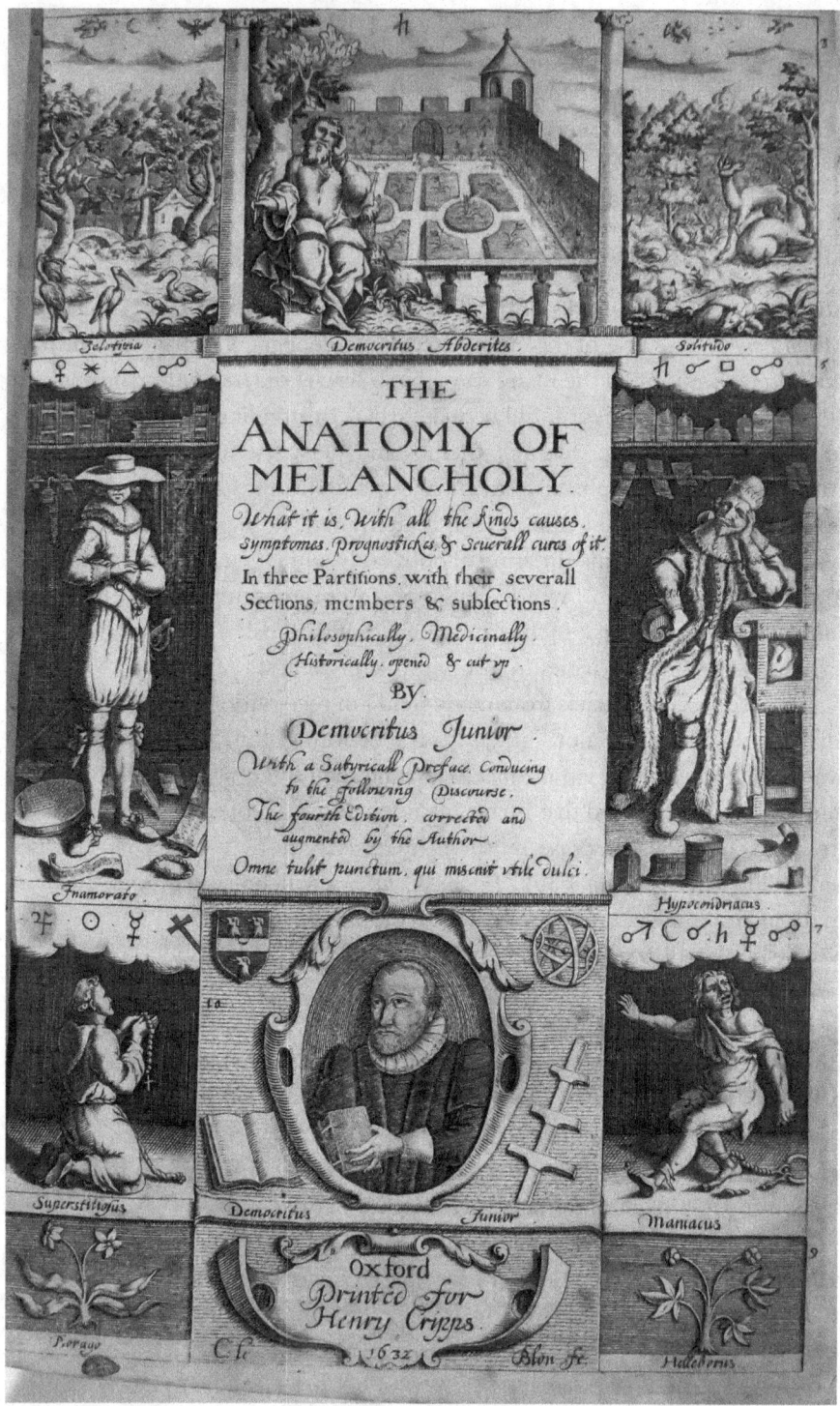

2. The frontispiece to the 1632 edition of Burton R., *Anatomy of Melancholy*, and Edward McKnight Kauffer's reinterpretation for the Nonesuch Press's edition in 1925.

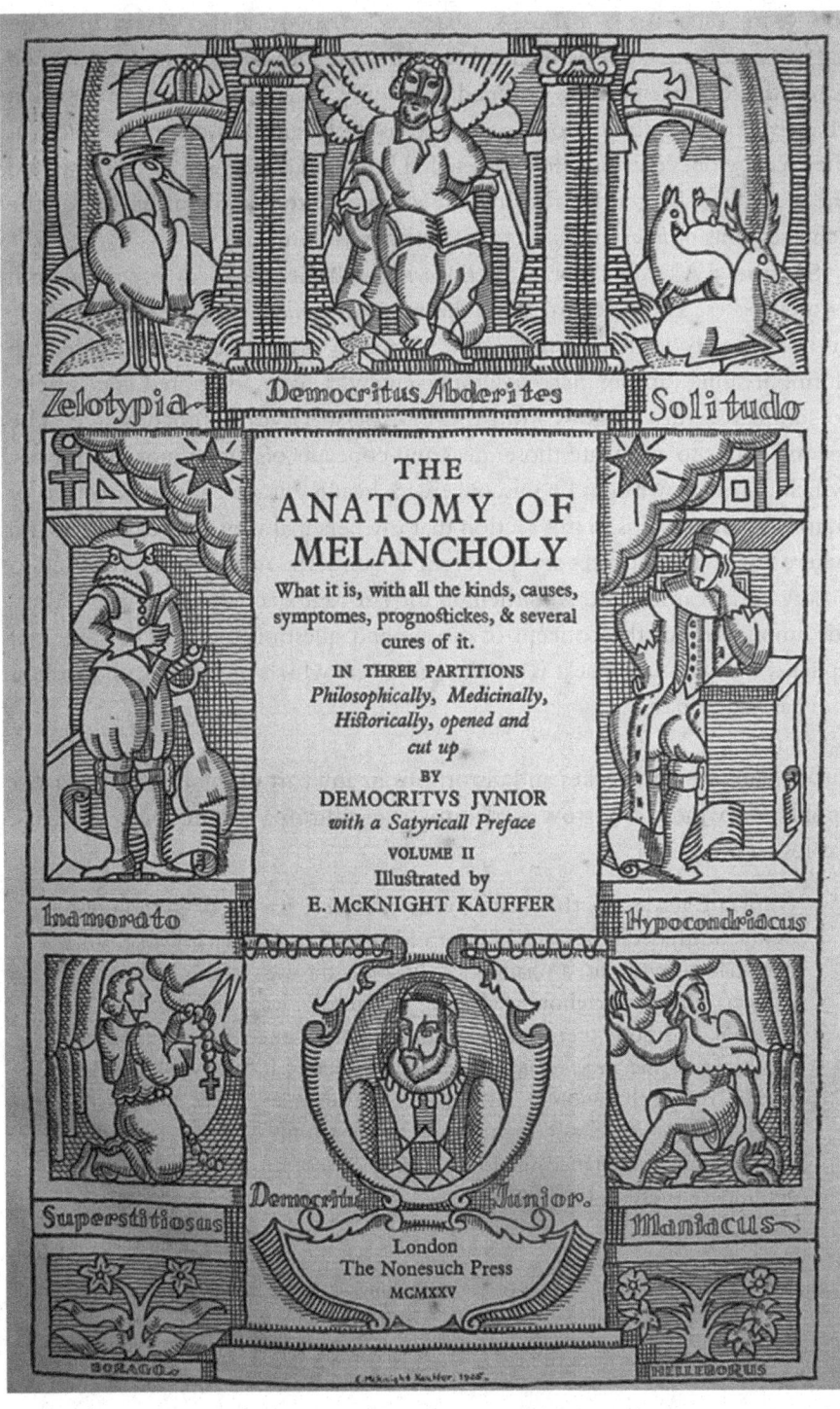

Zelotypia

Democritus Abderites

Solitudo

THE
ANATOMY OF
MELANCHOLY
What it is, with all the kinds, causes,
symptomes, prognoſtickes, & several
cures of it.
IN THREE PARTITIONS
*Philosophically, Medicinally,
Historically, opened and
cut up*
BY
DEMOCRITVS JVNIOR
with a Satyricall Preface
VOLUME II
Illustrated by
E. McKNIGHT KAUFFER

Inamorato

Hypocondriacus

Superstitiosus

Democritus Junior.

Maniacus

London
The Nonesuch Press
MCMXXV

BORAGO

HELLEBORUS

2. (cont.)

the years 1860–1914, 1914–45, 1945–70, 1970–95 and 1995–2020. This chronological narrative is detailed and divided into topics roughly mapped across the four perspectives outlined previously. As mentioned earlier, the last chapter, covering the period 1995–2020, is dealt with less comprehensibly as the recency of events precludes a detailed historical assessment. It is in this and the preceding chapter that the linked decision not to describe in any detail the achievements of *living persons* has its most obvious impact.

Section 3: A single chapter, the *Epilogue*, with its appendices, is written with two purposes. The first is to assess the progress *Epilepsy* has made since 1860, and to identify which of the many ideas and discoveries that bubbled up during its long journey *have endured* and why. I have attempted very briefly to summarise this progress from the four perspectives outlined above. The second aim is to articulate those ideas and concepts of contemporary epilepsy which in my view might be misconceived, heading in the wrong direction or frankly incorrect. It is in this section that my personal views are expressed and where my own prejudices and preferences trump the neutrality I have tried to ensure in the earlier text. And then, in the last pages, and briefly, I also address the ambiguities of the concept of disease and question the very existence of epilepsy – suggesting that it is an *idea* and a *term* which now holds up progress and has had its day.

Finally, and for all mistakes and distortions in any part of the book, I offer my apology – which I borrow verbatim from Burton, for no one can have expressed this better:

> GENTLE reader ... [If] I have overshot myself, have spoken foolishly, rashly, unadvisedly, absurdly, I have anatomized mine own folly. . . . [If] I have had a raving fit, a phantastical fit ... If through weaknesses, folly, passion, discontent, ignorance, I have said amisse, let it be forgotten and forgiven ... I hope there will no such cause of offence be given; if there be, *Nemo aliquid recognoscat, nos mentimur omnia.*[13] I'll deny all (my last refuge), recant all, renounce all I have said, if any man except, and with as much facility excuse, as he can accuse; but I presume of thy good favour, and gracious acceptance (gentle reader). Out of an assured hope and confidence thereof, I will begin.

---

[13] Burton translates this in a footnote as: 'let not anyone take these things to himselfs, thy are all but fictions'. (Burton, *Anatomy of Melancholy*, Nonesuch edition p. 78).

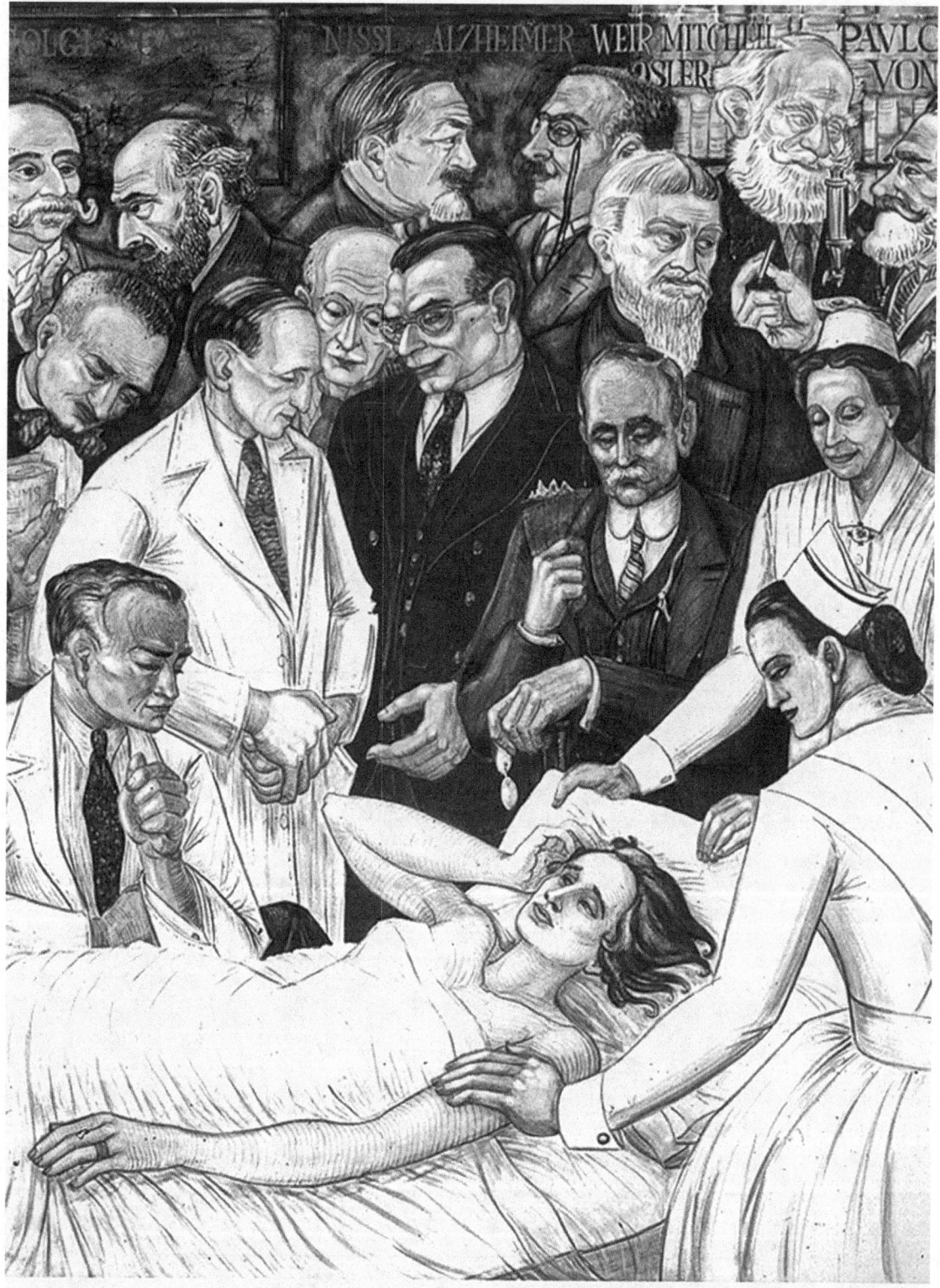

3. 'The Advance of Neurology' (1954). A detail from the painting by Mary Filer on the wall of the Montreal Neurological Institute, with Penfield and Jasper in the foreground, Mary Filer as nurse and patient, and many celebrated predecessors watching. In the back row (in this detail) are Golgi, Cajal, Alzheimer, Weir Mitchell, Osler, Pavlov and Von Monakow.

PROLOGUE

A NOTE ON THE CONCEPT – THE IDEA – OF EPILEPSY

THE CONCEPT (IDEA) OF EPILEPSY – IN OTHER WORDS, ITS DEFIN-
ition, meaning and signification – needs briefly to be considered before
launching into its history. I am not concerned here so much with the narrow
medical definition of epilepsy, but rather with what it implied to the generality
of citizens as well as to its sufferers, doctors and scientists, and how this changed
over the long twentieth century. This is explored in depth throughout the next
chapters and taken further at the end of this book. But it seems appropriate to
offer a brief outline here.

At first sight, it may seem surprising that the concept of epilepsy would
change much over time. Yet radical changes have occurred over the whole
course of this period, and it is absolutely the case that the idea of epilepsy in
2020 would be *completely unrecognisable* to any citizen, doctor or patient of 1860
or 1900 or indeed later. That is not to say that any of the *physical manifestations*
have altered at all; they have not, and were presumably the same in 2020 as they
were in 1860 or in 400 BC when the Hippocratic collection entitled *On the
Sacred Disease* was written. What has been utterly transformed in the twentieth
century is how the condition is conceived, what it signifies and what it means.
Any appreciation of its history, in the various periods considered in this book,
must be cognisant of this fact.

As with all aspects of its history, the concept of epilepsy will vary with
perspective, differing greatly, for instance, to the doctor, the scientist, the patient
or the everyman. Many aspects feed into how epilepsy has been conceived, but

at the centre are four distinct but closely interrelated issues which have played a particularly important role throughout the long twentieth century in moulding the idea of epilepsy, and which are relevant to all four perspectives:

- whether epilepsy is perceived as a *disease* (a unitary disease, or a heterogenous collection of diseases) or simply a *symptom*;
- whether epilepsy is explicable as a functional mental disorder or an organic neurological disorder;
- whether epilepsy has other inherent features apart from seizures; and
- the extent to which epilepsy is an inherited disorder.

The pendulum on each of these points has swung back and forth over the course of the century. With each reciprocating motion, the concept of epilepsy has changed, as has its meaning.

I remember lecturing some years ago to a huge gathering of epilepsy patients in India (organised by the indomitable Dr K. S. Mani). At the end of my talk, one person in the audience stood up to chastise me, enraged that I had 'referred to epilepsy as a disease'. 'It is not', I was told; 'it is a condition'. Ever since that time, with this encounter seared in my memory, this point has interested me, and by extension the question as to whether epilepsy is a disease (or condition) at all.

I do not think there is really any logical difference between a *condition*, *a disorder* and a *disease* from the scientific and medical perspective. I have yet to hear a coherent argument for differentiating the terms in these regards. But the person in the audience did have a point, for a distinction can be made on personal or societal grounds. To many individuals with epilepsy, calling it a disease implies something more serious, more biological and more fundamental. If I understood the basis of the complaint by my Indian interlocutor, it was that a condition implies that the entity is less damning and also more acceptable. The importance of terminology on framing the societal view is illustrated by this and other examples given throughout the book – not only in the use of those words now considered prejudicial but even in its their linguistic origins (for instance in the words for 'epilepsy' in some Eastern languages).

More fundamental than the semantic differentiation of disease/condition/disorder, and certainly more difficult, is the question of whether epilepsy is really a disease (or condition/disorder) at all. In other words, *does epilepsy as a disease entity actually exist?* And, if it does, what does it signify – what is its *meaning* – what is its *idea?*

THE CONCEPTS OF 'DISEASE'

One aspect of this question concerns whether there is any real distinction between epileptic seizures, the existence of which no one doubts, and epilepsy itself. In early history the question did not arise, for symptoms were considered synonymous with diseases (fever and skin rash, for instance). It was only after the work of Thomas Sydenham and others that a disease came to be seen as a characteristic constellation of symptoms and signs. By the nineteenth century, with the rise of the discipline of 'morbid anatomy' (pathology), the finding of pathological change had become a cardinal criterion of a disease. This criterion was supplemented after the invention of the microscope by finding histological abnormalities and then, as the twentieth century progressed, by identifying physiological, biochemical and, most recently, molecular and genetic changes. The identification of these *objective* abnormalities – loosely considered to be the *causes* of the illnesses[1] – became, in the mind of many doctors and scientists, a prerequisite for the designation *disease*. In parallel, in the last half-century molecular biology has elucidated numerous pathophysiological *mechanisms* of disease – explaining how a disease comes about. From these developments has evolved the modern *medical model* of disease in which three criteria are used to categorise an entity as a distinct disease: a unique constellation of symptoms and signs, a characteristic pathogenesis (set of mechanisms) and a characteristic causal pathology. Where no cause is found, the condition is sometimes considered 'idiopathic' (i.e. a disease unto itself, a *morbus per se*) signifying not that there is no cause but that the cause is as yet unidentified (most of these conditions are likely to have internal/congenital/inherited causes). Not all diseases fit this simple model, and boundaries can be blurred. For instance, some conditions are defined as disease because they deviate statistically from the norm (where health and disease are seen as being on a spectrum) – hypertension is one example. The greatest difficulties in applying the medical model of disease, however, relate to mental conditions (psychiatric disorders) where there is often no overt causal lesion nor clear pathogenesis, few physical signs, and where it is only subjective experience and behaviour that is considered abnormal. Accordingly, the idea that such mental phenomena are in fact diseases has been repeatedly challenged as arbitrary or even illusory (examples include the pronouncements of the anti-psychiatry movement in the 1960s, the contemporary arguments about the status of ADHD and other formulations of the DSM).

Of course, the medical model is not the only way to define disease (and again this topic is further discussed in the Epilogue of this book). Again, perspective is important. To the scientist, the condition is seen in molecular or mathematical terms, but to society the impact of epilepsy is often overwhelmingly construed in economic or legislative terms and in social and cultural attitudes. To the patients it is the fact of *being epileptic* which is often more important than just having seizures, with its effects on such aspects as social interactions, social relationships, marriage,

---

[1] The complexities encountered in defining 'cause' in epilepsy are discussed further on pp.606–7.

domestic life, driving, education and employment. Their concern is with epilepsy as an illness, not a disease in the medical sense, and their actions ('illness behaviours') are often utterly unrelated to any scientific or medical concern.

THE ORIGINS OF THE MODERN MEDICAL CONCEPT OF EPILEPSY: THE WORK OF HUGHLINGS JACKSON

As we shall see, like so much else in neurology, the modern history of epilepsy can be said to have begun with the work of John Hughlings Jackson in the 1860s and 1870s. When he started out on his studies, the nature of an epileptic seizure was completely unknown. It, and epilepsy, were still considered by some to be caused by supernatural or thaumaturgic influences and both were entangled with and hardly differentiated from hysteria. Other pathogenic theories existed and the more physiologically minded physicians considered seizures to be reflexes with an origin located in the medulla or even the spinal cord. Jackson utterly dismissed these (now seemingly prehistoric) concepts. With remarkable intuition, in 1873 he proposed that the physical manifestations of an epileptic seizure were caused by *a sudden and excessive discharge* of neurons in a *localised* area of the cerebral cortex (the superficial grey matter of the brain). He saw the physical manifestations of a seizure simply to be a reflection of this disturbed physiology.[2] In Jackson's view, the seizure was a 'symptom' of this abnormal physiology. It is this singular insight that can be said to have launched the topic of epilepsy into its modern era, and since Jackson the concept of the epileptic seizure has hardly changed. At the time, there was a titanic struggle between science and religion to provide an explanatory model for the world, and Jackson's lucid explanation of epileptic seizures was a signal example of the power of science. Although clearly defining seizures, Jackson however shied away from definitively defining epilepsy – one suspects because he saw the inherent logical difficulties in doing so. To Jackson, the term epilepsy was simply shorthand for the physiochemical mechanism of seizures; in other words, the two were almost synonymous and, indeed, throughout his oeuvre he used the term *epilepsy* largely interchangeably with that of *epileptic seizure*.

THE CONCEPTION OF EPILEPSY BETWEEN THE 1880s-1930s: EPILEPSY AS A PSYCHO-HEREDITARY MENTAL DISORDER

Another conception of epilepsy arose in the late nineteenth century, with the increasingly prominent idea that heredity was the primary cause of seizures. The view grew up that only idiopathic epilepsy was the true *disease* known as epilepsy. It

---

[2] Jackson called this abnormal cellular 'nutrition'; today, the same concept is called 'abnormal excitation' and explained in terms of molecular biochemistry and physiology.

was a disease that met the three criteria of a medical model of disease, with its spectrum of symptoms and signs (importantly, with symptoms extending beyond seizures), a clear-cut pathogenesis (degeneration) and a clear-cut cause (heredity). On the other hand, seizures occurring in other diseases, such as brain tumours, infections or trauma, were thenceforward considered as symptomatic seizures and not included within the rubric of epilepsy. This became the orthodox view and was held well into the 1920s.

The idea of what *Epilepsy* was had thus been transformed. It was thereafter universally considered by both medicine and the public at large to be an inherited mental disorder and a brain degeneration. The underlying inherited germ-plasm defect was known as the neuropathic trait, which was believed to cause not only seizures but also behavioural and personality failings such as criminality, amorality and sexual deviance. This was a toxic mix, and the disease engendered prejudice and hostility. In response, patients and their families sheltered in denial or conceal-ment. Epilepsy was a condition which signalled the possession of an inherent genetic weakness, and thus was not a condition which a family would willingly admit to having. The clinical practice of the time reinforced the idea that epilepsy was a mental disorder treated, as it was usually, by psychiatrists in an asylum setting.[3] To the public there was, in effect, little distinction between epilepsy and lunacy.

In the early twentieth century, the massive public interest in heredity led to a powerful eugenic movement and the eugenicists, considering epilepsy to be an inherited organic mental degeneration, focused their ire on the personality of sufferers, their psychological defects and social worthlessness. At the same time, psychoanalysis became the predominant theory of mind, and psycho-analytical theory considered epilepsy to be inherited but of a functional nature, with both seizures and the personality defects the result of the psychological mechanism of infantile regression. These theories, both euge-nical and psychoanalytical, were highly damaging. To the individual with epilepsy and to society at large in this period, epilepsy reared its head as a feared and stigmatised condition – and, furthermore, one which, because it was inherited, might overwhelm and degrade the moral fibre of Western society. In the materialistic and agnostic society of those times, the societal response was increasingly that of social exclusion and rejection. Fear that the defective germ plasm might weaken the fabric of a nation and resentment at the cost of caring for the mentally ill grew, especially in the war years. The consequences were dire; the rights of the individual with epilepsy were

---

[3] Neurology was in any event a young and small specialty, and its concepts converged to a great extent with those of the much larger and better-established specialty of psychiatry when it came to brain disorders. As Henry Maudsley wrote: 'Mental disorders are neither more nor less than nervous diseases in which mental symptoms predominate, and their entire separation from other nervous diseases has been a sad hindrance to progress'; Maudsley, *Body and Mind*, p. 41.

circumscribed, resulting in widespread involuntary institutionalisation and sterilisation, and in Nazi Germany, for some, in euthanasia.

THE CONCEPTION OF EPILEPSY BETWEEN THE 1930s–1980s: EPILEPSY AS A PHYSIOLOGICAL DISORDER

The 1930s were to prove a transitional decade for the concept of epilepsy, due mainly to the growing influence of the specialty of neurology which had begun insistently to stake its claim on the condition. The divide between neurology and psychiatry widened. Neurologists (and neurosurgeons) were in general impatient with both eugenical and psychoanalytical concepts of epilepsy, and proposed that seizures were due usually to an underlying cerebral pathology, even if it could not be identified, and, in parallel, considered inheritance to be a minor part of causation. To the advanced neurologists of the period, epilepsy was not a mental disorder but a medical condition. Furthermore, they rejected the concept of inherent personality defects or behavioural features, and considered epileptic seizures to be the main manifestation of epilepsy. Opinion gathered force that *idiopathic epilepsy* was not inherited but that its cause was simply unknown, and therefore that epileptic seizures in idiopathic epilepsy were not inherently different from any other symptomatic seizures. Idiopathic epilepsy was seen simply as a variant in which the underlying pathology had not yet been detected, and not in other ways distinctive; by implication, the idea that epilepsy was a distinct disease was rejected. Given the growing number of causes identified for epilepsy, it was increasingly held that restricting the term *epilepsy* to the idiopathic condition was illogical and that it should either be replaced by a plural form (i.e. *the epilepsies*) or abandoned altogether. In the definitive textbook of neurology of its time, Kinnier Wilson deliberately entitled the chapter on epilepsy 'The Epilepsies' and, given the heterogenous causation of seizures, pondered on whether it would not be better if the term *epilepsy* was replaced by *paroxysmal disorders* or *convulsive states* to indicate 'a series of diverse conditions distinguished by the occasional occurrence of "fits"'.[4] To emphasise his point, he placed his chapter within the section titled 'Disease Conditions of Uncertain Nature'.[5] To Wilson and many neurologists of the time, a seizure was now conceived as a *symptom* of an underlying pathology, of which there were many varieties. Putting the matter into a nutshell, the senior American epilepsy specialist of the time, William Cobb, identified sixty causes of seizures, and stated in 1941: 'Because … a great many different forms of interference with nervous

---

[4] Wilson, 'The epilepsies', p. 2.   [5] Wilson, *Neurology*, vol. 3, p. 1469.

integration may lead to the production of fits, and because the interfering factors are varied and even paradoxical, I believe that epilepsy cannot be called a disease ... it is a symptom of many cerebral diseases.'[6]

This was the state of play at around 1940, with the idea of epilepsy the subject of adversative opinions and unresolved debates. But then a tidal wave engulfed the seas of epilepsy and changed the concept of epilepsy again. This was the introduction of the electroencephalogram (EEG). It became suddenly possible, it seemed, to visualise the very physiological changes that Jackson had described and that occurred both during and between seizures. This radically shifted the interest to physiological theories of pathogenesis and, as Lennox famously put it, epilepsy was simply 'a cerebral dysrhythmia'.[7] Epilepsy had moved firmly into the organic neurological camp and because seizures whatever their causes seemed to have similar physiological signatures, it became a term which incorporated all conditions with seizures of any cause, not just idiopathic epilepsy.

In the aftermath of the Second World War, eugenics came to an abrupt end, discarded as an acceptable social policy. The idea that epilepsy was essentially an inherited disorder was also largely rejected (nor was there a shred of pathological evidence of an inherited lesion), as was the view that epilepsy was a mental disorder with inherent behavioural or personality features. The UN Declaration of Human Rights, coming on the heels of the Nuremburg trials, opened a new era of protection for minority groups and for disadvantaged individuals. For the first time, the voice of the patient began to be heard and lay organisations to be formed. An anti-asylum and then anti-psychiatry movement changed the public mood. In the more liberal atmosphere, societal attitudes towards epilepsy became more sympathetic. The rights of those with epilepsy began slowly to be asserted, in Western societies at least, as the condition became seen for the first time legally as well as culturally to be a medical condition like any other.

The prominence given to electrographic changes had moved the emphasis from aetiology to pathophysiology, and seizures of all causes were grouped into the single disease entity that was epilepsy. In actual fact, in this formulation (similar as it was to that of Jackson), epilepsy and seizures became again almost synonymous, albeit this time at a physiological and pathophysiological rather than clinical level. A classification of *epileptic seizures* arose in the 1960s based on both clinical and EEG appearance, and a confusingly similar *classification of the epilepsies* followed in 1989.

---

[6] Cited by Lennox as Cobb (1941, p. 196), although no complete reference is given (Lennox, *Epilepsy and Related Disorders*, vol. 1, p. 52).
[7] Lennox, *Epilepsy and Related Disorders*, vol. 1, pp. 51–3.

In the 1980s, in part because of the difficulties inherent in considering epilepsy as a disease, the concept of the epileptic syndrome arose, an entity falling somewhere between the symptom and the disease. A syndrome was defined as a specific constellation of symptoms, signs and EEG features, but unlike a disease it was without a fixed aetiology (and indeed cut across aetiological categories). The concept of an epilepsy syndrome filled the void between that of the epileptic seizure and that of epilepsy.

Two further developments then shifted the medical concept of epilepsy again. First was the introduction of neuroimaging; second, the rise of molecular medicine/genetics. With these new technologies, the focus turned again onto cause. Soon, hundreds of causative conditions were recognised, not just the sixty that Cobb had identified. Neuroimaging reasserted the importance of structure as well as function, thus weakening the idea that epilepsy was a purely physiological phenomenon and leading to the view, first expressed in the 1920s, that there was often (some even claimed always) a structural anomaly or pathological lesion underlying epileptic seizures. In parallel, with the rapid development of molecular science, a whole variety of molecular and cellular physiological and chemical changes and mechanisms were identified which it was found could result in epileptic seizures. The clinical EEG came to be seen as a summation of the physiological changes and as a *diagnostic biomarker* of these rather than anything more fundamental. Furthermore, the molecular physiological and chemical processes were found to be dynamic, changing over time in an individual as epilepsy evolved into a chronic state.

By then, public attitudes had become more supportive. Discriminatory or exclusional legislation was struck out, and more resources were allocated to epilepsy. Access to medical care for those with epilepsy was provided at an unparalleled level. Perhaps for the first time in history, too, individuals were emerging from the shadows and felt able openly and frankly to write about their condition. Realistic descriptions of epilepsy, and more sympathetic attitudes, began to appear in literature and film.

THE CONCEPTION OF EPILEPSY 1990s–2020

Much changed in these decades. The 'new genetics', as it became known, first surfaced in clinical epilepsy in the mid-1990s. By 2016, more than 700 genes had been discovered in conditions which included seizures in their pheno-type, and suddenly epilepsy was increasingly being conceptualised again as a genetic disorder, or at least a disorder with strong genetic influences. The old idea of the epileptic personality, which had been closely tied to the ideas of heredity, remained largely rejected, but in its place was the view that there were frequent psychiatric 'comorbidities' – actually a similar notion but with a different name. Epilepsy was again being conceived as a disorder with inherent and inherited behavioural and psychiatric associations in addition to seizures (and some even proposing epilepsy to be a 'spectrum disorder'). In these ways, the 'new' ideas about the inheritance of epilepsy were a modern reworking of the concept of the neuropathic trait. Furthermore, neurology and psychiatry grew closer together (united under the banner of neuroscience). And although epilepsy was still very much considered a neurological rather than a mental disorder, this distinction was becoming increasingly blurred.

And so by 2020 there were a number of conceptual parallels with epilepsy in the late nineteenth/early twentieth century. Of course, much also was different. The rights of the person with epilepsy were not infringed in 2020 as they were in the early twentieth century, and societal attitudes were not remotely as hostile (at least in Western societies). Stigma remained a problem in 2020, but of orders of magnitude less than in the pre–World War II years, and people with epilepsy were able to be far more open and less fearful about their condition. Nevertheless, the parallels should not be ignored. Without vigilance, one can see how easily eugenic concepts might creep again into epilepsy and how public attitudes may again harden. And although by 2020 the meaning of epilepsy was different from that at the beginning of this story, there is a clear sense of circularity; concepts have been recycled and ideas have re-emerged.

SHOULD EPILEPSY STILL EXIST?

A final thought, taken up again at the end of this book, is that, from the scientific and medical perspectives, because of the multiplicity of aetiologies and molecular abnormalities and mechanisms, and the great variation in the clinical symptomatology and context, the idea that there is a clear-cut disease called epilepsy has become increasingly untenable. Epileptic seizures have come to be perceived as a manifestation of myriad processes and causes, and no one doubts their existence. But, from the medical perspective, the only way in which a disease called epilepsy could be considered valid is to define it as a 'state' in which there was a 'propensity to have recurrent seizures' – a wholly circular and unsatisfactory way of conceptualising a disease, and one which meets none of the aforementioned criteria of the medical model.

It is from the societal and personal perspectives, however, that the use of the term epilepsy has more legitimacy, as a useful shorthand to signify those who suffer from seizures – regardless of cause or pathophysiology. The downside, of course, with this use of the term is that it comes with much historical baggage, prejudice and stigma.

Given that there is little justification for considering epilepsy to be a disease on medical grounds, might it not be better to dispose of the term *epilepsy* altogether; to refer to individuals simply as suffering from epileptic seizures and not as persons with epilepsy (or, worse, 'epileptics'). These are issues debated in the final paragraphs of this book.

It is with these thoughts in mind, framed by the contextual background of the shifting conceptions of epilepsy, that we approach the narrative history of epilepsy in the long twentieth century, the topic of the next section.

'A PLAGUE UPON YOUR EPILEPTIC VISAGE'

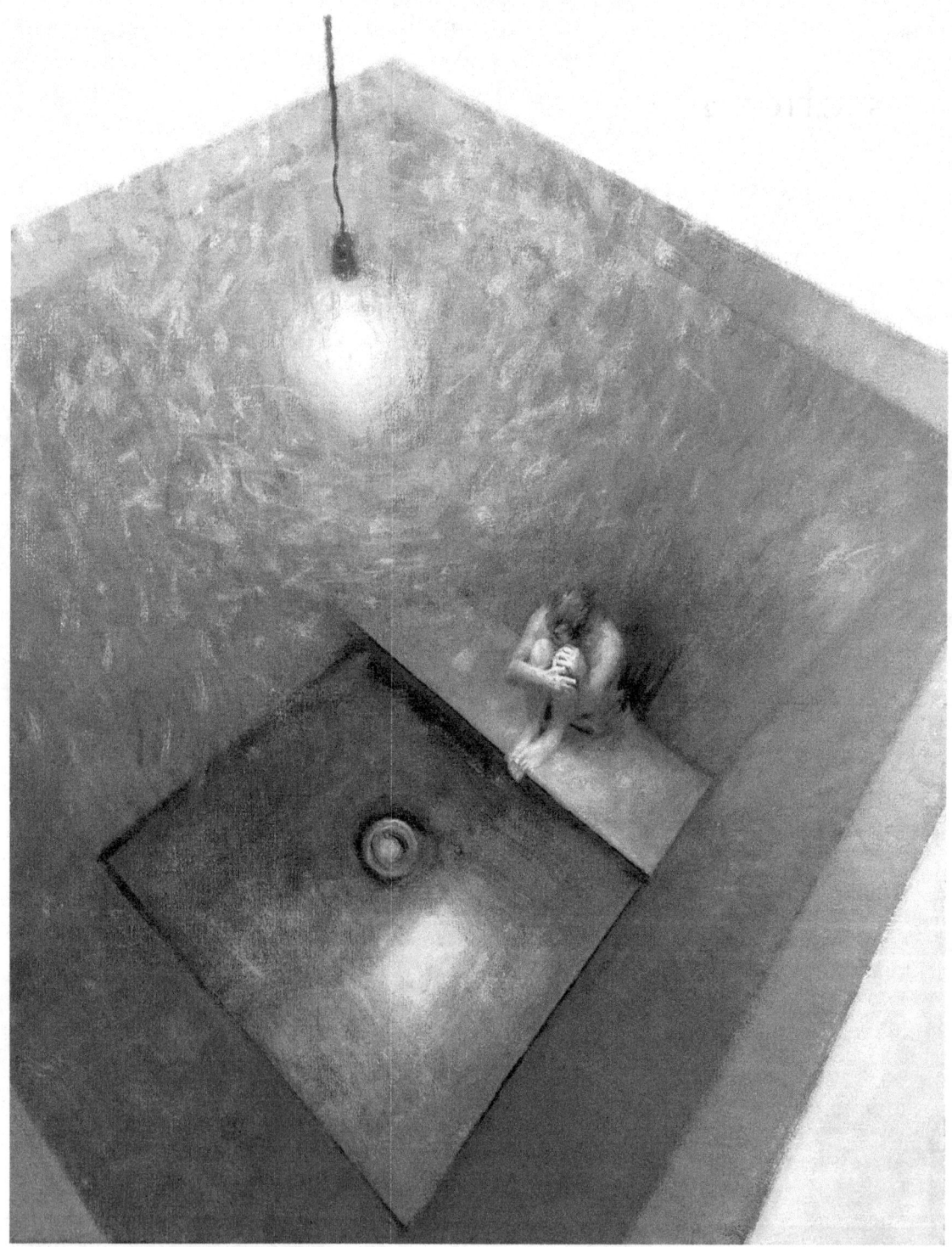

4. 'Isolation'. An interpretation of the social isolation and exclusion of those with epilepsy, 1860–1914. (Painting by David Cobley, 2021)

ONE

1860–1914: THE BIRTH OF MODERN EPILEPSY

EPILEPSY IS ONE OF THE OLDEST RECORDED DISEASES. IT APPEARED ON an Assyrian cuneiform and in ancient texts from a variety of civilisations before many other common conditions were recognised.[1] It is also an affliction to which special status was imputed – considered sacred by the ancients, or a sign of magic, evil or demonic (and sometimes divine) possession in many cultures and times.[2] In early-nineteenth-century Europe, epilepsy was still heavily stigmatised by its association with possession, lunacy, sorcery and witchcraft, as well as its signification as sin, its shocking loss of control and otherness, and the fear that it was contagious.

The modern conceptual framework of epilepsy, from both the medical and the societal points of view, dates only from the nineteenth century, and

[1] In Babylon, epilepsy is mentioned on the cuneiform Sakikku from around 1067–46 BC, and in China in Huang Di Nei Jing, a text dating from sometime in the first three centuries BC (Kinnier Wilson and Reynolds, 'Translation and analysis'; Lau et al., 'Announcement of a new Chinese name').

The pre-1860 history is most expertly covered by Owsei Temkin (*Falling Sickness*). The ancient literature contains many spiritual and magical references. William Spratling noted in *Epilepsy and Its Treatment* that the disorder was referred to by a remarkable variety of names, including *morbus sacer, morbus major, morbus Herculeus, morbus commitialis, morbus mensalis, morbus convivialis, mobus insputatis, morbus viridellus, morbus vitriolatus, morbus sonticus, morbus caducus, morbus unicatus, morbus foedus, morbus sideratus, morbus scelestus, morbus daemoniacus, morbus deificus* and *morbus astralis* (pp. 11–13).

[2] Beliefs which seem to have been present from the beginning of recorded history, and although challenged by such rationalists as Hippocrates, have persisted.

particularly the years after around 1860.[3] Medical and scientific activity in epilepsy over the succeeding few decades was by many measures more intense than at any previous time – and for a brief period epilepsy had its place in the sun. It was a time, in advanced circles at least, when the superstitious baggage weighing epilepsy down was largely disposed of, and when the ways in which the condition is now conceived were clearly formulated. This was a time notable for the rise of science – surely the most important cultural trend of the long twentieth century – and when science in epilepsy, as in other fields, began to release the stranglehold of religion. The rapid progress in the years after 1860 did not, of course, come out of the blue. In the preceding half-century, knowledge had increased incrementally, and several leading physicians and psychiatrists wrote on epilepsy, notably in France, Germany, Holland and England.[4] However, it was in the three decades or so after 1860 that epilepsy made the greatest progress. The organic concept of epilepsy changed fundamentally with the work of John Hughlings Jackson; its clinical neurology with that of William Gowers, Jackson, Otto Binswanger, Charles Féré and others; its functional anatomy with the work of Jackson, David Ferrier and Victor Horsley; its psychiatry with the work particularly of the French school of Bénédict Morel and his followers; and its treatment with the advent of bromide therapy and then of neurosurgery. Theories of brain function were formulated, not least based on the newly discovered principles of cerebral localisation. There was extraordinary scientific and medical progress, and epilepsy after 1860 bore only a tenuous relationship to its conception in earlier times. The same is not true of all diseases. In this sense, epilepsy was not only one of the most ancient but also one of the most modern of common medical conditions.

This was the period when neurology began to form as a medical specialty, arising from both general internal medicine and psychiatry. Although later in the twentieth century epilepsy came to be seen as a primarily 'neurological disease', for the entirety of this period it was very largely medically managed by psychiatrists, and conceptualised as a mental disorder within the psychiatric framework of mental deficiency and the socio-psychiatric concepts of inherited degeneration. This had enormous social and cultural implications. Linked to

---

[3] A similar dividing line between pre-modern and modern epilepsy was made by William Lennox (*Epilepsy and Related Disorders*), Temkin (*Falling Sickness*) and Walter Friedlander (*History of Modern Epilepsy*).

[4] The leading authorities who published books, theses or important papers on epilepsy in the decades before 1860 included: in France, Marie-Jean-Pierre Flourens, Jean-Étienne Dominique Esquirol, Louis Jean François Delasiauve, Antoine Baron de Portal, Bénédict Augustin Morel; in Britain, James Pritchard, Richard Bright, Marshall Hall, Robert Bentley Todd, Astley Cooper, Samuel Wilks; in Germany and Holland, Moritz Heinrich Romberg, Karl Friedrich Burdach, Adolf Kussmaul, Adolf Tenner, Wilheim Griesinger, Jacobus Schroeder van der Kolk.

personality defects and criminality, epilepsy was heavily stigmatised and, where possible, was concealed, kept hidden and denied. The majority of sufferers did not receive any medical care, but where this was necessary it was provided mainly in asylums, and then within the newly conceived 'epilepsy colonies'.

Then, around the turn of the century, the searchlight of medicine turned away from epilepsy. Two very different books were published which were to have an immense influence on the next decades and were examples of the divergent paths that neuro-medicine (neurology and psychiatry) was taking: Sigmund Freud's *Die Traumdeutung* (*Interpretation of Dreams*; dated 1900, although actually published in November 1899) and Charles Sherrington's *Integrative Action of the Nervous System* (1906). Freud, in all his work, challenged Charcot's theories of the degenerative, inherited and organic nature of hysteria and the fallacies of his concept of hystero-epilepsy (with its 'four stages'); in doing so, he launched psychiatry onto a distinctive path, focusing on internal unconscious psychological mechanisms, a form of scientific psychology that had utterly different premises from that of neurology. Sherrington's work, in contrast, established experimental neurophysiology as the dominant science of neurology.

Epilepsy was hardly mentioned in the work of either man, but despite this both were in later decades have profound indirect effects on epilepsy. In the decades prior to 1900, epilepsy had been at the centre of neurology and psychiatry, but in the first years of the twentieth century the ascendant intellectual thrusts of neuroscience and neuro-medicine moved to other areas.[5] As the paths of psychiatry and neurology divaricated, few clinicians or scientists carried out advanced research in epilepsy, and epilepsy would have to wait until the late 1930s to again occupy the centre ground.

SCIENCE AND SOCIETY IN THE LATE NINETEENTH AND EARLY TWENTIETH CENTURIES

Karl Polanyi called the nineteenth century 'England's century',[6] as it was there, in this period, that the benefits of the Industrial Revolution were most keenly exploited, and a prosperous middle class arose, educated and innovative. The other advanced countries of Europe were gripped by the revolutionary ferment of the *springtime of nations* which ushered in a period of new thinking and intense intellectual activity. It was in this context that the modern era of

[5] The number of papers on epilepsy in the neurological literature declined. Between 1900 and 1910, for instance, the leading neurology journal *Brain* published only five original papers primarily concerned with epilepsy (these included William Broadbent's Hughlings Jackson Lecture and William Turner's lectures on epilepsy). It seems only a relatively small amount of original basic or clinical research directly involved with epilepsy was carried out.

[6] Polanyi, *Origins*.

medicine was born, and it was then too that 'science' started to become pre-eminent as a way of thinking. Peter Watson, in his book *A Terrible Beauty* (2001), noted that the leadership of Germany in many areas of science was due to the mid-nineteenth-century restructuring of its universities.[7] This notwith-standing, most research in epilepsy in this period was conducted not in universities, but by individual clinicians outside the university setting, embed-ded either in their clinical practices or in animal experimentation with little organised infrastructure in what was an essentially amateur manner.[8] The idea that science held the key to modern clinical practice was born in this period, and the modern science of epilepsy advanced more in the period 1860–1900 than at any time before, and arguably since.

The tempo of epilepsy science in this period also illustrates another central thesis of modern history: that major scientific progress is not made by the slow incrementation of knowledge, a slow accumulation of small factual advances as researchers engage in a long journey to an ultimate understanding of the natural world ('normal science').[9] Rather, most progress is made by a series of discon-tinuities, fresh frameworks or new paradigms that replace much of the work of previous normal science ('paradigm shifts', 'scientific revolutions'). As we shall see, the science of epilepsy throughout the long twentieth century has pro-gressed by alternating periods of such normal and revolutionary science, with transitions often driven by social, political or economic forces. Their impact on medical science could not be illustrated better than by the example of epilepsy in the early twentieth century, when eugenics, anxieties about heredity and a fear that degeneration was leading to a decline of civilisation were at the forefront of the public agenda. In addition, epilepsy suffered from the intensely pronatalist stance of medicine in that period (very different from today), with a demand for healthy persons by industry, the military and (in Britain) the empire – and epilepsy, common in young people, was seen as a gross impediment.

Another dominant aspect of late-nineteenth-century social thought – the trend towards secularisation – also had a great impact on epilepsy. Charles Darwin's *Origin of Species* appeared in 1859 and, with justification, has been

---

[7] Watson, *The German Genius: Europe's Third Renaissance*, pp. 225–37.

[8] There were distinguished exceptions: for instance, the Brown Institution founded in London in 1871 (see Wilson, 'Brown Animal Sanatory Institution'), whose superintendents included John Burdon-Sanderson, Horsley and Sherrington); and the Obersteiner Institute founded in Vienna in 1887 (see Kreft et al., '125th anniversary'). In terms of basic medical research, Germany led the way. It has been estimated that in 1891, for instance, 500 scientists were focused on medical research in Germany, compared with 50 in the United Kingdom and very few in the United States (Brandt and Gardner, 'Golden age of medicine?'). Few, if any, non-clinical basic scientists, however, were involved in epilepsy. In the major medical schools of Europe, too, teaching in clinical medicine remained far more prominent than research and had much higher priority.

[9] Kuhn, *Structure*.

called the most important book of that century. It sparked a Herculean battle between modern secular science and traditional religious beliefs over the origins and position of humans in the natural world and their relationship to God. In the hostile debates that followed, science began to bore into the edifice of the church, whose defences started to crumble. This climactic transformation meant a great deal to people with epilepsy, whose lives up to that point had been mired in religious superstition and beliefs and who, as a result, were subject to exclusion and rejection on religious grounds. No one should underestimate the importance of this change. Science clashed with religion in many disparate areas of Victorian life. A small but instructive example, affecting epilepsy, was the dispute between the medical staff and the lay administration at the National Hospital for the Paralysed and Epileptic in London which simmered for several years and then burst into the public arena in 1899. The hospital had been founded in 1859 on a bedrock of philanthropy and the explicitly Christian ethic of care for the poor and disadvantaged. However, by the 1880s its medical staff were being lauded worldwide for their scientific work in epilepsy and for their role in the emergence of neurology as a scientific and clinical specialty. Increasingly disturbed by the perception that the doctors were more interested in science and novel treatment (not least in the field of neurosurgery), and in vivisection and animal experimentation, than in the welfare of their patients, the hospital governors tried to exert more control over medical practices. It was in essence a clash between religious conservative authority and secular medical science, and the row exploded onto the pages of the national press. R. Brudenell Carter, a hospital physician (and a seasoned journalist), published a polemical letter in *The Times* that concluded:

> The case lies in a nutshell. A proper reform of the constitution of the hospital would leave it in the very van of curative work in the growing science of neurology; while a victory for the board would reduce it to a receptacle of incurable paralytics and hysterical imposters, living in an establishment controlled by a secretary-director, and nominally under the medical care of weak or incompetent practitioners.[10]

Parliament weighed in, and an independent committee of enquiry vindicated the doctors; the board were thus forced to resign. New science had gained the upper hand over conservative religious philanthropy.[11] The events were, in microcosm, a sign of the direction that twentieth-century society was taking. It was to be a path travelled very much further in the course of the next 100 years.

[10] See *The Times*, 21 August 1900, p. 6. Letters and editorials appeared in other newspapers and journals, including *The Guardian, Westminster Gazette, Westminster Budget, Hospital, Echo, Christian World, Queen, St James Gazette, The Lancet, The British Medical Journal* and *Nursing Record*.

[11] The events are described more fully in Shorvon and Compston, *Queen Square*, pp. 45–50.

This having been said, science, did not have free rein. As society became more secular, politics and economics did have an increasing influence over the direction and the nature of science. This serves to emphasise the blindingly obvious which is that science was and is in no way absolute and hermetically sealed; and that it is as relative and interconnected as any other human activity. Paul Feyerabend's colourful view that the claims of science have many similarities to those of astrology, voodoo and alternative medicine is no doubt exaggerated, but it does underscore the impact of culture on science[12] and few can disagree that '[r]eason is, and ought only to be the slave of the passions'.[13] The science of epilepsy was (and still is) the mercy of contemporary societal norms of morality and human relations, distancing it from dry scientific logic.

EPILEPSY IN 1860: THE BOOKS OF SIEVEKING AND DELASIAUVE

Two influential books provide a snapshot of epilepsy around 1860 at the end of its 'premodern history'. The first was *Traité de l'épilepsie* by Louis Delasiauve.[14] The author was a French alienist, a modernist strongly committed to the republican movement and change in French society, to social welfare and universal education, founder of *Le Journal de médecine mentale* and the leading figure in the field of epilepsy in Paris at mid-century.[15] His book was based on his experiences, first among the epilepsy patients at the Hospice de Bicêtre, and then the ward for 'epileptics and adult idiots' at the Hôpital de la Salpêtrière. Opening with the words 'Humanity knows no infirmity more loathsome, more mysterious in its origins, more extreme in its manifestation than the cruel disease known as epilepsy',[16] the book goes on to review the work of the French alienist tradition in prior decades, and then presents Delasiauve's own observations based on more than 500 cases. He describes different types of seizures and their patterns and provides a long list of causes, including the multitude of diverse lesions found in post-mortem findings, and an equally extensive catalogue of contemporary therapies, of which he felt only valerian to be truly efficacious. Of critical importance to the history of epilepsy was his work on classification, which then, as now, was an issue that consumed much energy. Two different approaches had earlier developed that often mixed up one with the other. First, epilepsy was categorised by the visible form of the seizures (a 'seizure type' classification). Great advances had been made in describing the clinical appearance of seizures, particularly by the earlier

---

[12]   Preston, 'Paul Feyerabend'; Feyerabend, *Against Method* and *Tyranny of Science*. See also Lévi-Strauss, *Wild Thought*.

[13]   Hume, *Treatise*, II.3.3, p. 415.   [14]   Delasiauve, *Traité de l'épilepsie*, p. 1.

[15]   For an appreciation of the life and work of Delasiauve, see Walusinski, 'Louis Delasiauve'.

[16]   Translated from Delasiauve, *Traité de l'épilepsie*, p. 1.

French alienists, although it was then left to Jackson and to Gowers, Binswanger and others to provide truly comprehensive and modern descriptions (in my opinion, so good were these descriptions that very little of importance in this regard has been added since). Second, a classification by aetiology also had been sometimes proposed, although applied haphazardly, with causation divided sometimes into predisposing and exciting categories, sometimes into proximate and remote categories, and sometimes classified by anatomical site (e.g. spine, medulla or white matter). Terminology was a confusing tangle of overlapping categories, and by 1850 the classification of epilepsy had become varied, inconsistent and unsatisfactory.

The achievement of Delasiauve was to cut through the nosological brambles and to devise a logical system with precise boundaries. This was an important step in bringing epilepsy into the modern world. He divided epilepsy into three broad groups: sympathetic epilepsy – epilepsy due to bodily pathologies outside the brain ('and its dependencies'); symptomatic epilepsy – epilepsy due to brain lesions); and idiopathic epilepsy – epilepsy occurring in the absence of brain lesions or pathologies elsewhere.[17] He also recognised four different seizure types – '*absences, vertiges, accès intermédiaires, chutes* [or] *accès complets*' (p. 55; precursors of subsequent categorisations into absence, focal and generalised seizures). Delasiauve's classification was based on the early work of Jean-Étienne Esquirol,[18] but was less confused and ambiguous. It is notable, too, that he considered sympathetic, symptomatic and idiopathic forms all to be part of the disease 'epilepsy', and here he parted company with his successors John Russell Reynolds, Gowers and Turner, for instance; we shall return to this issue later. Delasiauve's book was a landmark in epilepsy history also for his critical review of French epileptology at a time when the study of epilepsy was wholly within the realm of psychiatry, and when the French school of psychiatry was a leading influence on the concepts of epilepsy. His humanity and zeal for social reform, in the spirit of his predecessor Philippe Pinel, further distinguished Delasiauve from most other French psychiatrists, at a time when psychiatry was

[17] Delasiauve, *Traité de l'épilepsie*, p. 37. The term *idiopathic epilepsy* was coined by Galen to designate epilepsy caused by a disorder of the brain itself – in contrast to sympathetic epilepsy. Auguste Tissot (1770) also recognised the existence of epilepsy occurring in the brain but without overt cerebral lesions and called it 'essential epilepsy'. To Delasiauve, idiopathic and essential epilepsy were synonymous terms. The term *primary epilepsy* is another synonym invented later and now used mainly in veterinary medicine.

[18] Esquirol, *Des maladies mentales* (1838). He divided epilepsy into essential, sympathetic and symptomatic categories. Essential epilepsy included seizures caused by external forces, cerebral lesions or moral affections (either on the part of the mother, nurse or patient). Sympathetic epilepsy could be caused by afflictions of the gut, blood (sanguine system), lymphatic system and organs of reproduction, or by external causes. Symptomatic epilepsy could be caused by delayed dentition, infections or cutaneous phelgmasiae. He separated epilepsy from demonomania (the delusion of demonic possession).

evolving into an oppressive social force, and when the profession was becoming increasingly materialistic and bureaucratic.[19]

The second book was *On Epilepsy and Epileptiform Seizures* by Edward Sieveking (1858).[20] Sieveking trained in Germany, France and Britain and was well acquainted with the advanced practice of epilepsy medicine across Europe. He became a celebrated London clinician (serving as physician to two generations of the British Royal family), and his book encapsulates the thought and mood of both continental and British epileptology. It is a scholarly work which surveys the contemporary literature, reflecting Sieveking's trans-European perspective and refined by his experience in earlier translating Moritz Romberg's *Manual of the Nervous Diseases of Man* (1853), a work cited respectfully in different sections of his book.[21] *On Epilepsy* opens with the observation that the strides in the science of physiology made in previous decades had not been matched by any in the therapeutics or pathology of epilepsy: 'The history of epilepsy, more than of other affections of the nervous system, until the most recent periods has been the history of one of the weakest sides of medical science.'[22] He bemoaned the widespread superstitions about the cause and nature of epilepsy (p. 1), one example of which was a belief in the influence of the moon, such that 'the three terms "epilepsy", "lunatic" and "demoniac" were in the eyes of many "convertible"' (p. 90); indeed, the book devoted seven pages to the 'demoniac controversy' (pp. 85–91).

Sieveking disagreed with Delasiauve over the question of classification. He saw epilepsy as a symptom and noted 'the impossibility of rigidly carrying out the distinction between essential and non-essential, idiopathic or symptomatic epilepsy', which he considered as sufficient reason for 'discarding such an arrangement' (pp. 162–3).[23] Moreover, knowledge of pathology was not sufficiently advanced to allow a sensible classification, and thus in his view all cases should be simply categorised as 'epilepsy'.

Of greatest influence on subsequent epilepsy theory, however, were not Sieveking's ideas on nosology, but his views on causation, heredity and

---

[19] For a study of the evolution of French psychiatry, see Goldstein, *Console and Classify*.

[20] Sieveking, *On Epilepsy*.

[21] Romberg's two-volume *Lehrbuch der Nervenkrankheiten des Menschen*, occupying over 800 pages, was translated into English in 1853. It is often considered the first true textbook of neurology.

[22] Sieveking, *On Epilepsy*. He specifically mentions Charles Bell, Marshall Hall, Pierre Fourens, François Magendie, Johannes Müller and Charles-Édouard Brown-Séquard 'who have illumined a field which before the beginning of the present century was enveloped in darkness' (p. vii), although it must be noted that none of their theories of epilepsy survived the next decades.

[23] Others in the period who held that epilepsy was a symptom and not a disease were William Hammond (*A Treatise on the Diseases of the Nervous System*, 1871) and Charles Féré (*Les épilepsies et les épileptiques*, 1890).

treatment. He followed the well-established practice of the time in dividing the causation of epilepsy into 'predisposing' and 'exciting' factors, and devoted separate chapters to each. A common predisposing factor was, in his view, heredity, as part of the 'neuropathic trait' or 'neurological taint' (discussed later). Other predisposing causes included various chronic diseases and also sexual derangements. Sieveking called the predisposition to epilepsy the epileptic 'diathesis', and he used the following rather vivid analogy: '[T]he diathesis may be compared to combustible material of greater or less inflammability, which differs in the facility with which it will take fire but will infallibly do so if a flame of sufficient intensity is brought into contact with it' (p. 158). He likened the exciting causes to the sparks that ignite this combustible material (just as a spark ignites gunpowder). Exciting causes included fright, mental work, anxiety, dentition, fever, pregnancy, various physical diseases and masturbation (which he considered both exciting and predisposing). This became the predominant framework for viewing aetiology in epilepsy. In terms of pathology and pathogenesis, Sieveking repeated the orthodoxies of the day (which were completely wrong) in proposing the medulla to be the seat of epilepsy,[24] and cerebral vascular disturbance the likely mechanism (proximate cause) of seizures. Sieveking's book too provides graphic descriptions of the state of therapeutics in epilepsy (described later in this chapter).

Sieveking, and to a lesser extent Delasiauve, both summarised the state of epilepsy knowledge in 1860, and in this sense looked backwards. The real revolution in epilepsy studies was to occur in the subsequent decades with the work of the next neurological generation.

PSYCHIATRY OF EPILEPSY

But first, to psychiatry. Despite the advances of neurology, epilepsy in the half-century prior to the First World War was treated largely under the purview of psychiatry not neurology, and largely in the setting of asylum practice. This reflected the predominant idea of epilepsy as a mental disorder entangled with concepts of progressive degeneration, heredity, mental handicap and the neuro-logical trait, concepts which coloured the societal attitudes to epilepsy and the experiences of those with epilepsy.

---

[24] Jacobus Ludovicus Conradus Schroeder van der Kolk was one of the first clinicians to take a physiological approach to epilepsy and was an important influence on Brown Sequard and the next general generation of clinical scientists. His book *On the Minute Structure and Functions of the Medulla Oblongata and the Proximate Causes and Rational Treatment of Epilepsy* was highly regarded. In his Sydenham Lecture of 1859, he stated: 'The first cause of epilepsy . . . is exalted sensibility and excitability of the medulla oblongata . . . These caused the medulla to be "liable to discharge upon itself" and these discharges caused spasms in blood vessels leading to hyperaemia followed by involuntary reflex movements . . ." Frequent or repeated fits caused inflammation of the cortex leading to "incurable dementia" due to "thickening and dilatation of blood vessels.'

Epilepsy As a Mental Disease

The number of persons with epilepsy who also have comorbid mental illness and/or mental impairment is today recognised to be relatively small. The reason this was not realised in the late nineteenth and early twentieth centuries was that all studies of epilepsy were conducted from asylums. Most 'normal' persons with epilepsy and their families kept the disease hidden owing to the stigma and hostility engendered by the condition, and many sought only occasional medical attention, if any at all. The selection bias thus introduced was the root cause of many false theories in epilepsy and is a striking example of how damaging it can be to see a condition from only one perspective. The problem was exacerbated by the fact that no real distinction was made at the time between mental deficiency and psychiatric illnesses – and the confusion caused by the mixing of the two continued well into the twentieth century.

The predominant school of psychiatric theory considered epilepsy to be a type of psychosis, and one in which psychotic, behavioural or personality abnormalities (not least violence and criminality) were *an inherent part of the condition*. So prevalent was this view that the standard textbook of psychiatry by Carl Friedrich Flemming, published in 1859, described epilepsy as one of the most frequent external forms of psychosis acting upon the central organs of the nervous system.[25]

Two French psychiatrists – Bénédict Morel[26] and Jules Falret, both directors of asylums – were prominent theoreticians of the time. Morel was, according to his fellow physician Charles Lasègue at the Pitié-Salpêtrière, interested particularly in the character of his patients with epilepsy and 'was one of the first to discern the epileptic within epilepsy' instead of simply describing the fits.[27] Morel noted irritability, anger and violence, among a long list of other typical characteristics, to be common in his patients, and in 1860 described these symptoms as masked or larval epilepsy' (*épilepsie larvée*). He considered these to be psychotic symptoms and, indeed, in occasional cases to be present without the occurrence of any definite 'orthodox' epileptic seizures. His ideas were shared by Falret,[28] who considered the psychiatric manifestations of epilepsy more important than the seizures and divided the psychiatric symptoms into those occurring in relation to a seizure, those occurring as part of the epileptic character and those taking the form of prolonged episodes of delirium (epilepsy insanity; *folie épileptique*). In the first category were cases which would later be called psychomotor seizures. The third category – 'epileptic insanity' – Falret divided into two groups: *petit mal intellectuel* and

---

[25] Flemming, *Pathologie*, pp.117–18.
[26] Morel trained as an assistant to Falret at the Salpêtrière.
[27] Temkin, *Falling Sickness*, p. 316.   [28] Falret, *Maladies mentales*.

grand mal intellectuel. Paul Samt (1844–75), a student of Wilhelm Griesinger,[29] also considered psychotic symptoms to be epileptic and introduced the concept of epilepsy equivalents. These were mental symptoms such as severe delirium, anxiety, hallucinations, violence, memory disturbance or stupor, and even religious ecstasy, which could be transient or prolonged. It is not clear to what extent Morel, Falret and Samt considered larval epilepsy, epileptic insanity and epileptic equivalents to have the same mechanisms as more orthodox epileptic seizures, and the distinction between these forms seems at times to be quite confused, but all three believed these examples of psychotic symptomatology to be characteristic of epilepsy. And all three contributed to the idea that persons with epilepsy had, almost inevitably, defects of character and personality which manifested in psychotic and behavioural symptomatology.

By 1900, great nosological debates were raging in the field of psychiatry, with some taking the traditional view that mental disorder was a unitary condition, exhibiting a spectrum of symptoms with varying degrees of severity and tending strongly to progressively worsen and ultimately end in dementia. Others, most notably Emil Kraepelin, introduced the idea that different mental disorders were discrete and distinct entities. Where this was the case, epilepsy was sometimes separated from the other conditions, although still considered to be primarily a mental disorder. In the first edition of Kraepelin's textbook, for instance, he treated epilepsy as one of the neuroses, but by the seventh edition (1903–4)[30] it had been assigned its own category as one of the three major psychoses (the other two being schizophrenia and manic depression).[31]

Epilepsy: The Theories of Degeneration and of the Neurological Trait

It was in the context of the study of mental symptoms in epilepsy that the theory of *dégénérescence* (degeneration) was proposed, again by Morel.[32] This was to prove a most egregious example of flawed science, and one which had profound consequences for epilepsy. The term was taken to indicate a tendency for complex forms of brain function, and higher levels of civilised behaviour, to

[29] Wilhelm Griesinger was the leading German psychiatrist of his times. He considered mental illness to be an organic unitary disorder. Of his students, Paul Samt was the one most interested in epilepsy. His work included a celebrated and detailed study of forty cases of epileptic insanity (Samt, 'Epileptische irreseinsformen').

[30] Kraepelin, *Ein Lehrbuch*.

[31] The unitary view of mental disorders continued to be influential, and later adherents included, for instance, Karl Menninger (*The Vital Balance: The Life Process in Mental Health and Illness*, 1963) and Henri Ey (*Études psychiatriques*, 1954). The Kraepelin approach can be seen as a precursor of the DSM classification schemes of the American Psychiatric Association.

[32] Morel's theory of degeneration in 1857 was detailed in his book, *Traité des dégénérescences physiques, intellectuelles et morales de l'espèce humaine et des causes qui produisent ces variétés maladives*.

disintegrate progressively into simpler and more primitive types. In the later decades of the nineteenth century and right through the early years of the next, this theory became a predominant narrative in many intellectual areas and extended far beyond mental illness. Degeneration, as the disintegration of complex structures and 'higher' behaviour, came to be seen as an explanation for a range of social, political, economic and moral as well as biological phenomena. As such, it was applied as an explanation for such disparate topics as urban poverty, criminality, alcoholism, and even the failure of the European armies in foreign adventures (for instance, the British army in the Boer War[33]) and a perceived decline in public standards of behaviour.

The theory acquired great traction in neurology, not least because it became linked to the question of inheritance. By then, August Weissman's theory that inherited traits were transmitted in 'germ plasm' contained in the gonads was widely accepted.[34] Cerebral degeneration was held to be one such inherited trait, variously named the *neuropathic trait*, the *neurological taint* or the *neuropathic taint*.[35] Many conditions were considered to be inherited together in this trait, including epilepsy, insanity, psychiatric disorders of various types, mental retardation, general paralysis of the insane and locomotor ataxy, moral degeneration such as was found in alcoholics or criminals, and degeneration in sexual behaviour evinced by masturbation, perversion and sexual excess.

Idiopathic epilepsy was considered a central symptom of the degenerative neurological trait. It was believed that the neuropathic trait manifested itself in different forms within a kinship, with some family members afflicted with epilepsy and others with disorders such as insanity, chorea, hysteria, alcoholism and immorality. This theory was widely accepted among those calling themselves neurologists as well as psychiatrists, and when other conditions were included as evidence of the trait, Manuel Echeverria reported an inheritability rate in 25% of those with epilepsy, Reynolds 31%, Binswanger 36%, Gowers 40%, Joseph Déjerine 67% and Turner 51% (Table 1.1).[36] In contrast, Jackson earlier had opposed the idea of mixing up conditions with, as he put it, 'no evident pathological connection'.

---

[33] War was widely considered to be a test of social fitness and manhood. Poor performance was taken as a worrying sign of degeneration of the national stock.

[34] Weismann's theories of germ plasm were in part derived from Francis Galton. The 'Weismann barrier' was a powerful counterweight to the then prevalent Lamarckism.

[35] The mechanisms of inheritance were, of course, unknown at this time. The predominant belief was that inheritance was mediated by germ plasm, which was transmitted from parents to offspring. The chromosome theory of inheritance was proposed in 1902, the term 'gene' coined as the Mendelian unit of heredity in 1909, and the fact that chromosomes carry genes was recognised in 1911.

[36] Echeverria, 'On epileptic insanity'; Reynolds, *Epilepsy*; Binswanger, *Die Epilepsie*; Gowers, *Epilepsy*; Dejerine, *L'hérédité*. The origin of the term 'neurologist' to define a physician specialising in the treatment of neurological disease arose at some point in the late nineteenth century – although its provenance is obscure.

TABLE 1.1 *The neuropathic trait: The proportion of epilepsy cases who have a family history of epilepsy, insanity, alcoholism, chorea or other features of the neurological trait*

	Gowers 1901	Binswanger 1899	Turner 1907
Epilepsy	41%	11%	37%
Insanity	14%	30%	5%
Alcoholism	Not stated	14%	3%
Chorea	2%	Not stated	Not stated
Other neurological conditions	Not stated	Not stated	5%
No known family history	60%	Not stated	49%

Gowers based on 2,400 cases
Turner based on 676 cases. His other neurological condition included chorea, 'nervousness', migraine, paroxysmal headache, suicide and deaf-mutism
(Derived from Turner, *Epilepsy*, pp. 23–7)

Morel proposed that the inherited tendency became progressively more severe over generations and eventually resulted in dementia and the extinction of the line. The theory was further fleshed out by Jacques-Joseph Moreau, who published an influential text titled *La psychologie morbide* (1859) in which he introduced the category of the 'neuropathic family', by Valentin Magnan, Jean-Pierre Falret and ultimately by Charles Féré,[37] who divided the neuropathic family into a psychopathological arm, which included epilepsy and the major psychiatric disorders, and a neuropathological arm, which included chorea, migraine and Parkinson's disease.[38]

Degeneration was considered to release the lower centres from the inhibitory control of the cortex, resulting in animalistic and atavistic traits, intellectual decline and aberrant behaviour – as Henry Maudsley put it, 'like the turbulent, aimless action of a democracy without a head'.[39]

The fact that these theories were completely devoid of robust evidence did not dim the enthusiasm for this idea or prevent their ubiquity and domination of mainstream neuro-medical theory from 1870 until at least into the 1920s.

As it was also considered that the presence of the degenerative germ plasm could be detected by physical stigmata, especially facial and cranial features,

[37] Leading French psychiatrists of the period.
[38] After Morel's 1857 book, the development of the theory of degeneration can be traced in Morel, *Traité des maladies mentales*; Moreau, *La psychologie morbide*; Falret, *Maladies mentales*; and Féré, 'La famille névropathique'.
[39] Maudsley, *Physiology of Mind*, p. 179. Henry Maudsley was an influential advocate of the theory of degeneration.

studies of physiognomy flourished.[40] The notion of degeneration was also linked to the concept of atavism, which had biological plausibility given the theory of recapitulation popularised by Ernst Haeckel in 1866 ('ontogeny recapitulates phylogeny').[41] Degeneration was thought to bring out atavistic characteristics (physical, behavioural and mental) which therefore were the physical signs of the degenerative tendency. Epilepsy was seen as one symptom of inherited degeneration, atavistic in nature and inevitably part of a progressive downward degenerative spiral.

Epilepsy, Criminality and the Epileptic Personality

Another important influence on the late-nineteenth and early-twentieth-century view of epilepsy was the work of Cesare Lombroso, the physician and criminologist who founded the Italian school of positivist criminology.

Using the prevalent scientific method of anthropometrics – the measurement and quantification of physical and mental attributes – Lombroso studied the inheritance of criminality and packed his writings with statistical and numerical tables. As his ideas evolved, he focused on the link between epilepsy and crime. His theories were most fully expressed in the fourth edition of *L'uomo deliquente*,[42] in which he proposed that there were 'born criminals' who inherited a criminal trait and possessed 'anomalies' – physical and psychological characteristics – which resembled those of primitive man and apes (p. 1) (Table 1.2). These traits were, in his words, 'atavistic throwbacks' to a more primitive stage in human evolution (p. 39). Epilepsy was one of these features, and Lombroso considered it to be a fundamental component of the 'criminal type'. He showed that criminals and people with epilepsy shared similar physiognomy, physical and psychological features, and moral deficiency, and produced long lists of features he had measured

[40] Physiognomy has a long history dating from ancient Greece. It was considered so subversive that it was banned from university study in England in 1551 by Henry VIII. As a topic of social and medical interest, it had a resurgence in the 1770s following the work of Casper Lavater, Sir Thomas Browne and Franz Joseph Gall who coined the term 'cranioscopy' (later known as phrenology) as a method of assessing intellectual and emotional characteristics from the shape of the skull. In psychiatry, an important landmark was the publication of *Des maladies mentales considerées sous les rapports médical, hygiénique et médico-légal* (1838) by Esquirol, who found that the insane and the retarded had specific physical appearances which reflected their degenerative taint. Moreau, Falret and Magnan developed these concepts further. The fashion for anthropomorphic measures was popularised by Francis Galton and Karl Pearson and these measures became fundamental anthropological tools. Later, they were, with IQ measurement, misappropriated by the eugenics movement and for Nazi theories of racial hygiene in their assault on those with epilepsy. Regrettably, in recent times anthropomorphic measures have had a resurgence as part of the 'new genetics'.

[41] Actually, the theory was said to have been first proposed by Antoine Étienne Renaud Augustin Serres.

[42] Lombroso, *Criminal Man (L'uomo deliquente*: the first edition was published in Italian in 1876). The fourth edition appeared in 1889 with a whole chapter entitled 'The epileptic criminal'. Epilepsy similarly strongly featured in the fifth edition of 1896–7.

TABLE 1.2 *Anomalies shared by epileptics and criminals, as published by Cesare Lombroso*

Skull	Abnormally large, microcephaly*, sclerosis*, asymmetrical skull (12–37%), med. occ. fossetta, abnormal cranial indices, large orbital arches*, low sloping forehead*, wormian bones*, simple cranial sutures*
Face	Overdeveloped jaw*, jutting cheekbones*, large jug ears*, facial asymmetry, strabismus, virility (in women)*, anomalous teeth*
Brain	Anomalous convolutions*, low weight*, hypertrophied cerebellum*, symptoms of meningitis
Body	Asymmetrical torso, prehensile feet, hernia*
Skin	Wrinkles*, beardlessness*, olive skin*, tattoos*, delayed grey hair/balding*, dark and curly hair*
Motor anomalies	Left handedness (10%)*, abnormal reflexes, heightened agility (16%)*
Sensory anomalies	Tactile insensitivity (81%)*, insensitivity to pain*, overly acute eyesight*, dullness of hearing, taste and smell*
Psychological anomalies	Limited intelligence (30–69%)*, weak memory (14–91%), hallucinations (20–41%), superstitious*, blunted emotions*, love of animals, absence of remorse*, impulsivity (2–50%)*, cannibalism and ferocity*, pederasty (2–39%)*, masturbation (21–67%)*, perversity (15–57%)*, vanity*, sloth*, passion for gaming*, mania/paranoia, delirium, dizziness, delusions of grandeur (1–3%), irascibility (30–100%), lying (7–100%), theft (4–75%), religious delusions (14–100%)
Causes	Heredity (of alcoholism, insanity, epilepsy, old parents), alcoholism

(% in epileptics). * = Attributable to atavism. In Lombroso's view, if conditions were not atavistic in origin, they were due to arrested development in most cases or in a few to other diseases or traits. (Derived from edition 4 and 5 of Lombroso, C. *L'uomo delinquente (Criminal Man)*, 1889 and 1896–7)

and correlated. He claimed that 26.9% of all epileptic men and 25% of all epileptic women have a 'full criminal type' from the physiognomic point of view (p. 248), and that a significant proportion of those with epilepsy exhibit mental characteristics that he also found in criminals.[43] He extended his theory and proposed that criminals exhibited '"hidden epilepsy" (*epilessia larvata*)' manifested by 'sharp, sudden outbursts ... [the] psychological equivalents of physical seizures, marked by unpredictability and ferocity', and that hidden epilepsy was responsible for criminal acts, especially acts of physical or sexual violence.[44] His ideas became widely accepted and were considered further confirmation of the existence of degeneration and the neurological taint.[45]

[43] Lombroso also wrote: 'As Gowers notes, epileptics frequently bark, meow, drink blood and devour live animals, including their fur' (p. 266). This was a misquote as Gowers only refers to these symptoms in hysteroid attacks, not genuine epilepsy (*Epilepsy*, p. 140).
[44] Lombroso, *Criminal Man*, pp. 11, 257. The concept of 'masked epilepsy' or 'larval epilepsy' (*épilepsie larvée*) derives from the work of Morel (Morel, 'D'une forme de délire').
[45] The classic book of the times, Max Nordau's *Degeneration* (*Entartung*, published in English in 1895), was dedicated to Lombroso. Lombroso initiated the 'schola positiva' of criminal studies in which criminality was attributed to inherited brain disorders, and criminal behaviour was

As part of his biological interpretation of personality, and perhaps embold-ened by the positive reception of his works on epilepsy and criminality, Lombroso produced, in 1888, a strange book: *The Man of Genius* (*L'uomo di genio*). In this, he took the view that epilepsy and genius shared many features:[46] a family history of alcoholism or insanity, an inclination to criminality, religi-osity, cranial anomalies, moral insanity, sexual and intellectual precocity, higher rates of suicide, a tendency to vagabondage, a double personality, delusions, a strange passion for animals and, particularly, the loss of a moral sense. He also noted a resemblance between epileptic seizures and moments of inspiration, and as an example quotes the famous conversation between Kirilloff and Shatov in Dostoevsky's *Possessed*:[47]

> 'There are moments ... and it is only a matter of five or six seconds – when you suddenly feel the presence of the eternal harmony. This phenomenon is neither terrestrial nor celestial, but it is an indescrib-able something, which man, in his mortal body, can scarcely endure – he must either undergo a physical transformation or die. It is a clear and indisputable feeling: all at once, you feel as though you were placed in contact with the whole of nature, and you say, 'Yes! this is true.' When God created the world, He said, at the end of every day of creation, 'Yes! this is true! this is good!' ... And it is not tenderness, nor yet joy. You do not forgive anything, because there is nothing to forgive. Neither do you love – oh! this feeling is higher than love! The terrible thing is the frightful clearness with which it manifests itself, and the rapture with which it fills you. If this state were to last more than five seconds, the soul could not endure it, and would have to disappear. During those five seconds, I live a whole human exist-ence, and for that I would give my whole life and not think I was paying it too dearly.'
> "You are not epileptic?"
> "No."
> "You will become so. I have heard that it begins just in that way'" (p. 339)

Lombroso postulated that epilepsy was a form of 'irritability of the cerebral cortex' (p. 336) which was also the basis not only of criminality and nervous disorders, but also of genius:

> It is sufficient, however, to recall to the reader the numerous men of genius of the first order who have been seized by motory epilepsy, or by that kind of morbid irritability which is well known to supply its place. Among these we find such names as Napoleon, Molière, Julius Caesar, Petrarch, Peter the Great, Mahomet, Handel, Swift, Richelieu, Charles V., Flaubert, Dostoïeffsky, and St. Paul. (pp. 337–8)

seen not so much as a social problem with its origin in societal deficiencies, but rather as a medical problem with biological roots.

[46] Lombroso, *Man of Genius*, pp. 336–52.   [47] Lombroso's transcription is not entirely accurate.

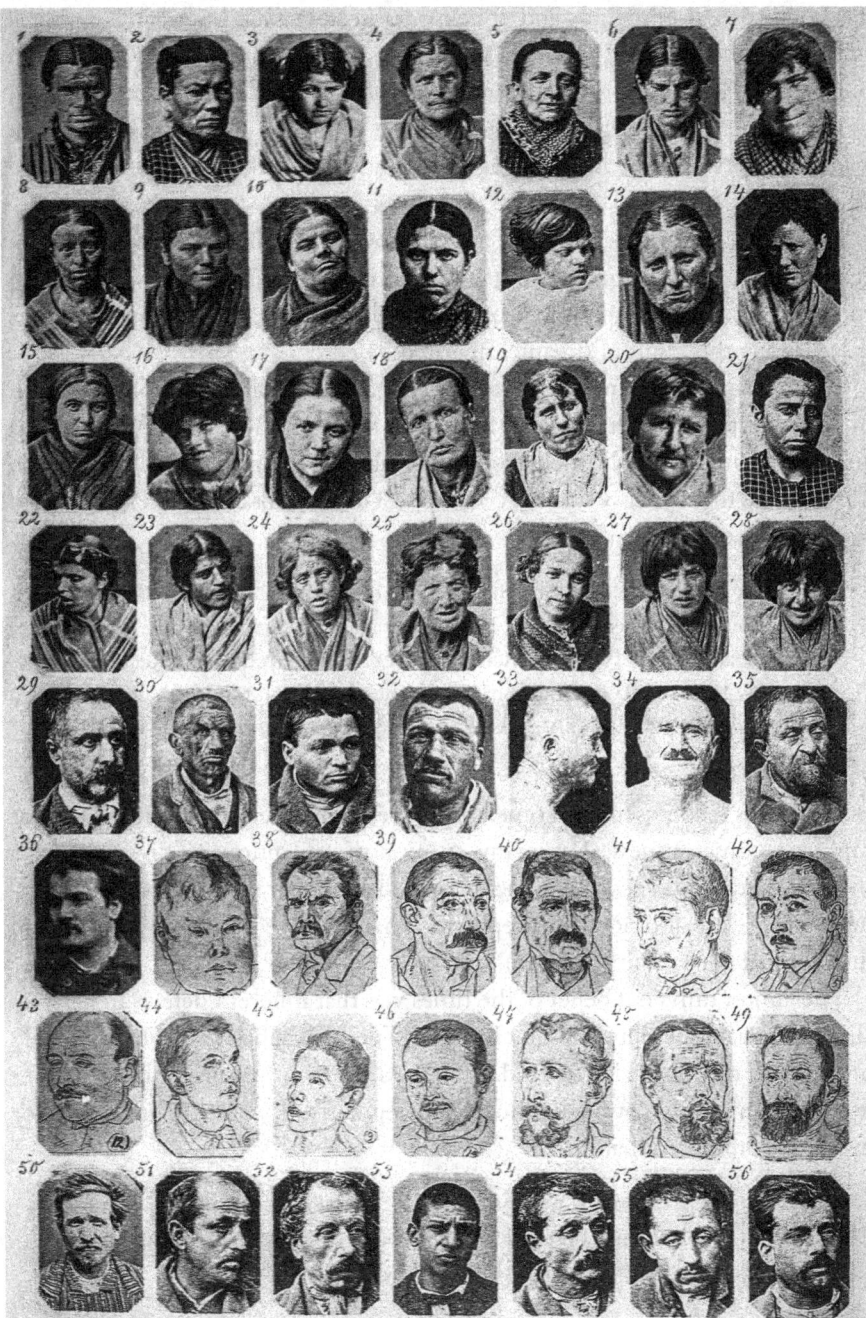

5. 'The Faces of Epileptics'. An illustration from *L'uomo delinquente* (1876) by Cesare Lombroso, purporting to show the physiognomy of epilepsy and its similarities with the faces of criminal types.

To Lombroso, both genius and epilepsy transcended the boundaries of banal normality, and the link between all three was their amorality: 'The greatest proof of all, however, is that affective insensibility, that loss of moral sense, common to all men of genius, whether sane or insane, which makes of great conquerors, even in the most recent times, nothing else than brigands on a large scale' (p. 337).

Lombroso's work had the effect of moving psychiatry further into an academic and intellectual setting, thereby raising its status. His work also stimulated the concept of biological determinism: the idea that mental disorders were largely the result of organic inherited defects.

Unfortunately, the universal acceptance that criminality was more common in those with epilepsy dragged the condition further into a maelstrom of stigma and exclusion, and unleashed a storm of abusive opinions. William Bevan Lewis noted that epilepsy was the commonest form of insanity which presented to the medico-legal expert:[48]

> Epilepsy is a disease to which the criminal class are peculiarly subject; it is the associate of intemperance, moral degradation, vicious bodily organisation, and the very varied heritage of criminal parentage; and, in the second place, of all cerebral diseases it is the one which tends to engender impulsive forms of insanity, as well as to degrade and brutalise the victim's nature. (p. 243)

Bevan Lewis recognised that some crimes were due to epileptic automatism or impaired consciousness, but many were not; epileptics, in his view, also showed character defects including incontrollable anger, impulsivity and sometimes mania. He also noted that epileptic seizures were 'frequently feigned by the criminal community' (p. 246).

The almost universal belief of the times was that inherent defects in personality and behaviour were constant features of epilepsy, and criminality was only one part of this. Psychiatrists and physicians drew up extensive lists of other features commonly found in those with epilepsy. In 1867, Griesinger, for instance, considered that:

> A very great number of epileptics are in state of chronic mental disease even during the intervals between the attacks. In order to appreciate to what extent this is the case, we must not confine

[48] Lewis, *Text-Book* (1889, with the same text repeated in the second edition of 1899). William Bevan Lewis was the highly respected medical director of the West Riding Pauper Lunatic Asylum in Wakefield, where Ferrier carried out his first experimental work. In this unlikely setting, under the inspired guidance of James Crichton-Browne, brain research flourished to an extraordinary extent. He wrote of Bevan Lewis's textbook that, forty years later, '[it] still in many respects holds its own . . . The *Text-Book* is much more than a textbook, being really a compendious system of psychological medicine' (Crichton-Browne, 'William Bevan-Lewis').

ourselves to the isolated cases met with in private practice, but we must study the question in the light of the results furnished by observations conducted in large asylums devoted to such patients. Thus, amongst 385 epileptic women observed by Esquirol, there were 46 hysterical, of whom many suffered from hypochondria and maniacal attacks; 30 others were maniacs; 12 were monomaniacs; 5 were idiots; 145 were dements ...; 50 were weak in memory or had exalted ideas. Sixty ... were free from intellectual derangement; but nearly all of these were irritable, peculiar, and easily enraged. The latter trait of character – a dominant, suspicious, discontented, misanthropic perversion of sentiment, sometimes even actual melancholia with suicidal tendency – is observed in a great many epileptics. This may, in great degree, originate from the sense of their sad and exceptional position, from the perception of the moral death to which their condition condemns them.[49]

Two decades later Gowers noted that deterioration of the mental state was one of the most dreaded consequences of epilepsy.[50] In its slightest form there were merely mild memory defects, especially of recent events, but its more severe degree was characterised by defective moral control, mischievous restlessness and irritability in childhood, which might develop into vicious and criminal tendencies in adult life. Bevan Lewis, based on his asylum population, found that only a small proportion of patients exhibited 'a perfectly normal state of mind'; others were 'moral imbeciles' whose faults were entirely in the affective sphere; 'the extensive class of those in whom the main feature is intellectual perversion; in whom delusional states are rife, and in whom the passions are violent and uncontrolled'; finally, there were patients with epileptic dementia: 'None of the insane arrive at a more degraded level than the epileptic dement; none of them exhibit more repulsive traits – more obnoxious passions.'[51] Across all types, Bevan Lewis noted a tendency to self-engrossment and hypochondriasis. He signalled out religiosity, but in the epileptic patient

> [H]is religious life fails in its *intellectual grasp*; it is essentially egoistic, shallow, selfish, and similar to the undeveloped phases of the religious life in a low grade of civilisation. The grossest animal passions find their gratification *pari passu* with this mock display of pietistic fervour ... The lower types of epileptics also exhibit a characteristic low cunning and deceit; they are treacherous in their dealings with their associates, thievish

---

[49] Griesinger, *Mental Pathology*, pp. 405–6. For Griesinger, mental illness was an organic disorder and not moral failure, and epilepsy was a 'complication' of insanity.

[50] Gowers, *Epilepsy*, p. 121. Gowers also recognised that mental deterioration was by no means inevitable, a fact that other later authors seemed to overlook.

[51] Lewis, *Text-Book*, pp. 240–1.

in their propensities, and when arraigned upon a charge of misconduct, will meet it with the coolest audacity, and lie to the bitter end. The epileptic shows a tendency, akin to that of the hysteric subject, to malingering. Both will falsely accuse of violence those with whom they are aggrieved; will treasure up a tooth, or wilfully pull out their hair by the handful and present it, to countenance their charge: and will cunningly call to their defence certain delusional notions to which they may be prone. (p. 242)

The range of adverse personality traits was broadened and extended by later researchers. In 1907, for instance, under the heading 'The Epileptic Temperament', the leading British epileptologist, Turner, wrote:

It is rare to find epileptics who do not present some form of mental obliquity, ... the possession of which is a feature of their hereditarily degenerative disposition ... self-opinionated and egotistical, and possess a conceit and assurance which is out of all proportion to their achievements; ... prolix and pretentious [conversation] ... tenacity, obstinacy, ... possess[ing] a religious fervour ... which contrasts strongly with their actions, which are often perverted, passionate and immoral. Their ideas of right and wrong are often vague ... habitual irritability ... Their judgement is feeble: they are frequently credulous and mystical, and given to superstitious ideas and fancies ... psychoasthenic.[52]

He also found abnormalities of emotion and feebleness of willpower and obstinacy. He concluded, however, that 'None of these last features should be regarded as in any way peculiar to epileptics, for they are the common attributes of most forms of mental degeneracy and deficiency' (p. 120). Intense religious imagery was thought to be another feature of the epileptic personality. This was particularly emphasised by Samt, who spoke of the 'god-nomenclature' of epileptic patients who thought they were in heaven. As he put it: 'Poor epileptics ... have the prayer book in their pocket, the dear Lord on the tongue, and are blaggards in body and soul.'[53]

Similarly, the most prominent American epilepsy doctor of the time, William Spratling, agreed, noting that the mental capacity in epilepsy is impaired to some extent in the great majority of cases.[54] He devoted a whole

---

[52] Turner, *Epilepsy*, pp. 119–20.

[53] 'die armen epileptisschen das Gebetsbuch in der Tasche, den lieben Gott auf der Zunge, aber den Ausbund von Canaillerie im ganzen Leibe tragen' (Samt, 'Epileptische Irreseinsformen', p. 147, cited in Temkin, *Falling Sickness*, p. 369).

[54] Spratling, *Epilepsy and Its Treatment*. According to Spratling, only 8–10% of cases suffer 'in the lighter degree only' (p. 462). Forty per cent of cases deteriorated to the state of 'feeble-mindedness, imbecility, idiocy, dementia and manic-depressive states', and it was an 'axiomatic' fact that 'every true epileptic convulsion destroys or impairs the integrity of the mental

chapter to the mental state in epilepsy, listing numerous defects and citing Richard von Krafft-Ebing's *Psychopathia Sexualis*[55] for examples of debased moral practices and sexual perversions widely thought to be more common among those with epilepsy. Other more random and arbitrary characteristics included '[t]ransitory ill-humour and simple loss of memory[,] pronounced adjuncts of the epileptic's mental peculiarities: emotional irritability, impulsiveness, moral anergia, and incapacity for any form of valuable productive occupation dependent upon the initiative in conception and consecutive activity'.[56]

All of this, today of course, is recognised to be nonsense, and explained in part by the selection bias introduced by asylum practice. This was responsible for another, equally erroneous thread woven into the dark tapestry of mental disturbance and epilepsy in this period – the universally accepted view that people with chronic epilepsy would almost inevitably suffer progressive dementia. This was attributed both to the progression of the inherited cerebral degeneration and also to the effect of repeated seizures. In Philadelphia, Martin Barr cited his own series of 800 cases, in which 565 had evidence of a 'grave neurotic heredity'; 'imbecility, idiocy and dementia' were found in '80 per cent of all epileptic communities'. He viewed epilepsy as a 'degenerated condition of tissue, nerve and nerve centers; by reason of which nervous energy from its very initial point of formation is tainted and corrupted in its production, transmission and elimination ... causing a gradual but certain deterioration of all the powers of the being – physical, mental and moral'.[57] Turner devoted twelve pages of his book to this topic, dividing his patients into those without mental impairment (13.6%), those with mild memory disturbance (31.6%), those with more widespread mental impairment (25.4%) and those with pronounced dementia to the extent they needed constant supervision (29.1%). Dementia was an 'integral feature of the disease, and, as such, a prominent symptom of the malady' and the result of the hereditary degenerative disposition, although cerebral damage due to frequent major seizures was also thought to play a role.[58]

---

facilities to some extent' (p. 438). He concurred with Turner that only about 10% of epileptics could be 'cured', that treatment in the early stages of the disease was effective, and that the longer seizures continued, the worse the prognosis (p. 293).

[55] Spratling, *Epilepsy and Its Treatment*, p. 462; von Krafft-Ebing, *Psychopathia Sexualis*, pp. 364–74.

[56] Spratling, *Epilepsy and Its Treatment*, p. 440.

[57] 'Philadelphia Neurological Society, November 24, 1903', pp. 104–5. Barr made his comments following the reading of a paper by M. A. Starr, 'Is epilepsy a functional disease?' Barr was superintendent of the Pennsylvania Training School for Feeble-Minded Children at Elwyn and a strong advocate of eugenic sterilisation. He was the author of the novel *The King of Thomond: A Story of Yesterday* (see p. 138).

[58] Turner, *Epilepsy*, p. 152.

Epilepsy and Mental Deficiency

Because of the focus on asylum practice, epilepsy was also widely conceived throughout this period as being intimately associated – indeed, coterminous – with low intelligence (feeble-mindedness or 'mental deficiency', as it was then known). Mental deficiency was considered a largely unitary condition, and the fact that it had many different causes was then not recognised. Epilepsy was part of the symptomatology of mental deficiency, and both epilepsy and feeble-mindedness were considered manifestations of the same inherited cerebral degeneration.

In the early twentieth century, psychology became imbued with a strong metric thread. This trend was set in motion by the quantitative hereditarian work of Galton and Karl Pearson, among others, in Britain, and the anthropomorphic work of Lombroso in Italy. Then, the most important boost to biometry was the invention of IQ scales in France in 1905 by Alfred Binet, developed with the aim of detecting mentally defective children, and the assessments of 'mental age' formulated by his colleague, Theodore Simon.[59]

The seemingly objective techniques of psychometric measurement led inevitably to categorisation which in turn stimulated changes in social policy. In Britain, earlier legislation – and particularly the Idiots Act of 1886 and the Elementary Education (Defective and Epileptic Children) Act of 1899 – had brought into law the need to provide care for idiots and imbeciles.[60] The legislation was largely philanthropic in spirit, and included the provision of institutions but also special day schools, especially for those who were in the feeble-minded range and considered at least partly educable. In 1904, a Royal Commission on the Care and Control of the Feeble-minded was set up to 'consider the existing methods of dealing with idiots and epileptics and with imbecile, feeble-minded or defective persons not certified under the Lunacy Laws'.[61] The commission's long (580 pages) and influential report was published in 1908 and became a landmark document in the field of mental handicap, leading to the passage of the controversial Mental Deficiency Act of 1913. The report found, as had Binet and Simon, that many people with mental deficiency were unknown to the system (0.46% of the British population – approximately 100,000 persons – were estimated to be mentally defective) and that they should be brought into touch with a 'friendly authority'. It was also considered that the majority of epileptics were 'insane' (i.e. exhibiting psychiatric disorders and/or mental deficiency). And although a chapter was devoted to the question of 'sane epileptics', defined as those 'not certified under the Lunacy Act of 1890', the report

---

[59] The Binet Simon IQ tests were refined by Lewis Terman and Charles Spearman and became known as the Stanford–Binet Intelligence Scale.

[60] It made no distinction between mental deficiency and mental disorder despite the fact that in Britain from around 1300 'born fools' (idiots, *fatuus naturalis*) were differentiated from lunatics (persons who 'hath had understanding, but by disease, grief or other accident hath lost the use of his reason', (see Bucknill and Tuke, *A Manual of Psychological Medicine*).

[61] *Report of the Royal Commission* on the Care and Control of the Feeble-Minded.

made it clear that 'it does not follow that a sane epileptic is not, in some degree, mentally defective. Many of them are . . . [No] epileptic escapes quite free from a certain amount of dullness. They have graduations from the simplest down to the severe. They require to be looked after by somebody' (p. 302–3). The report considered that the number of epileptic children who are otherwise normal was small and 'many who are classed as sane epileptics are but little removed from the mentally defective, so that probably during their life as workers and patients they may have to be transferred from one colony or institution to another as the epilepsy passes into mental defect and eventually becomes the lesser malady' (p. 303). In the report it was also noted:

> The children of the poor who are epileptics cannot be treated at home, and no serious attempt is ever made to save them from drifting into the hopeless condition of epileptic insanity. Prejudice, ignorance and poverty of many parents render treatment at home futile. Most of them only have medical aid for a month or two, or even less time than this, unless improvement is obvious; others have no treatment at all after the first convulsion and fright is over, as they are firm in their faith that the child will grow out of the disease, whereas the fact is they grow into it. (pp. 311–12)

It was unanimously agreed that the current provision for sane epileptics was unsatisfactory[62] and urged that special provision be made in the shape of farm and employment colonies, and special educational facilities.[63] Early treatment and early commitment to a colony were recommended, as '[t]imely intervention of the State has a splendid chance of saving the epileptic from the doom awaiting him' (p. 313). Children were a focus of the report, as late-onset epilepsy was considered by one witness 'as also always due to syphilis or alcoholism'. The report espoused the view that marriage between epileptics was to be avoided if possible, but there was no suggestion of certification, sterilisation or any absolute prohibition on marriage.

The 1913 act[64] embodied two key principles: separation and control (most clearly indicated by the name of the new regulatory body set up under

[62] 'As regards the present provision for epileptics it may be stated that large numbers of them are dealt with in lunatic asylums, large numbers in workhouses in surroundings which are generally described as ill-adapted for their requirements, a small number in certified epileptic schools, a small number in idiot asylums, and a certain number, not very large, in philanthropic institutions. Some of them are relieved by county councils as lunacy authorities, some by guardians as "lunacy authorities," some by boards of guardians as Poor Law authorities, others by county councils as education authorities, others by guardians as "education authorities," and others by philanthropy' (*Report of the Royal Commission*, p. 320).

[63] In Germany, similar proposals were made. See, for instance, Vogt, *Die Epilepsie des Kindesalters*.

[64] Mental Deficiency Act. Only three members of Parliament voted against it, among them Josiah Wedgwood: 'It is a spirit of the horrible Eugenic Society which is setting out to breed up the working class as though they were cattle' (Feeble-Minded Persons Bill). The act stated that for the mentally defective and pauper epileptics, housing in colonies should be provided,

the act – the Board of Control). A complex structure of detection, supervision, distribution and institutionalisation was inaugurated. The act empowered the state to take action by colonising both mentally deficient and epileptic individuals. The emphasis for children was still on education, and the colonies were run on educational lines by the mental deficiency committee of a local authority. Nevertheless, the act extended involuntary state-controlled measures which restricted as never before the rights of the mental handicapped.

It was in the United States that the metrical approach to mental impairment had the greatest impact on the field of epilepsy, and this was thanks in large part to the work of psychologist Henry Goddard. Goddard adapted the Binet–Simon tests and, beginning in 1908, applied them to inmates, including those with epilepsy, in the asylum in Vineland, New Jersey, where he had been appointed director of research from 1906 to 1918.[65] In 1912, he published *The Kallikak Family: A Study in the Heredity of Feeble-Mindedness*, a book which became a talisman for eugenics.[66] He introduced quantitative scales that also were to prove a valuable weapon in the armamentarium of the most important social trends of the time and which claimed the authority of science - that of *eugenics*.

Eugenics and Epilepsy

Heredity was (and is) the prototypical example of a subject in which science and societal attitudes were (and remain) intimately intertwined, an entanglement that was to prove injurious for people with epilepsy. It is difficult from the perspective of today to appreciate the extent of antipathy towards epilepsy that existed in the first years of the twentieth century, with stigma fuelled by hereditarian theories of degeneration, the association of epilepsy with mental derangement and its categorisation as a mental disease. These ideas led inexorably to the involvement of epilepsy

and for the others, the local authorities should be authorised to provide for accommodation, maintenance, care, treatment, education, training and control.

[65] There was a second epileptic colony in New Jersey, the Skillman Village, where IQ tests were also performed. David Weeks was the director at Skillman, and the tests were performed by J. E. Wallace Wallin, who became an important figure in American psychology. At Skillman, Wallin created the first clinical psychology laboratory of any epileptic colony. He compared his findings with those of non-epileptic residents at Vineland and concluded that the 'intellectual superiority of the epileptic defective is conspicuous' (Wallin, 'Eight months'). This must have been anathema to Weeks and Goddard. After eight months there, Wallin clashed with Weeks and was replaced by Edwin Katzen-Ellenbogen (see Nevins, *Tale of Two 'Villages'*, and Hermann, '100 years of *Epilepsia*'). The scandalous career of the unscrupulous Katzen-Ellenbogen is related by Nevins and Hermann.

[66] *The Kallikat Family: A Study in the Heredity of Feeble-Mindedness* was based on the family history of an inmate at Vineland. Of the 480 individuals in the family tree, three had epilepsy. Goddard also wrote a textbook of psychology, *Psychology of the Normal and Subnormal* (1919). In reading his work, one is struck by the authoritarian tone and the intense dislike he seems to have had for those with mental deficiency. His textbook does not mention epilepsy.

in eugenics. Epilepsy became the neurological disease most consistently singled out in eugenic texts, and a major eugenic target.

The term 'eugenics' was coined by Francis Galton in 1883, and the early eugenic concepts were developed in Britain.[67] It was a theory which was based on, and extended, Darwin's idea of the survival of the fittest, and had the original aim of encouraging the spread of favourable genes (positive eugenics) rather than restricting the reproduction of those with unfavourable genes (negative eugenics); however, this emphasis was to change in the next decades. The theories spread quickly around the world, and by 1910 eugenic research was most intensively carried out in the United States, which led this field not only in medicine but also in the public and political spheres. Engaging the public was key to the success of the eugenicists, and popularist eugenic movements arose in many countries. As the focus switched to negative eugenics, policies began to be enacted into legislation which prohibited marriage and enforced the segregation and/or sterilisation of those deemed to be carrying such genes. In the midst of this fray stood the stigmatised and disparaged disease epilepsy.

Probably the first example of an epilepsy in which eugenic methods were proposed was the very rare familial type of progressive myoclonic epilepsy which Heinrich Unveriicht had described in 1891. In 1903, Hermann Lundborg, for his doctoral thesis, studied the condition and traced one family back to the eighteenth century. He recognised its autosomal recessive nature and insisted that families with this taint were degenerate and should not reproduce[68].

Soon however eugenic attention turned to epilepsy in general. The first anti-marriage law targeting epilepsy was passed in 1895 in Connecticut. By 1939, eighteen other American states had prohibited marriage of those with epilepsy. At the first meeting of the Society for the Study of Epilepsy and the Treatment and Care of the Epileptic in 1901, Spratling wrote: 'I believe the time will come, and should come, when every State will enact laws to prohibit, if possible, the marriage and intermarriage of epileptics. I think such prohibition would be best for the epileptic, best for society at large, best for posterity, and best for the State for economic reasons.'[69] In 1904 he reiterated this position, except for cases in which the possibility of offspring was eliminated or where an older person developed seizures which were clearly not a sign of idiopathic epilepsy: 'But who can doubt the extreme rarity of these conditions? On the whole, it is better in every way that epileptics should not marry.'[70] The

[67] The first eugenics society, the Eugenics Education Society, was founded in Britain in 1904 and was to become an important influence globally.

[68] Lundborg, H. B. 'Die progressive Myoklonus-Epilepsie'. The condition now bears the name Unverricht–Lundborg Disease. Lundborg later became a keen advocate of racial hygiene, and in 1922 was the first Director of the Swedish state Institute for Racial Biology in Uppsala.

[69] Cited in Lennox, *Epilepsy and Related Disorders*, p. 981.

[70] Spratling, *Epilepsy and Its Treatment*, p. 353.

extraordinary venom the disease attracted[71] can be gathered from W. Duncan McKim's influential *Heredity and Human Progress*, published in 1900, which contained a long section on epilepsy.[72] McKim was an extremist in many of his views, and in regard to those with epilepsy he wrote:

> These afflicted beings live, for the most part, lives of great dejection and unhappiness; they are a menace to society through their tendency to violence and crime, and to themselves through the frequency of their accidents and the suicidal impulse to which they are prone; their existence, directly and indirectly, absorbs a large portion of the public wealth . . .; as progenitors, they transmit a very direful curse; and for these evils the best plan as yet devised can promise only mitigation. Shall we continue to impoverish and destroy many happy and useful lives that we may prolong the pitiable existence of the dependent epileptic? In the great majority of cases, epilepsy appears in early life: to these sufferers, and to those who have their welfare most at heart, an early death would be sweet relief. (p. 147)

He suggested a radical solution:

> The surest, the simplest, the kindest, and most humane means for preventing reproduction among those whom we deem unworthy of this high privilege, is a *gentle, painless death* [his preferred method was by inhalation of carbonic acid gas]; and this should be administered not as a punishment, but as an expression of enlightened pity for the victims – too defective by nature to find true happiness in life – and as a duty toward the community and toward our own offspring . . . The essential feature of the plan is the gentle removal from this life of such idiotic, imbecile, and otherwise grossly defective persons as are now *dependent for maintenance upon the State*, and of such criminals as commit the most heinous crimes, or show by the frequent repetition of crimes less grave, by their bodily and mental characters, and by their ancestry, that they are hopelessly incorrigible. But we may specify more minutely the individuals whom we should select for extinction . . . It is clear that all idiots would require such a decision; and of imbeciles by far the greater number, and especially those who while intelligent gave sure indication of *moral* imbecility. The majority of epileptics would require extinction; but those in whom the disease has apparently been caused by injury or by some removable condition, and whose families give indication of but little degenerative taint, should first be detained for a time, to profit perhaps through the chance of cure by treatment. (pp. 188, 189)

[71] The idea that epileptics were 'subhuman' was already well established. An example of the prevalent attitude was provided by Silvio Tonnini in 1891: the epileptic is 'one who is not master of his actions, who is affected by degenerative disease that possesses him entirely. And so his sweat, urine, skull, hair, genitalia, shape of the feet and hands, and internal organs are epileptic, non-human' (Tonnini, *Le epilessie*, cited in Salomone and Arnone, 'Care of epileptics').

[72] William Duncan McKim (1855–1935), American physician, Baltimore. On the title page is a quote from Shakespeare's Hamlet (I, ii, 133–7): ' 'Tis an unweeded garden / That grows to seed; things rank, and gross in nature, / Possess it merely.'

McKim's abhorrent book was based on laughable science but despite this was widely read, and many agreed with its sentiments.

In the early 1900s, efforts were being made to quantify the hereditarian aspects of epilepsy. A key organisation was the American Breeders' Association, which set up committees to study various aspects of human eugenics, including an epilepsy committee chaired by Charles Davenport, and with David Weeks and Everett Flood amongst the members.[73] From this evolved the Eugenics Record Office (ERO) in Cold Spring Harbor, which opened in 1910 under the directorship of Davenport, and was to become the most influential organisation in the field of human eugenics of its time.[74] It was from there that the first major study of the heredity of epilepsy in the eugenics era was published by Davenport and Weeks in 1911. This was a 30-page paper showing the results of an analysis of 177 families from among the inmates of the New Jersey State Village for Epileptics at Skillman.[75] In the established manner of ERO research, trained fieldworkers were sent in to interview patients and their families, and pedigree charts were constructed. Davenport was a recent convert to Mendelian explanations of inheritance, and he and Weeks analysed the pedigrees using what they termed the 'Mendelian method'. Davenport himself believed that most epileptic conditions were inherited by recessive processes (progressive myoclonic epilepsy being an exception). The researchers looked primarily for feeble-mindedness and epilepsy in the families, but also noted the presence of alcoholism, migraine, chorea, paralysis, neurosis and prostitution, and took the presence of these in the kinships as evidence of the same inherited defect (the neurological taint). After convoluted and at times (to me) incomprehensible commentary, Davenport and Weeks provided a summary of their findings. Epilepsy and feeble-mindedness were each due to the absence of a protoplasmic factor that determined complete nervous development; when

---

[73] Charles Benedict Davenport was the most influential figure in epilepsy genetics and eugenics of the period. He held various eugenical positions, including chairman of the Commission on Bastardization and Miscegenation. David Fairchild Weeks (1874–1929), an American physician, superintendent and medical director of the New Jersey State Village for Epileptics at Skillman, New Jersey, was president of the International League Against Epilepsy (ILAE) in 1912. Everett Flood was an American representative, with Weeks, at the founding of the ILAE in Budapest in 1909 and a member of the American National Committee of the ILAE.

[74] The American Breeders' Association was a eugenics association founded in 1903 by agricultural breeders and biologists. The ERO was to play a very important part in American eugenics, not least for the fieldwork it carried out.

[75] Davenport and Weeks, 'First study'. In fact, Weeks had presented abbreviated findings at the first Eugenics Congress in London in 1912 (it is notable that epilepsy was the only 'medical disease' which was the subject of a lecture at the conference). Amongst his conclusions were that 'the common types of epileptics lack some element necessary for complete mental development. This is also true of the feeble-minded; Two epileptic parents produce only defectives; Epilepsy tends in successive generations to form a larger part of the population; the normal parents of epileptics are not normal but simplex, and have descended from tainted ancestors'. *Abstracts read at the first International Eugenics Congress*, p. 10–12.

both parents were epileptic or feeble-minded, all of their offspring would be affected. Persons with migraine, chorea, paralysis and extreme nervousness carried some defective germ cells and were 'tainted'. When such individuals mated with other similarly affected individuals, 25% of offspring were defective and when they mated with defectives, about 50% of offspring were defective. That normal parents with epileptic offspring had tainted germ plasm was evidenced by the presence of nervous defects in close relatives. Although Davenport and Weeks recognised that there are other organic causes, they believed that in the overwhelming majority of cases epilepsy was due to an inherited predisposition. They further believed that the number of cases was multiplying in an alarming fashion: 'there is evidence that in epileptic strains the proportion of epileptic children in the latest complete generation is double that of the preceding ... Provided marriage matings continue as at present and no additional restraint is imposed the proportion of epileptics in New Jersey would double every thirty years' (pp. 669–70).

This flawed demographic prediction proved to be powerful propaganda and had an immediate and crucial impact on policymakers. Davenport and Weeks urged the segregation of epileptics of both sexes. They predicted that if this were successfully achieved, within fifty years those with epilepsy would be a small minority – though, '[o]f course, through immigration, through trauma, and through the chance union of defective germ cells of normal persons a thin stream would be maintained, but the State would have control of the situation and the expense would be ever diminishing instead, as now, ever increasing' (p. 669).

As a result of this work, segregation was then implemented in many asylums. Fairly quickly, however, it was recognised that neither the anti-marriage laws in the community nor the segregation in asylums were sufficient as ways of restricting reproduction, and from 1907 legislation regarding involuntary sterilisation of the mentally defective began to enter the statute books, first in the state of Indiana, to prevent procreation of confirmed criminals, idiots, imbeciles and rapists.[76] In March 1909, California, the most active among the states in this respect, passed the Asexualization Act. Initially, the act permitted sterilisation 'to the benefit ... of any inmate',[77] and after 1913 also for eugenic purposes (although it was still often carried out with the view that it would improve the individual's own quality of life).[78] In 1912, the president of Ohio's State Board of Administration 'declared that if a law for sterilization was not passed the State would be bankrupt within ten years by the expense of caring

[76] The 'Indiana Eugenics Law'. Epilepsy was not mentioned specifically mentioned but was inferred. In 1905, an earlier law in Indiana had prohibited the marriage of 'epileptics'.

[77] 'Act to permit asexualization'.

[78] Braslow, 'In the name of therapeutics'. The law again was not specifically enacted for epilepsy, but for those who have a mental disease 'that may have been inherited and likely to be transmitted to descendants' or 'those suffering from perversion or marked departures from normal mentality'. Epilepsy was conceived to be within these categories.

for the weak-minded'.[79] In New Jersey in 1911, Weeks spearheaded the drafting of an involuntary sterilisation law for the State Legislature, and the Act to Authorize and Provide for the Sterilization of Feeble-minded (Including Idiots, Imbeciles and Morons) Epileptics, Rapists, Certain Criminals and Other Defectives was passed into law that same year. It acted as a model template, and within ten years forced sterilisation of those with epilepsy was practised in many states.

A key element of Davenport's work was the use of 'pedigree charts' (p. 642) of defective families, displayed in the same way as in Goddard's book on the Kallikak family. The charts were visually very compelling. Other examples of large pedigree studies by the ERO were of the Nam and the Ishmaelite families. In these families, the same general approach was taken: epilepsy, feeble-mindedness, insanity, alcoholism and criminality were included in the charts, sometimes with other features, such as hysterical personality traits and deafness. Reading the descriptions of the pedigrees, the subjective biases and prejudices of the investigators are abundantly clear,[80] as is their lack of objectivity. But this does not seem to have tempered the enthusiasm with which these stereotypes were received. The case descriptions were sometimes backed by quantitative psychological and physical measures of intelligence, personality and physical characteristics, and these enhanced their apparent scientific credibility. Davenport and Weeks's Mendelian approach was conceptually fallacious, their methods sloppy and their analyses biased and inaccurate, and many scientists were critical of the studies. Nevertheless, they caught the public imagination, due partly to Davenport's campaigning zeal, considerable financial support (not least from Mary Harriman, wife of the railway magnate) and because Davenport's science chimed with traditional conservative American

[79] 'Ohio's many imbeciles'.
[80] The description of the Nam family is a case in point (Davenport, *The Nams: The Feeble-minded as Country Dwellers*; Estabrook and Davenport, *Nam Family: A Study in Cacogenics*). 'A great amount of consanguineous marriage has taken place. . . One "family" here which traces back to a single pair comprises over 800 individuals . . .In this community the study showed 232 licentious women and 199 licentious men, and only 155 chaste women and eighty-three chaste men. Fifty-four have been in custodial care either in asylums or country houses, twenty-four have received outdoor aid, and in addition private aid has been given them by charitable persons for years. Forty have served terms in state's prison or jail. There are 192 persons who use alcohol in extreme quantities, *i. e.*, are sots . . . [T]hey worked only when the mood o'ertook them, they remained poor. Their children did not attend school, and thereby grew up more ignorant than their parents, and in an environment where intemperance and harlotry were the leading evils . . . As one drives through Nam Hollow, he finds a settlement of ten huts and hovels. . . . The window panes are stuffed with rags in winter to retain the smoky heat of the one stove. The beds are, in general, piles of old rags and worn-out blankets. Means of sanitation are entirely unknown. Whole families live in one room . . . Such conditions as these can only lead to illegitimacy, inbreeding, and their attending evils of pauperism and dulness [sic] . . . a collection of hovels situated on a rocky and barren hill, and occupied by a group of degenerates all descended from the same person (See Chart B, Generation I 3.)' (Estabrook and Davenport, p. 2).

moralism. In was only in 1939 that the ERO was finally closed amid criticism from the US Congress and judged to be a 'worthless endeavour from top to bottom'.[81]

The first International Eugenic Congress was organised by the Eugenics Education Society and held in London on 24–30 July 1912.[82] There, Weeks presented further data on 397 patients with epilepsy from 388 families (which included the 177 pedigrees reported in the earlier paper). His conclusions, which even at the time should have been seen as obviously false, now included the view that neurosis and other tainted conditions were more closely related to epilepsy than feeble-mindedness, and that epilepsy was a recessive Mendelian factor. By then, eugenics movements were established around Europe, and the scene was set for the introduction of wider eugenic measures to prevent the propagation of epilepsy described in the next chapter.

THE NEUROLOGY OF EPILEPSY

Although epilepsy was still viewed generally as a mental disorder in the period under consideration, and treated largely in the arena of psychiatry, the new specialty of neurology had made its debut in the decades after 1850 and had made major contributions to an understanding of the condition. Neurology was progressively to gain more influence throughout this period, but it was only in the 1930s that it had become the medical specialty responsible for managing epilepsy, in Western countries at least, wresting medical control of the condition from psychiatry.

Specialisation in Medicine and the Birth of Neurology

Specialisation in internal medicine dated from the second half of the nineteenth century. The differentiation of neurological conditions from the amorphous mass of general medicine conditions and the birth of a new clinical specialty – neurology – underpinned the new 'scientific' interest in epilepsy. From the first stirrings of neurology, epilepsy was its preceptor and was at its very centre, at

---

[81] Cited in Sussman, *Myth of Race*, p. 195.

[82] It was an illustrious affair, with 120 delegates and celebrities. The president of the meeting was Leonard Darwin, the son of Charles. The vice presidents and general committee members were some of the best-known figures in medicine (including Thomas Allbutt, William Osler, Rickman Godlee, James Crichton-Browne, Frederick Mott, Henry Havelock Ellis, A, F. Tredgold), science (including Archibald Geikie), politics and aristocracy (including Winston Churchill, Ottoline Morrell) and law (the Lord Chief Justice), and prominent eugenicists, (including Max von Gruber, Auguste-Henri Forel, Alfred Ploetz, August Weismann, Alexander Graham Bell, David Starr Jordan, Bleecker van Wagenen). Those involved with epilepsy were also well represented, and included Auguste Marie, Charles Davenport, James Risien Russell, neurologist, representing the National Hospital, Queen Square and Penn Gaskell the National Society for Epileptics at Chalfont.

least in Britain and continental Europe.[83] And when, by 1900, neurology had risen to be considered a pinnacle of medicine, this was in no small part due to the work carried out in epilepsy.

To a significant degree, the great progress made in understanding the *scientific basis* of epilepsy – its physiology, anatomy and pathology – was due to the evolution of specialised epilepsy hospitals and epilepsy colonies. In London, between 1860 and 1878, three special hospitals were established for epilepsy,[84] the most prominent being the National Hospital for the Relief and Cure of the Paralysed and the Epileptic at Queen Square. In other cities, institutions acted both as hospitals and asylums. For instance, in Paris insane and epileptic patients were gathered at the Hospice de la Vieillesse-Femmes (L'hôpital de la Pitié-Salpêtrière; initially for females only) and the Hospice Bicêtre (initially for aged males and the insane), and in New York a hospital and asylum for the paralysed and epileptic was opened on Blackwell's Island in 1867. In Berlin, both neurology and epilepsy remained much more closely tied to psychiatry, and although Griesinger opened separate wards for neurology in 1865, these were placed within a psychiatric hospital in 1889.[85]

The Neurology of Epilepsy, 1860–1900: Reynolds, Jackson and Gowers

As mentioned earlier, both Delasiauve and Sieveking's concepts of epilepsy were essentially backward-looking, representing the culmination of the pre-modern period of epilepsy. A more forward-looking book, launching the process of metamorphosis of epilepsy into its modern form, was *Epilepsy: Its Symptoms, Treatment and Relation to Other Chronic Convulsive Diseases*,[86] by John

[83] The notable figures in the field of the neurology of epilepsy included: In Britain, David Ferrier, Victor Horsley, William Gowers, John Hughlings Jackson; in France, Jean Cruveilhier, Alfred Vulpian, Jean-Martin Charcot; and in the German-speaking countries, Moritz Romberg, Wilhelm Griesinger, Heinrich Obersteiner, Otto Binswanger, Emil Kraepelin, and the school of neuropathologists who worked on epilepsy (see later in this chapter). In the United States, neurology emerged with the work of Silas Weir Mitchell and William Hammond, and although both were held in high esteem among medical circles and set neurology on a high trajectory, neither made any particular contribution to epilepsy, possibly because American neurology was oriented less closely to psychiatry than was the case in Britain and Europe.

[84] The National Hospital for the Relief and Cure of the Paralysed and Epileptic (founded in 1860), the London Infirmary for Epilepsy and Paralysis (founded in 1866) and the West End Hospital for Diseases of the Nervous System, Paralysis and Epilepsy (founded in 1878).

[85] The close link between neurology and psychiatry in Germany remained well into the post–Second World War period

[86] Reynolds, *Epilepsy*. Sir John Russell Reynolds was an English physician at University College Hospital and the National Hospital, Queen Square and later professor of the principles and practice of medicine at University College London. One of the most celebrated physicians of his generation, he wrote extensively on neurological topics and edited the five-volume *System of Medicine* (1866–1979).

Russell Reynolds, a physician appointed to the National Hospital Queen Square in 1863.[87]

Although published in the same year as the second edition of Sieveking's book (1861), the two volumes are quite different. Reynolds's work pointed to the future and proved highly influential on his two great successors: John Hughlings Jackson, who quoted extensively from it, and William Gowers, who dedicated his own work on epilepsy to Reynolds, 'whose example has stimulated and friendship encouraged the work'.[88] Reynolds, like Jackson and Gowers, took a very neurological view of epilepsy, and his book can be seen as a staging post in the process of separation of neurology from psychiatry.

His book opens with a long section on the question of what constitutes a disease, and we shall return to this question again at the end of the book. In Reynolds view, when it comes to considering epilepsy, only idiopathic epilepsy was the genuine form of the disease, the *morbus per se* (a disease in and of itself). In conditions in which convulsions were due to some other identifiable pathology, the convulsions should be considered symptoms of these other conditions and the term 'epilepsy' should not strictly speaking be applied to these forms. He recognised that it was an 'organic' disease of the brain, but one in which the underlying physiochemical cause was as yet undetected. This idea, that the term 'epilepsy' should be narrowly applied only to its genuine form, 'idiopathic epilepsy', was adopted by both Gowers and Turner and remained the dominant view at least until the 1920s.

Reynolds considered that the 'cause' of epileptic seizures could be divided into proximate and remote categories. The proximate cause was 'an abnormal increase in the nutritive changes of the nervous system' (very similar to today's conception if the word 'nutritive' is substituted by 'excitatory'). Remote causes were those that triggered this nutritional change, such as a tumour, stroke, trauma or infection. He recognised that the remote causes could be insignificant in some people and overwhelming in others, and also that sometimes

---

[87] The name of this hospital has an interesting history, bound up in changing social trends. At its foundation in November 1859, the hospital was referred to in documents as the National Hospital for the Paralysed and Epileptic or the National Hospital for Paralysis and Epilepsy. By March 1860, its official name was the National Hospital for the Relief and Cure of the Paralysed and Epileptic. In 1926, the first formal name change occurred, to the National Hospital, Queen Square, for the Relief and Cure of Diseases of the Nervous System, including Paralysis and Epilepsy. The name was then often abbreviated to the National Hospital for Nervous Diseases, not least as the inclusion of epilepsy and paralysis was deemed a 'deterrent to the public'. Then in 1948, at the time of incorporation into the NHS, the name changed to the National Hospitals for Nervous Diseases. In 1980, the fund-raisers of a new building campaign urged a change in name in view of the fact that, to the public, nervous diseases were the same as neurotic disorders, and the name became the National Hospital for Neurology and Neurosurgery. This too is a clumsy name, and to many around the word, it is still known either as the National Hospital or the National Hospital, Queen Square or simply as Queen Square (from Shorvon and Compston, *Queen Square*, pp. 3–4)

[88] The dedication in Gowers, *Epilepsy* (1881).

severe disease resulted in insignificant epilepsy. He also held that different types of seizures were due to differing anatomical locations of the abnormal nervous centres. In all these points, he anticipated Hughlings Jackson. In passing, it is also notable that Reynolds considered the emphasis on masturbation as a cause of epilepsy (an idea popularised by Tissot,[89] and perpetuated, for instance, by Delasiauve and Sieveking) to be mistaken, as were the ideas of 'some mysterious entity taking possession of the body', a theory 'long since passed' (p. 6).

In terms of classification, Reynolds proposed a variation on Delasiauve's scheme, splitting sympathetic epilepsy into two (Table 1.3). Thus, he categorises conditions in which seizures occurred into four categories: *idiopathic epilepsy* (the genuine form of epilepsy), defined as an 'internal cause', a *morbus per se*, in which he included eclamptic seizures and the '"idiopathic convulsions" of children'; *eccentric (or sympathetic) epilepsy*, in which a convulsion was due to an external irritation, such as a head injury (this category has some similarities with the current concept of 'acute symptomatic seizures' and reflected the work of Marshall Hall, who had divided epilepsy into centric and eccentric categories); *diathetic epilepsy*, in which the nutritive change caused seizures due to the effect on the brain of general systemic diseases and toxaemias;[90] and *symptomatic (centric) epilepsy*, a term used for epilepsies in which there was a more or less contiguous structural brain disease (pp. 13–27).

Reynolds described the symptoms of epilepsy in great detail and considered the medulla and upper spinal cord to be the seat of the loss of consciousness, respiratory and other changes, and the convulsive movements in epilepsy.

In relation to the mental state of his patients, Reynolds cites and dismisses what he called the 'powerful remark' of Morel namely that: 'It is in the nature of nervous disease to imprint on the physical and moral idiosyncrasy of patients a very special character; and without being able to say conclusively that all the elements which formed their previous intellectual and moral qualities completely disappear, one can, however, affirm without exaggeration that such patients share a common character.'[91] Morel called this the *epileptic character*, but Reynolds entirely disagreed, finding around a third of his own cases of idiopathic epilepsy free from any mental failure and a further third with only slight memory problems (pp. 40–5). He also noted that the absence of intellectual

---

[89] Tissot published his book in 1758 first in Latin (*Tentamen de morbis ex manustupratione*), then in French (*L'Onanisme*). The English translation (*Onanism*) was published in 1776.

[90] Diathetic epilepsy was a new category, in which the nutritive change was the result of a general systemic disturbance caused by toxaemia or cachexia. The causes of cachexia he listed included tuberculosis, scrofula, rachitis, syphilis, pyaemia, anaemia, alcoholism, lead poisoning, typhus, variola and other exanthemata and diseases which alter nutrition, such as pneumonia, carditis and pericarditis.

[91] Translated from Morel, *Études cliniques*, vol. 2, p. 316. Reynolds also cites Esquirol's opinion that of the epileptic women in the Salpetrière, four-fifths were insane, and the remaining one-fifth had 'something of a singular personality'.

TABLE 1.3   *The classification of epilepsy devised by J. Russell Reynolds 1861*

Category	Comment
1. Idiopathic epilepsy	An internal cause – a *morbus per se*. This may have a basis in heredity or conditions operating after birth.
2. Eccentric epilepsy	(Synonyms: secondary epilepsy; sympathetic epilepsy) Epilepsy due to some systemic disturbance, or 'change in the organism', which when cured will result in the cessation of seizures. Reynolds accepted that 'eccentric convulsions' can be exacerbated by a predisposing tendency, and he proposed that they had a 'reflex' basis.
3. Diathetic epilepsy	Epilepsy in which the convulsions are part of another illness. Examples are cachexia or toxaemia, and in which the nervous system is 'involved in that general nutrition-change which is the essential element of the cachexia itself' and have their basis in a general not specific remote cause. These can include patients with an existing predisposition (or not) and other existing symptomatic causes.
4. Symptomatic epilepsy	Epilepsy in which convulsions are due to 'more or less contiguous structural disease of the brain. Thus, an intracranial tumour, a chronic inflammatory condition of the meninges, softening or disintegration of the brain substance, or any other structural change in the nervous centres . . . may set up that peculiar interstitial or molecular change which is the immediate cause of convulsion.'

(From: Reynolds, *Epilepsy*, pp. 13–29)

failure did not imply the non-existence of a hereditary predisposition, but that although deterioration could occur, it was by no means the rule, and he wasted no ink at all on the question of the 'epileptic personality'. As we shall see, the battle over the existence of the 'epileptic personality', of which this was an early skirmish, was to carry on for the next 100 years. But Reynolds's formulation was far closer to today's than any others of his time. In all these points, he took a position at striking variance to the previous orthodoxy.

In relation to either the pathophysiology of seizures or their treatment, Reynolds had nothing particularly new to say. But this was not the case in the subsequent works of his younger colleagues: John Hughlings Jackson and William Gowers.

We should start with Hughlings Jackson. To frame the new neurology, the basic organisation of the nervous system needed to be understood. Many added to this area of knowledge, but by far the greatest contribution was that of John Hughlings Jackson, who is now not without reason named the father of neurology. Temkin considered Jackson the founder of modern epilepsy, and this too is an opinion few would question. Born in Yorkshire and educated and apprenticed in York, Edinburgh and London, he received his university degree from St Andrews, and in 1859 was appointed to the Metropolitan Free Hospital in London. He was subsequently recruited to the London Hospital and then the National Hospital for the Paralysed and Epileptic ('the National Hospital, Queen Square') and the Royal London Ophthalmic Hospital. It was at Queen Square that his interest in epilepsy and neurology flowered. He worked there for more than thirty years, forming the 'epilepsy quadrumvirate' with Ferrier, Gowers and Horsley.[92]

Influenced by the philosopher Herbert Spencer, Jackson proposed a scheme of organisation of the nervous system in hierarchical and evolutionary terms. He saw brain structure arranged in a compartmentalised manner, with different functions located in different areas but integrated into a hierarchical configuration. He considered that evolution had resulted in the formation of the higher centres, which differentiated man from lower animals, and any disease which damaged the highest structures resulted in the release of lower functions of a more primitive nature (he called this dissolution). He saw the brain as a 'sensorimotor machine' functioning to a large extent via neural reflexes. He differentiated between function and structure, positive and negative symptoms, and explained loss of function and consciousness. He disputed the distinction between brain and mind and rejected the concept of the unconscious. His conception of the architecture and hierarchy of neurological structure and function constituted a paradigm shift in brain science, and his writings and influence have proved enduring and far reaching.[93]

Jackson wrote on many aspects of neurology and psychiatry, all in a fascinating, complex prose style in which his thoughts are ringed with conditional thoughts and diversions much like that of Proust. But it was the work on epilepsy that was at the forefront of his enduring influence.[94]

With singular intuition, Jackson defined the epileptic seizure as 'an occasional, an excessive, and a disorderly discharge of nerve tissue on muscles'.[95] This was an extraordinarily perceptive thought given the completely unknown nature of neuronal function; it is the definition that still applies today, and which has dictated the course of the science of epilepsy ever since. It was seventy years later, with the introduction of electroencephalography (EEG), that it became possible to 'visualise' the electrochemical changes in a seizure, and the brilliance of Jackson's conception of a disorderly discharge was then

[92] See Shorvon and Compston, *Queen Square*.
[93] See York and Steinberg, *Life and Work of John Hughlings Jackson*.
[94] Between 1870 and 1895, Jackson had 1,453 inpatients under his care at the National Hospital – including 371 cases of epilepsy that he documented in great detail, in addition to larger numbers in his private practice and at his practice at the London Hospital, and this caseload formed the basis of his ideas of epilepsy. Lekka: The Neurological Emergence of Epilepsy.
[95] Jackson, 'Study of convulsions'. Reynolds had referred to a seizure as an explosion, and Sieveking had used the analogy of a spark igniting gunpowder, but no one before Jackson had proposed that a seizure was due to a discharge of hyperexcitable neurons.

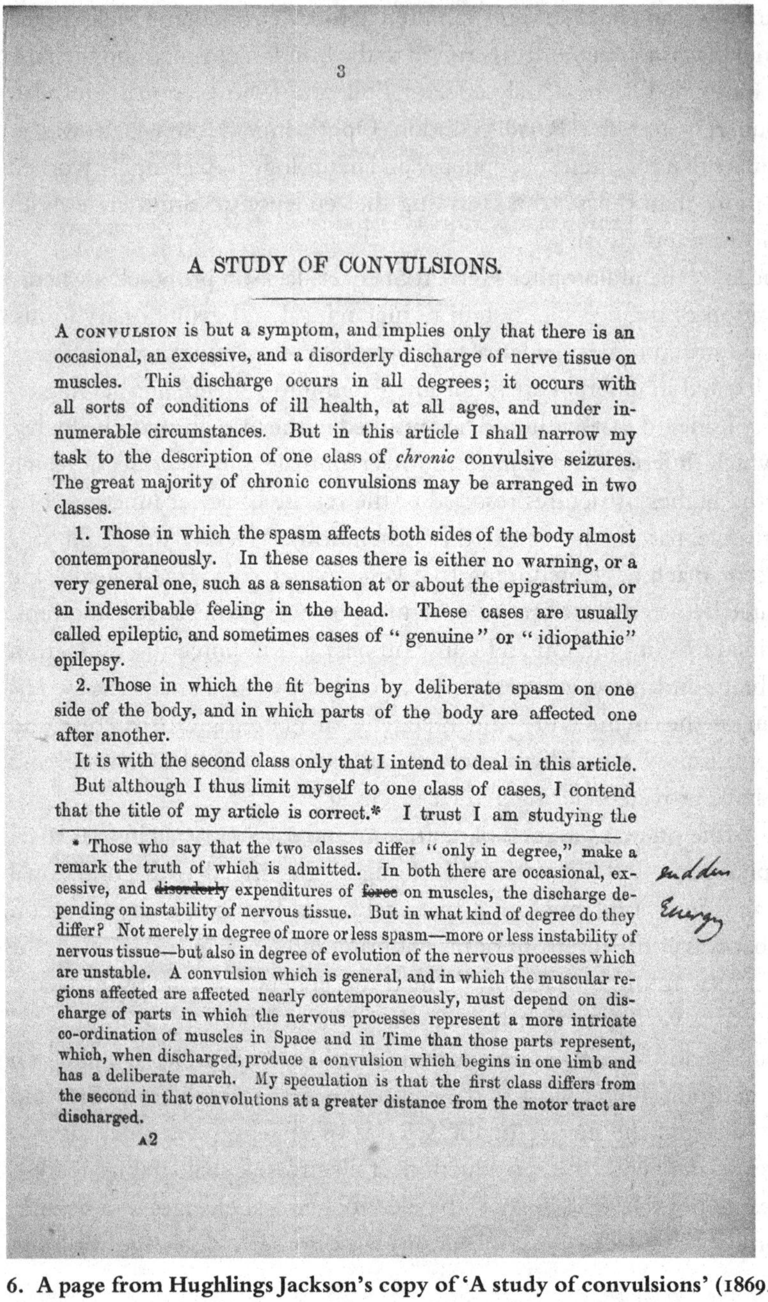

3

A STUDY OF CONVULSIONS.

A CONVULSION is but a symptom, and implies only that there is an occasional, an excessive, and a disorderly discharge of nerve tissue on muscles. This discharge occurs in all degrees; it occurs with all sorts of conditions of ill health, at all ages, and under innumerable circumstances. But in this article I shall narrow my task to the description of one class of *chronic* convulsive seizures. The great majority of chronic convulsions may be arranged in two classes.

1. Those in which the spasm affects both sides of the body almost contemporaneously. In these cases there is either no warning, or a very general one, such as a sensation at or about the epigastrium, or an indescribable feeling in the head. These cases are usually called epileptic, and sometimes cases of " genuine " or " idiopathic " epilepsy.

2. Those in which the fit begins by deliberate spasm on one side of the body, and in which parts of the body are affected one after another.

It is with the second class only that I intend to deal in this article.

But although I thus limit myself to one class of cases, I contend that the title of my article is correct.*   I trust I am studying the

---

* Those who say that the two classes differ " only in degree," make a remark the truth of which is admitted. In both there are occasional, excessive, and ~~disorderly~~ expenditures of ~~force~~ on muscles, the discharge depending on instability of nervous tissue. But in what kind of degree do they differ? Not merely in degree of more or less spasm—more or less instability of nervous tissue—but also in degree of evolution of the nervous processes which are unstable. A convulsion which is general, and in which the muscular regions affected are affected nearly contemporaneously, must depend on discharge of parts in which the nervous processes represent a more intricate co-ordination of muscles in Space and in Time than those parts represent, which, when discharged, produce a convulsion which begins in one limb and has a deliberate march. My speculation is that the first class differs from the second in that convolutions at a greater distance from the motor tract are discharged.

A2

[handwritten margin note: sudden Energy]

6. A page from Hughlings Jackson's copy of 'A study of convulsions' (1869/1970). In this page is a version of his famous definition of a convulsion. This copy shows Jackson's own handwritten post-publication revisions.

completely vindicated. As Jackson developed his ideas about brain structure and function, he went further and placed the seat of epilepsy firmly in the cerebral cortex, writing in 1873: 'Epilepsy is the name for occasional, sudden, excessive, rapid, and local discharges of grey matter.'[96] Prior to this, most authorities held that epilepsy was a form of reflex with its origin in the medulla or the upper spinal cord, a view strengthened by the experiments of Jackson's colleague at the National Hospital, Eduard Brown-Séquard.[97]. In his Lumleian Lectures of 1890,[98] Jackson defined the nervous discharge as the liberation of energy by nervous elements, and the epileptic discharge as 'sudden, excessive and temporary' (p. 736) and 'of a highly explosive character ... [a] physiological fulminate [like the fulminate used with] gunpowder in a cannon'. The explosion in the 'mad part' detonates the surrounding 'sane cells' (pp. 735–6). Just as gunpowder can store energy that is liberated when firing the gun, so the energy stored in nerve cells could be explosively liberated in an epileptic discharge.

For Jackson, most seizures arose from a local starting point in the cerebral cortex, and therefore the *first* symptom of a seizure indicated the location, within the cerebral cortex, at which the seizure originated. Indeed, it was partly through his clinical observations of the epileptic fit that he evolved his theory of cerebral localisation. As he wrote: 'There is nothing more important than to note where a convulsion begins, for the inference is that the first motor symptom is the sign of the beginning of the central discharge'; 'The mode of onset is the most important matter in the anatomical investigation of any case of epilepsy'; and 'One of the most important questions we can ask an epileptic patient is, "How does the fit begin?"'[99] He also realised that the discharge could spread to neighbouring cells, calling the cells of origin a mad part (he later called these 'bastard cells') spreading to sane cells that are made to 'act madly'. He thus was the first to suggest the existence of an *epileptic focus*, and coined the term *epileptogenic zone* – a concept which led directly to the idea that neurosurgical resection of the epileptic focus might cure the seizures.

Jackson provided superlative descriptions of focal and generalised seizure types. Although based on his own minute observations of seizures, they were similar to the earlier descriptions. Terminology, however, was then quite confused. Jackson used the terms *grand mal* and *petit mal*, which were time-honoured names. However, in relation to the more 'minor' forms of epilepsy, *les petit maux*, numerous terms were extant. These included partial seizures (about which James Pritchard had written extensively), *vertiges* (Esquirol), *absence* (Calmeil), *accès incomplet* (Herpin), *psychic epilepsy*, *larval* or *masked* epilepsy (Morel) and *petit mal intellectuel* (Falret, whose excellent descriptions were of what are now called psychomotor seizures). Other, more prolonged epileptic states were also sometimes described that overlapped with some of

---

[96] Jackson, 'Anatomical, physiological'.
[97] Charles-Édouard Brown-Séquard (1817–94) was perhaps the most celebrated medical physiologist of the period (see Aminoff, *Brown-Séquard*).
[98] Jackson, 'Lumleian lectures'.   [99] Jackson, 'Notes'.

these categories: hallucinations, reveries or the more prolonged *furor épileptique*, *folie épileptique* and epileptic delirium. Automatic movements without awareness, automatisms or unconscious cerebrations had also been recognised.[100] The term 'aura' also changed meaning in the nineteenth century from its original usage, which was confined to the ascending 'breeze'-like feeling to all 'warnings' of an impending convulsion – a change attributed to Pritchard. To Reynolds, the term 'epilepsy' should be reserved for those attacks which were associated with convulsions and loss of consciousness. Jackson sometimes used the term 'epileptiform' to refer to other types.

Jackson's contribution was to provide a logical framework within which the various seizure types could be placed, based on their location and position in the hierarchical structure of the brain. This anatomical localisation had the effect of clearing the fog that surrounded the multitude of clinical forms. Jackson went on to describe two novel types of seizures and to ascribe their cerebral location. First was the focal motor seizure, now known as the Jacksonian seizure.[101] Jackson identified its origin in the motor cortex of the brain. He subdivided the seizures into those that began in the foot, the hand, the face and the tongue, and described the evolution of motor features (now known as the Jacksonian march), using this to make inferences about the functional organisation of the motor cortex. Jackson speculated that the recruitment of muscle groups in the Jacksonian march represented activation of adjacent parts of the cortex that therefore must subserve different movements, a supposition confirmed, as we shall see, by the experiments of Gustav Fritsch and Julius Hitzig, Ferrier and Horsley.[102]

Jackson also defined what became known as the psychomotor seizure and its origin in the temporal lobe.[103] Jackson's descriptions of this seizure type were complete and comprehensive. He postulated that it arose from the temporal lobe, and specifically from the uncinate gyrus (though with great prescience in these days of neural networks, he wrote: 'This was on the hypothesis that the discharge

[100] For instance, by Jules Baillarger in his essay *Théorie de l'automatisme*, written in 1945 and included in *Recherches sur les maladies mentales*, vol. 1, pp. 494–500; Carpenter, *Principles*; Höring, *Über Epilepsie*.

[101] Charcot is said to have been first to name the unilateral focal motor seizures 'Jacksonian seizures'. He and Jackson referred to the earlier descriptions of Louis François Bravais (1801–43), physician at the Bicêtre, who described the clinical phenomenon in his medical thesis titled *Recherches sur les symptômes et le traitement de l'épilepsie hémiplégique*. But Bravais did not assign the origin of the seizure to the central cortex, nor did he investigate the pathology or pathophysiology. He did suggest therapy using a seton (for assessment of the work of Bravais, see Eadie, 'Louis François Bravais').

[102] Fritsch and Hitzig, 'Über die elektrische Erregbarkeit'; Ferrier, 'Experimental researches' and 'Cerebral localisation'; Beevor and Horsley, 'Electrical excitation of the so-called motor cortex'.

[103] Earlier authors had described the features of 'incomplete attacks', including loss of awareness, automatisms and dream-like perceptual changes, including Griesinger and John Cheyne. Falret gave a particularly good account (see Falret, 'De l'état mental').

lesions in these cases are made up of some cells, not of the uncinate group alone, but of some cells of different parts of the region of which this gyrus is part – a very vague circumscription, I admit – the uncinate region').[104] In his first paper on this 'particular variety of epilepsy' in 1880, Jackson described the clinical semiology in a patient (a medical doctor with the pseudonym 'Querens'), who committed suicide ten years later and came to post-mortem. In the second paper, Jackson wrote that 'he begged his colleague Walter Colman to search the taste region of Ferrier on each half of the brain very carefully'. He did so and found 'a very small focus of softening in the uncinate gyrus of the left half of the brain'.[105]

Jackson also hypothesised about the difference between a local attack and a generalised attack (a convulsion) and considered that it was the extent and spread into lower structures of the brain that characterised the latter. The symptoms of the generalised seizure were due, in his view, to the release of lower nervous system levels from the control of the higher regions.

It is also notable that, although he described aetiologies and seizure types in detail, he avoided any synoptic classification of epilepsy.[106] He made the fundamental point that there are two different types of classification. The first he called a gardener's classification, which he viewed as a utilitarian scheme based on facts of practical value. This he contrasted with a botanist's classification, which was a scientific classification based on a listing of natural classes for instance of species, genera and phyla.[107] Jackson bemoaned the fact that only gardener classifications existed in the field of epilepsy, as knowledge had not proceeded far enough to devise a coherent botanist's scheme – a situation which, as we shall see, still applies some 150 years later.

Finally, Jackson's idea of causation in epilepsy is of great interest and, as ever, reflected his deeply intellectual approach to medicine. Closely following the example of Reynolds, he differentiated between cause at the level of the cell (i.e. the molecular changes which result in a seizure, and which he called the proximate cause), and, at the level of gross anatomy, the downstream 'remote' cause which might trigger the molecular changes (for instance, a brain tumour or abscess).[108] As he wrote, in his characteristically discursive style:

> The confusion of two things physiology and pathology under one (pathology) leads to confusion in considering 'causes'. Thus, for example, we

[104] Jackson and Stewart, 'Epileptic attacks'.
[105] Jackson, 'On a particular variety'; Jackson and Colman, 'Case of epilepsy'. The context of these cases is described, and Dr Z identified, in a brilliant piece of detective work by David Taylor and Susan Marsh ('Hughlings Jackson's Dr Z').
[106] In fact, with great foresight, he also avoided a clear definition of epilepsy, considering epileptic seizures to be simply 'symptoms' of physiological changes in cortical cells.
[107] Jackson, 'Classification and methods'.
[108] In fact, Reynolds had made a similar point, so Jackson was not the first to suggest this; but the idea was more deeply explored by Jackson.

hear it epigrammatically said that chorea is 'only a symptom' and may depend on many causes. This is possibly true of pathological causation; in other words it may be granted that various abnormal nutritive processes *may lead* to that functional change in grey matter which, when established, admits occasional excessive discharge. But physiologically, that is to say, from the point of view of Function, there is but one cause of chorea – viz., instability of nerve tissue. Similarly in any epilepsy, there is but 'one cause' physiologically speaking – viz., instability of grey matter, but an unknown number of causes if we mean pathological processes leading to that instability.[109]

Jackson defined the term 'physiology' in the narrow and specific meaning of 'the departure from the healthy *function* of nerve tissue. That function is to store up and to expend force . . . [I]n epilepsy . . . the cells . . . store up large quantities and discharge abundantly on very slight provocation: there is what I call increased instability, or shortly, instability, or what is otherwise spoken of as increased excitability'.[110] By the term 'pathology' he meant the 'coarse' conditions which precipitate this physiological change. To Jackson, the fundamental cause was the physiological change. He considered the instability of the nervous tissue to be due to abnormal nutrition, and one leading possibility in his mind was the substitution of phosphorus with nitrogen and thus an 'over-azotised' (p. 356) state of the grey matter; he advised his patients to avoid eating meat for this reason. As for the changes that could result in this defective nutrition, Jackson recognised that there were many widely differing conditions and that in cases without gross pathology there might be local arterial, venous or capillary thrombosis at the epileptic focus. He thought that the plugging of vessels (or the irritation caused by a tumour) at the site of the epileptic focus might result in hyperaemia[111] and he dismissed the idea that the nutritional defect was due to cerebral anaemia – another theory recurring on and off until the 1940s.

These were just some of the novel concepts Jackson brought to epilepsy. He wrote numerous papers (537, according to the standard bibliography; and approximately 250,000 words on the topic of epilepsy in his selected writings[112]) and gave many published lectures. Through these it possible to dissect the evolution of his views on epilepsy. His earliest work was within the tradition of his times, and it was after 1864 that he began to strike out into uncharted territory. His novel theories of epilepsy were formed mainly in the late 1860s and 1870s, and thereafter his ideas matured and broadened (this evolution of thought explaining the sometimes contradictory nature of his early and later work). Unlike most of his contemporaries, he never published a book – a curious and unexplained omission at a time when a book was the main

[109] Jackson, 'Classification and methods'. (In Taylor, *Selected Works*, Vol. 1, p. 218).
[110] Jackson, 'Scientific and empirical investigation'.
[111] Jackson, 'Anatomical, physiological'.   [112] York and Steinberg, *Introduction*.

vehicle for clinical communication and advancement. One can only muse on the fact that had a book been written in the late 1880s on epilepsy, when his ideas had been most fully fleshed out, this would have been an extraordinary work. Despite this, he was revered by his colleagues and, after a period of neglect, is again being fully acknowledged. If there is one person who could claim to have made the greatest contribution to epilepsy in the whole of the modern era, then surely it is he.

Jackson's younger colleague, and a student of Reynolds, William Gowers is the second person of supreme importance in epilepsy of this period. Gowers (that 'brilliant ornament of British medicine'[113]) was a prolific author and, as was the case with Jackson, epilepsy was at the centre of his oeuvre. Gowers and Jackson were different, though, in most other ways. In striking contrast to Jackson, Gowers's writing was clear and concise. Gowers was no theoretician, but an entirely practical person; he was not interested in philosophising about the nature of the brain. Both, though, shared a sharp eye for detail and minute observation, and Gowers's *Manual of Diseases of the Nervous System*[114] was the outstanding neurology textbook of the period, widely known as 'the bible of neurology'. Forty of its 1,350 pages are devoted to epilepsy and eclampsia, and are a concise summary of his thought, but it was his monograph *Epilepsy and Other Chronic Convulsive Disorders*[115] which was his greatest contribution to epilepsy. Temkin described the work as 'the most important contemporary book written in English on the cause, symptoms and treatment of epilepsy'.[116] Indeed, no other book at the time, in any language, approached Gowers's work in terms of the scope and brilliance of its technical description. One is tempted to add to Temkin's eulogy that this book has had no equal at any time since – with the possible exception of William Lennox's work of 1960.

Gowers agreed with Reynolds, to whom the book is dedicated, that the term 'epilepsy' was best confined to the idiopathic disease (a *morbus per se*) and purported to restrict most of his consideration to such cases, which, as he put it, were 'functional' as opposed to those with seizures due to identifiable organic disease. This was the age of clinical description, and of unscrambling, in clinical medicine generally, and particularly so for disorders of the nervous system. Previously, neurological conditions were jumbled together and their

---

[113] Osler, 'Address', 11. Sir William Richard Gowers (1845–1915) matriculated from University College London and worked throughout his long career at the National Hospital for the Paralysed and Epileptic and University College Hospital.

[114] Gowers, *Manual*.

[115] Gowers, *Epilepsy*. The content of the two editions is very similar, the main difference being the statistical analysis of cases. There is also a final chapter on surgical treatment in the second edition

[116] Temkin, *Falling Sickness*, p. 350. Gowers later wrote another book of importance to epilepsy titled *The Border-Land of Epilepsy: Faints, Vagal Attacks, Vertigo, Migraine, Sleep Symptoms, and Their Treatment* (1907).

mechanisms misunderstood; the signal achievement of Gowers was to dissect, describe and order neurological disease. In the first edition of his monograph on epilepsy, he reported the findings of 1,450 cases of epilepsy personally observed during his years of practice at the National Hospital; the second edition (1901) provided an additional 1,500. Based on this clinical experience, he described all the main clinical forms of epileptic seizures and of epilepsy, set them into a rational framework and defined the clinical course and prognosis of the disorder. In the words of Macdonald Critchley, Gowers brought to the bedside all his skill as a natural historian:

> To him the neurological sick were like the flora of a tropical jungle, and his keen eye and collector's flair enabled him to identify, arrange and classify. He learned to recognise the diverse modifications of the banal or everyday material, while he quickly detected the rarities. Furthermore, he was able to pick out a species which had not previously been described or labelled. To his botanist's bent he added the virtues of diligence and orderliness, probably to an obsessive degree.[117]

In terms of aetiology, Gowers divided causes of seizures into exciting and predisposing categories.[118] To him the exciting cause operated mostly at the time of the first seizure, as

> the malady is self-perpetuating. This first fit leaves behind it a tendency to recurrence, which is, indeed, often an increase in the primary disposition ... The search for the causes of epilepsy must thus be chiefly an investigation into the conditions which precede the occurrence of the first fit. (1901, pp. 1–2)

To Gowers, the predisposition was largely inherited, and in this sense he was in full agreement with the psychiatrists and most other neurologists: 'There are few diseases in the production of which inheritance has more manifest influence, and the traceable influence is always far less than that which exists' (1901, p. 3). In this statement, Gowers emphasised that he accepted the then orthodox view that epilepsy (i.e. idiopathic epilepsy) was inherited as part of the 'neuropathic tendency' (the neurological trait) which was manifested mainly as epilepsy but also as insanity, chorea, migraine, hysteria and other chronic diseases of the brain and spinal cord. In families, he noted that the neuropathic tendency could assume the form of any one of these conditions, although epilepsy and insanity were the most common ('Epilepsy and insanity are interchangeable in families; they are certainly correlated', p. 5). In terms of 'exciting causes', which Gowers considered to be generally less important than heredity (Gowers used the same analogy of the spark and gunpowder as

---

[117] Critchley, *Sir William Gowers*, p. 30.   [118] Gowers, *Epilepsy*.

Sieveking, Reynolds and Jackson), he listed 'teething', mental emotion, trauma (including exposure to the sun), acute disease (such as scarlet fever), reflex causes (most notably gastrointestinal) and miscellaneous causes such as asphyxia, lead poisoning, anaesthetics, disturbed menstruation and pregnancy (pp. 19–36). Gowers also included a chapter on organic epilepsy (i.e. symptomatic epilepsy), in which he noted that many organic diseases of the brain cause convulsions during their 'active stage' and then are followed by attacks which recur over many years. 'They are usually partial and local in commencement, but may be general when severe, and often resemble idiopathic epilepsy in another feature – the occurrence after a time of minor attacks … the tendency to discharge is established by repetition. The ultimate course resembles that of idiopathic epilepsy'. It is for this reason that he included these cases in his survey of the idiopathic condition (1901, p. 154).

The chapters concerned with descriptions of seizures ('symptoms', as Gowers put it) are masterworks of clinical observation. He considered the prodromata and then the auras – reaffirming Jackson's view that the symptom of the aura can indicate in which part of the brain the seizure arises. Gowers realised that true idiopathic epilepsy occurred without an aura, and the aura was indicative usually of an organic cerebral cause. He divided auras into the following categories: unilateral, including sensory symptoms and head and eye versions; general or bilateral auras; auras referable to certain organs, notably visceral auras (recognising that epigastric auras were sometimes associated with fear); vertigo and allied sensations, including cephalic auras; sensations of the head and pain; psychical auras; and special sensory auras. All the descriptions were detailed and meticulous, as were the descriptions of the motor autonomic and systemic features of various forms of convulsions. And frankly, very little has been added to these in subsequent years. He also described partial seizures without convulsions, including the dreamy state of Jackson (the psychomotor seizure). He provided detailed descriptions of myoclonic jerking, including of cases which are clear examples of what is now known as juvenile myoclonic epilepsy. Finally, there were excellent descriptions of the after-effects of the various types of seizures.

In relation to mental symptoms, Gowers struck out in new directions. He divided the symptoms into 'paroxysmal mental disturbance', for instance epileptic mania and also what is now known as post-ictal psychosis,[119] and the interparoxysmal mental disorders. Included in the latter, was intellectual failure which he considered in most cases likely to be due to the underlying cause of the epilepsy rather than the epilepsy itself – a position which is

---

[119] Gowers, *Epilepsy*. '[o]ccasionally, after a fit, or, more frequently, after a series of fits, an attack of mental disturbance may come on which lasts for several days. It may be simply a demented state, or there may be hallucinations, with irritability and even violence' (1881, p. 143). A good example of his typically accurate, spare and precise observation.

accepted now but which then was at striking variance to the psychiatric orthodoxy. He did note that intellectual decline was strongly correlated to the duration of epilepsy and the frequency and nature of the seizures, but recognised that this relationship was not necessarily causal. He also pointed out that many patients have no mental deterioration, citing cases of petit mal in which forty attacks occurred a day for twenty years 'with no defect of mental power – not even of memory' (1881, pp. 120–126). Again, in marked contrast to the psychiatrists, he paid no attention to the concept of an 'epileptic personality' – a term which fails to receive any mention at all in his book. In all this, Gowers was many years ahead of his time.

His comments on the pathology of idiopathic epilepsy have also stood the test of time. He dismissed minor changes noted by others (that of induration of the cornu ammonis (hippocampal sclerosis) is described on pp. 89–90). In regard to the 'seat of epilepsy', he cited the work of Jackson and also Ferrier, Luigi Luciani and Vladimir Bekhterev[120] that it was in the grey matter of the cerebral hemispheres that the seizure commences and there was no longer any reason to implicate the medulla or other structures. He also dismissed the idea that seizures were due to vascular spasm and, again with great prescience, showed more interest in the biochemical changes.

Gowers was also one of the earliest to address the question of prognosis in great detail, devoting a chapter of his book to this topic. He noted that the 'danger to life was not great' and that the prospect of spontaneous cessation of epilepsy was 'an event too rare to be reasonably anticipated in any given case' (1901, p. 249). As for the chance of cure or remission on treatment, Gowers was of the opinion that this was particularly likely for epilepsy of short duration, for those with an inherited predisposition or whose epilepsy started after the age of twenty, for those without mental changes, those with infrequent seizures, for those with seizures without aura, and for those whose seizures did not occur during both sleep and wakefulness. The chances of remission were unaffected by the nature of the exciting cause. He also noted that if low doses of bromide were sufficient to stop seizures, then a good ultimate prognosis was more likely than in those requiring higher doses. He stressed that treatment was needed for two to three years, and that 'premature cessation of treatment is certain to involve recurrence, and the fresh start is harder than the first. There is no short

---

[120] Vladimir Mikhailovich Bekhterev was the most celebrated Russian neurologist of his time, a prolific researcher (publishing more than 1,700 papers) and a pioneer of neuroscience in Russia. He was the first to identify that the hippocampus had a role in memory. Although epilepsy was not his primary field he made contributions describing different forms of epilepsy and the surgical treatments of epilepsy. He died suddenly and in unusual circumstances, widely believed to have been poisoned by Stalin. Luigi Luciani was a renowned Italian physiologist, trained in medicine and known for his novel ideas on cerebral localisation, his work on the functions of the cerebellum as well as his work on epilepsy. Both Bekhterev and Luciani were founding patrons of *Epilepsia*.

road to a cure, and the prognosis must be largely influenced by the presence of the necessary patience and wisdom' (1901, p. 255) – conclusions which still largely apply.

This was the last period of history in which clinical science outpaced basic science. Slowly thereafter, laboratories replaced the clinics as the primary location of science. Although never himself a laboratory scientist, Gowers predicted this shift. After attending Santiago Ramón y Cajal's Croonian Lecture at the Royal Society in 1895, Gowers considered the histological findings to be the greatest discovery of his time, and one which would foster the 'new neurology'[121].

In the half-century after 1850, other important monographs[122] devoted solely to epilepsy were published, although none were a match for Gowers. In France these included books by Théodore Herpin (1852; heavily cited by Jackson), Jules Voisin (1897) and the monumental 635-page book by Charles Féré (1890). Charcot, too, wrote on epilepsy, but was most interested in its link with hysteria and the concept of hystero-epilepsy – a cul-de-sac and diversion which has continued to plague the topic. It is true to say that, despite his enormous contribution to other areas of neurology, Charcot added little of enduring value to epilepsy, except perhaps in his descriptions of epileptic fugue. In contrast to this, in Germany, Otto Binswanger's *Die Epilepsie* (1899) was an immense synthesis of the work in that country that reflected the close links between German neurology and psychiatry and pathology. Other important German contributions were by Hermann Nothnagel, who wrote an influential chapter in the *Cyclopaedia of the Practice of Medicine* on epilepsy but no book on the topic.[123] In Russia, Aleksei Kozhevnikov and Bekhterev published important papers devoted to epilepsy (both clinical and experimental), but not books.[124] In the United States, the main contribution in epilepsy was the book by Manuel Echeverria, a New York alienist who had trained at the National Hospital in London and whose book shows the strong influence of his erstwhile colleagues Gowers and Jackson.[125]

---

[121] Gowers, 'New neurology'.

[122] Herpin, *Du prognostic*; Delasiauve, *Traité de l'épilepsie*; Sieveking, *On Epilepsy*; Reynolds, *Epilepsy*; Echeverria, *On Epilepsy*; Gowers, *Epilepsy*; Féré, *Les épilepsies*; Voisin, *L'épilepsie*; Binswanger, *Die Epilepsie*; Taylor, *Selected Writings*.

[123] Nothnagal, 'Epilepsy and Eclampsia'. Binswanger's book *Die Epilepsie* (1899) was a standard German-language work on epilepsy.

[124] Epilepsia partialis continua was described by Kozhevnikov in Russian as 'spring-summer encephalitis' and is sometimes known as 'Kozhevnikov's epilepsy'. Aleksei Yakovlevich Kozhevnikov, based in Moscow, was considered to be the first academic psychiatrist appointed in Russia.

[125] Manuel Echeverria, *On Epilepsy*. He had also published another book, *De la trepanation dans l'épilepsie*, in Paris in 1842, and when at Queen Square continued to treat patients with epilepsy by trepanation.

The Theory of Cerebral Localisation

The physiological theory of cerebral localisation[126] was perhaps the most significant neuroscientific advance of the age, providing the anatomical under-pinning of the discipline of neurology and acting as midwife to the birth of clinical neurosurgery. It was to prove of fundamental importance to the clinical concepts of epilepsy over the whole of the twentieth century, and for this reason it is worth particular emphasis here.

The theory had its origin in the early 1800s. After carrying out stimulation experiments and focal resections of the animal brain, Marie-Jean-Pierre Flourens[127] concluded that the cerebral cortex was involved in perception, motor activity and judgement; the cerebellum in equilibrium and motor coordination; and the medulla in respiration and circulatory functions. However, he also believed that, within the cortex, intellectual and perceptual functions were not localised. This was known as the theory of equipotentiality, and it was supported by many renowned physiologists throughout the century, notably Friedrich Goltz.[128] Equipotentiality though was challenged by the landmark contributions of Eduard Hitzig and Gustav Fritsch who in 1870 localised motor action by cortical stimulation, Paul Broca who in 1871 showed that expression of speech was localised in the left inferior frontal gyrus, Carl Wernicke who in 1874 localised language comprehension to the left superior temporal gyrus and Hermann Munk who in 1881 showed that resecting a dog's occipital lobe would cause blindness.

The crucial research on cerebral localisation, from the point of view of epilepsy, however, was the work of David Ferrier[129] and his colleague Victor Horsley. Both carried out extensive studies, by electrical stimulation and focal

---

[126] The concept of localisation applied to many branches of medicine in addition to cerebral neurology, underpinning the general development of surgery. See Lawrence, *Medicine*.

[127] Jean Pierre Flourens was a pioneer of experimental brain science and also anaesthesia. He was known as a creationist and opponent of Darwinism.

[128] Friedrich Leopold Goltz served as Professor of Physiology at the University of Halle, and then the University of Straßburg. He was also known for his 'hydrostatic concept' of the function of the semi-circular canals in the inner ear.

[129] Sir David Ferrier (1843–1928) was a Scottish neurologist who graduated from Edinburgh University and was appointed physician to King's College Hospital and the National Hospital, Queen Square. Ferrier gave the Croonian Lectures at the Royal Society in 1874 and 1875. He summarised his work in a monograph, *Functions of the Brain* (1876; extensively revised in 1886), which he dedicated to Hughlings Jackson, 'who from a clinical and pathological standpoint anticipated many of the more important results of recent experimental investigation into the functions of the cerebral hemispheres. This work is dedicated as a mark of the author's esteem and admiration'. Ferrier delivered the Gulstonian Lectures of the Royal College of Physicians in 1878 and published them that same year (Ferrier, *Localisation*). He also gave the 1890 Croonian Lectures at the Royal College of Physicians (Ferrier, *Croonian Lectures*). It was on the basis of these lectures that Charles Sherrington became interested in neurophysiology. He dedicated *Integrative Action of the Nervous System* (1906) to Ferrier.

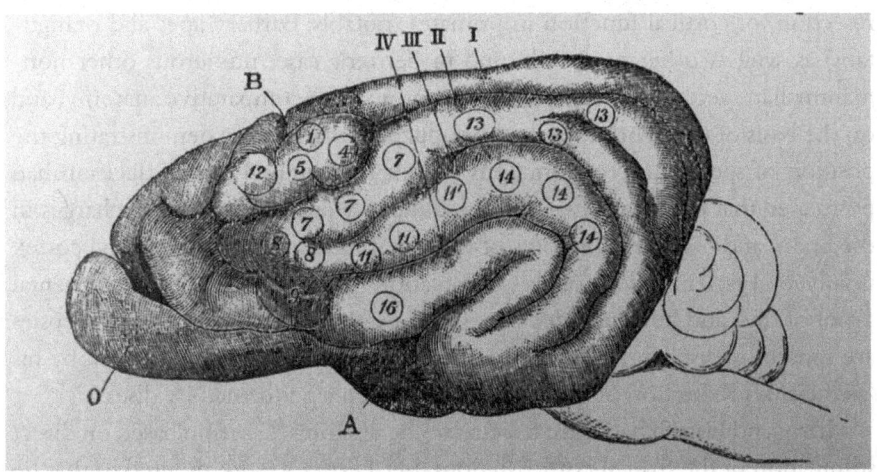

7. A page from David Ferrier's book _The Functions of the Brain_. The illustration is of one of his functional maps from the brain of a dog (note how similar these are to the functional maps of today). The circled numbers reflect different functions. He notes, for example, that stimulation at position 1 induces flexion of the opposite hind leg, as in walking, and at position 3 induces lateral wagging of the tail.

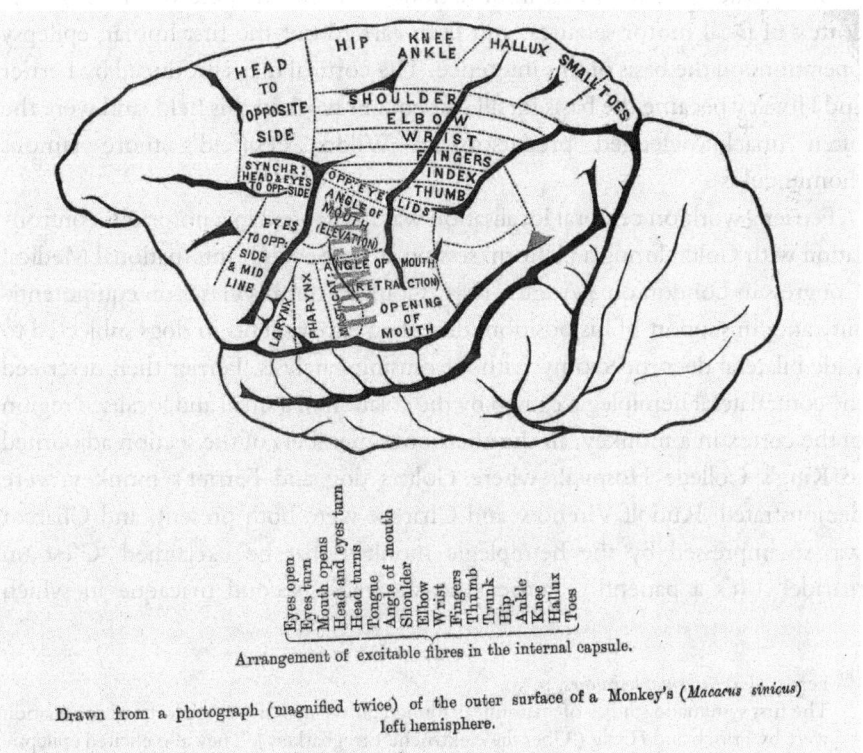

Arrangement of excitable fibres in the internal capsule.

Drawn from a photograph (magnified twice) of the outer surface of a Monkey's (_Macacus sinicus_) left hemisphere.

8. A page from the Philosophical Transactions of the Royal Society, illustrating the detail of Horsley's experimental work. Horsley's meticulous experiments used stimulation with minimal current every 2mm across the motor areas of the brain (of a Bonnet Monkey in this example). (C. E. Beevor and V Horsley, _Philosophical Transactions of the Royal Society_, 1890).

resection, of cortical function in primates (notably Barbary apes and orangutans) as well as other mammals, and in Ferrier's case, numerous other nonmammalian species too. These were masterpieces of comparative anatomy, and on the basis of this work they both produced cortical maps demonstrating the position of specific motor functions within the cerebral cortex. Jackson had postulated that the symptoms of focal epilepsy were due to focal discharges in the brain, and that the symptoms of the seizure reflected the part of the cortex involved. Ferrier undertook his stimulation work to provide experimental proof of this, and he concluded that Jackson's theory that 'unilateral epilepsies are caused by discharging cortical lesions' was correct, as demonstrated by his 'artificial reproduction of the clinical experiments performed by disease'.[130]

Hitzig and Fritsch had been the first to localise muscle action based on direct stimulation of the frontal cortex in dogs, but Ferrier's work differed in that he used long-duration faradic stimulation, which allowed complex movements to be observed (not just spasm).[131] He also examined more areas of cortex and with greater degrees of sophistication. Horsley also used electrical stimulation to catalogue the anatomical position of the motor symptoms ('functions') in primates. He transposed his findings onto the human brain by analogy with the primate structures, used this information to predict the site of origin in the cortex of focal motor seizures, and then carried out the first human epilepsy operations on the basis of this inference. The cortical maps produced by Ferrier and Horsley became the basis for all subsequent work in this field, and were the often unacknowledged precursors of Wilder Penfield's more famous 'homunculus'.

Ferrier's work on cerebral localisation was challenged in a notorious confrontation with Goltz during a platform session at the Seventh International Medical Congress in London on 4 August 1881. Goltz set out his views on equipotentiality and, in support of his position, described experiments in dogs subjected to wide bilateral decorticectomy without causing paralysis. Ferrier then described the contralateral hemiplegia caused by the ablation of a small and localised region of the cortex in a monkey. In the afternoon, members of the section adjourned to King's College Hospital, where Goltz's dog and Ferrier's monkey were demonstrated. Rudolf Virchow and Charcot were both present, and Charcot was so impressed by the hemiplegic monkey that he exclaimed 'C'est un malade!' ('It's a patient!'). Ferrier also showed a second macaque in which

[130] Ferrier, *Experimental researches*, p. 30.
[131] The first systematic studies of anatomical-topographical analysis using electrical stimulation were by Fritsch and Hitzig ('Über die elektrische Erregbarkeit'). They also elicited epileptic seizures through longer tetanic stimulation, demonstrating a cortical origin. When Ferrier attempted to publish his own work, the Royal Society held an inquiry into whether he had sufficiently acknowledged their precedence and concluded that he did not. Ferrier bitterly contested the decision.

bilateral resection of the superior temporal region had rendered the animal totally deaf such that it ignored a pistol shot fired close to the head. Ferrier considered Goltz's experimental technique to be flawed as he had obliterated brain matter using a jet of water, rather than by careful excision, an imprecise method which made it impossible to know exactly which structures had been damaged. Both Ferrier and Goltz consented to examination of the two animals' brains. On 9 August 1881 the examining committee reported that the brain lesions in Goltz's dog were not as extensive as claimed, with portions of the motor and sensory areas preserved, whereas Ferrier's monkey had, as Ferrier had predicted, a small and well-defined lesion in the motor area. This conclusion was widely publicised and proved an enormous boost to the localisationalist school.[132] Indeed, it was this event, more than any other, that demonstrated the validity of cerebral localisation in the minds of clinicians and, with Horsley and Rickman Godlee[133] in the audience at the congress, led directly to the birth of neurosurgery, the major therapeutic advance of the time.[134]

Ferrier's work may have been at the vanguard of clinical science, but it outraged influential figures in London society. Ferrier and Horsley were already being demonised by anti-vivisectionalists and the demonstration of a lesioned monkey was a step too far in the eyes of the popular and already powerful antivivisection movement. Ferrier was then accused under the Cruelty to Animals Act (1876) of performing 'frightful and shocking experiments on monkeys for which he did not have a licence'.[135] Court proceedings were held in November 1881. The prosecution excited passion and worldwide interest, and Jackson, Joseph Lister, John Burdon-Sanderson and Charcot were among those who attended the hearing; the proceedings were published in the *British Medical Journal*.[136] The opening address of counsel was thought by the *Boston Medical and Surgical Journal* to be 'the prosiest and poorest twaddle that could have been tolerated in the support of the feeblest case';[137] and in the proceedings that followed the charge was thrown out – albeit on a technicality. Samuel Wilks wrote an excoriating letter in *The Lancet*, warning against the

---

[132] The theory of equipotentiality, although wounded, experienced something of a revival in the twentieth century. Karl Lashley (1890–1958), an American psychologist, proposed the principle of mass action, suggesting that the amount of brain damage is directly proportional to decreased memory function. But, as Lashley himself concluded, equipotentiality is not total but regional, and is present only to a limited extent.

[133] Sir Rickman John Godlee performed the first resection of a brain tumour for epilepsy at the Hospital for Epilepsy and Paralysis, Regent's Park. He was the nephew of Joseph Lister, whose biography he wrote.

[134] Although another Queen Square surgeon, Sir Charles Ballance, claimed '[i]t was Ferrier, not any surgeon, who was the originator and founder of modern cerebral surgery' (cited in Gibson, 'Sir Charles Sherrington').

[135] 'Charge against a vivisectionist'.   [136] 'The charge against Professor Ferrier'.

[137] Cited in Spillane, 'A memorable decade'.

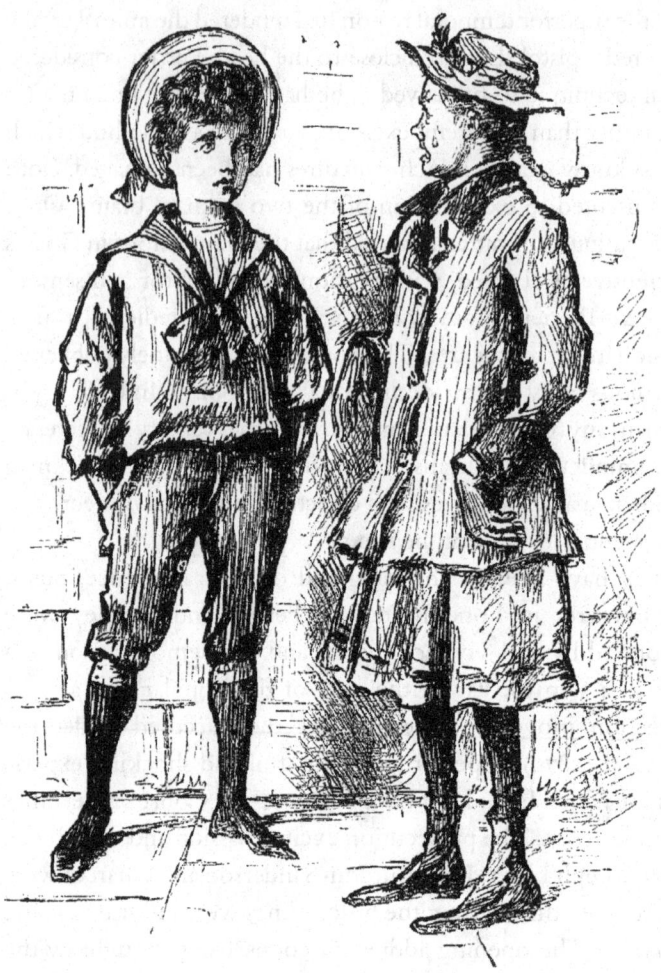

9. Animis Cœllestibis Irae [transl. Anger in the minds of the Gods]: a modern scientific discussion.

It wasn't only David Ferrier who was pursued by antivivisectionists. This is a cartoon from the satirical magazine, *Punch*, dated 5 November 1892, poking fun at the public row between Sir Victor Horsley and Ms Cobbe, a vocal antivivisectionist. The title is a quote from the *Aeniad*. The caption to the cartoon reads:

Miss Fanny (a gentle and most veracious child): '*Yah! You cruel coward! You and your friends shinned a live frog.*'
Mister Victor (an industrious but touchy boy): '*You're a liar! The frog was dead, and you know it!*'
Miss Fanny: Boo Hoo!. Whether it was dead or not, you have no right to call me names: 'Cos I'm a girl and can't punch your head!
Mister Victor: 'It's just because you're a girl that I can't punch yours! You should have thought of that before you called me a coward!'

dangers of the antivivisectionists, and the proceedings were deemed to have been a 'dishonour to the English nation in the eyes of the world'. Wilson wrote later: 'Only a few of his friends are aware of the personal abuse which this line of investigation brought [Ferrier] or of the extremes to which his opponents went in their endeavour to discredit his achievement.'[138]

The Neurology of Epilepsy 1900–1914: The Books of Turner and Spratling

In the first decade of the twentieth century, two leading physicians published books on epilepsy which summarised the current knowledge of that period. The most important was *Epilepsy: A Study of the Idiopathic Disease* (1907) by William Aldren Turner, a physician at the National Hospital for the Paralysed and Epileptic, King's College Hospital and at the Chalfont epilepsy colony. He was the key figure in anglophone epilepsy during the first two decades of the century (and, incidentally, also an authority on shell shock). As J. Kiffin Penry put it in 1973, Turner's book was 'a classic text to be placed alongside the works of Gowers and Jackson'.[139] This is perhaps an overstatement, but there is little doubt that, among almost all other books and papers of this period, Turner's work proved the most significant and innovative. His text is notable for its clarity of thought and concision, and for his plain, clear and precise writing style. He covered a wide range of clinical topics related to epilepsy and there are indeed aspects, for instance on prognosis and classification, now forgotten which would benefit from rediscovery. For the first time, too, statistical methods were applied in the study of prognosis and the effects of treatment. As a monograph, the book's format and style set the standard for all that followed up to the present day.

The second book of note was William Spratling's *Epilepsy and Its Treatment*,[140] published in 1904. This was the first significant book on the topic of epilepsy to emerge from the United States.[141] Spratling's book, like Turner's, was heavily influenced both in format and content by Gower's work published some twenty years earlier, and none of his descriptions are particularly innovative. His account

[138] For details, see Shorvon and Compston, *Queen Square*, pp. 143–4.
[139] Citation from the foreword to the facsimile edition of Turner's book, published by Raven Press in 1973.
[140] Williams Spratling's interest in epilepsy was stimulated whilst he worked with Dr Frederick Peterson who was a psychiatrist and psychoanalyst, Professor of Psychiatry at Columbia, President of the New York State Commission in Lunacy, and a key figure in establishing the Craig Colony. Spratling was appointed assistant physician in the State Hospital for the Insane in Morris Plains, New Jersey, and subsequently as superintendent at the Craig Colony for Epileptics in New York State. He was president of the National Association for the Study of Epilepsy. In his book, the word 'epileptologist' may have been used for the first time. He was a leading figure in the (albeit small) field of epilepsy in the United States. He died in a hunting accident, in which he was said to have tripped over a wire fence and to have shot himself accidentally with his own shotgun (Fine, Fine and Sentz, 'Importance of Spratling').
[141] The only previous book on the topic of epilepsy from the United States was Echeverria's *On Epilepsy: Anatomo-pathological and Clinical Notes* (1870). Echeverria was born in Havana and partly trained at the National Hospital, Queen Square and at Bedlam in London before moving to New York to become physician in chief at the New York Hospital for Epileptics and Paralytics and visiting physician at the Charity Hospital (originally named the Penitentiary Hospital) on Blackwell's Island. His book was heavily influenced by those of Reynolds and Sieveking.

is more rambling, and at times quite inaccurate. But, like Turner's work, Spratling's was well backed up by an excellent survey of the literature as well as his personal experience: a practice based mainly in an asylum, the Craig Colony for Epileptics, where Spratling was medical superintendent.[142] One senses in Spratling's work, though, a contempt and dislike of his epilepsy patients, in marked contrast to Turner's more kindly and humane attitude.

In the preface to his 1907 book, Turner thanked Hughlings Jackson for 'his great interest in the preparation of the work', but dedicated the book to David Ferrier, under whose tutelage he began his career in the field of epilepsy. From the perspective of today, however, the precursor of Turner's work was surely neither Jackson nor Ferrier, but Gowers, and particularly his *Epilepsy and Other Chronic Convulsive Disorders*. Both books share clear and simple prose, both are intensely practical and clinically oriented, and both are utterly embedded in the authors' clinical practices – in Turner's afforded by the great number of outpatients seen at the National Hospital and at the Chalfont Centre for Epilepsy.

It is important to realise that the concept of epilepsy in 1900 was very different from that of today. Questions regarding definition did not revolve only around whether the term should refer purely to the idiopathic condition, but also around whether it should be restricted to the occurrence of seizures or should more broadly incorporate the associated psychological disturbances and social aspects of the condition. Spratling declined to define epilepsy at all, noting: 'It is exceedingly difficult to define a disease in which changing conditions of mind are prominent and essential features – like insanity, for instance – and it is even more difficult to define a disease that is partly mental, partly physical; more the former at one time, more the latter at another.'[143] Turner was more forthright. He (like Reynolds and Gowers before him) restricted his book to idiopathic epilepsy, which he considered to be the 'disease' epilepsy, and which had specific features and followed a specific course,[144] and he provided an altogether more penetrating definition of (idiopathic) epilepsy than any of his predecessors:

> Epilepsy is a chronic progressive disease of the brain, characterised by the periodic occurrence of seizures, in which loss of consciousness is an

---

[142] In one bizarre and distressing section on the effect of race on epilepsy, Spratling cites 'Searcy' of the Alabama Bryce Insane Hospital, who in 1902 found that negroes in Alabama were thirteen times more likely to be in an asylum than was the case thirty years earlier. Spratling blames this on degenerating lineage, of which 'epilepsy and insanity are but indications and results' (Spratling, *Epilepsy and Its Treatment*, p. 56).

[143] Spratling, *Epilepsy and Its Treatment*, p. 14. He did, however, cite the definitions of Gowers, Thomas Allbutt, Russell Reynolds and Echeverria.

[144] However, in his Morison lectures of 1910, he states: 'The term "epilepsy" refers to a symptom; it is the clinical expression of a group of diseases ... They may be divided into four primary divisions: ... 1. The organic epilepsies ... 2. The early epilepsies ... 3. The late epilepsies ... 4. Idiopathic epilepsy.' He calls idiopathic epilepsy (genuine epilepsy) a 'chronic disease of the brain' (Turner, 'Morison Lectures').

essential feature; commonly associated with convulsion, and frequently accompanied by psychical phenomena of a well-defined type; occurring generally in persons with a hereditary neuropathic history, which shows itself in signs, or stigmata, of degeneration; running its course uninterruptedly, or with remissions, over a number of years; and terminating either in a cure, in the establishment of the confirmed disease, in delusional insanity, or in dementia. (p. 1)

To Turner, as to others of this period, the psychical aspects of epilepsy were considered integral to the disease: 'In earlier days the convulsion, or fit, was regarded as the sole element of importance in the clinical study of epilepsy; but in more recent years the psychical factor has come to be looked upon as of almost equal importance, and both are regarded as manifestations of a predisposition associated with inheritance' (p. 2).[145]

Turner then moved to classification. He divided seizures into minor seizures, major seizures and psychical seizures. He also recognised that minor and major seizures might have an aura (the *prélude* of the French writers), be incomplete ('minor fit'; the *accès incomplets* or *vertige* of the French writers) or be complete ('major fit'; the *crise* of the French writers). Citing the influential approach of Herpin,[146] Turner discussed the evolution from aura to incomplete attacks – for instance, a dreamy sensation followed by a fall without convulsion; and the evolution of an aura into a complete attack, the major convulsion, which would now be called secondary generalisation, recognising too that many major convulsions occur without any aura. Turner also provided a detailed definition of the prodromata of an epileptic seizure – changes in affect or temperament, myoclonic jerking or brief sensory disturbances – as well as the various types of aura. Although the terminology has changed periodically in subsequent years, his descriptions of clinical phenomena have hardly been bettered. Original also was his emphasis on the pattern of attacks over time. Sections of his book are devoted to such categories as epilepsy in which only a

---

[145] According to German Berrios, prior to the neurological advances of the mid-nineteenth century the psychological aspects were considered an integral part of epilepsy, but with the work of Jackson, Gowers and others this connection was lost (Berrios, 'Epilepsy and insanity'), although Turner's definition of epilepsy makes it clear that this was not the case. Turner also cited G. Aschaffenburg as stating that 'periodic fluctuations of the psychical equilibrium' might indicate epilepsy even if there was no history of overt seizures. Turner himself noted that 'psychical equivalents' were examples of the psychosis that occurs around seizures (*Epilepsy*, p. 5).

[146] Herpin, *Des accès incomplets d'épilepsie* (1867), published posthumously. Herpin suggested that incomplete (partial) seizures could sometimes evolve into generalised tonic–clonic seizures (the basis for the current concept of secondary generalisation) and, furthermore, that the clinical phenomenology at the onset of a seizure is always or nearly always identical for individual patients. Contrary to much received opinion, he hypothesised that when symptoms started in the periphery or the viscera, their origin was in the brain. He also considered that epilepsy might be curable if treated early. Herpin also provided an early description of what is now called juvenile myoclonic epilepsy.

few episodes occurred (now sometimes called oligoepilepsy), epilepsy with a diurnal pattern and senile epilepsy.

A further contribution originating with Gowers and expanded upon by Turner concerned pathogenesis. It was his view that the epilepsy, once initiated, evolved. 'The cardinal principle' was that the cause of epilepsy is the cause of the first fit, and that 'the instability of the brain, once induced, becomes embedded, so that when further epileptic convulsions appear, they may, and do, recur quite independently of the original or any other obvious exciting cause'. In this way, the epileptic state, or constitution, becomes 'established'[147], and seizures persist even after the exciting cause has been removed (p. 64).

Turner recognised two categories of idiopathic epilepsy: one in which heredity was the predisposing cause, and a second, smaller category of epilepsies due to 'various exciting, or accidental phenomena' (p. 41), although even these cases involved a significant contribution from an inherited predisposition (p. 64). Turner went on to explain that what is inherited is a 'family neuropathic degeneration' – here again following Morel and the nineteenth-century French school. In his series, evidence of a hereditable factor was manifest by the presence of an 'ancestral history of epilepsy' in 37% of his cases and of insanity, alcoholism and other nervous disorders in a further 14% (pp. 26–7). The physical stigmata of degeneration were present in 66% of cases (p. 38). He noted the frequent occurrence of febrile seizures and also the fact that although 'epilepsy and insanity are the two main elements of the psychopathic hereditary degeneration', there were also examples of hysteria, chorea, drug habit and migraine in the families of epileptics indicative of the neuropathic diathesis (p. 29). He also subscribed to the 'law of progressivity', by which this taint worsened through generations and the conditions became more severe. The various physical stigmata taken to indicate the presence of the neuropathic trait included such features as facial deformities and asymmetry and abnormalities of dentation, eyes, ears or limbs, pathological changes in the brain, and even astigmatism and stammering (pp. 30–8).[148]

By 1900, it seems that the grip of the theories of the neurological trait and of inherited degeneration was almost total even in advanced neurological circles. There were few contemporary neurologists or psychiatrists who did not accept these tenets (although, as we have seen, a notable exception was Jackson). Another leading physician, Joseph Arderne Ormerod, gave the 1908 Harveian Oration entitled 'Heredity in relation to disease', in which he divided the

---

[147] Turner, *Epilepsy*, p. 41.

[148] The idea that those with epilepsy have a specific physical appearance or anthropometric structure has never fully died out. See, for instance, the theories of the Kretschmer school and Karl Westphal in the 1930s (Westphal, 'Körperbau und Charakter') and occasional writings today.

inherited conditions into two categories. First were the neuroses, which included 'epilepsy, insanity, hysteria, neurasthenia, tics, alcoholism, etc. characterised ... by perverted nervous action rather than by coarse structural disease'. These conditions were the expression of the neurological trait and 'varied and inter-changeable *inter se* of some one underlying nervous defect'. They represented 'an ill-timed or inappropriate response of a nervous system which adapts itself badly to its surroundings' and were distinct from the second group of diseases in which there was a clear family history, such as Friedreich's ataxia, Strümpell's spastic paralysis and periodic paralyses.[149]

Spratling avoided classification, and instead subdivided his seizure types in a random fashion, giving detailed descriptions of each.[150] In terms of aetiology, he too accepted the primacy of heredity. However, he also emphasised that, in the majority of cases, both predisposing and exciting causes interact, and he quantified this assertion succinctly, if rather quaintly, by supposing that, if the point at which a seizure occurs 'is represented by 100 [, i]f there are already present 60 of these points from, we will say, *a predisposition due to heredity*, there will remain but 40 points to be supplied by some exciting cause to bring the disease to light'; and that, similarly, if the predisposing cause amounted to only 40 points, 'it will require 60 points of the exciting cause' (pp. 58–9).

Turner's account opens with the demographic features of epilepsy, and he used national statistics to establish a prevalence of epilepsy of 1–3/1000. This is one of the first serious published analyses of prevalence and thus a landmark in epilepsy epidemiology. He then considered aetiology, pathogenesis and prognosis, extending the concept of epilepsy in several innovative ways. First, he emphasised the importance of dividing the epilepsies into categories according to the duration of the illness. Basing his work on an analysis of 1,000 patients seen by him at the National Hospital, Queen Square and the epilepsy colony at Chalfont, he concluded that with proper treatment, new-onset cases carried the chance of cure; conversely, in confirmed or established cases, extended remission or cure was generally not possible. He postulated that as epilepsy continued, it triggered pathological and functional changes in the brain - in other words, he saw epilepsy as a dynamic and progressive process. He conceptualised epilepsy as an organic disease of the brain in which the progressive

---

[149] Ormerod, *On Heredity*, pp. 34–5, 39. By then it was recognised that heredity was mediated by chromosomes, although how this was achieved was not known. Mendel's laws had been rediscovered by Bateson, and Ormerod was aware of these, as well as the controversy over the inheritance of acquired characteristics, of Galton and Pearson's statistical work, and of the evolving science of eugenics. William Bateson coined the term 'genetics' for the study of inheritance and of variation. His book *Materials for the Study of Variation* (1894) was a foundation work in genetics.

[150] His subdivisions comprised grand mal, petit mal, psychic, Jacksonian, serial attacks, reflex epilepsy, epileptic equivalents, partial epilepsy, tetanoid epilepsy, hystero-epilepsy and myoclonus epilepsy.

character of the 'paroxysmal' and 'interparoxysmal' symptoms was a sign of organic change demonstrable, for instance, histopathologically. Following the lead of Gowers, Turner examined the prognostic factors associated with long remission, demonstrating that the shorter the duration of the illness, the absence of a neuropathic family history, the type of seizures (major attacks alone), a low frequency and the presence of long remission were all good prognostic signs; a 'cure' was encountered in 10–12% of cases (pp. 220–3).

Spratling's book is notable for long stretches of text on the psychiatry and mental states of epilepsy, supporting enthusiastically the concept of the 'epileptic personality', but his most original chapter covered the medico-legal aspects of epilepsy. Here he breaks new ground, differentiating crimes committed during a seizure (or in the post-ictal state) and those unrelated to seizures, taking the view that the epileptic has no responsibility for the former. There was no epilepsy defence equivalent to that of 'guilty but insane' and Spratling argued this lack should be remedied. He was an experienced expert witness in court, and the chapter has a series of instructive but chilling legal case reports.

The chapter on status epilepticus was by L. Pierce Clark and reiterates his prize-winning papers with Thomas Prout published the year before.[151] These were definitive statements on status epilepticus and are described later.

Both Turner and Spratling devoted much attention to the aetiology of epilepsy and both adopted the by then well-established practice of dividing causes into predisposing and exciting categories, with both agreeing that the main predisposing cause was heredity. However, their lists of 'exciting causes' varied and included: dentition, sleep, menstruation, infections, alcohol, toxins, sexual aberration, psychological factors and other reflex triggers.[152]

Many authors had noted that seizures often seemed to occur with no obvious exciting factor, and various other wild theories were proposed to explain their precipitation. Although almost always clothed in scientific explanation, these theories were in fact predicated on prevailing fashion and have been now largely discarded; two examples demonstrate this well. The first is the 'reflex theory of epilepsy'. Reflex action as an explanation of cerebral mechanisms had

---

[151] Clark and Prout, 'Status epilepticus'.

[152] It is interesting to note that the distinction between the categories of predisposing and exciting causes was held well into the 1930s. In 1935, a variant on this idea was proposed by V. M. Bascaino (of Catania), who divided 'the causative factors of convulsive attacks of the epileptic type into four principal groups: predisposing, precursory, facilitative, and exciting (*déchainantes*). The first included hereditary influences; the second, cerebral lesions; facilitative factors included variations of pressure and atmospheric electricity, menstruation or pregnancy, spasm of the subcortical vessels, the state of vagotonia, alkalosis, strong emotion and so forth; and the exciting factors were those which provoked epileptic attack by a physico-chemical mechanism, such as the presence in the circulation of placental products (eclampsia) or renal products (uraemia)'. He thought that in the same patient, 'the attacks might thus have different origins' ('International Neurological Congress in London').

a long pedigree, being articulated in detail by Marshall Hall[153] and supported by the authority of Jackson. As a mechanism of epilepsy, it was believed that irritation outside the brain resulted in vascular congestion or exhaustion of the brain's inhibitory processes, which led to discharge of the nerve cells, or that peripheral irritation influenced the cells at the base of the brain and upper cord, in time altering their nutrition so as to create a 'morbid excitability'. According to Walter Friedlander,[154] the eleven most frequently mentioned sites of irritation were the periphery (injuries to peripheral nerves, skin scars, etc.); eyes (eye strain); ear, nose and throat disorders; teeth (caries); digestive problems; constipation; worms in the gastrointestinal tract; rectum; reproductive organs; genitals (including that due to phimosis). Even as late as 1917, in the gynaecological textbook of James Craven Wood, a chapter on epilepsy links reflex seizures to pathological changes in the womb.[155]

The reflex theory led to an assortment of unlikely treatments, ineffective at best but often positively harmful. The surgical excision of traumatic lesions of the peripheral nerves, removal of a tight prepuce in boys, treatment of coexistent diseases of the ears or nasopharynx and removal of foreign bodies, adenoid growths and polypi were all recommended. Turner also subscribed to the view that errors of refraction should be corrected and glasses worn, in view of the dramatic results reported by Féré and others – although one senses his lack of zeal about this utterly pointless therapy.[156] Wood considered that catamenial epilepsy was most likely to indicate a utero-ovarian origin, but surgery was needed before the 'habit' of epilepsy had become set. He was, however, 'compelled to admit that the sum total of cures resulting from radical work upon the genital or abdominal organs is not encouraging, but it is sufficiently so to justify the correction of such lesions … The discouraging results have been due in the past largely to our lack of knowledge in selecting suitable cases.'[157]

---

[153] Marshall Hall also published a book devoted to epilepsy: *On the Threatenings of Apoplexy and Paralysis; Inorganic Epilepsy; Spinal Syncope; Hidden Seizures; the Resultant Mania; etc.* (1851) – a strange mixture of ideas about the early signs of a seizure, notably trachelismus. He also wrote on 'hidden seizures', which occurred without obvious convulsion and may occasion 'a monomaniacal tendency to suicide or homicide. *Crime* may be committed, and no proof of previous insanity exist. Of such a case, the Law, hitherto, equally with Medicine, has taken no cognizance. This crime may be one involving loss of property, honour, life.' (p. 77). He also described post-seizure hemiparesis before Todd, whose name is usually associated with this phenomenon.

[154] Friedlander, *History*.

[155] Wood, *Clinical Gynecology*, which included a chapter on epilepsy, perhaps a hangover from earlier links between hysteria and the womb and the idea that hystero-epilepsy was caused by a wandering womb.

[156] Turner, *Epilepsy*, p. 54.

[157] Wood, *Clinical Gynecology*, p. 138. Exactly the same reason is given for failures of epilepsy surgery today!

Another widely accepted theory, now discredited, was that seizures were caused by 'autointoxication'. According to this concept, epileptic seizures (and various mental disorders) were the result of toxins produced within the person's own body – an echo of Galen's theory of humours. In 1907 Turner took the view that this was a likely cause of serial epilepsy, status epilepticus and fits associated with acute mental symptoms, as evidenced by the 'general somatic disturbances' which accompany them, but again likely only in those with an inherited predisposition.[158] The gist of the most widely accepted theory was that 'autotoxins' were produced in the gastrointestinal tract and then acted on the brain.[159] The cause was often thought to be constipation or the slow passage of food through the gastrointestinal tract, resulting in over-fermentation or putre-faction. This concept included the belief that occult infections in the bowel caused epilepsy. In 1916, Charles Reed believed that he had identified the bacterium, *Bacillus epilepticus*, in the blood of epileptic patients.[160] Uric acid was another, often postulated, causative toxin, and Donáth believed that the toxin was choline. A range of exotic radiographic and sigmoidoscopic studies purported to show anatomical variations (now recognised to be entirely spuri-ous) in the colon and, as a result, colectomy became a recognised and quite widely used treatment.[161] One extreme advocate of the toxin theory of mental diseases was the alienist Henry Cotton, superintendent of the New Jersey State Hospital at Trenton, a residential institution for the mentally ill. He began a programme of surgical therapy of extraordinary proportions, largely for psych-otic but also for epileptic inmates.[162] In one 12-month period, 6,472 dental extractions were performed, as well as 542 tonsillectomies and 79 colon resec-tions, as well as resections of spleens, gall bladders and ovaries. Between 1918 and 1925, 2,186 major operations were carried out.[163]

In a variant of the autointoxication theory, Carlo Ceni,[164] a leading figure in the growing field of Italian neurology, treated epilepsy with serum from other

[158] Turner, *Epilepsy*, p. 199.

[159] Is it too fanciful to see echoes of this in the currently fashionable concept of the 'microbiome'?

[160] Reed, 'Bacillus epilepticus'. Charles Alfred Lee Reed (1856–1928) was a physician in Cincinnati and one-time president of the American Medical Association.

[161] See Axtell, 'Acute angulation', and Clark and Busby, 'Value of roentgen analysis'. The same theories were advanced to explain psychosis: Nevins, *Tale of Two 'Villages'*.

[162] Cotton, *Defective, Delinquent*. Cotton presents case studies, including patients, and provides case reports of seizure control in a six-year-old as well as in a forty-year-old man with nocturnal convulsions which were cured by colectomy. Cotton (played by John Hodgman) featured in the TV drama *The Knick* (2014), a fictionalised account of the goings-on at the Knickerbocker Hospital in the 1900s, where Cotton removes his wife's teeth to treat depression.

[163] Cotton became a national figure, lauded publicly for his remarkable cure rates. In 1921, the president of the American Medical Association declared that Trenton State was one of the country's 'great institutions . . . a monument to the most advanced civilisation' (details are taken from Nevins, *Tale of Two 'Villages'*).

[164] Carlo Ceni won the Craig Colony award in 1909 for his experimental work on epilepsy.

patients on the basis that epilepsy was due to an autocytotoxin, latent in blood cells and released in a convulsion, and that the serum contained an antiauto-cytotoxin which had therapeutic benefits (in fact, not totally dissimilar to recent immunological theories).[165]

Most experimental work of the period was devoted to physiological studies in animals of cortical excitability, and the observation that excitability could be changed by toxins or altered chemical parameters was considered strong confirmation of autointoxication. Support for the theory of blood-borne toxins was also provided by iinfluential experiments in which the injections of blood from epileptic patients into guinea pigs and rabbits produced violent convulsions.

The Neuropathology of Epilepsy

When the modern science of epilepsy first surfaced in the latter decades of the nineteenth century, pathology was the predominant scientific discipline in medicine.[166] Neuropathology was one of the few 'laboratory' sciences available to clinicians. Indeed, most clinicians did post-mortems on their own patients, laying the groundwork of gross morbid anatomy although contributing little to theories of pathogenesis of idiopathic forms of epilepsy. During those early years, the discipline had made great strides, boosted particularly by the theory of the cellular basis of disease.[167] In parallel, histopathology developed,[168] which depended on developing technologies, including improvements in microscopy, hardening of tissue by fixation, embedding of tissue in paraffin wax (introduced around 1870 in Germany) and the invention of the microtome.[169]

Virchow had recognised (and named) glia, but the most important neuropathological advances had to await methods of staining nerve tissue that

[165] Other treatments based loosely on toxin theories included hot-air baths, predicated on the idea that the 'sweat of epileptics' was poisonous (Cabitto), and various forms of organotherapy, for instance with sterile emulsions of brain (Babes), cerebrine (Lion and Poehl) or ovarian substance and tauriceine (Toulaux and Marchand) (see 'An Epitome of current medical literature').

[166] It is notable how proficient physicians were in neuropathological examinations at that time. The leaders in the field of neuropathology were the neuropsychiatrists in the Austro-German tradition (including Meynert, Bratz, Wilhelm Sommer and Binswanger).

[167] The theory was consolidated by Rudolf Virchow in his magnum opus, *Die Cellularpathologie in ihrer Begründung auf physiologische und pathologische Gewebelehre* (1858). Virchow's work finally buried the view that disease is due to an imbalance of the four humours, and it formed the basis for all modern pathology. It was a paradigm shift of enormous importance in many fields of medicine.

[168] The earliest histopathological work is perhaps that of Johannes Müller (1801–58): *Über den feineren Bau der krankhaften Geschwülste* (1838).

[169] Landmarks included fixation by Müller's fluid in 1860 and by formalin in 1893; the introduction of various microtome technologies, including the Cambridge rocker in 1885, developed by Horace Darwin, the son of Charles; haematoxylin and eosin, introduced in 1876 by A. Wissozky on the basis of Paul Erlich's earlier studies; and frozen sections of biopsy material by François-Vincent Raspail.

allowed the differentiation and investigation of different cell types. In 1873, the Italian pathologist Camillo Golgi invented the silver stain, which rendered neurons intensely black in colour and showed that they had a profusion of branching and interconnected elements as well as long axons covered in myelin (Virchow's term). Subsequently, Santiago Ramón y Cajal, a Spanish neuro-pathologist, improved the methodology further by producing a series of exquisite drawings illustrating the three-dimensional structure of the brain. Golgi posited that neurons were fused together, forming a network of con-nected cells; however, Ramón y Cajal evolved the 'neuron doctrine', which stated that the cells were all discrete entities – in close proximity but not joined to each other.[170] Battles between these two theories of nervous structure raged, with celebrated pathologists on either side. Only later was the debate resolved in favour of the neuron doctrine, not least through the work of Charles Sherrington, who reasoned that contact between discrete cells was made at synapses (his term).

Whilst microscopy and histopathology were to prove vitally important in epilepsy in later years, in this early period what was striking to Gowers, and to all who followed him, was the absence of any gross neuropathology in idio-pathic epilepsy. As Gowers put it, 'Great as is the aid which . . . the microscope has afforded in the investigation of the structural changes which underlie or constitute many diseases of the nervous system, it cannot be said to have thrown much light on the nature of idiopathic epilepsy.'[171]

Following Jackson's theory that epilepsy arose in the cortex, and not the medulla or other subcortical structures, pathologists began to look critically at the histology of the cerebral cortex. Amongst the first was W. Bevan Lewis, who examined the brains of epileptic patients dying in the West Riding Lunatic Asylum.[172] He observed that the first change in epilepsy was change of shape, fatty degeneration and then vacuolation of cells in the second cortical layer which he considered to be cells that inhibited the motor (Betz) cells in lower layers. These then degenerated and died, and he considered that epilepsy was caused by the loss of inhibition. He was the first to show microscopic pathology in the cerebral cortex and this helped confirm Jackson's view that the cortex was the seat of epilepsy.

In 1893, Ira Van Gieson showed neuroglia changes.[173] Luigi Roncoroni found a decrease in cells in the fourth cortical layer and an unusual abundance of neurons in the subcortical white matter, and Philippe Chaslin demonstrated widespread gliosis.[174] Even then, there were dissenting voices about the origin of the observed

---

[170] Golgi and Cajal shared the Nobel Prize in Physiology or Medicine in 1906 for their work on the microscopic structure of the nervous system.
[171] Gowers, *Epilepsy*, p. 199.   [172] Lewis, *Mental Diseases*.
[173] Van Gieson, 'Traumatic epilepsy'.   [174] Cited in Binswanger, *Die Epilepsie*.

changes, with Hermann Oppenheim,[175] for instance, regarding the glial changes in the outer cortical layer and in the cornu ammonis to be the consequence not the cause of epilepsy – this was to be a debate which continued through much of the century. By 1900, the cortical origin of epilepsy had become the orthodoxy of advanced medicine. The mechanisms of epilepsy though remained obscure. Elmer Southard, professor of neuropathology at Harvard, postulated that it was the increased glia density (gliosis) which caused the discharging lesion.[176] Turner recognised gliosis, engorgement of blood vessels, and loss of ganglion cells and atrophy, but reasoned these were the 'result of epileptic fits' and not their cause.[177] He believed these changes to be due to intravascular clotting and thus hypoxia of the cortical cells, in a brain 'hereditarily and structurally predisposed to instability and convulsion' (p. 184). But he considered the alterations in cell shape and vacuolation reported by Bevan Lewis, and in the nucleus and nucleolus reported by Clark and Prout (who did not cite Lewis's work), to be signs of the inheritance of a degenerative nervous system.

How a seizure spreads from the epileptic focus was another concern of pathologists. Heinrich Unverricht proposed a 'law of irradiation' by which the discharge originated in the focus and spread through the motor cortex like the waves caused by dropping a stone into water. This was disputed by others, including Binswanger. Prus felt that a fit was a 'complex reflex' and its spread followed extrapyramidal pathways, and Clark and Prout came to the conclusion, as had Prus, that epilepsy was primarily a sensory phenomenon involving a highly organised sensori-motor reflex of the cerebral cortex.[178]

It was not only the cerebral neocortex which attracted the attention of pathologists in epilepsy, but also the hippocampus (or Ammon's horn, as it was frequently referred to), which was recognised to be often gliotic and hardened. This pathological change, known as Ammon's horn sclerosis, was known to be a common finding in autopsy brains of epileptic patients following the first description by Camille Bouchet and Jean-Baptiste Cazauvieilh in 1825. In 1880, Wilhelm Sommer[179] reviewed all the reports and estimated that about 30% of epileptic brains showed the pathology. Sommer noted that the pyramidal cell loss was limited to what became called 'Sommer's sector' (now known as the CA1 region) and postulated that this might be the site of origin of seizures. In 1893 Ramón y Cajal[180] and in 1899 Emil Bratz[181] provided detailed and accurate descriptions of Ammon's horn sclerosis. Bratz noted the relative lack of cellular loss in what is now called the

---

[175] Oppenheim, *Lehrbuch der Nervenkrankheiten*.   [176] Southard, 'On the mechanism'.
[177] Turner, *Epilepsy*, p. 165.   [178] All cited in Clark and Prout (paper 3).
[179] Sommer, 'Erkrankung'.
[180] S. Ramón y Cajal, *Uber die feinere struktur des Ammonshornes*. Z Wissen Zool 1895 565:613–663. (Translated as *The Structure of Ammon's Horn*, with a forward by Paul D. MacLean. Springfield: Charles C. Thomas, 1968).
[181] Emil Bratz was born in Poland but trained and worked in Germany, becoming a leading figure in German psychiatry.

CA2 region. He estimated that Ammon's Horn sclerosis was found in 50% of epileptic brains, yet did not consider the lesion to be a cause of epilepsy but rather the result of seizures. Gowers noted that this was not found in what he called 'idiopathic epilepsy' writing:

> It is more than doubtful whether any importance is to be ascribed to the induration of the cornu Ammonis (*pes hippocampi*), to which so much weight has been attached by Meynert and others. Although changes of trifling character (atrophy and induration with wasting of the cells) have been described as present in one half of fifty cases of epilepsy examined (Bratz. 'Berlin. Gesellsch. f. Psych.,' Dec., 1897), they cannot be regarded as significant, being found apart from epilepsy. All physiological and pathological considerations render it improbable that the lesion has any direct relation to the disease. In the cases of epilepsy which I have examined, the cornu Ammonis was perfectly healthy, and in the two cases in which the structure was diseased, the patients had never suffered from convulsion or epileptic symptoms.[182]

In contrast, of the 115 cases of epilepsy which Turner had examined pathologically in detail, 50% showed Ammon's horn sclerosis, which he attributed to interference of the vascular supply. He also noted gliosis, angiomas (and what are now known to be cavernomas), cerebellar atrophy and changes in the long tracts of the medulla and spinal cord, all of which he believed to be the result of seizures.

By 1914 histopathology had thrown up a variety of other relatively minor changes, with little agreement about their relevance to pathophysiology. In his summary of the pathological changes delineated in the previous fifty years, James Wood spoke for many when pointing to the lack of evidence and their utterly random nature. He listed: 'increased weight of the brain (Echeverria); reduced weight of the brain (Meynert); dilatation of the vessels of the superior portion of the cord; aneurysm and atheroma of the blood vessels; sclerosis of the cornu ammonis; anaemia of the brain; an increased quantity of the cerebro-spinal fluid; tumours and thickening of the meninges of the brain; great redness and vascular tension in the fourth ventricle (Schroeder van der Kolk); alteration of the pineal gland; abnormal thickness and abnormal thinness of the cranial bones; perivascular and vascular changes in the cerebral cortex (Bloch and Marenesco); neurological proliferation (Chaslin); hypertrophy of the neurological bundles lying between the pia and outermost nerve bundles (Bleuler); persistent chymus and large intestinal glands (Ohlmacher); increased blood coagulability and fatty degeneration of ... the medulla ... Indeed, the changes recorded by pathologists are so various that it is utterly impossible to construct an explanation of the paroxysms upon a pathological basis'.[183] Most of these observations and ideas have not endured.[184]

---

[182] Gowers, *Epilepsy*, p. 214.   [183] Wood, *Clinical Gynecology*, p. 139.
[184] Wood, *Clinical Gynecology*, p. 139.

Another view, commonly expressed, was that idiopathic epilepsy had a developmental basis. Minor abnormalities which were taken to represent small developmental defects were reported by such authorities as Roncoroni, Theodor Kaes, Chaslin and Alois Alzheimer, for instance. This idea then fell out of fashion and was hardly discussed in the interwar years, but was revived during the 1960s by Vieth,[185] who found what he termed 'microdysgenesia' in 40% of epilepsy cases and considered these to be developmental causes of epilepsy. Their presence is still thought by many to be largely illusory and their significance remains contentious.

As no gross anatomical abnormalities were found in the idiopathic condition, theories of pathogenesis fell back onto functional change. These included vascular congestion (following Jackson) or, alternatively, vascular insufficiency (or 'brain anaemia'), toxic or metabolic changes and reflex disturbances. It was then that the concept of an altered balance between excitation and inhibition became the leading explanation of epilepsy; expounded, for instance, by reflex theorists who held that inhibition was due to the sensory side of reflex action and excitation due to the motor nerve activity. As we shall see, although theories of cerebral reflexes are now to a large extent dismissed, this theory of an imbalance between excitation and inhibition remains a predominant explanation of epilepsy right up to the present day.

Status Epilepticus

Status Epilepticus was a manifestation of epilepsy in which particular progress had been made, in the form of a series of three remarkable papers, published in 1903/4, by L. Pierce Clark, first assistant, and Thomas P. Prout, pathologist and second assistant, at two state asylums for the insane in New York and New Jersey.[186] Clark was to go on to a career as a neurologist specialising in psychoanalysis and epilepsy, but his work on status epilepticus stands above his other contributions. This trio of papers formed the first serious study of status epilepticus since the latter part of the nineteenth century, and won the prestigious Steven's Triennial Prize of Columbia University for Original Research.

The term 'status epilepticus' (*état de mal*) is thought to have been coined by the inmates of the Salpêtrière, and was first used in the medical literature by Louis Calmeil in his doctoral thesis of 1824.[187] The most significant previous

---

[185] Veith and Wicke, *Cerebrale Differenzierungsstörungen*.

[186] Clark and Prout, 'Status epilepticus'. L Pierce Clark was an important, intriguing and eccentric figure in American neurology and psychiatry. (see Shorvon *Enigmatic figure*). His psychoanalytical theories are described in the next chapter.

[187] Calmeil, *De l'épilepsie*. Louis-Florentin Calmeil (1798–1895) was a French psychiatrist who succeeded Esquirol as director of Charenton, the lunatic asylum in Charenton-Saint-Maurice. He is also credited with introducing the term *absence*.

studies of status epilepticus were those of Désiré-Magloire Bourneville in 1876[188] and Friedrick Lorenz in Kiel in 1892, but it was the papers of Clark and Prout that brought the topic firmly into the twentieth century.[189] Their definition of the condition as 'the maximum development of epilepsy, in which one paroxysm follows another so closely that the coma and exhaustion are continuous between seizures' (vol. 60, p. 295) remained essentially unchanged for the rest of the century. They recognised that major convulsions (grand mal) or psychic (partial) or focal motor forms of epilepsy could all evolve into status epilepticus and, as Bourneville had previously recorded, that during an episode of convulsive status epilepticus, the condition evolves into a non-convulsive (stuporous) form. They also noted a prodromal stage (Bourneville had called this *état de mal de passage*) in which serial seizures of escalating frequency preceded the status as 'stepping stones' (p. 296). They described the neurological and systemic effects, focusing, as Bourneville did, on the temperature (the fever curve), and also noted petechial haemorrhages and other dermatological effects. Status epilepticus was a common cause of death among epileptics in the asylum, wrote Clark and Prout, and they pronounced it, in fin-de-siècle fashion, as the 'true climax of the disease and less a chance termination which by proper treatment could be avoided; certainly, chance plays no part as agent in the production of the status. An epileptic is fore-doomed to die of the status as the maximum development of the disease' (p. 294).

They waded into the debate about whether idiopathic epilepsy was the only disease to which the term 'epilepsy' should be applied, noting that true status epilepticus occurred not only in idiopathic epilepsy but also in symptomatic epilepsies ('dependent upon gross organic brain lesions, as abscess, tumor, etc.'), which they considered particularly likely to end fatally in status epilepticus; thus, in their view, 'the different manifestations of status resulting from differ-ent brain lesions must bear a certain close relationship to true status epilepticus' (p. 297).

They saw no value in subdividing status into seizure types nor in drawing a distinction between status and serial seizures, noted that convulsive and non-convulsive status merged into each other, and made a number of acute observations about the factors influencing the occurrence of status and its frequency.

Of great interest were their views on prognosis: 'the inherited instability of the cerebral cortex is the real basis of the causation of epilepsy', they wrote,[190] and each seizure increases and accentuates the abnormality, setting in train a

---

[188] Bourneville, 'L'état de mal', in Bourneville, *Recherches cliniques*; Lorenz, 'Über den Status epilepticus'.
[189] For this history, see Shorvon, *Status Epilepticus*.
[190] Clark and Prout, 'Status epilepticus', vol. 61, 94.

series of degenerative changes whose logical termination is the last episode of fatal status epilepticus:

> Generally one attack of status paves the way for another, and in fact, there is no limit to the number of status periods that may occur before death supervenes. Although Bourneville and Lorenz state that a patient cannot have more than three or four periods of status, several of our cases showed four or five, and one case had six status periods under our personal observation before death resulted from the seventh. As a general rule, two or three status periods in idiopathic epilepsy cause death, while innumerable periods of status epilepticus unilateralis may occur in hemiplegic epileptics and death not take place. (p. 301)

As status epilepticus was the natural termination – the climax – of these processes of idiopathic epilepsy, there was no need to search for other causes. Nonetheless, Clark and Prout did recognise that metabolic disturbances and intercurrent illness, especially the sudden withdrawal of bromide, were powerful precipitating factors. The clinical features and the progression of status through various stages reiterate Bourneville's work and are valuable descriptions today of the course of status in unventilated and untreated patients. Clark and Prout gave accurate and detailed accounts of the convulsive stage, then the stuporous stage and, in those with focal motor status, transient post-status hemiplegia. They went on to describe the neurological and systemic effects.[191] Most of their cases continued for two to nine days and, in addition to convulsive status epilepticus, they also described other forms, including statuesque attacks, general clonic spasm, status myoclonicus, status hystericus and non-convulsive states. Of the non-convulsive cases, they described one patient (whose status would now be categorised as complex partial) who had 760 seizures in 12 hours, and also noted that whilst convulsive status often ended in death, psychic status did not. Clark and Prout laid out the diagnosis and differential diagnosis before moving to prognosis, which was 'necessarily grave, since it is recognized as the severest form of the epileptic state' (p. 664).

The pathological findings were also presented in great detail in the third paper and in Clark's chapter in Spratling's textbook, in the hope (unrealised) that these might shed light on the underlying pathogenesis of idiopathic

---

[191] An interesting observations, now rather lost, was that the: '*tâche cérébrale* of Trousseau, the meningitic streak of Bourneville, or better the dermographism of Féré and Lamy is always an accompanying symptom of severe status. As is to be expected from the real nature of the phenomena its intensity and persistence in status depends upon the degree of exhaustion of the vaso-motor apparatus which, as we before observed, is the real index to the general vascular exhaustion ... The white and blue oedema of Sydenham and Charcot are said to be occasionally accompaniments of the status epilepticus, but as such conditions are of particularly common occurrence in the status hystericus, one is led to doubt the diagnosis of the form of status in which these peculiar oedemas are said to be found' (pp. 653–4).

epilepsy itself. Clark and Prout also dismissed sclerosis of the cornu ammonis as the essential lesion and cerebral anaemia as the cause of convulsions – both had 'practically no advocates' (p. 666). There follows a masterly, critical account of the various pathological changes previously described, including vacuolation, minor anomalies of the cortex, and gliosis and 'neuroglial hyperplasia' (vol. 61, p. 81). This account then led to a detailed discussion of Clark and Prout's own pathological findings, which were the subject of their third paper examining the morbid anatomy and histology of seven cases.[192] They found striking changes in the nucleus and nucleoli of the cortical cells, gross chromatolysis, vacuolation, destruction of pyramidal cells particularly in the third cortical layer, infiltration of the cortex by leucocytes and proliferation of the neuroglia. Most of these changes are now fully accepted.

They reviewed microscopic changes, including Ammon's horn sclerosis, and attributed the damage largely to diseased sensory cells (as suggested by Bevan Lewis, whose work they did not cite). The cause was unidentified toxic or autotoxic agents 'engrafted upon a cortical organic cellular anomaly which is induced largely by a faulty heredity, the exact anatomic nature of which is not known'.[193]

For the first time since Bourneville's work three decades earlier, this series of papers defined all aspects of the condition and was unparalleled in its detail and originality. Indeed, little more needed to be said, and subsequent reports published over the next half-century added little to these classical studies. Further real advances had to wait until the current era of molecular science.

The treatment of status epilepticus was also studied. In his celebrated case of 'Marie Lamb' in 1874, Bourneville had used poltices, purgative enema and quinine sulphate to no effect.[194] Amyl nitrate was used in 1876, and Gowers recommended bromides and morphia. An editorial on the treatment of status epilepticus in 1905[195] summarised contemporary therapy, which included the advice to administer bromide if the status was caused by an abrupt withdrawal of bromide. In general, Clark and Prout took what seems a most sensible and effective approach based on the stages of status (and one with echoes of that used today): a rapid increase of the dose of bromide in the premonitory stage, with opium and chloral supplementation; then inhalation of chloroform in the convulsive phase, given up to complete anaesthesia in severe cases. Chloral and the intrathecal administration of bromide could also be tried at this stage, along with numerous other remedies, including cold baths and venesection. In the stuporous stage, stimulants were needed and treatment with strychnine, digitalis and whisky. Abundance of nutritious food and careful nursing were considered essential. Turner in 1907 recommended a very similar regimen.

[192] Clark and Prout. 'Status epilepticus' (paper 3)
[193] Prout and Clark, in Spratling, *Epilepsy and Its Treatment*, p. 334.
[194] Bourneville, 'l'État de mal'.   [195] 'The treatment of the epileptic status'.

HEALTHCARE OF EPILEPSY 1860–1914

It is easy to forget how different the practice of medicine in 1860 was from that of today. Neither the prominence and power of medicine today nor the well-developed systems of care 'from cradle to grave' existed; the cradle-to-grave journey was much shorter, in any event.[196] Medicine was directed mainly at acute conditions, with little in the way of effective therapy available for most chronic conditions. Epilepsy was a disease for which there were few existing facilities, and what was available depended on the patient's social class.

The majority of he population of Western countries fell into the category of the 'deserving poor'. Their general medical and surgical hospital care was provided by general hospitals financed by charity and philanthropic donations. These hospitals were places of last resort, and the majority of people entered them with little expectation of survival. In Britain, most (possibly all) hospitals refused to admit patients with epileptic seizures on the grounds that they would disturb or even infect other patients,[197] and it is likely that similar interdictions applied in other countries. If inpatient care was needed, the public lunatic asylums run by local authorities were the only option, and were directed by psychiatrists (alienists) who were outside the medical mainstream. Their function was not so much medical as social. Of those of this class who did not require incarceration, most were untreated except for an occasional visit to the local general practitioner. When therapy was obtained, drugs such as bromide and other antiepileptics could be bought over the counter, without a prescription or any forma medical advice.

For the better-off, those from the small middle and upper classes, consultations were conducted in private consulting rooms or in patients' own homes. Few from these classes would contemplate admission to any general hospital[198] let alone a public asylum. Even surgery was performed out of hospital, and Cushing gives a graphic description of Horsley performing neurosurgery in a

---

[196] In Britain, life expectancy (male, female) in 1870 was about 41–4 years and had risen to around 51–5 years by 1910; today life expectancy is 79–83 years (figures from the Office for National Statistics).

[197] The thought that a person seeing an epileptic fit might develop epilepsy was strongly held even among leading psychiatrists of the period, such as Emile Kraepelin and Eugen Blueler. In lunatic asylums, epileptic patients were separated from other inmates in the hope of preventing worsening of their symptoms and protecting them from the persons with epilepsy (see Esquirol, *Des maladies mentales*).

[198] In the United Kingdom census of 1861, only 157 of the 10,414 inmates in voluntary hospitals were classified as professional people (most were government officers, teachers or clergymen), and only 14 as 'persons of rank or property not returned under any office or occupation' (*Census of England and Wales*, pp. xcviii–xcix).

patients' kitchen.[199] When inpatient care was needed, admission was invariably into a private asylum or sanatorium of varying luxury and sophistication depending on what could be afforded.

At the other end of the spectrum, the only medical care available for the destitute (the undeserving poor) was in the workhouse, a system best developed in Britain but in existence throughout Western Europe and North America. There, medical care was free but notoriously rudimentary.

In the later decades of the century these arrangements began to change, a process fuelled by general public unease about many aspects of medical care, by improving finances, and by the rising power and influence of the medical profession. Epilepsy was a specific and prominent concern, and in Britain, for instance, an editorial in the national daily newspaper, *The Daily Telegraph* complained:

> Few persons can have been long familiar with the streets of any great European city without having observed, more or less frequently, a desolate wretch writhing on the ground foaming at the mouth, hissing between the teeth, lacerating the tongue by frenzied clampings, drawing up all the limbs convulsively and then, perhaps smitten into rigidity, as if suddenly petrified. They have been told it was an epileptic patient, and have passed on . . . is it credible that none [i.e. no institution] exists for the cure or alleviation of the epileptic and paralytic?[200]

As prosperity increased, two new types of epilepsy facility began to be formed, supported by public philanthropy – the specialist hospital and the epilepsy colony. In Britain, as an example, small specialist hospitals, dedicated to a specific condition (or group of conditions), began to be opened, especially in London, in a trend known as the voluntary hospital movement. One of first hospitals to be so established was the National Hospital for the Relief and Cure of the Paralysed and Epileptic.[201] The hospital provided inpatient and outpatient care for epilepsy, and such was the demand that it expanded from a single terraced house with 17 beds in 1860 to a new, purpose-built hospital with 175 beds in 1888 (in which year 26% of admissions and over half of the outpatients were for epilepsy[202]). At this time, patients were drawn from the deserving poor and care was free; as the hospital's fame grew, private beds for paying patients were later introduced.

---

[199] In Fulton, *Harvey Cushing*.

[200] *Daily Telegraph*, 2 November 1859. Publication of this editorial was in all likelihood inspired by the fund-raisers of the National Hospital, an early example of product placement.

[201] Shorvon and Compston, *Queen Square*, pp.100–102.

[202] In this period, only 'sane epileptics; were allowed admission. Amongst epilepsy cases excluded from the hospital were those with epileptic mania or 'imbecile' epileptics (Shorvon and Compston, *Queen Square*, p. 341).

The rise of these specialist hospitals was not always welcome, and opposition came mainly from the senior physicians in the general hospitals, no doubt concerned about the threat they posed to their practices. In Britain, a common claim was that many such institutions were set up by doctors to increase their referral base, with self-interest masquerading as philanthropy or scientific advance. *The Lancet*, for instance, commenting on the foundation of three such hospitals (the Galvanic Hospital,[203] a Dispensary for Ulcerated Legs and a Dispensary for Disease of the Throat and Loss of Voice) was vituperative: 'These excrescences are being reproduced with all the prolific exuberance characteristic of malignancy, and soon the metropolis threatens to swarm with nuisances of this kind ... Next may come a Quinine Hospital, an Hospital for Treatment by Cod-liver Oil, by the Hyophosphites, or by the Excrement of Boa-Constrictors.'[204] This having been said, the arrival of the National Hospital for the Relief and Cure of the Paralysed and the Epileptic was universally welcomed. In Germany too, specialisation and 'physicians for white or red blood corpuscles' were mocked and disparaged, and the special small private hospitals were often established by outsiders such as Jews who were excluded from university careers. By around 1900, only 12% of German physicians were specialists (nearly half in ten cities) and even by 1930, very few specialist departments existed, with these only in the largest hospitals.

The always conservative medical establishment could not stem the tide, though, and by 1900 the case for specialisms such as neurology, and for specialised neurological facilities, had in Britain been won. By the early twentieth century specialist units were opening even in the general hospitals. The first neurology unit opened in a general hospital in 1907, and others followed, but in many European countries dedicated neurology clinics appeared only decades later. In the United States, the first hospital dedicated to neurological patients, the Neurological Institute of New York, opened in 1909.[205]

Asylums and Colonies

Another feature of the political and societal climate of the nineteenth century was the escalating tendency to institutionalise the mentally ill, not least in an attempt to remove them from the public gaze. This led to one of the most

---

[203] Rivett suggests that the London Galvanic Hospital (opened in 1861) was among a group of 'special hospitals' that were 'little more than brothels', and it certainly did not survive long (Rivett, *Development*, p. 49).

[204] 'March of specialism', *Lancet*.

[205] The earliest neurology clinics were in London, at the National Hospital, in Paris, at the Salpêtrière, and in Vienna, where Theodor Meynert (1833–92) founded a neurological department in the Universitätsklinik für Psychiatrie und Neurologie in the 1880s. In Germany, although neurology wards were opened in Berlin in 1875, these were then subsumed under psychiatry in the 1880s.

striking medical phenomena of the nineteenth century, the growth throughout the Western world in the number of public and private lunatic asylums.[206] In Britain, for instance, the number of asylum inmates grew from 10,000 at the beginning of the century to around 100,000 by the end, and in the United States asylum inmates numbered 150,000 by 1904. Patients with epilepsy who required incarceration were admitted into these asylums, but it was at the same time widely accepted that for the 'sane epileptic' (those without psychiatric disorders or intellectual disability) this was often not an appropriate setting. As the nineteenth century drew on, pressure to find an alternative gave rise to what became known, with imperialist overtones, as the epilepsy colony movement. These new centres were established with the purpose of providing shelter, medical care, education and employment for people with epilepsy in a residential setting but outside the system of lunatic asylums.[207]

By the end of the century, the colony movement had become widely supported. The early epilepsy colonies were not state institutions but rather private initiatives of the church, and the role of philanthropy was crucial. Almost all were founded on religious principles and were imbued with Christian ideals. The philanthropist Andrew Reed, who founded the first 'asylum for idiots' in England, reflected feelings held by many god-fearing Victorians when he wrote of the inmates that they were: 'fellow creatures who were separate and alone, but [had] the Divine image stamped upon all'.[208] As a broad generalisation, the colonies in Catholic countries were primarily focused on the religious care of individuals but in protestant countries, the religious imperatives were complicated by wider concerns about the woes of society and also the personal responsibility of the individuals seeking help. The British Charity Organisation Society and the German Inner Mission, for instance, were active in creating colonies. They did so on the basis not only of their godly credentials but also dismay at the pauperism, social decay and criminality that accompanied the move from a rural agrarian to an urban industrial economy. Both believed in self-help and the duty and responsibilities of citizens, and both deplored state intervention. Led by a philosophy inspired by Kant and others, and by a moral earnestness which emphasised duty and conscience, both were evangelical and austere. The charitable societies focused particularly on the 'deserving poor' – those who through no fault of their own were in straightened circumstances – but excluded those who because of immoral or intemperate behaviour impoverished themselves. There was then a strong and widely held belief that the church, and not the state, was the proper agency for poor relief.[209]

---

[206] In Britain, public mental asylums were established after the passage of the 1808 County Asylums Act and in the United States through legislation passed in 1842.

[207] Similar colonies existed for other diseases, such as asthma and diabetes, and for the deaf and the dumb.

[208] The Park House asylum, Highgate, in London (cited by Penrose, *Mental Defect*, p. 2).

[209] Henderson, 'Rise of the German Inner Mission'.

What was possibly the first residential centre for epilepsy had been established at La Teppe in Tain-l'Hermitage in France and was originally the project of a private individual (Count Louis de Larnage).[210] From 1859 it was taken over by a Catholic congregation (the Company of the Daughters of Charity). In 1848, La Force near Bordeaux was opened by John Bost[211] for a community of the disabled; in 1862 it was extended to provide homes for those with epilepsy. Bost emphasised the importance of country air, writing that he had

> This vision of a simple religious life in the country became the pattern for all the continental colonies where the residents were to be cared for kindly and treated with respect, and which were entirely non-medical.

In 1865, Dr Albert Moll[212] of the asylum Auf der Pfingstweide, addressed the second German Conference of the Inner Mission on the topic of unsatisfactory state of care of those with epilepsy in the public asylums and workhouses:

> For the epileptics, all asylums are closed. He is lonelier than the mentally insane, the blind, the deaf and the cretin; he cannot find any asylum, which opens for him a human idea. He has to pass on the palaces, which were created by humanity for the insane, but he is not allowed to enter them in the same way as they are opened to the blind and to the deaf! He doesn't have the right to seek help under the roof of such institutions where the loneliest of all would have been sheltered as the most common neglected individual. The only places which remain open to him are the most neglected corners in a house for the poor or a mad house in which he is deprived due to the hard-heartedness of humans to everything on which a disease has a natural right.[213]

Two years later, in 1867, the Bethel colony in Bielefeld, was founded as the Pflegestätte für epileptische Knaben and supported by the von Bodelschwingh Foundation of Bethel[214] to provide shelter and employment and a caring

---

[210] It is often written that in the fifteenth century, the Priory of St Valentine in Rufach (Alsace) was the first residential sanctuary for epilepsy. But it seems likely that the monks there primarily provided outpatient treatment rather than refuge. There was an earlier monastery in Rome dedicated to St Bibiana which also offered treatment, in the form of hulwort (a herb).

[211] Jean Antoine Bost (1817–81), a Swiss Calvinist pastor.

[212] Johann Christoph Albert Moll founded the Heil- und Bewahranstalt für Epileptische auf der Pfingstweide in Meckenbeuren and other hospitals.

[213] Moll and Balke. *Die Fürsorge* (translation supplied by Eugen Trinka).

[214] The colony started life as a small farmhouse, under Pastor Simon from Bensburg. It was then taken over and enormously expanded by the visionary Friedrich von Bodelschwingh, a strong advocate of the Inner Mission, and after him by his son Friedrich (Fritz) von Bodelschwingh. The latter played an important part, during the Nazi period, in protecting his charges from transportation and murder. This is described by Karl Stern in *Pillar of Fire*: 'when the Nazis carried out the slaughter of all mental patients, Pastor Bodelschwing insisted that he would be killed along with his inmates. It was only on the basis of his international fame that the politicians let him get away with it, and let him and his inmates live. This was a kind of as a "last-ditch" stand of Christianity' (p. 127).

environment. It was this colony at Bethel that acted as a model for all subsequent institutions in Europe and elsewhere.[215] Almost all these asylums catered for varying degrees of mental handicap, but equally almost all excluded those with psychiatric, conduct or behavioural disorders and for whom the only recourse remained the lunatic asylum. Similar facilities sprang up in other countries, including Meer in Bosch in Holland (1885); the Swiss Epilepsy Center in Zurich (1886); Chalfont Centre for Epilepsy (1884) near London and the Maghull home[216] in Liverpool (1888); and the Saxon Epilepsy Centre, Kleinwachau, an 'asylum for epileptics' close to Dresden (1889). In 1892, the Heil- und Pflegeanstalt für epileptische Kinder in Kork opened its doors for children with epilepsy. The Asylum for Epileptics in Tersløse Dianalund in Denmark (later renamed the Philadelphia Colony) was founded in 1897, and the colony Vaajasalo Kuopio in Finland in 1898 (later renamed Vaajasalo Sanatorium). In 1906, William Quarrier opened the Colony of Mercy at the Bridge of Weir near Glasgow, and in 1911 the Sandvika colony was founded outside Oslo.[217] Almost all catered for varying degrees of mental handicap, but equally almost all excluded those with psychiatric, conduct or behavioural disorders and for whom the only recourse remained the lunatic asylum or workhouse. Most had little medical input and were focused on care and education. For instance, at Meer & Bosch medical input remained limited to a visiting general physician and the institute was run by a minister, aided by nursing staff; only around 1920–30 did medicine became more prominent and a medical director was appointed.[218]

By the turn of the century, however, colonies were also being set up by local and governmental bodies, especially in the United States.[219] These were far more secular and although publically sporting a 'Christian ethic' were far less

[215] In 1891, Miss Burdon-Sanderson from England visited the epilepsy colony at Bethel. She reported there were 3,000 persons in the colony, of whom 1,000 were epileptics of all age groups, social classes and mental and physical abilities, and was highly impressed. This visit was one factor which led to the foundation of the Chalfont Centre.

[216] The Maghull home was run by Dr William Alexander, who was one of the first to write a book entirely devoted to treatment and focusing on epilepsy surgery (Alexander, *Treatment of Epilepsy*, 1889) – especially cervical sympathectomy and trephining – as well as considering medical and hygienic therapies.

[217] Which institution qualifies as an epilepsy centre or colony is difficult to define. Meinardi considered that prior to the First World War there were only thirteen centres in Europe, but others cite larger numbers. Turner, for instance, listed ten in Britain alone: Maghull, Meath, Chalfont, Lingfield, Quarrier, Ewell, David Lewis, Monyhull, St Lukes and the Glasgow epilepsy colony (Turner, 'Statistics'). Different authorities give different dates of foundation for some of the epilepsy institutions, sometimes reflecting the date of their building, their fund-raising, their founding articles, first patient or the date when an institution was transformed into a facility for epilepsy.

[218] Personal communication from Walter van Embe Boas

[219] There were exceptions, such as the *Emmaus Asyl für Epileptiker und idioten* opened by the German evangelical Synod of North America in Missouri in 1893. In Britain an early example was the Ewell Epileptic Colony, established by the London County Council in

tied to religious authority than the earlier European institutions. The first established was the Ohio Hospital for Epileptics at Gallipolis, which opened in 1893 and by 1901 had 1,060 patients – the largest institution dedicated to the care of those with epilepsy.[220] By 1914 there were 13 colonies in America, 11 of which were state institutions.[221] Crucial in their development was the National Association for the Study of Epilepsy and the Care and Treatment of Epileptics, which was conceived in 1898 and held its first meeting in 1901. Designed to promote the establishment of epilepsy colonies in the United States and to share information among them and from the existing European colonies, the national association became an important force and lobby.[222] William Pryor Letchworth was its co-founder and president.[223] He was an indefatigable figure who spent several years travelling around Europe and the United States visiting asylums, initially for the insane and then later for patients with epilepsy. He campaigned tirelessly to improve the condition of those with epilepsy and wrote influential books and tracts; his descriptions of the conditions of patients before the establishment of colonies were heartrending.[224] As he concluded:

1903, consisting initially of 9 villas and 326 inmates. In Germany, in the early decades of the century, most patients were supported by the *Armenkasse* (a poor relief fund).

[220] The Gallipolis hospital was initially the Asylum for Epileptics and Epileptic Insane. The evolution of care at the Ohio colony from a place of shelter and sanctuary to a site of eugenics experiments is well described in Kissiov et al. in 'Ohio Hospital'.

[221] Graves, 'Baltimore-Meeting'.

[222] By 1906, the Craig Colony's objectives were to promote the general welfare of sufferers from epilepsy; to stimulate the study of the causes and methods of cure of the disease; to assist the various states in America in establishing a proper system of care for epileptics; and to advocate the care of epileptics in institutions designed to meet their special needs. The colony counted more than 100 members and associate members, including well-known figures in the field of epilepsy such as Spratling, Gowers, Turner, Alan McDougall, Clark and Prout, Davenport and Muskens, as well as several lay members.

[223] Letchworth was a major figure in American epilepsy. He was President of the National Boards of Charities which helped manage all of the State Institutions. He was a Quaker who made his fortune in business, not least in the manufacture of rifles for the Union side in the American Civil War. He then devoted his life to charitable works in asylums and was particularly interested in epilepsy. His two authoritative and detailed books reporting on his travels were to be highly influential: *The Insane in Foreign Countries* (1889) and *Care and Treatment of Epileptics* (1900). He founded an annual journal devoted to epilepsy (possibly the first in the world): the *Transactions of the National Association for the Study of Epilepsy and the Care and Treatment of Epileptics*. He gave his 2,000-acre estate to the State of New York, now known as Letchworth Park. The institution for the mentally disabled, Letchworth Village, was opened in 1911 and named in his honour.

[224] Letchworth cites reports of a Dr Byers of the Ohio State Board of Charities who in 1876 found a 'stout colored man in the Stark County Jail, whose scalp was bared in several places, and whose face and body were fearfully bruised by falling and beating against the strong, rough iron bars of his prison-cell. He was held simply for restraint', and another 'case of a poor boy who had fallen, in an epileptic fit, into the fire ... This poor boy's head and the upper portions of his body were entirely denuded, and portions of the facial muscles had been destroyed. There had been, apparently, no effort of nature toward healing, and, with sightless eyes and raw and bleeding flesh, I found him lying, as he had lain for six months, a hideous spectacle of human suffering, without the possibility of any alleviation of his condition.' In

'Any attempt to describe in written words must fall equally short of conveying an idea of the utter and abandoned wretchedness of very many of this class now (if of quiet disposition) simply supplied with food and clothing, or (if dangerous) caged and chained in the narrow, dark, damp, and dirty cells of the ordinary infirmary, jail, or madhouse.' Letchworth and Oscar Craig negotiated the purchase by the state of a former Shaker Colony at Sonyea, and on this site established the Craig Colony for Epileptics in 1894.[225] This institution incorporated many of Letchworth's ideas about the benefits of custodial care in epilepsy colonies elaborated in his *Care and Treatment of Epileptics*, published in 1900. William Spratling was appointed superintendent and would later cite the Craig Colony as exemplifying the ideal aims of a colony: to wit, to provide a simple and elemental home life, to preserve individuality (which was lost in large asylums) and to provide vocations for all who required them. Colonies should be sited at a distance from centres of population ('the defectives who live in them have no place in the strenuous life').[226] In a glowing review of Letchworth's book and the association's transactions of 1902, W. Aldren Turner, a foreign member of the association, asserted that the 'system [of colonies had now] "come to stay"'.[227]

As they developed, most colonies became in effect self-contained 'villages', providing work, sport, education and religious and social activities. Usually the patients were in small 'houses', with a house mother or father responsible for a small 'family' of patients. This had much therapeutic value and encouraged a family spirit, and many patients 'found an intelligent sympathy and understanding of their problems'.[228] The colonies were felt to differ from asylums because epilepsy caused difficulties in living independently that were distinct from those due to mental handicap or psychiatric or behavioural disorders.[229] Provided that

---

Ohio at the time it was reported that of 646 people with epilepsy, 10% were incarcerated in county jails. These reports led to the foundation of the State Hospital for Epileptics at Gallipolis (Letchworth, *Care and Treatment*, pp. 64–5).

[225] Oscar Craig (1836–94) succeeded Letchworth as President of the New York Board of Charities. He died in an accident (his carriage overturned) before the colony was opened. An influential line of physicians worked at the colony, including Spratling and Shanahan (its first two medical directors), Pierce Clark as assistant and James Frederick Munson as its resident pathologist. At the colony detailed records were kept of all seizures occurring, sometime 50,000 a day, and social workers complied detailed geneology charts.

[226] Spratling, *Epilepsy and Its Treatment*, p. 341. The care and treatment regimens at the Craig Colony are given in detail in Spratling's book and in a paper given in 1901 (Spratling, 'Ideal colony', 1901). His care regimes included daily exercise, work, diet, abstinence from alcohol, strict regimes for sleep, showers and not baths.

[227] Turner, 'Reviews'.   [228] Letchworth, *Care and Treatment*, p. 64.

[229] The particular problems of epilepsy were considered by Spratling to include: medical issues (seizures, injuries, drug treatment), undermining of confidence and identity caused by transient loss of consciousness, the effects on personality development and relationships, parental overprotection, popular prejudice and a failure to meet potential.

the colonies avoided admitting patients with severe mental handicap or psychiatric disorders, they could focus on these specific epilepsy issues. It was felt that '[t]he patient, removed from the isolation in the home, was given much freedom and, after being considered an outcast from society, was a part of a community'.[230]

David Lewis's epileptic colony near Manchester was a prototypical example of an advanced institution of the early twentieth century. Founded in 1904 on 113 acres of land, with a large farm at the centre, the colony was described in detail in a paper in *Epilepsia* by its director, medical doctor Alan McDougall:[231] 'Only epileptics are admitted. They come and remain of their own free will' (p. 132); they could leave whenever they wished. Patients who were insane or dangerous were not admitted. There was accommodation for men, women and children, and 'for the rich and for the poor' (p. 133). By 1909 the facilities were full, with 220 colonists housed in villas. It was a non-medical facility, in which the female attendants were called sisters, not nurses; there was no resident doctor; and the inmates were called colonists, not patients. Work was provided on the farm and in the laundry and stables.

The Craig Colony housed patients in 6–10 bedded houses (males and females in different houses, whose locations were separated by a large river!) attended by a resident family, parents and children. An emphasis was placed on teaching an occupation: farming and carpentry for men, and dressmaking and such like for women. The purpose was to train the inmates, who were often previously isolated, in sociability and good manners and, where possible, to provide an occupation. Black and white inmates were mixed at a time when separate wards existed in many American hospitals. The Skillman Village for Epileptics in New Jersey was a similar institution. It opened in 1898, when acting governor Foster M. Voorhees signed a bill into law establishing the institution. It was designed to be a self-sustaining agrarian community, where those with epilepsy could live together in a wholesome environment, learn trades, receive medical treatment and leave the alms houses, insane asylums and prisons in which they had been previously contained. Its sprawling grounds included a farm with chickens, cows and pigs; fields for growing fruits and vegetables; a power plant; a firehouse; and even a theatre where the residents staged operettas like the *Pirates of Penzance*.[232] Many colonies were intended to be self-sustaining through their farms and workshops. Such arrangements were typical of the style of colonies which had spread across Europe, the United States and countries in the British Empire.

---

[230] Collier, 'Social implications'.   [231] McDougall, 'David Lewis'.

[232] The fortunes of the Skillman colony evolved over the twentieth century in a fashion typical of many colonies. Its facilities declined dramatically in the harsh social environment of the Great Depression of the 1930s and the Second World War, and the colony became known as 'the snake pit of New Jersey'. In 1953 it was transformed into a psychiatric treatment centre focusing on alcoholics, drug addicts, emotionally disturbed children and people with cerebral palsy, and in 1983 into a centre for developmental disabilities. Skillman closed in 1998 (see 'Princeton State Village for Epileptics').

(a)

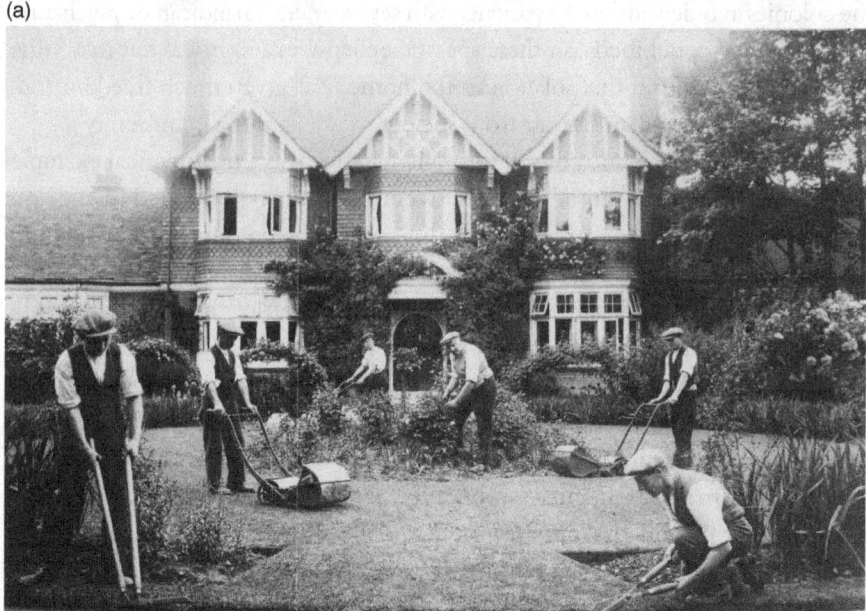

(b)

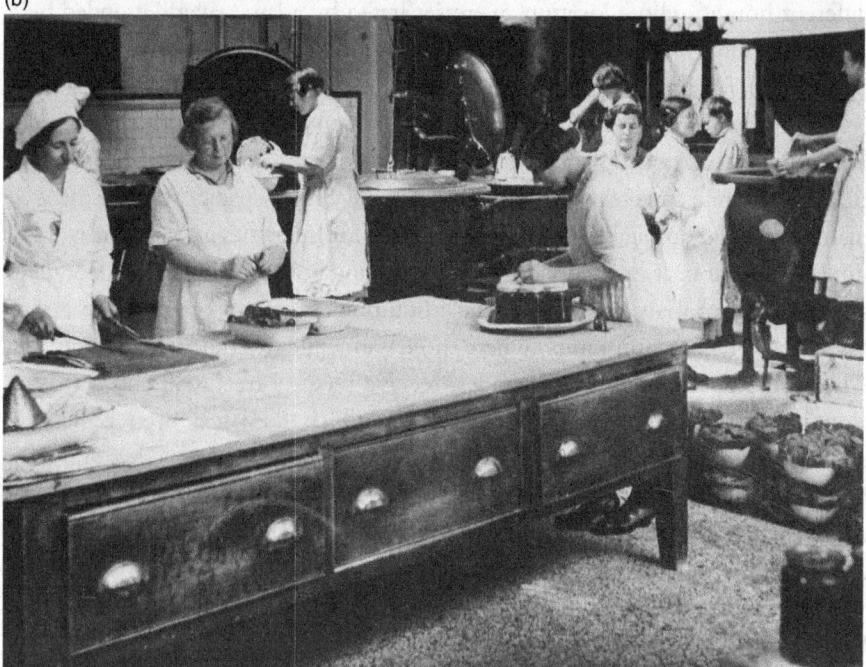

10a,b. Colonists engaged in various employments at the Chalfont Colony around 1900
(from the archives of the National Society for Epilepsy)

The enthusiasm for setting up the colonies in the years between 1890 and
1914 has several explanations. The principal stated motive in all cases was
undoubtedly a desire to improve the control of epilepsy, and there was a

universally accepted medical opinion that the hygienic regimen which colonies offered might cure or alleviate seizures. But removal of epileptics from the streets of large towns was also welcomed by citizens who disliked the sight of disability and who also, to some extent, feared that epilepsy might be contagious. The colonies were paradigmatic examples of the way epilepsy was viewed in those years: primarily as a social rather than a medical problem.

Exactly what percentage of patients with epilepsy was found in these various settings is not fully known. Turner calculated that 1,649 epileptics were admitted to asylums in Britain (epilepsy accounting for 7.6% of all admissions), 1,481 to the five English epilepsy colonies, 680 on the outpatient register of the National Hospital Queen Square and 51 cases among the British troops (0.9/ 1000). He pointed out that there was no data for the general prevalence of epilepsy in the population; indeed, in the asylums 'epilepsy ... is so closely related in the early years of life to idiocy and imbecility and then in later years to dementia that it is almost impossible to separate these for statistical purposes'.[233] The numbers admitted to workhouses or general hospitals, unrecognised or concealed in the population, or with epilepsy due to gross lesions or bodily disease was entirely unknown, as was the number attending private doctors or hospital outpatients in general hospitals.[234] Turner concluded, '[I]t is therefore obvious that it is impossible to give even an approximate estimate of the number of epileptics in England'. He also cited figures from other countries with prevalence rates varying from 0.4–2.5/1000. Turner spoke for all physicians in the field of epilepsy when he wrote that admission to such institutions was 'a satisfactory method of treating epileptics both in the early and later stages of their disease'.[235]

Although medical input to the early colonies was mostly slight or nonexistent, this began to change as the number and reputation of the colonies grew. Neurologists and psychiatrists were soon involved in the establishment of colonies and their management. For instance, in America Frederick Peterson and Spratling were instrumental in setting up the Craig Colony for Epileptics. In England, Ferrier in collaboration with other physicians at the National Hospital was the driving force behind the founding in 1882 of the National

[233] Turner, *Epilepsy*, p. 12

[234] These statistics were gathered as part of the 'Special Project of the International League Against Epilepsy' and reported in *Epilepsia*. Assuming a prevalence rate of 5/1,000, the number of persons with epilepsy in Britain in 1907 would have been in the region of 200,000, which is an indication of how few persons with epilepsy were identified.

[235] Turner, *Epilepsy*, p. 251. Turner was unusual in having a practice in an asylum (the Chalfont Colony), a neurological hospital (the National Hospital), a general hospital (King's College Hospital) and a private outpatient practice, and so had a unique perspective on the potential value of the colonies.

Society for the Employment of Epileptics which established the Chalfont Centre in 1884.

As doctors assumed a more central role in the colonies, care became increasingly medicalised. Inevitably, tensions arose between the lay ideal of 'care' and 'welfare' and the medical ideals of research and treatment, resulting in clashes in various institutions. An example, at Chalfont, was the showdown in 1908 between doctors and administrators, much as happened eight years earlier at the National Hospital, Queen Square. A large donation had been received by the charity from C. A. Tate, a sugar baron. The doctors wanted to use it for a hospital building and the appointment of a resident medical officer, but the lay board members wanted to construct more homes. A bitter row ensued, which the lay members won. When a subsequent demand for the appointment of a medical superintendent was turned down, Turner and the medical committee resigned and the medicalisation of the centre came to an abrupt end. This was a bruising encounter that turned the centre into what was essentially a care home with very little medical input for the next four decades. It also demonstrated that although medical power and influence had risen enormously, at the start of the twentieth century it was not unchallenged.

By the turn of the century, the medical involvement in colony care had not only grown, but had also became more authoritarian. As Spratling wrote, in the treatment of epilepsy '[c]ontrol of the [p]atient [was] most [e]ssential ... *The more absolutely the physician is permitted to control the patient in every respect, the more promising the hope of amelioration or cure.*'[236] Incarceration in a colony was an ideal method of exerting such control. Spratling's authoritarian approach was harsh and seems to reflect his disdainful attitude to many of his epileptic patients:

> In many cases the family can give the attention required, though oftentimes, especially if there are other children in the family, the patient is a constant source of solicitude and anxiety. Irrespective of the influence of the invalid child on its immediate associates in other ways not desirable, the danger from assault by the patient is sometimes great, making him a constant and positive menace in the home. This, to be sure, is not always the case, but it often is; and when we recall the essentially explosive nature of the disease, we can understand the risk every home assumes in keeping an epileptic among its members. (p. 338)

Spratling emphasised that colonies were settings where 'wholesome discipline' could be applied: 'The final and most satisfactory plan of securing full control of the patient is to place him in a colony designed for all types, except the insane, or in one for selected cases only' (pp. 338–9). The Bethel and Craig Colonies were examples of the former, and the Chalfont Colony the latter. Spratling recognised the value of providing a 'home life, simple and elemental in form'

---

[236] Spratling, *Epilepsy and Its Treatment*, p. 337 (italics in original).

and also employment and education; 'The epileptic, the chronic insane, and the feeble-minded can all be successfully colonized.' The system could be adapted to meet the peculiar needs of these three classes, although the 'fundamental features are the same . . . To modify these would be fatal to the system itself' (pp. 340–41).

The National Association for the Study of Epilepsy and the Care and Treatment of Epileptics remained the driving force in relation to policy for epilepsy care in America in the pre–World War I period. As it evolved, the mood changed, and by 1910 its brand of medical paternalism began to be crystallised around the eugenic movement.

As eugenic policies gained traction, public attitudes to the handicapped became less sympathetic. The secular American epilepsy colonies proved an ideal environment in which to pursue eugenic experimentation and practice, and moreover this could be conducted without consent, oversight or much regulation of any sort. Many of the early superintendents were medical eugenicists, including leading ILAE figures such as William Shanahan, Weeks and James Frederick Munson.[237] The superintendents were in a powerful position and colonies became fertile ground for eugenic research and methods of control. No contradistinction was seen between eugenic treatment and Christian ethics. Everett Flood, superintendent of the Monson Hospital for Epileptics in Palmer Massachusetts, established in 1895 and which by 1905 housed 700 inmates, illustrates this well. On the one hand, he saw the role of the colony as: to remove the sufferer from undue mocking from the populace; to allow weaning from overdose of bromide and avoidance of chronic bromism; moral training and discipline – no self-indulgence; to prolong life; to control diet; to protect against injuries in seizures; to give 'him happiness in a world of his own; to assure him work; it is a Christian way of doing things'.[238] At the same time, he was an enthusiastic advocate and 'tester' of eugenic sterilisation ('asexualisation') of the inmates in his colony. Procedures included castration, vasectomy and tubal ligation, and these became widespread in American state institutions. Martin Barr[239] reported in detail on the effects of castration in children, not only on sexual appetite but also on their behaviour and epilepsy, citing Flood's work at Monson:

> Dr Everett Flood, superintendent of the Hospital for Epileptics at Palmer, Mass., reports 26 cases in which asexualisation was performed, some being circumcised at the same time, with no bad results. With 24 the cause for

---

[237] Spratling, superintendent of the Craig Colony, discouraged marriage but did not advocate sterilisation. His wife, however, was a leading eugenicist.

[238] Flood, 'What has been gained?' See also Kaelber, 'Eugenics'.

[239] See Barr, *Mental Defectives*, for a detailed history and survey of the development of institutions in Europe and America.

operating was epilepsy and persistent masturbation. One-half were under fourteen, two over twenty, and the remainder about fifteen years old, the mental and moral condition being good in 2, fair in 9, but poor in the others. Observation for some years after operation, noted mental condition improved in only 3 cases, and moral condition in only 4 – 2 kleptomaniacs reformed, one who was salacious improved, and one who was solitary acquired a more social disposition. The temper was improved in all but 4 cases. The sexual appetite seemed to disappear in all but 2 cases, and appeared in these only periodically. The effect upon the epileptics was favorable; with some the attacks ceasing altogether or returning, as in a single case, after immunity of two years. (p. 196)

The eugenic tendencies in colonies, focused on preventing reproduction, were mirrored by similar developments and legislation in the wider American community. For instance, in Connecticut a law approved in 1897 stated:

No man and woman either of whom is epileptic, or imbecile, or feeble-minded, shall inter-marry, or live together as husband and wife when the woman is under forty-five years of age. Any person violating or attempting to violate any of the provisions of this section, shall be imprisoned in the state prison not less than three years ... Every man who shall carnally know any female under the age of forty-five years who is epileptic, imbecile, or feeble-minded, or pauper, shall be imprisoned in the state prison not less than three years. Every man who is epileptic who shall carnally know any female under the age of forty-five years, and every female under the age of forty-five years who shall consent to be carnally known by any man who is epileptic, imbecile, or feeble-minded, shall be imprisoned in the state prison not less than three years. (p. 189)

Although operative procedures in colonies and asylums on account of epilepsy was often carried out under the radar,[240] attempts soon began to be made to pass laws allowing asexualisation of asylum inmates for eugenic purposes. The first attempt to legislate in this way occurred in Michigan in 1897, which failed, but then laws were successfully passed first in Indiana in 1907, and soon after other states followed suit.

TREATING EPILEPSY

It has been said that it was only somewhere between 1910–12 that 'a random patient with a random disease, consulting a doctor chosen at random had, for the first time in the history of mankind a better than fifty-fifty chance of profiting from the encounter'[241]. This perhaps over-cynical view did probably

---

[240] Lombardo, *Three Generations*.
[241] An aphorism attributed to Lawrence Henderson by Blumgart in 'Care for the patient'.

apply to most disorders of the brain – but not to epilepsy. Epilepsy had the distinction, from 1860, of becoming the first neurological condition to have specific and somewhat effective therapy in the form of bromides and, as we shall see, epilepsy continued to lead the way in neurological therapeutics for most of the long twentieth century. But before then treatment was indeed a curious mixture of herbal, hygienic and frankly harmful remedies, even in the hands of the best physicians (Table 1.4)

Hygienic Treatment

From the perspective of today it is perhaps surprising to note that drug therapy had not, at least until the late interwar years, gained a dominant position in the treatment of epilepsy. In the period between 1860 and 1914, medication was generally considered only one small part of the treatment approach. This was partly because epilepsy was widely considered to be a mental disease, because drugs had limited effectiveness and also because much greater attention was then paid to preventing deterioration and other deleterious aspects of epilepsy. This broad approach incorporated what was known as 'hygienic treatment'.

The term hygiene encompassed many aspects of general lifestyle, including a nutritious but restricted diet, encouragement of physical exercise, productive employment (especially outdoors), avoidance of stress, therapeutic baths, a quiet lifestyle that avoided overexcitment or overstimulation, abstinence from alcohol and sexual excess, and education within the mental capacity of the sufferer. It was felt important not to stress or mentally tire. Loosely defined, hygienic therapy aimed both to reverse and to prevent the external factors

TABLE 1.4 *Delasiauve's categories of treatment for epilepsy*

Category of treatment	Treatment
1. Debilitating treatment	Bleeding, tepid baths
2. Evacuants	Emetics, purgatives, exudatives – vasicatories, cautery, setons, moxas
3. Sedatives	Calmatives (not specified), lime flower water, chocolate, camphor, ether
4. Specifics	Valerian, asafoetida, garlic, rue, musk, castor, opiates, stramony and belladonna, digitalis, squil, oxide of zinc, sulphate and valerianate of zinc, quinine, iron, indigo, nitrate of silver, cantharides, nux vomita, pepper, intravenous injection of a purgative mixture, malarial infection, trephining

leading to poor health, to promote mental well-being and aspects of living that enhance good health. Initially introduced as public health measures, hygienic approaches focused at first on physical disorders. But by the mid-nineteenth century they were extended to and became an integral part of the treatment of many mental disorders, so much so that in the early and mid-twentieth century associations of mental hygiene were set up in many countries.[242]

Most medical authorities of the period emphasised strongly the importance of physical and mental hygiene – a notable exception being Gowers – and many authors went into great detail on specific measures.[243] Attitudes were summarised by Turner in 1907: '[E]pilepsy is, in the majority of cases, a progressive degenerative malady, and ... the object of treatment does not lie only in an attempt to combat the convulsions by sedative medicinal remedies, but to prevent by every possible means the tendency to mental deterioration, which is so important a clinical feature of the disease'.[244] He favoured early hygienic treatment, to be applied as soon as possible after the onset of epilepsy as there was a chance of cure if used quickly; and it was for this reason that he favoured admission to colonies for early as well as chronic cases.

Hygienic treatment was at the centre of the regimes adopted in the epilepsy colonies. According to Shanahan, assistant physician at the Craig Colony and leading American epileptologist, 'the three great essentials in the management of epilepsy are the diet, hygiene and occupation, and ... it is only after these have been arranged to the best possible advantage of the patient that medical treatment is to be considered'.[245] Turner advocated a comprehensive approach, dividing treatment in colonies into prophylaxis of epilepsy in a neuropathic child (one who had inherited the neuropathic trait but had not yet developed epilepsy); treatment at the onset of the disease; hygiene of the epileptic; education of epileptic children; care of the 'confirmed epileptic' (i.e. one whose disease had become established);[246] and surgical treatment. Of these, hygienic therapy was central. His recommendations included physical exercise (one regime included violent exercise for 20–30 minutes three times a week, followed by a cool bath); warm baths, spinal douches and massage to improve

---

[242] Clifford Whittingham Beers founded the mental hygiene movement in America. He became mentally ill himself and was institutionalised for three years. He later wrote *A Mind That Found Itself: An Autobiography* (1908) based on his experiences of maltreatment and abuse in the asylums to which he was committed. This is one of the few early eyewitness accounts from a patient's perspective and was very influential in promoting the movement. He fell ill when his brother developed epilepsy and became obsessed with the thought: '[W]hat was to prevent my being similarly afflicted? ... Doomed to what I then considered a living death' (p. 9).

[243] See, for instance, Sieveking, Delasiauve, Féré, Binswanger and Spratling, all of whom devoted extended chapters or sections of their books to hygienic measures. A notable exception was Gowers.

[244] Turner, *Epilepsy*, p. 227.   [245] 'Therapeutics. Epilepsy'.   [246] Turner, *Epilepsy*, p. 260.

the peripheral circulation; hot baths to promote skin excretion; occupation, preferably outdoors or, for the 'frailer epileptic', semi-sedentary work; for epileptic girls, the avoidance of dancing; avoiding excessive excitement and promotion of a 'simple life'; total abstinence from alcohol, and use of tobacco in moderate amounts only; and avoidance of marriage. He also considered education of children, according to their individual mental capacities, to be vitally important. He noted studies showing that 17% of epileptic children could attend normal schools, 27.5% were best educated in special classes and 40% required education in residential schools or colonies. Only 15.5% were ineducable.[247]

Diet was considered of great importance, especially the avoidance of constipating food and of toxins. As Spratling opined: 'It is essential that he [the epileptic] be properly guided in his food habits . . . especially in cases in which the disease is autotoxic in origin.' Patients needed to be free of gastrointestinal disorders of any kind (constipation, flatulence, indigestion), and Spratling even listed those items of food which were 'suitable for epileptics'. He suggested dietary approaches which included regularity, moderation and proper chewing ('every morsel . . . should be thoroughly masticated before it is swallowed. Epileptics of inferior grades are prone to bolt their food almost wholly unmasticated').[248]

Turner noted that 'epileptics are notoriously big eaters, and, being habitually subject to constipation, are prone to overload the digestive tracts and organs'.[249] Accordingly, two principles had to be borne in mind when considering dietary management: first, nervous energy is fuelled by the albuminous and nitrogenous contents of food (as suggested by Hughlings Jackson) and so these should be restricted; second, toxins introduced with food and formed in the digestive tract or by the liver can precipitate seizures. Diets were useful ancillary treatments, especially in early stages and when bromides were proving ineffective, requiring increased doses. Turner cited authorities who extolled the benefits of limiting red meat (e.g. Konrad Alt, who recommended a mixed milk and vegetable diet without meat) and 'salt-starvation', especially when combined with bromides. He dismissed the farinaceous and nitrogenous diets recommended by others. His main emphasis, though, was on a diet free of 'purin bodies', which existed in meat extracts, thymus or pancreas, some vegetables and tea, coffee and cocoa (p. 246). He found this of 'remarkable benefit' in controlling grand mal seizures, but not always myoclonus or absence seizures. A largely random collection of other foodstuffs was routinely prohibited by doctors of the

---

[247] Turner, *Epilepsy*, pp. 247–51.   [248] Spratling, *Epilepsy and Its Treatment*, p. 354–5.
[249] Turner, *Epilepsy*, p. 244.

period, and Turner's approach had at least some biochemical justification. He also saw diet as a way of mitigating the adverse effects of bromide.

Medicinal Treatments

Up until the introduction of bromides, the medicinal treatment of epilepsy was arbitrary and unsatisfactory, and the writings of many early physicians were steeped in pessimism. Treatment was largely by herbals and often entirely empirical. In a standard work on physic, published in 1813, therapies advised included antispasmodics (digitalis, valerian, castor, musk, ether, oil of amber, oleum animale, oleum cajeputae, auric montana, belladonna, hyoscine and opium), astringents (mistletoe) and tonics (cinchona, metals especially iron, copper and zinc, silver and arsenic) – all therapies which continued to be used until the end of the century.[250]

After 1850 some authorities took a more positive view of prognosis, notably Herpin, who considered epilepsy curable. He particularly recommended zinc oxide, which he found had terminated seizures in two-thirds of 42 cases, and milk parsley (*Selinum palustre*), which did so in 4 of 10. He also mentioned the ammoniuret of copper, the salts of valerianic acid, wormwood, hyoscyamus (henbane), ammonia and the boiled flesh of the mole (which had a high reputation).[251] Delasiauve divided his medicinal treatment into four categories, as was the fashion of the time (see Table 1.4). Sieveking, too, felt that epilepsy could be cured but that there was no purpose in listing all the individual drugs that had been tried: 'In fact, there is not a substance in the materia medica, there is scarcely a substance in the world, capable of passing through the gullet of man, that has not at one time or another enjoyed a reputation of being an antiepileptic' (p. 299). He did, however, record the common practices of the time, which included non-specific treatments such as purgatives and turpentine, salts of iron, zinc, and specific drugs such as opiates, other narcotics, hyoscyamus, conium, belladonna, hydrocyanic acid, chloroform, indigo, *Cotyledon umbilicus*, valerian, silver, nitro-muriatic acid, digitalis, iodides, belladonna and mistletoe.

Others speculated on potential mechanisms, an example being Jonathan Osborne, the leading Irish physician of his time (and president of the Irish College of Physicians), who was particularly in favour of a combination of digitalis and cantharides - the crushed up remains of the blister beetle, known also to be a potent aphrodisiac. He tried the drug on the basis that sleep and epilepsy have 'points of resemblance' and that sleep is due to turgescence of the choroid bodies, and cantharides was well known to stimulate erectile tissue;

---

[250] Thomas, *Modern Practice*, pp. 317–23.
[251] Herpin, *Du prognostic*. Théodore Herpin had perhaps the greatest influence on subsequent epilepsy work (and especially on Jackson) than any other mid-century French physician.

also, that this and digitalis 'produc[ed] a beneficial change in the capillary circulation belonging to the seat of the disease'.[252]

Physical therapies were also popular, both for the acute treatment of seizures and also as a long-term therapy. These included cupping, the use of setons and ligatures, section of peripheral nerves, baths, enemas, cauterisation, galvanism, induction of fever, blood-letting and leeches and, finally, castration or circumcision.

Then in 1857 a new and powerful drug entered the fray which, within a few years, was to become the principal treatment of epilepsy worldwide – bromide. It is worth pausing to describe the bizarre nature of its entry into the treatment of epilepsy. On 1 May 1857, at the Royal Medical and Chirurgical Society in London, Sieveking presented a paper describing in detail fifty-two patients with epilepsy. He focused on masturbation as a particular cause of epilepsy, finding that in nine of the cases 'the sexual system was in a state of great excitement, owing to recent or former masturbation' (p. 129). He also noted the influence of the menstrual cycle in females. The paper was then opened for discussion, with Sir Charles Locock, a fashionable London obstetrician and accoucheur to Queen Victoria (he attended the births of her nine children) in the chair. Locock, commenting on the influence of onanism and menstruation on epilepsy, reported that as bromide caused impotence he had tried it on a girl with hysteria, and then hysterical epilepsy, and found it highly effective: 'Out of fourteen or fifteen cases treated by this medicine, only one had remained uncured.' Locock's comment is worth recording in full, showing how misconception piled on misconception resulted in a remarkable discovery:

> A great number of cases of epilepsy, both in boys and girls, arose from the practice of onanism. This was a cause very frequently overlooked, and might account for the great increase in the disease of late years. There was a form also of hysterical epilepsy connected with the menstrual period, and as periodic as that function. This form of the disease was very difficult to treat. The attacks only occurred during the catamenial period, except under otherwise strong exciting causes. He had been baffled in every way in the treatment of this affection. Some years since, however, he had read in the *British and Foreign Review*, an account of some experiments performed by a German on himself with bromide of potassium. The experimenter had found that when he took ten grains of the preparation three times a day for fourteen days, it produced temporary impotency, the virile powers returning after leaving off the medicine. He (Dr. Locock) determined to try this remedy in cases of hysteria in young women, unaccompanied by epilepsy. He had found it, in doses of from five to ten grains, three times a day, of the greatest service. In a case of hysterical epilepsy which had occurred every month for nine years, and had resisted every

kind of treatment, he had administered the bromide of potassium. He commenced this treatment about fourteen months since. For three months he gave ten grains of the potassium three times a day. He then gave the same dose three times a day for fourteen days before the menstrual period, and latterly had only ordered it in the same dose, three times a day, for a week before the expected catamenia. This patient had had no epilepsy since the commencement of the use of the potassium bromide.[253]

Thus was bromide therapy announced to the medical world – for misdiagnosed patients on the basis of a total false aetiology and mechanism; however, apart perhaps from his contribution to the preservation of the European monarchy, it was to be Locock's lasting achievement.[254] In the next few months, Sieveking himself tried the new drug, but was not impressed. In the first edition of his book (1858) he wrote: 'I have since prescribed the bromide, but have not as yet obtained any definite results which would justify the expression of an opinion.'[255] In the second edition (in 1861), he was more positive: '[T]hough I have not enjoyed the same amount of success, [I] have found it decidedly beneficial. In one case, where the irritation of the sexual apparatus was very marked, a permanent cure seemed to be attributable to it.'[256]

Exactly how bromide exerted its antiepileptic action was unknown, and theories included a sedative action, vasoconstriction of the sympathetic nervous system, effects on reflexes or as an anti-toxin. Whatever its action, it was soon apparent that, for the first time in history, there was a truly effective antiepileptic drug – and over the next few decades, bromides were enthusiastically promoted.[257] Uniquely among neurological disorders, it seemed that an effective drug treatment for epilepsy had been discovered, and the excitement this engendered, palpable in the papers of the period, no doubt contributed to the elevation of epilepsy into the neurological spotlight.

Having said this, not all authorities were enthusiastic. Jackson hardly mentions drug treatment at all in any of his writings and one senses that the empirical state of therapy carried no intellectual challenge or interest for him. Even by 1888, in a British Medical Association lecture on 'the diagnosis and treatment of diseases of the brain', Jackson mentioned only bromides, belladonna and nitrogycerine. Bromides he thought as an 'empirical therapy' that exerted its action possibly by 'substitution nutrition' stabilising nervous matter. He expanded at more length on the avoidance of nitrogenous foods, eating less and exercising more, and being content 'to live on a

[253] Sir Charles Locock (1799–1875), an English obstetrician. Sieveking, 'Medical Societies'.
[254] A revisionist view is that Samuel Wilks was the first person to try bromide in epilepsy, on the basis that iodide was effective. See Friedlander, 'Who was "the father"?'
[255] Sieveking, *On Epilepsy*, p. 222.   [256] Sieveking, *On Epilepsy*, 2nd edn., p. 292.
[257] Early citations were: Duckworth Williams, *Efficacy of the Bromide of Potassium in Epilepsy*, Crichton-Browne, 'Bromide of Potassium upon the Nervous System'.

lower level'. The patient should '"avoid excitement". But in young people we may err in being too strict; we may narrow a young epileptic girl's life too much by forbidding the amusements proper to her age. If she have a fit soon after a hearty game or a dance, it is, I think, only the premature development of a fit nearly due.'[258]

Gowers, more practical and less philosophical, however, devoted fifty pages to medicinal treatment in his 1881 monograph on epilepsy, including an entire section on bromides, which he endorsed as the standard treatment:[259] '[Bromide] has almost superseded other drugs in the treatment for the disease. The signal benefit which, in the majority of cases, attends its use, has rendered the administration of bromide and the treatment of epilepsy almost equivalent expressions ... In the majority of cases it is influence is far greater than that exerted by any other known agent' (1881, p. 252). As a result, toward the end of the nineteenth century, nearly two tonnes of bromides – mainly in the form of the potassium salt – were being prescribed annually through the pharmacy at the National Hospital in Queen Square (Table 1.5).

By then, new formulations of bromides began to multiply, and eventually at least forty-five different bromide preparations were on sale. Gowers came down strongly in favour of potassium bromide. By 1901, and the second edition of his book, he had had experience with the bromide of sodium, strontium, nickel, camphor, the combined bromide of rubidium and ammonium and of zinc. He reported on the effects of bromides with the addition of arsenic to stop bromide skin lesions, a formulation called bromalin, which was said to produce formaldehyde when administered and act as a gut antiseptic on the 'doubtful theory' that bromide's 'inconveniences' were due to gastrointestinal derangements', and bromipin, in which sesame oil was combined with bromide and praised 'on the continent' for not causing a rash or mental depression (1901, p. 273). Bromides, he thought, could usefully be combined

TABLE 1.5 *The quantity of bromides prescribed at the pharmacy of the National Hospital in 1899*

Bromide of potassium	3,664 lbs
Bromide of sodium	313 lbs
Bromide of ammonium	114 lbs
Bromide of strontium	6 lbs
Bromide of lithium	3 lbs
Total bromide	4,100 lbs

From Gowers (1901), p. 265.
(4,104 lbs is therefore approximately 2 imperial tonnes or 2,000 kgs)

[258] Jackson, 'Remarks'.   [259] Gowers, *Epilepsy* (1881, 1901).

with other antiepileptics such as belladonna, atropine, digitalis, zinc (especially in hysteroid convulsions), cannabis and opium. Variations on the theme included the idea of Paul Flechsig from Leipzig of giving large doses of opium for six weeks, then suddenly withdrawing it and substituting bromide.

Gowers also introduced borax as a therapy.[260] The first extended report of the therapy dated from 1890 in which it was concluded: '[W]e may say that we do not wish in any way to compare borax to bromide in the treatment of epilepsy, but consider it well worthy of a trial, especially in those cases where bromide has failed or is badly borne.'[261] Gowers also elaborated on how to dose, in adults and in children, and how to withdraw therapy – policies which remain valid to this day.

A wide variety of other drugs remained in use, and Gowers evaluated each in turn, in often disparaging terms (Table 1.6), as well as the physical therapies of counter-irritation, trephining, castration and circumcision. By the time of writing of the second edition, Gowers emphasised even more the role of bromides, with other drugs listed only as useful adjuncts.[262] These included borax, digitalis, belladonna, gelsemium, zinc, nitroglycerine and cannabis. Other authorities published similar lists, varying in detail more than substance. In Germany, for instance, the leading authority Otto Binswanger (1899) rated bromides and opioids as his preferred medicinal therapies.[263] For status epilepticus, he recommended chloral, chloroform, morphia, amyl nitrite and the hydrobromate of hyoscine, maintaining the 'strength' of the patient and reducing temperature by the use of ice (ideas which have parallels with the treatment today).

Gowers's authority was such that few disagreed with his opinions, but nevertheless a range of largely useless therapies were mentioned by others, some strange and exotic, such as hemlock (conium), strychnine and picrotoxin (although Gowers pointed out that this triggered convulsions), antisepsis of the

---

[260] Gowers, 'Gulstonian Lectures'.

[261] Risien Russell and Taylor, 'Treatment of epilepsy'. This view was enthusiastically endorsed in a subsequent letter in which it was stated: 'There can be no doubt that when the bromides, administered either alone or in conjunction with belladonna, fail to relieve convulsive seizures, biborate of soda is the most likely drug to be of service. And I would also point out that boracic acid, so far as I have tried it, appears to be quite as efficacious as its alkaline salt' (Bury, 'Treatment of epilepsy').

[262] Most other authorities of the time place a similar emphasis on bromide. Binswanger devoted thirty pages of his textbook *Die epilepsie* (1899) to bromide, and only ten pages to other medicaments and only ten pages to hygienic therapy. Nothnagel complained about the poor advances in treatments, and concluded that 'Bromides are not an infallible sovereign antiepileptic, but are able to have more effects than any other' (1877; p. 313).

[263] Binswanger realised that bromides were effective only in some cases, and warned against overestimating their efficacy. He also noted that there was considerable reluctance among patients and doctors to prescribe bromides due to their significant side effects (*Die Epilepsie*, pp. 372, 382).

TABLE 1.6 *Anticonvulsant drugs listed by Gowers in 1881 and 1901*

Drugs of definite benefit	Drugs of doubtful benefit
Bromide: Ammonium	Bromide: Aluminium
Potassium	Rubidium
Sodium	Nickel
Lithium	Bromalin
Strontium	Bromipin
	Hydrobromic acid
Digitalis	Potassium iodide
Belladonna/atropine	Opium/morphia
Strophanthus	Mistletoe
Stramonium	Turpentine
Cannabis	Cocculus indicus/picrotoxine
Gelsemium sempervirens	Chloral
Borax	Nitrate of silver
Zinc	Sulphate of copper
Iron	Benzoate of soda
Amyl hydrate	Nitroglycerine
Hyoscine	Piscidia erythrina
	Codeia
	Calabar bean
	Ergot
	Sclerotic acid
	Nitrite of Amyl
	Camphor
	Osmic acid
	Curare
	Hydrastin
	Chinolin
	Resorcin
	Antipyrine
	Acetanilide
	Aconite
	Hydrocyanic acid
	Osmic acid
	Thyroidin

[For status epilepticus: bromide, chloral hydrate, hydrobromate of hyoscine, morphia]

gastrointestinal tract and intestinal irrigation, rattlesnake venom (crotalin) and biological therapies such as anti-rabies vaccine and serotherapy. Some recommended the induction of infectious diseases such as erysipelas. Although Gowers himself considered that drug therapy to terminate acute seizures was not needed as the attacks were self-terminating, others used inhalations of ammonia, lavender, camphor, musk or asafoetida, or even injection of curare. Gowers – rather alone on this point – seemed little interested in 'general management', finding diet on the whole useless. Nonetheless, he did

recommend the avoidance of meat and emphasised the need to avoid constipation, and provided sound advice on occupation and marriage.

Within a few years therapy across the continent of Europe seems to have
become very similar, demonstrating the remarkable rapidity with which medical developments, then communicated largely through books and personal
contact, were translated into clinical practice. Although bromides were widely
recognised to be a breakthrough, many of the other therapies prevalent at the
beginning of the nineteenth century were still considered valid adjuncts. In
France, Féré – trained by Charcot and in 1887 appointed chief physician to the
Bicêtre – provided similar advice to Gowers in both his monumental *Les
Épilepsies et les Épileptiques* (1890) as well as in a shorter version in the series
Encyclopédie Scientifique des Aide-mémoire (1892).[264] He favoured bromides
above all else, taking the view that they both decreased the excitability of the
nervous centres and reduced vascular congestion, but also mentioned camphor,
opium, valerian, atropine ether, chloroform, belladonna, nitrate of silver,[265]
zinc oxide, borax, porphyrised copper and ammonium copper sulphate (1892,
pp. 174–82). Physical treatments seem to have been especially popular in
France, and Féré included hydrotherapy, galvanism and, reflecting Charcot's
influence, the use of bitemporal compressors, as well as his own invention, a
double-wall cap of fabric filled with lead shot (1892, pp. 183–7). He also
recommended lukewarm baths, purgatives, cautery and the use of blisters. He
mentioned too that the Chinese used acupuncture, the first mention of this for
epilepsy in any major European text.

Binswanger's *Die Epilepsie* was the standard German-language work on
epilepsy at the end of the century. Of its 470 pages, 120 were devoted to
therapy. In his view, too, bromides had pushed all other drugs into the
background, but treatment still had to be individualised and great patience
was required:

> How many bitter disappointments are caused to the doctor and patient
> when hasty conclusions are drawn from temporary improvement. How
> often have treatment methods been touted as a panacea for epilepsy,
> which here or there, if used quite accidentally, temporarily improved
> the condition! As far as completely harmless curative methods are con-
> cerned, besides loss of money and time they only cause the patient wasted
> effort and renewed disappointment. It is much more worrying when
> intrusive or even life-threatening medical and operative treatment
> methods are prematurely trumpeted into the world without an exact

[264] Féré, *Épilepsie* (part of a series titled *Encyclopédie scientifique des aide-mémoire*, edited by M.
Léauté).

[265] Interestingly, silver nitrate was said to give the skin a blue colouration (not dissimilar to the
modern drug retigabine) – for instance, in the character Oscar Dubourg in Wilkie Collins's
novel *Poor Miss Finch*.

and careful examination based on numerous and long-term medical observations being carried out beforehand. The epileptic eagerly grasps everything new that promises salvation in his gloomy, desperate situation. (p. 352)

He followed Gowers in warning that therapy can appear effective when in fact improvement was due to spontaneous remission, the use of hygienic treatment or the effects of suggestion. Other treatments he considered to have shown some effectiveness included valerian, radix artemisiae, belladonna and atropine, hyoscine, digitalis, cannabis, opium, morphine, pilocarpine, picrotoxin, simulo, curare, chloral hydrate, amylene hydrate, nitroglycerine, anti-malarials, anti-pyrexials, sodium nitrite, zinc and zinc salts, borax, lithium and bismuth.

Although bromides had become the standard treatment of epilepsy through-out the Western world, their side effects caused concern. 'Many are yearly declaring against [the use of bromide therapy]', wrote L. Pierce Clark in 1900: 'Its abuse has been great, and the routine treatment of all cases by bromides is not only poor therapy, but actual, culpable negligence.'[266]

Turner (1907) had a more balanced view. Noting that bromides were effective for young patients at the onset of their disease, with remission of seizures in more than 50% of cases and long-term cure in 23%, he felt that bromides should be given as early as possible. But in chronic (established) cases, the medicament had 'relatively little value'.[267] At the time, a variety of formu-lations were available – bromide of aluminium, ammonium, potassium, sodium, lithium, strontium, nickel, camphor, rubidium and ammonium, iod-ine, chlorine, bromaline (bromethylformin), bromapin (bromine and sesame oil), hydrobromic acid and Gélineau's formula. To Turner, many of these were 'quack remedies' (p. 227), and none had been subjected to any sort of com-parative trial. Nevertheless, physicians of the period had their favourites. Turner followed Gowers in taking the view that the sodium and potassium salts of bromide were more efficacious than the strontium or lithium salts, and to obscure the taste, he opined that 'the syrup of Virginian prune could be added' (p. 232).

Bromism was a horrid condition which must have made the lives of many patients miserable. Gowers devoted 4 pages to this topic, Féré included graphic pictures of the skin condition, and Turner provided a vivid textural description:

This condition is characterised by a blunting of the intellectual faculties, impairment of the memory, and the production of a dull and apathetic state. The speech is slow, the tongue tremulous, and saliva may flow from the mouth. The gait is staggering, and the movements of the limbs feeble and infirm. The mucous membranes suffer, so that the palatal sensibility may be abolished, and nausea, flatulence, and diarrhoea supervene. The

---

[266] Clark, 'Digest of recent work'.   [267] Turner, *Epilepsy*, p. 234.

action of the heart is slow and feeble, the respiration shallow and imper-
fect, and the extremities blue and cold. An eruption of acne frequently
covers the skin of the face and back. (p. 230)

When fully developed, the lesions on the skin took the form of boils, pustules
and weeping sores, a condition known as bromoderma. Gowers had noted that
co-medication with arsenic prevented and also removed the rash, but if the arsenic
was discontinued, the rash returned. Disinhibition, self-neglect, irritability, violent
behaviour, emotional instability, depression, a schizophrenia-like psychosis and
hallucinations were among the cognitive and psychological symptoms caused by
bromide and were sometimes severe. Turner stated correctly that the side effects
mainly occurred when the dose was too high and condemned the cavalier manner
in which the drug was often given. If treatment was cautious, side effects could be
minimised. Nonetheless, bromide-soaked individuals in the back wards of asylums
became synonymous with epilepsy, adding to its stigma. Spratling was more
scathing and, citing others, considered bromide a drug of last resort: 'I know of
no drugs save those which produce habits such as opium and cocain, that are so
universally abused as the bromids . . . The question naturally arises, Does the good
they accomplish in this way more than counterbalance their injurious effects in
other ways? In the majority of cases the answer is, No; in some, Yes.'[268]

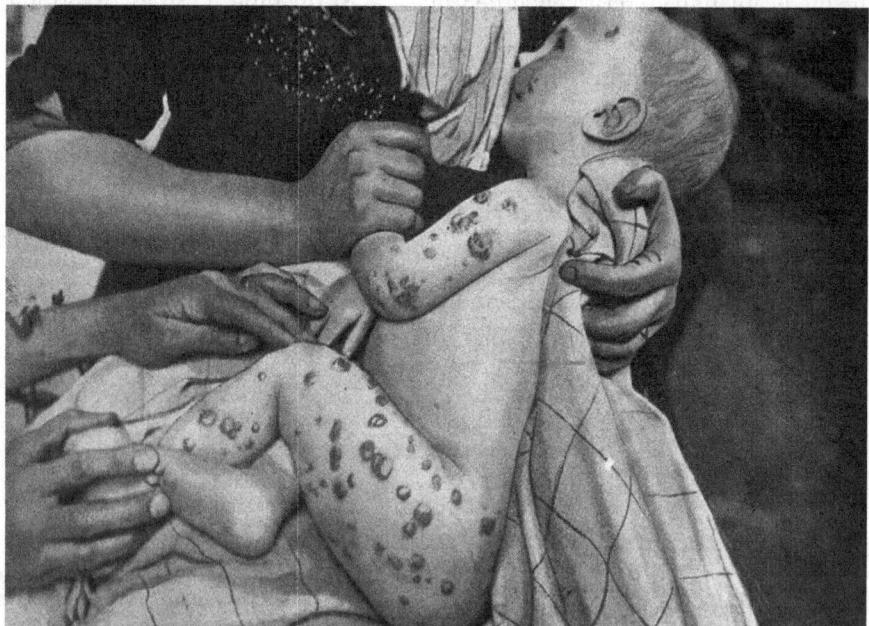

11. **Bromoderma in an infant.** The appalling skin lesions of bromide therapy were amongst
its worst systemic features. Image from Norman Purvis Walker, (1905) *An Introduction to
Dermatology* (3rd ed.) (William Wood and Company).

[268] Spratling, *Epilepsy and Its Treatment*, pp. 365–6.

Herbals had by the turn of the century largely disappeared as first-line therapy – after several millennia of constant use. Nevertheless, although Turner considered bromide to be the mainstay of drug treatment, he also recommended other drugs, in order of general usefulness: belladonna, atropine, zinc salts, opium and strychnine (Table 1.7). He rejected the use of bowel

TABLE 1.7 *Treatments listed by Turner in 1907 and Spratling in 1904*

Turner (1907)	Spratling (1904)
Drugs of definite or limited benefit	**Drugs of benefit**
Bromide: Potassium	Bromid: Potassium
Sodium	Sodium
Ammonium	Ammonium
Lithium	Strontium
Strontium	Bromapin
Gelineau's formula	(sometimes combinations of potassium, sodium
Bromipin	and ammonium bromide with bicarbonate
Bromalin	of soda and liquor potassii arsenitis)
Bromocarpine	
Chloral hydrate	Opium
Digitalis	Codeine
Glycerophosphates	Borax
Borax	Chloral hydrate
Belladonna (Atropine)	Amyline hydrate
Zinc salts (oxide, valerianate, lactate)	Nitroglycerin
Opium	Zinc
Strychnine	Chloretone
Chloride of calcium	Urethan
Calomel (mercurous chloride)	Solanum Carolinense
	Simulo
	Iron peptonate and magnesium
Treatment of no benefit	**Treatment of no benefit**
Monobromate of camphor	Borate of soda
Eosinate of sodium	Trional
Chloretone	Coal tar derivatives (antipyrine, phenacetin, acetanilide)
Antipyrin	Chloroform
Intestinal antiseptics:	Serum treatment (of Ceni)
Sulpho-carbolate of soda	
Salol (phenyl salicylate)	
Beta-naphthol	
Salicylate of bismuth	
Organotherapy, Serotherapy	Electricity, hydrotherapy, relief of eye strain, induction of infectious disease

antiseptics, eosinate of sodium and chloretone, as well as the bizarre fashion for organotherapy. Spratling too cited chloral, amylene hydrate, nitroglycerin, chloretone, urethan, sodium carolinense, simulo, trional, iron, coal tar derivatives and chloroform. Apart from choral and chloroform, which he favoured for status epilepticus, the other drugs on Spratling's list were given at best dismissive and passing mention by Turner.

Of all the other drugs, borax, a naturally occurring salt and carrying with it the authority of Gowers, was perhaps the most popular remedy. Turner found borax on its own to be ineffective. Prescribed in combination with bromide, it could be of benefit, but its value was limited by troubling side effects. With Gowers's imprimatur, its use soon spread rapidly, with reports from Italy, Germany and the United States; endorsements of borax purificatus 7.5 grains, or sodium biborate in combination with potassium bromide, were published as late as 1935.[269] Gowers attributed the effects of borax to its antispasmodic action, and others later to its antiseptic effect on toxins in the gut.[270] Spratling also favoured borax, but he found the gastrointestinal and dermatological side effects too severe to allow long-term treatment in most patients.

Many other diverse and spurious treatments remained in use, justified by poor science and jargon. For instance, Charles Hughes, superintendent of the Fulton Insane Hospital in Missouri and editor of *Alienist and Neurologist*, a leading journal in the field, enumerated in 1904, seemingly without irony, an impressive range of pathophysiological and therapeutic twaddle:[271]

> [Epilepsy can arise from] the condition and mechanism of the cerebral circulation, such as irregular, anaemic or other blood impress or pressure states, as from cardiac irregularity (cardiac epilepsy so-called), traumatisms, autotoxic and other toxaemic states, as from external sources like camphor or other narco stimulants, external psychic and autopsychic impressions transmitted periphero-neural impressions and similar exciting intestinal sources of peripheral irritation ... [Epilepsy was] influenced in its paroxysmal display by sanguineous hyperchlorinization, as ... in excessive meat eaters and eaters of other forms of highly salted seasoned food ... [Treatment sought to] restore the integrity and physiological equipoise of the epileptic neurone wherever in the epileptogenic zone

---

[269] See, for instance, McCartney, 'Further notes'; 'Compounds of boron and potassium in epilepsy'; Wilson, 'Treatment in general practice'.

[270] Borax remained popular as a washing powder, but had a decidedly slow death as a pharmaceutical. In 1922 Hans Jacob Schou, when appointed director to the Dianalund Kolonien Filadelfia in Denmark, reintroduced borax there at a dose of 3–6 g/day. It was used in use there until 1950, often added to barbiturate, bromide or hydantoin. The fashion for the drug in the 1920s was attributed to its championship by Pierre Marie, although its effectiveness seems to have been low. John P. A. Jensen examined 300 random charts of the 5,492 patients with epilepsy in the colony between 1898 and 1948 which suggested that less that 5% experienced a 50% or more reduction in seizures (Jensen, 'Rise and fall of borax').

[271] Hughes, 'Quarter and semi-decade treatment'.

impaired neurone integrity permits the characteristic periodic and paroxysmal morbid display . . . To accomplish this we must maintain a persistent impression on the morbid and abnormally acting cerebral neurones especially involved. (pp. 326, 329)

Hughes believed that therapy should '[restore] the normal state of integrity of physiological nutrition [with] rebuilding of the damaged epileptoid neurones' (p. 330). To this end, given the multitude of causes, treatment must be 'unremittingly kept up for years', consisting of bromides, along with hypophosphites, lecithin and nerve tone rebuilders, cerebral galvanisation, reduction of meat in the diet, intestinal antiseptics and digestives, and prolonged 'hours of brain tranquilization and sleep'. In addition to this regimen, 'an active anti-malarial, anti-rheumatic or anti-syphilitic course is essential to the cure of some cases' (pp. 330–1).

A mixture of science, common sense and nonsense typified the general standard of writing about epilepsy in this period. Even by 1916, Edward Twitchell[272] could write that '[e]pilepsy has so long been one of the opprobria medicorum that we welcome anything new of promise' (p. 483). He went on to list the 'more important' published papers in the field of cause or treatment of epilepsy in the preceding three to four years. These make dismal reading. His list included: A. Leroy's view that 'asthma and epilepsy were manifestations of the same disease'; H. Aimé's belief that 'haemophiliacs . . . never . . . become epileptics [due to] the delayed coagulation time of the blood' (obviously unaware of the case of the Duke of Albany); Donáth's theory that choline was the cause of epilepsy; Bolten's view that essential epilepsy was due to parathyroid hypofunction; Ammon's statement that '62% of all epileptics die directly from the disease' and '42% die in an attack' (p. 484); and the view of many authorities that the neurococcus was the cause of epilepsy, causing constipation, which could be cured by colectomy. Other treatments he mentioned were intraspinal injection of 2% calcium chloride, intrathecal injection of spinal fluid from one epileptic into another, salvarsan and iodides.

Phenobarbitone

The antiepileptic phenobarbitone had been newly introduced into practice by the time Twitchell noted that the combination bromide-dietetic treatment was 'the prop of the great majority' and that '[t]hose who condemn as worthless or harmful the bromide treatment are apt to be those who have discovered marvellous new remedies which relegate all others to oblivion' (p. 483), a

[272] Twitchell, 'Recent work in epilepsy'.

philippic one suspects aimed at phenobarbitone. But his arrow was misdirected, for phenobarbitone turned out to be by far the most important step in the medicinal therapy of epilepsy of this period, and perhaps in the whole of the twentieth century. By the 1920s it dominated drug therapy, and did so for decades to come. It is still one of the most widely used antiepileptics in the world.

Although its effects were discovered by chance, it was nonetheless the first useful compound in epilepsy to have resulted from the growing science of synthetic chemistry. Barbituric acid was first synthesised in 1864 (on St Barbara's day, hence its name) in a Belgian laboratory by Adolf von Baeyer, research assistant to the celebrated August Kekulé,[273] by the condensation of urea and malonic acid. The first clinically useful barbiturate derivative, barbitone (Seconal), was synthesised in 1902 by two German chemists working at Bayer – Emil Fischer and Joseph von Mering – and found to be a useful hypnotic. By 1904 Fischer had synthesised several related drugs, including 5-ethyl-5-phenylbarbituric acid – phenobarbital (Luminal) – which was then launched onto the market as a hypnotic and sedative. By 1912 it was widely used for these purposes.

In mid-February 1912, Alfred Hauptmann,[274] then a clinical assistant in Freiburg, gave phenobarbital to his epilepsy patients as a tranquiliser and observed that their epileptic seizures were suppressed.[275] Whether apocryphal or not, the story is that Hauptmann was sleeping above the ward and was kept awake by the nocturnal epileptic attacks. He prescribed Luminal to put his patients to sleep, and then noticed serendipitously that it abolished the noisy seizures. His monumental article is an excellent example of meticulous medical observation.[276] He reports that following his first chance observation, he began systematically to examine the potential for phenobarbital. He selected epileptic patients who had been at the clinic for many years due to the severity of their illness, who had been unsuccessfully treated with high-dose bromides and for whom there were good records of seizure frequency. He conducted his

---

[273] Friedrich August Kekulé von Stradonitz (1829–96), a German, was the most prominent organic chemist of his generation. Three of the first five Nobel Prizes in Chemistry were awarded to his students, including Jacobus Henricus van 't Hoff Jr (1852–1911), Hermann Emil Louis Fischer (1852–1919) and Johann Friedrich Wilhelm Adolf von Baeyer (1835–1917).

[274] Hauptmann, 'Luminal bei Epilepsie'; Hauptmann, 'Erfahrungen aus der Behandlung'. Alfred Hauptmann (1881–1948) had a chequered career. He distinguished himself in service in the First World War, for which he was awarded the Iron Cross and the Knight's Cross. After the war, he returned to academic work in 1918, and in 1926 Hauptmann was invited to the position of chair of psychiatry and neurology as well as directorship of the nerve clinic at the Martin Luther University of Halle-Wittenberg in Halle an der Saale. In 1935, as a Jew, he was forced to resign and cease work as doctor, then was imprisoned for a period in the Dachau concentration camp before fleeing to Britain and then the United States, where he died in 1948.

[275] Kumbier and Haack, 'Pioneers in neurology'.   [276] Hauptmann, 'Luminal bei Epilepsie'.

observations over many months to avoid random fluctuation of seizures. He prescribed up to 300 mg/day (100 mg a.m. and 200 mg p.m.), which was a lower dose than that used for night sedation (often up to 600 mg in Hauptmann's clinic). He presented one case history of a patient for whom Luminal was substituted in the place of bromide. In this patient, the seizures lessened in frequency and severity, mental agility was enhanced and the 'state of nutrition and strength improved to a quite extraordinary degree' (p. 1908). He concluded that Luminal was indicated mainly for the severest cases of epilepsy, which were beyond the influence of even the heaviest doses of bromide. Cases of medium severity could be rendered seizure-free with doses between 150 and 200 mg/day; more severe cases never required more than 300 mg/day. He noted that harmful side effects were absent, that Luminal could replace bromide in less severe cases and that the drug did not 'cure' epilepsy but acted by reducing the sensitivity of the cerebral cortex and thus suppressing attacks. Hauptmann observed also in passing that his findings did not support the theory that suppressing seizures simply leads to increased irritability.

Despite its evident effectiveness, the drug was not rapidly taken up in international practice. This was perhaps in part due to the outbreak of the 1914–18 war, which disrupted international medical communication and exchange in the field of epilepsy.[277] In striking contrast, for instance, to the speed at which bromide before and phenytoin afterwards were adopted into routine practice, phenobarbital therefore had to wait for its value to be widely appreciated.

Surgical Treatment of Epilepsy

The development of epilepsy surgery depended intellectually on the recognition that function was localised anatomically in the human brain and that the symptomatology of the seizures could indicate the anatomical site, and practically on the development of orotracheal intubation, chloroform anaesthesia and Listerian antisepsis.[278]

The pioneer was Victor Horsley[279] in London, who the world's first true neurosurgeon and also an experimentalist who had helped define the

[277] A few sporadic reports of phenobarbital therapy in epilepsy were made in continental Europe during the war years, and mention made of its use in the German military during the war. See Pecheux and Lotte, '"Le Luminal"'; Fuchs, 'Epilepsie und Luminal', 'Die Wirkung des Luminals'; and Kutzinski, 'Luminalbehandlung bei Epilepsie'.

[278] Horsley himself was involved in developing the first two, and on one occasion nearly expired whilst experimenting with chloroform anaesthesia on himself. He was also meticulous in regard to Listerian antisepsis. Nevertheless, surgery was still hazardous and required great skill; Horsley's complication rates were remarkably low and unmatched by others.

[279] Sir Victor Alexander Haden Horsley (1857–1916) was a British surgeon. Educated at University College London, he initiated brain surgery at the National Hospital for the Paralysed and Epileptic. He also held the chair of pathology and then chair of clinical surgery at University College London, and was professor-superintendent of the Brown Institute in

localisation of function in the primate brain in extraordinary detail. This primate research was one the landmarks of nineteenth-century neuroscience. With colleagues who included Edward Sharpey-Schäfer,[280] David Ferrier and other physicians at Queen Square, he carried out a series of investigations on the simian brain, mapping function in 4 mm² areas by electrical stimulation using a very weak current and electrodes placed 2 mm apart, and by ablating small ('minute' as Horsley put it) areas of cortex. This work was published in eight celebrated articles in the *Transactions of the Royal Society*, amounting to 525 pages with 33 pages of plates. It included studies on functions of the motor regions, the internal capsule, the various and sometimes complex movements produced by electrical stimulation of the motor areas, and was complemented by briefer investigations of the occipital and temporal lobes.[281] Detailed cortical maps were produced linking function to anatomical structures, and these formed the basis for his human epilepsy surgery.

The theory behind his epilepsy surgery was simple: the clinical symptoms at the beginning of the seizure indicated the location (the 'epileptic focus') within the cerebral cortex, from which the seizure ('the excessive neuronal discharge') arose; by transposing his maps of function from the simian on to the human brain he could identify the cerebral location responsible for the clinical symptoms; removing this portion of brain (the 'epileptogenic zone', as Jackson described it) to a depth of just over 2 cm would cure the epilepsy. Until the introduction of EEG in the 1940s and neuroimaging in the 1970s, this method of clinico-anatomical correlation remained essentially the only way of identifying the site of the seizure. As a result, epilepsy surgery at the time was largely restricted to resection in the motor areas of the brain, except in cases in which there was ancillary evidence.[282]

London. In addition to conducting the first resective surgery for epilepsy in the modern era, and a variety of other neurosurgical firsts, he pioneered different neurosurgical techniques and invented a variety of instruments, bone wax and also a stereotactic frame which was the prototype of all that followed. He also pioneered studies of the thyroid gland and established that myxoedema could be treated with thyroid extract, and he was involved with a successful policy for rabies vaccination. He was a social reformer and stood for the British parliament on a radical platform. He was a vocal supporter of woman's suffrage and the temperance movement, had celebrated rows with antivivisectionists (see Figure 9), and campaigned against poverty in various forms. He had a distinguished war record, and died in active service in Mesopotamia. Osler considered him 'by far the most distinguished medical victim of the war, whether among our own troops or with those of the allies . . . he was the outstanding British surgeon of his generation' (Osler, 'Sir Victor Horsley').

[280] Sir Edward Albert Sharpey-Schafer, amongst the most celebrated physiologists of his time, was a key collaborator of Horsley.

[281] This body of work included remarkable descriptions of comparative brain anatomy in different primate species and other animals, including the kangaroo.

[282] In fact, the very first intracranial operation in the modern era was based on such ancillary evidence and not on the concepts of cortical localisation. The procedure had been performed by William Macewen in Edinburgh in 1879. The patient had previously had an extracranial orbital tumour removed, and then returned to Macewen with focal motor seizures. He decided to operate on the basis that there was a local recurrence of the tumour, which indeed

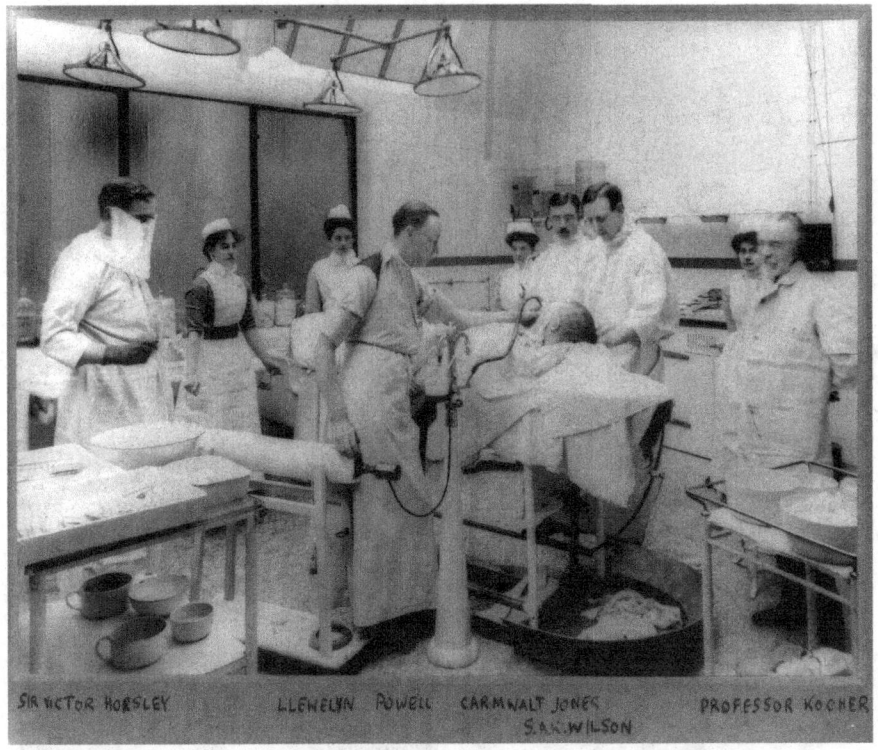

12a. A photograph of Horsley (gowned and masked on the left) operating at the National Hospital in about 1906. In the theatre are Dr S. A. Kinnier Wilson (at the back), Prof Emil Kocher from Berne (on the right; a close friend of Horsley and later a Nobel Prize Laureate) and the renowned anaesthetist Llewellyn Powell using the newly developed Vernon-Harcourt anaesthetic inhaler. Horsley was bandaged up under his gown as he was said to be having an elective appendicectomy in the days after this surgery.

12b. Four pages from his 1886 operation notes on patients with epilepsy., This casenote shows Horsley's own operative sketch and also his early use of clinical photography (from the Queen Square archive).

In 1886, supported by a letter of recommendation from Charcot, Horsley was appointed as assistant surgeon at the National Hospital for the Paralysed and Epileptic in London, and it was from this position, on 25 May 1886, that he carried out one of the first neurosurgical operations worthy of the name. His first patient had post-traumatic epilepsy, caused fifteen years earlier by a

proved to be the case. Macewen resected the recurrent lesion, which had extended intracranially (but not into brain tissue). The second intracranial operation involved resecting a tumour within the brain and was carried out in 1884 by Rickman Godlee at the West End Hospital in London. The location of the tumour was predicted on the basis of the seizure symptoms according to the theory of cerebral localisation by neurologist Hughes Bennett with the assistance of David Ferrier. The operation was a success, but the patient died of wound infection and Godlee performed no further brain surgery. Unlike Horsley, neither Macewen nor Godlee had performed experimental work nor had any special knowledge of neuroanatomy.

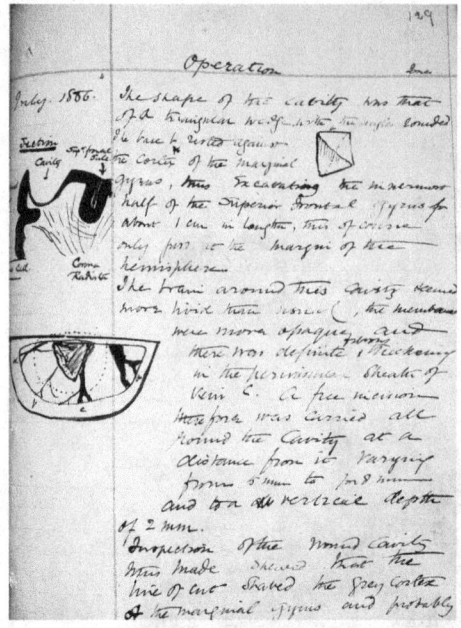
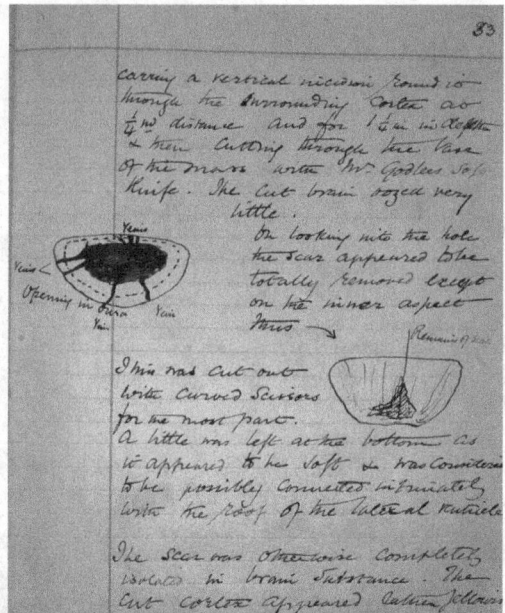
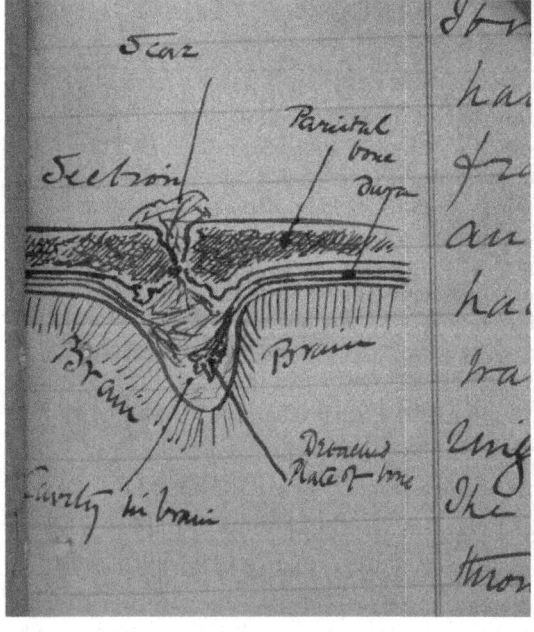
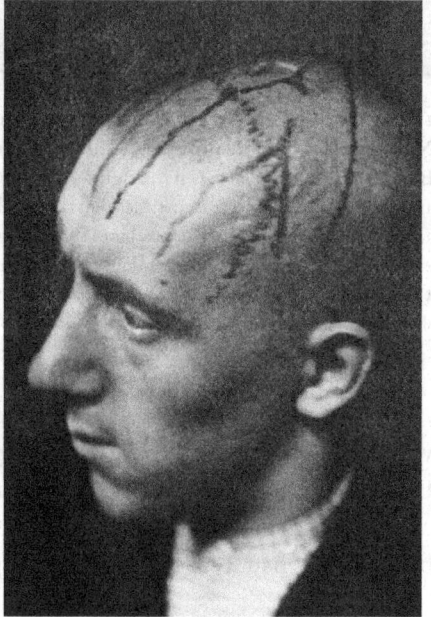

12b. (cont.)

depressed fracture of the skull. His seizures started with jerking in the right leg and spread to involve the right arm and face, with turning of the head and eyes to the right. On the basis of the symptoms, Horsley predicted the site of the epileptic focus and found a traumatic scar at the site. He excised the scar and the patient's seizures resolved completely. An operation on a second patient on 26

June 1886 was perhaps more audacious in the sense that there was no skull fracture to provide ancillary localisation information. The patient was a 20-year-old man who had recently developed epilepsy. Horsley predicted the site based on the motor seizures, operated and found a tuberculoma (a mass of tissue infected by tuberculosis) in the expected position. He completely removed the lesion and also used an induction current to carry out what was in fact the first case of peroperative electrical cortical mapping.[283] At a meeting of the British Medical Association in Brighton in October 1888, Horsley gave a lecture describing, in great detail, his first three operations, all involving epilepsy.[284] Heralding as it did the birth of neurosurgery, this was a landmark in the history of medicine. As reported in the *British Medical Journal*, the president of the section identified its outstanding merit, announcing that 'it would be difficult to overrate the interest of Mr. Horsley's paper, which he might characterise as pure science applied to the advancement of practical surgery' (p. 674). Charcot, who was in the audience (as were Jackson and Ferrier, and E. P. Thuring from New York, who had been present at the third of Horsley's operations), stated that 'British surgery was to be highly congratulated on the recent advances made in the surgery of the nervous system. Not only had English surgeons cut out tumours of the brain, but here was a case in which it was probable that epilepsy had been cured by operative measures.'

Many of the principles of modern neurosurgery were founded by Horsley, and by the end of 1886 he had completed ten operations for epilepsy, nine of which were deemed successful, and later operations on the spine and brain for many other conditions. One of his subsequent patients was his own son, Siward, who developed convulsions as a teenager. His work was celebrated worldwide and earned him the universally acknowledged title of 'Father of Neurosurgery'. Although his initial operations were on epilepsy, he focused his energies subsequently on other types of surgery, as seizures tended to recur months or years after the operations. It is said that by 1897 that he had ceased operating on epilepsy altogether due to the disappointing longer-term results.[285].

[283] As Horsley wrote: 'October 19th, 1886. Trephining over "facial centre," and removal of cortex composing that centre as determined by faradism at the time' (Horsley, 'Remarks on ten consecutive cases', [case number 5]).

[284] Horsley, 'Brain-surgery'. Horsley's use of the peroperative induction current in the second operation was to identify the 'centre of the thumb-area'. He considered this to be the centre of the 'epileptogenous focus' on the basis that the first symptom of the patient's focal seizures was 'clonic spasmodic opposition of the thumb and forefinger'. Horsley's work on the orangutan brain had shown this movement to be elicited by minimal stimulation of the 'ascending frontal and parietal convolutions at the line of junction of their lower and middle thirds' (p. 673).

[285] Letter from Wertheim Salomonson (1898), cited by van Emde Boas and Boon, *Epilepsy Surgery in the Netherlands*.

His work initially prompted a flurry of surgical interventions around the world,[286] but by 1910 enthusiasm for surgical treatment of epilepsy had, except in cases of post-traumatic seizures, significantly waned. It seems likely that in the hands of less skilful surgeons, the operations both failed to control seizures and were associated with unacceptable morbidity. The same applied to other areas of neurosurgery, and indeed, until the 1930s, only a handful of surgeons in the world had the suitable knowledge or expertise to operate on the brain for any indication, let alone epilepsy.

Reporting on the state of surgery in 1899, Otto Binswanger cited 146 cases of post-traumatic epilepsy operated on in the series of Paul Graf, which provides an interesting snapshot of then current practice. Forty-four per cent were simple trepanations, with or without opening the dura; the rest involved cortical resection of the scar tissue or drainage of cysts (on the basis of the theory that raised intracranial pressure caused seizures). At one year, the epilepsy in the cases with cortical resection was said to have improved in 15% and to have been cured in 23% of cases (in 35% of cases it was considered too early to judge). At three years, cure rates were only 6.5%. Binswanger concluded that the disappointing results were due either to the fact that, once established, seizures could arise in areas of the brain distant from the initial injury or that they were caused by the surgical scar.[287] Similarly, Harvey Cushing – the father of American neurosurgery – who visited Horsley in 1906 and subsequently engaged in a wide range of neurosurgical procedures, was not impressed by epilepsy surgery, which he had 'dropped ... for things I thought I could do better'.[288]

In 1907 Turner wrote: 'The favourable anticipations of the treatment of epilepsy, formed during the early years of Cerebral Surgery, have not been fulfilled.'[289] He (rightly) considered that surgery was ineffective when there was an inherited element to the epilepsy, therefore recommending that surgery should be avoided in anyone with a family history or any neuropathic degenerative stigmata. Spratling took exactly the same view. Both Turner and Spratling also cited the opinion of the Philadelphia surgeon William Keen[290] that surgery should be carried out as soon as possible after the onset of seizures to prevent the epilepsy becoming chronic. Turner summarised his own opinion of resective surgery by saying that it had some value in post-traumatic

---

[286] These included operations by J. A. Guldenarm and others in the Netherlands under the direction of Cornelius Winkler, who had expressed his intention to follow the example of Horsley, and Louis Muskens, a neurologist who also tried his hand at epilepsy surgery, albeit with a singular lack of success.

[287] Binswanger, *Die Epilepsie*, pp. 412–70.   [288] Preul and Feindel, 'Art is long'.

[289] Turner, *Epilepsy*, p. 253.

[290] William W. Keen worked with Silas Weir Mitchell on nerve injury and then studied for two years with Guillaume Duchenne in Paris and Rudolf Virchow in Berlin. He was 'America's first brain surgeon', and the first to employ Listerian antisepsis in the United States. John F. Fulton considered Keen to be 'Cushing's principal predecessor in neurosurgery in this country' (Whiteley, 'Department of Neurosurgery').

epilepsy in which 'a depressed fracture, a haemorrhagic cyst, or local encephalitis is present, and then only if it is carried out within a short time of the onset of the fits'. In generalised convulsions, in genuine idiopathic epilepsy and in cerebral birth-palsies, resective surgery was, he decided, 'useless'.[291]

Other modes of surgery were also undertaken in these years, indeed far more commonly than cortical resection. Trepanation (or trephining, as it was sometimes known) had been performed since prehistoric times, and was widely used for a variety of conditions well into the nineteenth century. At the National Hospital, Queen Square, the neurologist Manuel Echeverria was recorded as performing it in cases of epilepsy in 1868. In 1883 the results of 686 cases were reported from St Bartholomew's Hospital in London for the treatment of cranial injury and epilepsy.[292] In 1904 Spratling was still recommending it, especially in cases of traumatic epilepsy, as soon as possible after the first attack. Both Spratling and Turner also mentioned peripheral operations to remove 'irritations' (exciting causes) which triggered reflex seizures, correction of urethral strictures, relief of eye strain and astigmatism, bilateral resection of the cervical sympathetic nerves, treatment of caries and removal of adenoid growths and polyps – although Spratling was more enthusiastic about such treatments than Turner. Both endorsed the insertion of setons for counter-irritation with greater fervour. Turner dismissed vertebral artery ligation, mentioned by Spratling. Their greatest difference in opinion related to operations involving the abdomen and female generative organs. Spratling devoted eleven pages of his book to a detailed description of abdominal surgeries such as oophorectomy and hysterectomy, and concluded that '[a]s a general rule – one subject to modification in especial cases – operations on epileptic women for the removal of the reproductive organs may be done if the attacks came on about puberty in the first instance, and occurred thereafter in close conjunction with the menstrual epoch'.[293] The social and political struggles to control and dominate women were seemingly gladly reflected in the fashionable medicine of the period.[294] Turner is to be commended for rejecting this approach: 'The old procedure of removal of the ovaries, or other portions of the female

---

[291] Turner, *Epilepsy*, p. 259.

[292] Report by W. J. Walsham in 1882–3, cited in Ferrier, 'Cerebral localization'. Echeverria published his first book on trepanation (*De la trépanation dans l'épilepsie par traumatismes du crane*) in 1878.

[293] Spratling, *Epilepsy and Its Treatment*, p. 437.

[294] In Britain, the position of women in society had become a political issue. The suffragettes were active, and were aided by several doctors – notably Victor Horsley, who was outspoken in their support. He was a political activist who took on many left-wing causes, including better housing for the poor, better prison conditions for women and the abolition of alcoholism, which he recognised to be a cause of much domestic abuse. The political views of Turner are not known, but his attitudes on many social issues seem to have been advanced and liberal.

generative organs, was based on an entirely mistaken view of the nature and cause of epilepsy.'[295] Another operation, still practised in 1860 but which seemed to have died out by 1900, was section of peripheral nerves (or even amputation) in the arm or leg where a Jacksonian march was first experienced, or where 'reflex' seizures were thought to be caused by a peripheral lesion or irritation.

STIGMA AND THE EXPERIENCE OF HAVING EPILEPSY

This was an age when the patient's voice was silent, and for obvious reasons. Stigma was enormous and, to many with epilepsy, was more devastating and had more profound consequences than the condition itself. The previous 'religious' belief that epilepsy was due to demonic possession was replaced by 'scientific' theories which were in many ways more damaging to sufferers. The links with the scientific theories of degeneration, inheritance and insanity made epilepsy a feared and deeply unattractive prospect. It was perceived as a forbidding and hostile condition by the public, patients and doctors alike, and keeping one's counsel about the disorder was the only sensible option.

Epilepsy in good families was also hidden away to prevent the suggestion of an inherited degenerative trait becoming attached to the family's reputation. One example was the elaborate effort made to conceal the disease of Queen Victoria's epileptic son, Prince Leopold of Albany, who died aged 31 years in 1884.[296] Where the disease could not be concealed, the sufferer was withdrawn from view, as happened to Prince John, Leopold's grand-nephew and the epileptic fifth son of King George V, who was kept in virtual isolation until his death aged 13 in 1919.[297] Equally excluded from everyday society were those of lesser birth, who where possible were confined to home. For the poorest who could not afford this, there were only asylums for the insane and, for the destitute, the workhouses.

In view of this, it is perhaps not surprising that remarkably little was published by individuals with epilepsy about their experience of the disease. The biographies of famous people with epilepsy provide some peripheral information – for instance about medical consultations – but the personal effect that 'being epileptic' has was hardly documented.[298] Similarly, for those with

---

[295] Turner, *Epilepsy*, p. 255.   [296] See Zeepvat, *Prince Leopold*.

[297] Another royal princess, Maria-Anna Karolina of Austria, died of epilepsy. Her condition was also hidden from the population.

[298] A remarkable exception was the autobiographical account of Karl Wilhelm Ludwig Friedrich von Drais von Sauerbronn, an aristocratic Austrian who published a book under the nom de plume Diætophilus (a book with a hypergraphical title): *Physische und psychologische Geschichte einer siebenjæhrigen Epilepsie. Nebst angehaengten Beitraegen zur körperlichen und Seelendiaetetik für Nervenschwache. Erste Hælfte. Reine Geschichte in chronologischer Ordnung. Zwote Hælfte. Beurtheilende Zergliederung und Ergænzung der Thatsachen.* This is perhaps the

epilepsy in asylums or workhouses, virtually no personal testimony exists. In part no doubt this was because many were illiterate and few would have had access to publication, but even private diaries seem absent. Regardless of class or wealth, the hiding or denial of epilepsy was the usual response, and one senses that epilepsy was considered wholly out of the bounds of civilised debate. The leading doctors, too, seem to have been more interested in disease per se than in its effects on the biography of patients.[299]

The private records of even the most celebrated individuals known to have had epilepsy were also remarkably silent on the topic. The diaries and letters of Edward Lear (1812–88) can be taken as an example. Lear developed focal seizures at around the age of seven, and in his boyhood was severely affected – with 10–15 attacks a month and sometimes several a day. He was able to hide these as he sensed the onset of a seizure in time to remove himself from public view. In his diaries, as a code, he placed an 'X' next to the dates he had seizures and a score of between 1 and 10 to mark their severity. He described himself as '[coming] to awful grief'[300] at times and being prone since childhood to depression partly because of his seizures. Yet his letters, which were numerous and sometimes very personal, hardly if ever mention his epilepsy and very few of his friends or acquaintances knew about it; and there was no mention at all of the condition in his large published oeuvre. Lear's attitude was not uncommon. He referred to his condition as 'the Demon' and wrote as an adult that the seizures 'would have prevented happiness under any sort of circumstances. It is a most merciful blessing that I have kept up as I have, and have not gone utterly to the bad mad sad.'[301] Nevertheless, Lear spent much of his life abroad, possibly in an attempt to flee from the stigmatising effects of the condition. Another writer with epilepsy was Gustave Flaubert, who also hid his epilepsy from all but his closest friends and family, and whose seizures were said to have led to intellectual decline.[302]

---

first truly autobiographical account of epilepsy. Sauerbronn had a history of sixty-five grand mal seizures and described the auras in detail, and then cured himself with diet. In the preface he wrote: 'I present to you, for your opinion, a cosmopolitan wish. Potentates and private founders have formed institutions for the instruction of the deaf and dumb. Establishments for the cure of the epileptic would be much more useful.' He estimated the number of epileptics in Germany to be around 10,000, and concluded: 'How little light has yet fallen from madhouses on the bodily and mental functions of man!'

[299] The tenor of the practice of medicine in the late nineteenth century was harsh. Lennox, for instance, correctly observed that Jackson's writing did not reflect 'a "human" interest in his patients', there was 'little concern for the patient as a person' and '[t]he reader does not see the patient, but only his disease' (Lennox, *Epilepsy and Related Disorders*, pp. 714, 787). Lennox did not mention that Jackson wrote very little about treatment.

[300] Lear, *Edward Lear Diaries*.   [301] Cited in Bevis and Williams, *Edward Lear*, p. 307.

[302] There has been much debate about whether Flaubert's seizures were epileptic or hysterical (pseudo-seizures), and about the idea that they were responsible for his cognitive deterioration. Both ideas have been strongly contested by Henri Gastaut (Gastaut et al., 'Gustave Flaubert's illness').

One indication of how epilepsy might have felt comes from the fictional works of the period. Great literature can serve as a surrogate for the daily lived experience of a sufferer and is perhaps our most reliable guide to the idea of epilepsy at the time.[303] The picture painted is not pretty. In late-nineteenth-century works, epilepsy was portrayed by numerous writers as a metonym for violence, impulsiveness, criminality, immorality and insanity. [304] As always, though, the interchange between medicine and society was bidirectional and cultural attitudes coloured medical opinion. This was evident from the way that the medical descriptions of the epileptic personality mirrored the wider anxieties of social order, economic progress and national fitness, and owed much to Max Nordau[305] and other literary figures of the time. A strange example was the view of the psychiatrist Henry Maudsley who, following Lombroso, described 'epileptic neurosis' as being characterised by 'a singularly vivid imagination, which is apt sometimes to occupy itself with painful or repulsive subjects. Probably the invention of the modern sensation novel, with its murders, bigamies, and other crimes, was an achievement of the epileptic imagination.'[306]

The novels of Charles Dickens[307] feature a number of characters with epilepsy (or possible epilepsy). His depiction of the male characters is clearly influenced by the theories of hereditary neurological taint. Bradley Headstone (in *Our Mutual Friend*, 1865) is like an 'ill-tamed wild animal', a crazed, slow-thinking individual whose convulsive seizures can be seen as a metaphor of mental anguish and murderous thoughts. His raw and uncontrolled emotion and his polyvalent sexuality are other features of the epileptic personality in the Victorian mind. It has been suggested that his 'secret vice' was masturbation, another sign of the degenerate nature of his epilepsy.[308] Monks, in *Oliver Twist* (1837–9), was the product of a degenerate marriage, and unremittingly evil, violent and cowardly, met his end in an American jail. He was also physically monstrous, with an appearance which carried the stigmata of epilepsy: '[Y]ou, who from your cradle were gall and bitterness to your own father's heart, and in

---

[303] Many have focused on the verisimilitude of descriptions of epilepsy in the works of great writers. But this seems to me to miss the point. Their real value is not accurate description but the portrayal of the meaning of the condition.

[304] Of course, there were exceptions and honest and admirable characters also exist. Oscar, in Wilkie Collins's *Poor Miss Finch*, is an example (albeit with epilepsy which was post-traumatic rather than inherited). But these were very much in the minority.

[305] Although Nordau hardly mentions epilepsy by name in his work.

[306] Maudsley, *Responsibility in Mental Disease*, p. 243.

[307] It has been claimed that Dickens himself had childhood epilepsy, although the claim is strongly contested. Dickens was familiar with the medical literature on epilepsy and was interested in medicine and doctors, of whom he had a generally poor opinion.

[308] Mason, *Secret Vice*.

whom all evil passions, vice, and profligacy, festered till they found a vent in a hideous disease which had made your face an index even to your mind', and 'His lips are often discoloured and disfigured with the marks of teeth; for he has desperate fits, and sometimes even bites his hands and covers them with wounds.'[309] It has been suggested that Dickens used this to imply the epilepsy was due to syphilis, and there is an interesting parallel here with the lines from Shakespeare 'A plague upon your epileptic visage'.[310] The work of Dickens was a commentary on contemporary culture and lives, and often a parody of it. No reader at the time would have failed to recognise the contrast between Oliver (righteousness) and Monks (degeneracy), and the association of epilepsy with Monks' degenerate nature.[311]

A novelist whose depiction of epilepsy owes most to its conceptual link with crime was Émile Zola. His descriptions of Roubaud and Lantier in *La Bête Humaine* (1890) as degenerate, atavistic persons – violent, criminal, jealous and immoral, and with the physical stigmata of epilepsy – are firmly based on the writings of Lombroso and in the concept of the neurological trait. Lantier, a serial murderer and the human beast of the title, was born into an alcoholic family. At a point early in the tale, Zola describes Lantier's attempt to understand himself:

> He was beginning to think that he was paying for the others, for the fathers and the grandfathers who had drunk, for the generations of drunkards of whose blood he was the corrupt issue, that he was paying the price of a gradual poisoning, of a relapse into primitive savagery that was dragging him back into the forest, among the wolves, among the wolves that ate women.

The characters carry physical stigmata of criminality, and their epilepsy is a symbol of their social degeneration and violence.[312] Females with epilepsy are portrayed in rather different ways, often as being simple, dreamy and uncontrollable (e.g. Guster in Dickens's *Bleak House*) or childish, shallow, volatile and sexually abandoned (like Lucetta Templeman in Thomas Hardy's *Mayor of Casterbridge*, 1886). Another aspect of having epilepsy was the limitations this

---

[309] Squires, 'Charles Dickens'. There is an interesting parallel here with Shakespeare's lines
[310] King Lear, Act 2 Scene 2, line 79, Kent's rant to Cornwell (the spelling in the original text is 'A plague vpon your Epilepticke visage'). See also Betts and Betts 'A note on a phrase in King Lear', where it is suggested that this phrase refers to the facial marks of syphilis, which was probably then a not uncommon cause of epilepsy. Tim Betts was a long-serving president of the British branch of the ILAE, a liberal and an indefatigable advocate for epilepsy.
[311] Dickens, *Our Mutual Friend*, vol. 2, p. 97; *Oliver Twist*, vol. 3, pp. 232–3.
[312] Zola, *La Bête Humaine*, p. 53. Although first numerically quantified by Lombroso, the view that epileptics were violent has a long history in medicine and literature (for instance, as Desdemona facing death pleads to Othello: 'And yet I fear you; for you're fatal then / When your eyes roll so' (Shakespeare, *Othello*, V, 2, 37).

placed on marriage, and it is an interesting point that in the nineteenth-century literature, for instance, of Dickens, Zola, Hardy and Dostoevsky, none of the epilepsy characters are allowed to procreate.[313]

Dostoevsky, perhaps the most celebrated nineteenth-century author to feature epilepsy as a central theme in his novels, suffered himself from epilepsy, which he did not deny but equally did not write about in the first person.[314] His work adds a further dimension to the public perception of epilepsy – that of mysticism and revelation. It is not difficult to see that for Dostoevsky, writing about epilepsy had a cathartic element. His novels predate the writings of Lombroso, but he was known to have read Herpin, Esquirol, Trousseau and Romberg. Quite a number of the characters in his novels have epilepsy,[315] including three who were crucial to the stories: Smerdyakov (*The Brothers Karamazov*, 1879–80), Prince Myshkin (*The Idiot*, 1868–9) and Kirillov (*The Possessed*, 1871–2).[316] Pavel Fyodorovich Smerdyakov has many of the stereotypical characteristics of the public perception of 'an epileptic'. He exhibited inherited degenerative features, being the illegitimate son of 'Stinking' (Smerdyastchaya) Lizaveta', a mute, defective dwarfish vagrant woman and daughter of an alcoholic, and Fyodor Pavlovich Karamazov, in whose employ he was a servant.[317] Smerdyakov was an atheist, unlikeable, disloyal, unreliable, cunning, violent, prone to outbursts of anger and a murderer, and who in the end committed suicide. Plotting the murder he used faked seizures as an alibi, and it has been pointed out that Dostoevsky would have known better than others how easy this was to do.

In contrast to Smerdyakov, Myshkin is 'perfectly good', even Christ-like: honest, forgiving, handsome and attractive, though lacking in sensuality. Other characters in the novel refer to him as an 'idiot', misreading his intelligent, moral and spiritual nature for innocence and naïveté. Some have stressed a darker side to Myshkin, interpreting his epilepsy as a metaphor representing these contrary elements – bringing him by its ecstatic nature close to the sublime and the Kingdom of God, yet also to darkness and madness and evil. An epileptic seizure occurs at places in the book where the contrary elements in Myshkin's personality are in crisis. Myshkin degenerates, perhaps inevitably, and at the end is returned by his epilepsy to a sanatorium. The link between epilepsy and the Christian experience is a

---

[313] This was noted by Stirling, *Representing Epilepsy*, p. 37.
[314] Although ever since Freud wrote that Dostoevsky's epileptoid seizures were 'a self-punishment for a death-wish against a hated father', a veritable industry has arisen in trying to decide whether the epilepsy was genuinely organic or psychogenic (Freud, 'Dostoevsky and parricide').
[315] A full list can be found in P. H. A. Voskuil, 'Epilepsy in Dostoevsky's novels'.
[316] NB: *The Possessed* is sometimes translated as *The Devils* or *The Demons*.
[317] Dostoevsky, *Brothers Karamazov*. Smerdyakov in Russian implies 'son of the stinking one' (p. 87).

theme which permeates Dostoevsky's characterisations, often in a contradictory and complex manner. Kirillov is an atheist who plans to kill himself in
order to counter man's fear of death and to raise human consciousness to a
stage where there is no God other than human will. Yet, like Myshkin, he is
depicted as a Christ-like figure, and he shares with Myshkin an interest in
religious prophecy. His epilepsy – the existence of which he denied – took
the form of an ecstatic aura in which there is a moment of eternal harmony, a
transcendent moment which, ironically, was seen as confirming the existence
of God. Another element in the stories of Kirillov and Myshkin was their
sense of being outsiders, travelling extensively abroad, exiles from mainstream existence – like Dostoevsky and Lear in real life. In all these aspects,
it is easy to postulate that Dostoevsky reflected the complexity of his own
experiences of and reactions to epilepsy, its social and personal impact.

Other prominent leitmotifs in fictional descriptions of people with epilepsy include loneliness and isolation, denial of epilepsy and withdrawal,
dysfunctional sexuality and uncontrollable emotions. It is also clear that,
because the condition is 'hidden', persons with epilepsy are particularly useful
to novelists. The sufferers are disabled, but not in any physical sense. They can
function normally in most life settings for most of the time. Nonetheless, they
have an occult disease which confers on the sufferer abnormal personal
characteristics and can give the plot events of great dramatic moment. They
are, in effect, 'secret agents' who can be used imaginatively in plot and
narrative design.[318]

Another theme in nineteenth-century literature is the transformation of a
personality in the epileptic seizure and the use of the epileptic seizure as a
'threshold'. This is evident in *The Idiot* but is taken to its extreme in gothic
novels. Many nineteenth-century readers believed that violent and criminal
acts, often with sexual overtones, could be carried out in seizures and outside
the control of the sufferer. Figures such as Dracula did not have overt epilepsy,
but their transformations would, in the public's mind, be in accord with
behaviour during a seizure. In Dracula's case, for instance, the transformation
was brought on by the full moon, as epilepsy was often considered to be.
Similarly, Frankenstein's monster was the epitome of the stereotype of an
emotional, violent, sexually perverted epileptic personality. In a similar vein,
Álvaro[319] argues that Mr Hyde in *The Strange Case of Dr Jekyll and Mr Hyde*
(1886) was a manifestation of degeneration and epileptic fits (although
Stevenson never explicitly states that Hyde had epilepsy). Hyde was the

---

[318] These and other aspects are explored in the PhD thesis of Jessica Groper *She must have brought
reason.*
[319] Álvaro, 'Dr Jekyll and Mr Hyde'.

personification of evil and amorality, subject to episodes of aggressiveness and unprovoked violence and criminal behaviour. Episodes were preceded by vocalisations and facial changes, the experience of falling, loss of consciousness, jerking or twisting movements, and associated perceptual changes and amnesia. Álvaro also suggests there was a trend towards increasing frequency of the episodes when triggered by sleep or fever. The concept of the 'furor epilepticus', during which patients might even commit murder, was well established in the work of Esquirol, Portal, Morel and Lombroso.[320] Martin Barr's *The King of Thomond: A Story of Yesterday* (1907) was another strange science fiction, in which the director of an insane asylum creates a wax doll with machinery inside her to mimic human form, mixing up madness, romantic love, dream and fantasy. The main protagonists have epilepsy in their family and, although epilepsy is not a main theme, it can be seen as part of their inherited psychosis. Barr was himself superintendent of an asylum, and wrote extensively on epilepsy, favouring the eugenic sterilisation of 'feeble-minded epileptics'.[321]

The social stigma of epilepsy was recognised in medical circles, but not considered a matter of medical attention – and the adverse negative attitudes to epilepsy were shared as much by doctors as by the public. Descriptions of the life of inmates in the Craig Colony give some idea of how such patients were perceived and treated:

> Epilepsy is without doubt the worst disease that can afflict a human being ... The presence of the disease creates sympathy for the afflicted one, and sympathy tends to aggravate the disorder either through the person being granted improper privileges of many kinds, or by virtue of the fact that the individual is a 'skeleton in the family closet'. They must remain in the background, debarred from the family life, denied social pleasures, and not infrequently an epileptic child in a family where there are other children is a *positive menace* to the physical safety of such children ... If a patient desires to go on a visit ... [w]e can advise against it, but that is all. After a patient has been at the Colony two or three years, has acquired certain habits of living, has grown accustomed to certain forms of treatment, has become acquainted with Colony life in all its phases, and his d[i]sease, maybe, has been brought largely under subjection, if not wholly arrested, he sometimes becomes restless of the restraints it is needful to impose on him for his good, and wants to break away from them. *Invariably* when he does this and goes on a visit, his condition is usually as bad on his return to the Colony – and often worse – than when he first entered the Colony ... Recently a disturbed epileptic left the Colony without our knowledge and consent. On being returned to the

---

[320] Portal, Observations, p. 11; Esquirol, *Mental Maladies*, p. 284; Morel, *Études cliniques*, vol. 2, p. 702; Lombroso, *Criminal Man*, 4th edn.
[321] Barr, *Mental Defectives*, p. 17.

Colony, and when about to be taken from the train, he resisted and had to be removed by force. He drew a knife and stabbed an express messenger in the arm . . . To care for epileptics is far more dangerous than to care for the insane; the epileptic commits deeds of violence under great impulse. The insane is more stealthy and cunning, and there is more opportunity for self-defense.[322]

Others were kinder, an interesting example being Georges Clemenceau, future French prime minister, who was an intern at the Bicêtre:

> I know nothing more revolting that the sight of the physiological and social death of children. I lived, for a whole year, amongst the little epileptics of the Bicêtre. I saw them arrive, full of gaiety and intelligence, eager for pleasure and joy, but then they darken, as the dreadful seizures were repeated, become stupid, fall into idiocy where just enough of material life survives for the Creator to feast at His leisure on His creature's suffering. Well, when they come, one presents the inevitable, one struggles. Who knows? One may win.[323]

Jack London provides a unique perspective on life in the asylum in his short story 'Told in the drooling ward'.[324] The narrator, Tom, is a 'highgrade feeb' (feeble-minded person; his term) who has resided for twenty-five years in a Californian institution. It is a remarkable and successful attempt to get inside the head of an inmate, told with brutal directness. One house in the asylum is where the 'high grade epilecs' reside:

> They're stuck up because they ain't just ordinary feebs. They call it the club house, and they say they're just as good as anybody outside, only they're sick. I don't like them much. They laugh at me, when they ain't busy throwing fits. But I don't care. I never have to be scared about falling down and busting my head. Sometimes they run around in circles trying to find a place to sit down quick, only they don't. Low-grade epilecs are disgusting, and high-grade epilecs put on airs. I'm glad I ain't an epilec. There ain't anything to them. They just talk big, that's all. (p. 2)

For all this bombast, this short story is in fact tender, sensitive and warm. The inmates are heroes not villains, and worthy of respect and affection – in striking contrast to the messages of the eugenical movement that were all around him.

Two other novelists in the early twentieth century suffered from epilepsy and wrote epilepsy into their work, heavy with symbolist melancholy and depression. *Mot kveld* (*Towards Evening*, 1900), a novel by the Norwegian writer Tryggve Andersen, offers a bleak world vision wherein life is a constant

---

[322] *Craig Colony for Epileptics*, p. 29.
[323] Translation of G. Clemenceau, *La Mêlée sociale* (1913), p. 37.
[324] Jack London, *Drooling Ward*.

'confrontation with darkness' and death, miserable and absurd, and where humankind is helpless and doomed to suffer without knowing the cause. The prelude to the last scene is 'a spectacular storm of lightning', as if 'the sea is burning'. It is not difficult to see this intensely pessimistic life-view as reflecting the author's epilepsy and the storm as a metaphor for his seizures. Similarly, the oneiric novel by the symbolist writer Alfred Kubin, *The Other Side* (1909), is set in a dreamland in which Patera, the creator and ruler, becomes subject to epileptic seizures. The social structure of the kingdom begins to disintegrate into a degenerate and amoral morass in which sexual perversity, violence and cannibalism take hold. The seizures are viewed as proof that Patera is a lunatic, and epilepsy a curse which leaves destruction in its wake. The novel is Kafkaesque in its pessimism and claustrophobic vision. Kubin led a disturbed life, suffering nervous breakdowns and withdrawing to his family estate, and suffering from psychomotor seizures. His novel depicts epilepsy as something degrading and catastrophic. An effect magnified by his own dark and disturbing drawings which he used to illustrate the book. Kubin also provided lithographs for *The Golem* (1914/15) by Gustav Meyrink, another oneiric story in which the hero, Pernath, suffers epileptic seizures in a sexual scene involving a degenerated 14-year-old Jewish prostitute. The influence of Lombroso is strong in the novel, with degeneration, sexual deviancy, criminality and immorality running through the Wassertrum family. It was also made into a film, likewise entitled *Golem* (1980).[325]

Film was in fact a technology immediately adopted for epilepsy, perhaps not surprisingly given that epilepsy is a disorder of movement to which the medium might seem ideally suited.[326] At the Craig Colony in 1905, under the supervision of Spratling, the Boston neurologist Walter Greenough Chase filmed twenty-one epileptic seizures – probably the first complete cinematic case studies of epilepsy.[327] Chase called these his 'epilepsy biographs' (p. 56). Spratling wanted to record every epileptic seizure that occurred at the colony

---

[325] Andersen, *Mot kveld*, citations from pp. 154 and 148 of Schiff, 'Tryggve Andersen's novel'.

[326] Earlier, still photography had similarly focused on epilepsy, not least by Lombroso in his studies of physiognomy and stigmata, and Charcot in the celebrated *Iconographie photographique de la Salpêtrière* (Bourneville and Regnard, 1870–80) and *Nouvelle iconographie de la Salpêtrière* (1888–1918), in which epilepsy and hysteria are sometimes depicted in an overly sexualised form.

[327] Details from Cartright, *Screening the Body*, pp. 56–71, citing the 'Twelfth Annual report to the State Board of Charities, Craig Colony at Sonyea, New York, 1905' (pp. 177–8). An earlier film had been compiled by the celebrated neurologist Francis Xavier Dercum (1856–1931) of a nude artist's model who was asked, under hypnosis, to maintain a series of difficult postures. When she tired, she developed jerks and muscle spasms which Dercum claimed (erroneously) were equivalent to artificially induced epileptic seizures. The voyeuristic sexualised nature of this episode, which cannot have escaped the audience of Dercum's films, is reminiscent of Blanche Witman's hysterical performances under hypnosis by Charcot.

and for the attendant to write down the time, type of seizure and its duration. The film presented many practical problems, and to succeed, Chase wrote,

> we had some one hundred and twenty-five male patients from the infirmary assembled in a convenient spot out of doors on a warm summer day. The clothes were removed and the patients covered with blankets, so that, a seizure occurring, the blanket could be readily dropped and the subject, within a very few seconds, placed in the range of the camera. (p. 59)

The men were filmed having seizures, some nude, lying on the ground outdoors, some with ictal-induced penile erections, against a dark canvas backdrop.[328] Occasionally an attendant or physician stepped in to change the position for filming. One patient with status epilepticus was filmed. Women were also photographed, but clothed and in a more decorous fashion. These films give the impression that in the study of epilepsy, the sufferers were conceived as simply objects, scarcely human and certainly not worthy of respect – reflecting, no doubt, the attitudes of the alienists in whose charge the patients were placed.

That the stigma of epilepsy had severe economic effects was highlighted by Spratling, who found that 47% of a sample of his 1,322 cases (although it is not clear from where these numbers were drawn) were unemployed and 15% were housewives. Epilepsy, he pointed out, 'often impairs or completely destroys the usefulness of its victim in the commercial and social world, without any appreciable impairment of mind or body, the knowledge of the presence of epilepsy, no matter how mild or infrequent the attacks may be, sufficing to make the epileptic's presence undesirable'.[329]

THE BIRTH OF THE INTERNATIONAL LEAGUE AGAINST EPILEPSY

The rapid exchange of knowledge and the extensive professional contacts of medical practitioners across nations were notable features of medicine in this period. The growing wealth of the medical profession, the rise of easy transport by rail and boat, and the communication possible through a well-organised and effective system of medical journals and books led to an explosion of international activity. Its most glamorous symbols were the international congresses, and in particular the International Medical Congresses. From relatively humble beginnings in Paris in 1867, these gatherings took place at irregular intervals until 1913. They became increasingly grand affairs, led by the medical profession, graced by the presence of royalty, government ministers and other luminaries, and attracting national press coverage. They reflect the growing status of medicine as it emerged into the scientific age.

---

[328] See Sterling, *Dirty Work in a Laundry*.   [329] Spratling, *Epilepsy and Its Treatment*, p. 57.

From the point of view of epilepsy, the 16th International Medical Congress in Budapest, held between 29 August and 2 September 1909, was of singular importance. It was a spectacular and extravagant affair.[330] More than 5,000 delegates filed into the Redoute for the opening ceremony. The entrance of his Royal and Imperial Highness the Archduke Joseph triggered the singing of the Hungarian national anthem and a great many speeches. Every congress member was given a generous packet of literature and guidebooks, a ticket for free use of the local baths, as well as a bronze medallion designed by the sculptor György Vastagh.[331] The welcoming reception was something of a zoo, teeming with 'males . . . not too wrapped up in the affairs of science . . . who did not hesitate to push and struggle, to climb and crawl . . . to arrive at the refreshment tables'.[332] The congress served up a rich menu of entertainment, consisting not least of a number of soirees and a performance at the national theatre of Imre Madách's *Tragedy of Man* (an apt choice given the course of European civilisation in the next few decades).[333] The plenary addresses dealt with cancer; artificial parthenogenesis; tropical diseases; inheritance, selection and hygiene; and the 'climatic, geological and scenic peculiarities of the valley of the Vag and the high Tatra'.[334] Harvey Cushing's diaries paint a vivid picture of the events and personalities:

> Sunday, Aug. 29th. Budapest ... Opening of the congress in the Redoute. Very gorgeous but piping hot affair. Too 'much' people, too 'many' noise to hear or see. The Grand Duke in his swell uniform – Count Apponyi, Müller and the delegates. The Russians in their heavy fur uniforms must have melted. The Redoute a fine place for such a reception – the great staircase lined by gaily appareled guards – one Major-domo in particular most gorgeous. Henry Head in his Cambridge scarlet and pink gown much admired ... Monday, Aug. 30th. To the Congress to register – very well-arranged affair – with much literature gathered at separate stands. The Neurological Section and discussion of Frankl-Hochwart's paper. All very cordial. Showed the slides prepared for the surgical section. Oppenheim, Jendrássik, Levi et al. Dinner with Henry Head, the de Sarbós and 'Sir Museum Radishes' [Eugène de Radisics] at the Hungaria. To the Lord Mayor's reception with them in the Redoute. Crowded and hot. Later to the garden for 'citron'. Most amusing evening with Sir Malcolm Morris and Mr Jessop –

---

[330] The medical and national press were out in force. *The Lancet* and the *British Medical Journal*, for example, published elaborately detailed accounts of the goings-on. See 'The Sixteenth International Medical Congress', pp. 482–3, 691–766, 907–76 and 'The Sixteenth International Congress of Medicine', pp. 706–9, 797–801, 887–90.

[331] One of these medallions was bought for a song by the author in a junk shop recently, a sad ending for the distinguished object.

[332] 'Sixteenth International Medical Congress', p. 706.

[333] 'Sixteenth International Medical Congress', p. 887.

[334] 'Sixteenth International Medical Congress', p. 798.

who did not pay for their citrons. H.H. rather bored at Sarbó's threat to charge Edw. VII ... Tuesday, Aug. 31st. Luncheon at the Herczels at 1.30. Rovsing, Ceccherelli and others and wait until nearly 3 when Macewen, son and daughter stroll in. I tried to get away as the paper was booked for 3 but no – 'Macewen first and the meeting postponed until 4 &c' so we dallied with the elaborate lunch and coffee & cakes on the porch overlooking the garden until 4 and were late. Saw Fröhlich on entering and he said I had been called on twice and would not be again. Krause was reading and after he had finished, they called [on] unprepared me. It was late and most of the people had gone. Eiselsberg however there and spoke kindly of the work ... Wednesday, Sept. 1st. Dined at the Hungaria with the Thayers and was dropped by W.S.T. as Musser gave the signal to leave for the Court. Absurd arrangement with large red ribbons, smaller red ribbons and white ones. The first to be spoken to, the 2nd shaken hands with and the 3rd bowed to – this the most exclusive court in Europe. Rovsing and another big Dane finally picked me up and we drove over to be presented – line of carriages a mile long. Stunning entrance to the receiving rooms – great staircase with red uniformed creatures having great eagle plumes in their hats and carrying halberds lined the steps on either side. An impossibly hot room considering the character of the people and we entered and waited in the 3rd class room while his Grand Dukeship talked hours with Musser et al. of the large red ribbons. De Sarbó finally rescued me and after one look at the Duke we left for the outer world. A beautiful view by moonlight of the 'Escalier' and of the monument to the 'saint' of Budapest. Thence to a café with the Langes and other bearded orthopaedists and their wives where we were missed by K.C. and Mrs Thayer, they having gone to the theatre after the dinner ... Thursday evening, Sept. 2. The Dollingers' dinner at the Hungaria. A beautifully served and enjoyable feast for 200 guests, followed by speeches by representatives of the various countries. Prof. 'Chusching' got out of replying for America and Dr. Robert Lovett did finally respond. The dinner broke up after Prof. Ceccherelli of Parma threatened with all Italian violence an inoffensive old man from Fiume who had dared to address the assemblage in his mother tongue – Italian, Ceccherelli himself having responded for Italy in French, the official language.[335]

In the midst of this melange, two events in the field of epilepsy occurred which were to prove of immense significance. The first was the foundation of the ILAE. The second was the adoption by the ILAE of *Epilepsia,* the only scientific journal devoted to epilepsy. These were both essentially pan-European initiatives, with several key figures pushing them forward.

The idea of establishing a scientific journal in the field of epilepsy seems to have surfaced around 1905. Correspondence between Louis Muskens in

[335] Fulton, *Harvey Cushing,* pp. 294–5.

Amsterdam and Turner in London refers to the creation of a journal, to be published in Haarlem, which had 'the approval from almost all well-known scholars in this subject'.[336] In 1907, five renowned figures agreed to be patrons of the future journal: Jackson, Binswanger, Bekhterev, Fulgence Raymond and Konstantin von Monakow.[337] Then, in 1909, an editorial committee was set up consisting of Muskens, Turner, Spratling, Gyula Donáth, Ludwig Bruns and Henri Claude.[338] Donáth was appointed as editor, and the first issue appeared in March 1909. In September 1909, at its founding meeting, the ILAE took over ownership of the journal. Whether this was the plan at the time of the journal's foundation is not entirely clear, but the same figures involved in the journal were also involved in the foundation of the ILAE, and the two ideas were intimately connected.

The original conception of the ILAE was modelled on other organisations which had been founded in the previous few years, and notably the International Commission for the Study of the Causes of Mental Diseases and Their Prophylaxis, which shared personnel with the ILAE and had similar goals.[339] At a side meeting in a small room – the Salle Donau – in the Hotel

---

[336] L. J. J. Muskens to Jan Cornelis Tadema, 11 September 1905 (Special Collections, University of Leiden Library). Louis Muskens studied medicine in Utrecht, spent time in the USA with Dana, and in Britain with Sherrington in Liverpool and at the National Hospital, Queen Square where he served as a clinical clerk to Gowers, Jackson and Horsley. He returned to Amsterdam to run a clinic and was a lecturer at the University of Amsterdam. He was an important figure in the history of epilepsy, but his difficult personality alienated him from many of his colleagues. He was an experimentalist and clinician, involved in the foundation of the ILAE, served as its first secrétaire-général, was involved in the establishment of *Epilepsia*, dabbled in epilepsy surgery and was author of *Epilepsy: Comparative Pathogenesis, Symptoms* (1926; English translation, 1928), an important work on epilepsy from the 1920s.

[337] Otto Binswanger co-authored a textbook of psychiatry (*Lehrbuch Der Psychiatrie*, 1904) which was highly influential, and his book *Die Epilepsie* (1899) was a standard reference work on epilepsy. Fulgence Raymond succeeded Charcot as Chair of Neurology in the Faculty of Medicine in Paris. Konstantin von Monakow was Director of the Brain Anatomy Institute in Zurich and founding editor of the *Schweizer Archiv für Neurologie und Psychiatrie*.

[338] Donáth was a leading Hungarian neurologist, appointed to St Rochus. He was active in the post–First World War eugenics movement. Ludwig Bruns was Professor of Neurology in Hanover and co-author of the *Handbuch der Nervenkrankheiten im Kindesalter*. Henri Claude was Chair of Mental illness and Brain Diseases at the Hôpital Sainte-Anne.

[339] The International Commission for the Study of the Causes of Mental Diseases and Their Prophylaxis was founded in Milan in 1906. Marie, in his opening address at the foundation of the ILAE, referred to the ILAE as the daughter of this organisation, in which Tamburini was heavily involved, and also to the Office International de L'Hygeine Publique, which was founded in Paris in 1909 and which was a forerunner of the World Health Organisation. (See Shorvon, Weiss and Goodkin, 'Notes on the origins', and Shorvon et al., 'The International League Against Epilepsy, Centenary History'.)

Bristol on 30 August 1909, the ILAE met for the first time, with forty-six persons (mostly leading alienists) present.[340] At the meeting Augusto Tamburini[341] offered the support of the Commission, of which he was president and which had already created an epileptic colony in Rome. According to Auguste Marie, the ILAE was set up on the initiative of himself, Muskens, Donáth and Jacob van Deventer. Marie and Tamburini chaired the first two meetings and outlined what were the exceedingly ambitious aims of the organisation: to gather detailed data from all countries and then devise an international programme for epilepsy concerned with finding a cure, prevention, aid, social rehabilitation and wide-ranging experimental research.[342]

Marie[343] laid the marker for the ILAE, at its inauguration, in the following statement. The proposed ILAE was to act as

> an international action committee charged with centralizing all data related to the problem of epilepsy, its history, causes, and various manifestations in different countries. The data would be consolidated, then checked and compared, and a comprehensive inventory of regulations, laws, and private and public aid organizations could be created. Establishing what has already been done will make it easier to see what remains to be achieved; and on the basis of comparisons, we can come up with a programme … Carrying out this data-gathering exercise will necessarily involve official contacts with public authorities. One can also imagine the need for a central clearinghouse arising before too long … The comparative data could be made the subject of comprehensive reports by an international commission that would divide up the work and would publish results, analyses, and comparative tables. We can even envisage a permanent office, and for that, government support would eventually be indispensable … We wish to set up something analogous to the International Office of Hygiene [an early predecessor of the World Health Organization] or to the international psychological institute currently being created in Rome, under the patronage of the Italian government. Indeed, why should these existing entities not extend a hand to their daughter organization, the International League Against Epilepsy? … Obviously, such a vast and ambitious programme has the potential to engage the interest of philanthropists and intellectuals the world over … Madness generally is governed by laws, national and international regulations, public and private aid organizations, in other

[340] Among those present were Konrad Alt, Otto Hebold, Adolf Friedländer, Vladimir Bekhterev, Fulgence Raymond, Louis Landouzy, Robert Sommer, Wilhelm Weygandt and Augusto Tamburini.

[341] Augusto Tamburini was a celebrated Italian psychiatrist, later chair of psychiatry in Rome, and an early worker on cerebral localisation with Luciani. The events that resulted in his resignation from the presidency of the ILAE in 1911 are not known.

[342] Marie, 'Ligue international contre l'épilepsie'.

[343] Auguste Marie was an alienist at Villejuif and earlier at the colony of Dun-sur-Auron, where he was renowned for his humanity and sympathy for the inmates.

words, it has codes and statutes. We would like to do the same thing for a class of unfortunates who up to now have been denied the benefits of society. Epilepsy may be a problem of heredity, or result from a variety of acute and chronic infections. Its associations span all the way from criminality to the limits of human genius. One hundred years after [Philippe] Pinel and his followers elevated prisoners to the dignity of patients, society must make for epileptics the same allowances and the same salutary efforts as it does for other disenfranchised persons.

The ILAE was

to devote itself to special projects on behalf of epileptics, and to finding a cure and means of prevention, as well as providing aid and social rehabilitation. Nor will the League neglect experimental research and comparative physiopathology, or laboratory work, which are essential for elucidating a series of problems as complex as those raised by the origin, evolution and nature of seizure disorders, with their attendant range of somatic and psychic complications.

The primary method for achieving its aims was to obtain statistical information, and to do this the ILAE was to set up national committees, reporting to the central committee in Budapest, and to create questionnaires to standardise data collection. This collection of statistics remained at the centre of League activity and, in this early stage of its development, the ILAE was at heart bureaucratic, and not primarily concerned with scientific or clinical issues.

By the time of the second meeting of the ILAE in Berlin[344] in 1910, Tamburini had been elected president, and Donáth first secretary. Statistical reports were presented from two countries (England and Holland). The British report was compiled by Turner[345] and documented the number of epileptics in asylums and registered houses, attending the National Hospital, Queen Square, in the epilepsy colonies, in the British army in India, as well as the number of deaths due to epilepsy. The figures updated those in Turner's 1907 book and provided the most detailed analysis then available. The third meeting was held in Zurich. Tamburini was not present and sent a letter regretting that events constrained him to resign his presidency. He was replaced by the American David Weeks. The American Association for the Study of Epilepsy and the Care and Treatment of Epileptics had applied to associate with the ILAE and the application was accepted. William Shanahan presented a draft 'Object' of the ILAE, which proposed setting up an international committee, national committees, individual membership (with members all receiving a copy of *Epilepsia*) and annual meetings. This was a

---

[344] The meeting was held in conjunction with the International Congress on the Care of the Insane, and the ILAE session scheduled two lectures, titled 'Criminality amongst epileptics' and 'Physiopathological research in epilepsy'.

[345] Turner, 'Statistics from England'.

well-constructed administrative plan and to this day remains the basis of the ILAE's organisation (albeit with significant modifications).

The third meeting of the ILAE was held in Zurich in 1912 (no meeting was held in 1911, for reasons which are not clear) in conjunction with the international congress for psychology and psychotherapy. David Weeks lectured on the institutional work at the New Jersey Institution for Epileptics, from which he and Davenport produced their notorious paper on the hereditability of epilepsy. In all, fifteen lectures were due to be delivered on a range of epilepsy projects. The meeting was notable for its approval of the 'Objects' of the ILAE – its statutes and structure. In 1913, the ILAE met in London for their fourth meeting, in conjunction with the 17th International Medical Congress with its 7,000 delegates visiting the city. It was another glittering congress, with delegates received by Prince Arthur of Connaught, the grandson of Queen Victoria, at the Royal Albert Hall, and suffragettes picketing outside and trying to gatecrash the meeting.[346] Amongst the events was an operation by Harvey Cushing, a clinico-pathological demonstration at the National Hospital Queen Square of hereditarian diseases and Bateman's disparagement of American eugenics. ILAE members were amongst the speakers in the main sessions. The ILAE meeting itself was held on the 13 August at the Royal Society of Medicine but was sparsely attended. A handful of talks were given, most on international statistics and visits were arranged to the epilepsy colonies in Epsom and Alderley Edge.

Despite its modest origins, the ILAE was beginning to expand. By 1914 there were 17 national committees, more than 100 members, a well-written constitution and statutes, and a well-defined programme of work. Annual meetings had been held in conjunction with other International Congresses, and the League owned and published its own journal. Sadly, all the promise of the ILAE and the potential gains for epilepsy were suddenly ruptured when, on 28 June 1914, Europe was plunged into crisis and then war. The fifth annual ILAE meeting had been planned to be held on 5–7 September 1914 in Theodore Kocher's clinic in Bern, but it never took place. During the famously beautiful summer of 1914, few believed the war would last long. A brief note published in *Epilepsia* read: 'Because of the European war, the meeting of the International League Against Epilepsy has been adjourned until the summer of 1915.'[347] This proved wildly optimistic and the ILAE disappeared from view. For the next twenty years, no similar international activity or cooperation materialised.

---

[346] Cushing gave a very entertaining description of the congress (Cushing, *The Life of Sir William Osler*, pp. 366–8). For descriptions of the ILAE meetings between 1909 and 1914, see Shorvon et al., *The International League Against Epilepsy 1909–2009*, pp. 1–23, 217–224.

[347] 'Nouvelles'.

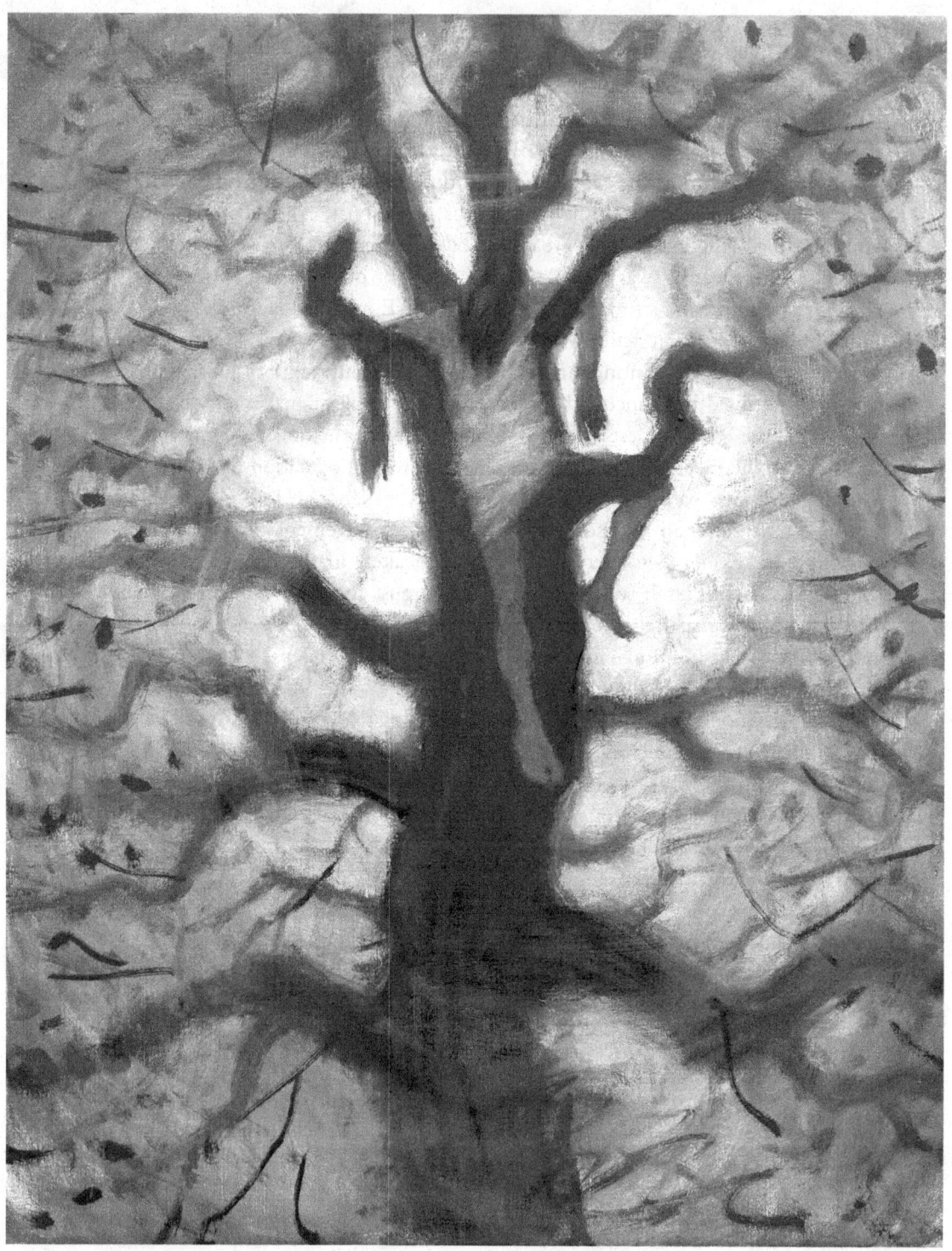

13. **'Entangled on the tree of eugenics.'** (A painting by David Cobley, 2021)

TWO

1914–1945: EPILEPSY IN THE AGE OF CATASTROPHE

CATASTROPHE

The two world wars and the years between them were, in Eric Hobsbawm's phrase, an age of catastrophe.[1] As the old-world order began to crumble, the First World War ushered in massive social upheaval, the fall of four empires and the rise of fascism and communism. Global power was rearranged, and the years were punctuated by the Russian Revolution, other revolutionary struggles in Europe, an influenza pandemic, the Great Depression and the even greater devastation of the Second World War. The world economies were on a roller-coaster ride, with periods of economic and national depression vying with episodes of decadence, and philanthropic support of routine healthcare and of epilepsy suffered grievously. In Europe and America uncertainty and a sense of impending crisis plagued the interwar years. Indeed, the very collapse of society was predicted by many; as Albert Schweitzer wrote in 1922 'It is clear now to everyone that the suicide of civilisation is in progress.'[2] The Great War had dealt an additional blow by destroying the idea that Western civilisation was moving in a continuously upward direction and the belief in its inherent righteousness. The rise of Nazism marked a low point in the previously trumpeted moral rectitude of European culture. Societal gloom hoed the ground on which the seeds of eugenics were planted and flourished. It was because of this, particularly, that this period was to prove disastrous for the

---

[1] Actually 1914–50. So named in Hobsbawm, *Age of Extremes*.
[2] Schweitzer, *Decay and Restoration*, p. 3.

disabled and those with epilepsy, in terms of both stigma and societal oppression.

It was also a period when medical and biological ideas entered popular culture as powerful metaphors for society and in turn, social trends influenced the course of medicine. Social structures were seen as 'organisms' needing diagnosis and treatment.[3] The American sociologist Talcott Parsons[4] stressed the similarities between biological organisms and societies in terms of integration and adaptation and a tendency to homeostasis (later, in 1951, he would introduce the concept of the sick role). Evolutionary principles were applied to social issues and psychological principles to social constructs such as industrial efficiency. Diseases were linked to social ills, and both nurtured pessimism about the 'morbid' state of Western society. Epilepsy became entangled in this confusion – seen as much as a social as a medical condition. Societal concerns also influenced medical beliefs particularly in the field of genetics and psychoanalysis, putting pay to the naïve idea held by some scientists that their disciplines were on a higher plane and isolated from the normal influences of social life.

Science gathered pace, but its influence proved in part a siren call. As we shall see some scientific developments were truly beneficial but others were to have a doleful effect on people with epilepsy, whose lives were as much battered by erroneous scientific theories as by war or religion. Progress in four areas had a particular impact on epilepsy: psychiatry and heredity (both of which had markedly negative effects), and neurophysiology and neuro-pharmacology (generally positive effects). These contradictory currents form major themes in this period, bracketed by the calamity of the two most devastating wars in human history. But, as has been observed by many, ironically it was war itself which stimulated many of the advances of medicine, including some which were to benefit epilepsy.

Scientific medicine developed strongly, especially in the later interwar years.[5] New investigations were introduced, notably in radiology and clinical pathology, and medical specialisation advanced, led by America.[6] Of greatest importance to epilepsy was the introduction of EEG: this was, in the subsequent decades, going to change the whole conceptual basis of epilepsy. Funding of clinical medicine and research enjoyed a boost, and that provided

---

[3] An influential intellectual group exploring this idea was the 'Pareto Circle' of academics at Harvard in the 1930s.

[4] See, for instance, Parsons, *Structure of Social Action*.

[5] In America, the number of hospital beds rose from 400,000 in 1909 to more than a million in 1932. 'Modernism' was a strong trend, with an emphasis on efficiency and hospitals were described as 'health factories' or 'health manufacturing plants' (see Lawrence, 'Continuity in crisis').

[6] The rise in medical specialisation and its impact on epilepsy is described in more detail in the next chapter.

by the Rockefeller Foundation in America was particularly relevant to neurology and psychiatry.[7] In the increasingly secular and industrialised world, medicine was claiming new territory and began to impinge on social policy relating to housing, nutrition, welfare and many aspects of human behaviour. In short, for the first time, medicine, and its science and social impact, were seen as central to the condition and culture of a nation. In parallel, governments became increasingly involved in healthcare decisions, with the result that the medical care of epilepsy became bound up with politics and economics to an unprecedented extent.

To picture medicine as uniform and science-based, though, would be wrong. Throughout this period, there was also a strong 'holistic' tendency amongst those who considered modern medicine to be too atomised.[8] Hygienic treatment was strongly emphasised. Antivivisectionist movements continued to exert a powerful influence.[9] Psychiatry throughout this period clung to its position as the primary medical specialty for epilepsy. Its theories, though, had a dire effect on the generality of persons with epilepsy by the linking of epilepsy to mental deficiency and by the impact of the psychoanalytical concepts of the epileptic personality and of epilepsy itself. Psychology, too, with the widespread usage of psychometric scales, reinforced the public perception that epilepsy was a form of mental defect. Perhaps largely because of psychoanalysis, neurology began strongly to differentiate itself from psychiatry, and the neurology of epilepsy turned to the strictly organic aspects of causation and pathophysiology. The drug treatment of epilepsy began to improve: at the beginning of this period with the introduction of phenobarbitone, and at its end with the discovery of phenytoin. The greater application of the science of medicinal chemistry and the introduction of new treatments increased the power and influence of the medical profession and led, especially in neurology, to a harder, more authoritarian and elitist stance amongst doctors in their dealings with epileptic patients.

In the early interwar years, the social and medical concepts coalesced in regard to ideas of degeneration, mental disorder, and inheritance. These were essentially medico-cultural phenomena which had gathered force throughout the first decades of the century. It was to be in Nazi Germany and its satellites

---

[7] The Rockefeller foundation had a great influence on the development of epilepsy, not least by its training fellowships and its funding of many leading epilepsy figures. In 1932, the foundation transformed psychiatry and mental health with the launch of a programme spending $60 million on infrastructure and research in epilepsy and other psychiatric disorders.

[8] An example was that of Germany in the Nazi period. There medicine, linked as it was to racial hygiene, lauded mawkish and holistic values and anti-specialist ideologies.

[9] The first legislation concerning the use of animals in research was the British 1876 Cruelty to Animals Act. As we saw in the previous chapter, the antivivisectionists clashed with the epilepsy researchers in the nineteenth century, and were to clash repeatedly in later years.

that the greatest damage from these concepts occurred. But in almost all cultures, the stigma of epilepsy remained, bringing shame to the families of sufferers. As in earlier decades, where possible, epilepsy was concealed or denied. It is with this dismal prospect that this chapter in the history of epilepsy opens.

EPILEPSY AND THE FIRST WORLD WAR

World wars scarred the beginning and end of this period and had a variety of consequences for those with epilepsy. Social isolation was reinforced by the prohibition on persons with epilepsy from serving on the front line or in advanced positions. This was not necessarily because of the risk of seizures but also because deficient moral fibre was widely assumed to be part of the condition and because of the notion that fits might be contagious or cause copycat hysterical behaviour. This was faintly ironic, as the advances in military weaponry resulted in many open head injuries, with epilepsy a not uncommon sequel.

The flood of wounded soldiers from the battlefields of World War One boosted the status and perceived importance of neurosurgery and led to great improvement in the acute treatment of head injury with knock-on effects on epilepsy. The leading anglophone neurosurgeons Victor Horsley, Percy Sargent and Harvey Cushing each published guidelines for the treatment of head injury in military practice[10], and a detailed analysis of the outcome of modern practice was subsequently published by William Adie.[11] All guidelines emphasised the advantages of early surgery, the importance of wound debridement, removal of bone and missile fragments, good surgical drainage, strict antisepsis, the creation of a large skin flap, copious irrigation and meticulous post-operative nursing. These practical measures unquestionably improved the outcome of head injury and also lowered the risk of post-traumatic epilepsy.

Interesting differences of emphasis characterised the approach of Anglo-American and German military medicine. German surgeons took a more conservative stance, both in defining indications for surgical intervention and in limiting the extent of primary surgery at the front.[12] The German view seems to have been that most such injuries were fatal and that a period of delay before

---

[10] For a review of the contribution of Horsley and Sargent to military neurology, see Shorvon and Compston, *Queen Square*, Ch.9. Cushing's contribution is discussed by Carey, 'Cushing'; see also Cushing, 'Study of a series'.

[11] Adie and Wagstaffe, *Note on a Series*. Adie analysed 656 cases of gunshot wounds to the head admitted to the British Military Hospital No. 7 in Saint-Omer between 1916 and 1917. Of these, 415 died as a result of the injury and almost always with cerebral infection or abscess. Five per cent of the survivors developed epilepsy. Adie was a neurologist at the National Hospital, Queen Square and Moorfields Eye Hospital.

[12] This approach was expanded upon in a report of the Second German Surgical Congress in 1916: Eiselsberg, 'Report on gunshot injuries'. Eiselsberg gave a detailed account of his war years in his memoir titled *Lebensweg eines Chirurgen* (pp. 233–59).

surgery would help determine its advisability. As a result, post-traumatic epilepsy was said to be more common in survivors. There was also debate in German circles about whether to leave a skull defect open in cases of epilepsy and whether surgery for epilepsy per se should be delayed, if carried out at all. Interestingly, phenobarbital was recommended for epilepsy only in the German military (along with bromides and a salt-free diet), perhaps a demonstration that Hauptmann's landmark discovery was better known in Germany than in France, Britain or America.

The First World War provided the opportunity to advance knowledge about the clinical features and frequency of post-traumatic epilepsy.[13] In a sample of 26,000 British military personnel receiving a pension due to a head injury, studied by Peter Ascroft, 34% of those with gunshot wounds to the head had developed epilepsy,[14] with epilepsy twice as common (45%) after penetrating injury than after wounds with no dural penetration (23%). In the German military, Lene Credner followed 1,980 head-injured soldiers for more than 5 years and 331 for more than 10 years after a severe head injury; 38% developed epilepsy.[15] Charles Symonds was the first to point out that there was a 'latent period' before the development of epilepsy, with the peak at eight months after the injury, and that a few cases occurred years later (one case after a delay of 16 years).[16]

Another effect of the First World War was the 'epidemic' of hysterical symptoms including non-epileptic attacks, probably more frequent on the battlefield than genuine epileptic seizures. These were one manifestation of what came to be known as *shell shock*, a condition which appeared in the French, British and German armies within a few months of the launch of hostilities on the Western Front in France. As the number of cases rapidly increased, a debate ensued about whether this seemingly new condition was a form of blast injury or concussion (commotional injury), or psychoneurosis. In December 1914, the epilepsy specialist William Aldren Turner was dispatched by the British War Office to investigate the growing epidemic of cases. There he met the neurologist Gordon Holmes and physician-psychologist Charles Myers, and together they engaged upon a series of analyses and interventions. The term 'shell shock' was coined by Myers in a paper in *The Lancet* in which he described three examples, concluding that the relationship of these cases to hysteria was 'close'.[17] A less sophisticated and less kind view was taken by

[13] See Sargent, 'Observations on epilepsy'; Ascroft, 'Traumatic epilepsy'; Credner, 'Klinische und soziale Auswirkungen'; Symonds, 'Traumatic epilepsy'; Denny-Brown, 'Clinical aspects'; Foerster and Penfield, 'Structural basis'.

[14] Ascroft, 'Traumatic epilepsy'.   [15] Credner, 'Klinische und soziale Auswirkungen'.

[16] Symonds, 'Traumatic epilepsy'.

[17] Myers, 'Shell-shock'. Later he regretted using the term and suggested that it be dropped – a suggestion adopted in a 1922 Commission report on shell shock. Myers was a close associate of W. H. R. Rivers, and both were important figures in wartime neurology (see Shephard, *Headhunters*).

almost all the Allied military authorities, who considered the symptoms to be 'pure funk' and the affected soldiers to be 'scrimshankers'. Similarly, in Germany, Emil Kraepelin took the view that the cause was not so much the environment of industrialised warfare, but more a sign of poor 'heredity' and degeneracy that resulted in these 'severe neurasthenic states'.[18] This strand of medical opinion was typified by Charles Wilson (Lord Moran), later to be Winston Churchill's personal physician, who wrote that war neurosis was a form of degeneracy linked to urbanisation:

> Such men went about plainly … unable to stand this test of men. They had about them the marks known to our calling of the incomplete man, the stamp of degeneracy … just a worthless chap, without shame, the worst product of the towns … [sent to] a shell-shock hospital with a rabble of misshapen creatures from the towns.[19]

Although initially Turner and Myers had planned to evacuate the shell-shocked soldiers back to Britain, the number of cases increased so rapidly as to make this impractical. Furthermore, it became accepted that early treatment close to the front line had the best chance of success. So forward treatment centres were created, and only the most recidivist cases were sent home. A variety of treatment approaches were taken just behind the front lines, including hypnotism, massage, rest, drug-induced sleep and a programme of graduated exercise and route marches. The soldiers who were returned to the United Kingdom were sent to various specialist centres, including Craiglockhart War Hospital, where W. H. R. Rivers famously treated Siegfried Sassoon with his psychoanalytic approach, and the National Hospital for the Paralysed and Epileptic[20] in London, where Lewis Yealland and Edgar Adrian employed 're-education' and 'counter-suggestion' using electrical shocks.[21]

Broadly comparable numbers of cases developed in the German trenches, where a similar pattern of care and range of treatments was employed.[22] In Germany, resistant cases were admitted to hospitals such as the Charité in Berlin (whose director then was Karl Bonhoeffer; 1,043 cases during the war)

---

[18] Kraepelin, *Psychiatrie*, p. 39.   [19] Wilson, *Anatomy of Courage*, pp. 20–1.

[20] During the First World War, up to 100 of the hospital's 270 beds were occupied by wounded soldiers, and a total of 1,272 servicemen were treated there.

[21] Yealland and Adrian, 'Common war neuroses'. Yealland and Adrian devised a form of therapy based on the power of suggestion and re-education, methods which hovered between persuasion and punishment. Yealland's *Hysterical Disorders of Warfare* (1918) contains detailed descriptions of the feigned 'fits' in shell shock and the mode of therapy. Edgar Douglas Adrian was awarded the 1932 Nobel Prize for Physiology or Medicine, jointly with Sherrington, for work on the function of neurons.

[22] Details taken especially from the work of Stephanie Linden. See Linden and Jones, 'German battle casualties'; Linden, Hess and Jones, 'Neurological manifestations'; Linden and Jones, '"Shell shock" revisited'. Of course, the effect of selection bias is an alternative explanation for the differences.

and Jena (under the direction of Binswanger; 2,275 cases during the war). The intriguing observation that non-organic seizures were a more common manifestation of shell shock amongst German than among British troops has been made on the basis that only 7% of the shell-shock cases admitted to Queen Square were due to non-epileptic seizures, compared to 28% admitted to the Charité, providing (albeit weak) evidence that the form the functional illness took was related to societal influences.[23] Both the German and British sides concurred that non-epileptic seizures were an unsavoury and particularly untreatable manifestation of war neurosis.[24]

In Britain, a War Office Commission was appointed in 1920 which heard exhaustive evidence. The commission's final report is the definitive statement on the condition.[25] It was concluded that treatment close to the front should be offered where possible, and every effort should be taken to prevent affected soldiers from leaving the battalion or divisional area. Better screening of personnel prior to recruitment was recommended, and under the influence of Holmes and the military authorities, it was also agreed that no soldier should be allowed to think that loss of nervous or mental control could provide an honourable avenue of escape from the battlefield, and only in exceptional circumstances would individuals be returned to the United Kingdom. In hospitals, the sufferers should be housed separately from other sick or wounded men. It was also recommended that these policies should be made widely known throughout the services. When cases were sufficiently severe to necessitate more scientific or elaborate treatment, they ought to be sent to special neurological centres. It is notable, too, that in the German guidelines for treatment (written in December 1916), neurotic soldiers classified as 'unfit for military service' or 'fit for home duty' were discharged without a military pension.[26]

In 1939, in preparation for the Second World War, it was made widely known that there would be no war pensions for psychological disorders. As a result of this, as well as new strategies of prevention and management and better screening on recruitment, shell shock and non-epileptic seizures were much less of a problem. It seems the lessons of the Great War had been learned.

PSYCHIATRY OF EPILEPSY

The battlefield neuroses in the First World War may have contributed to another remarkable and perhaps surprising development in the militarised culture of the times: the elevation of psychology and psychiatry to the status

[23] Linden, Hess and Jones, 'Neurological manifestations'.
[24] For an interesting description of alternative views of war neurosis in Germany at the time, see Eissler, Freud as an Expert Witness.
[25] Report of the War Office, p. 92.   [26] Linden and Jones, 'German battle casualties'.

of serious scientific disciplines. In the field of epilepsy this had a profoundly negative impact in three particular ways: first, the consolidation of the link between mental deficiency to idiopathic epilepsy and its inherited nature; second, the rise of psychoanalysis, which viewed epileptic seizures to be the result of psychological mechanisms; and third, the bolstering of opinion that people with epilepsy had a specific defective personality structure.

Psychology, Mental Defect and Idiopathic Epilepsy

The blanket term 'mental disorder' had in the nineteenth and early twentieth century included those with defects of intelligence (then called mental defi-ciency and now learning disability) as well as those with defects of behaviour, conduct and mood (for instance insanity or psychosis, now referred to as psychiatric disorders) and those who developed cognitive impairment in later life (now referred to as dementia). No clear distinction was made between the three quite distinct entities,[27] and all sufferers were bundled together in lunatic asylums. As Lionel Penrose put it, the word 'mental' described the whole class of conditions which exonerated 'the average medical practitioner ... from having to probe further into the matter'.[28] Idiopathic epilepsy was included in this mix and itself considered a mental disorder in which defects of behav-iour, conduct, mood and intelligence were inevitable components (as Turner had written in 1907 'psychical phenomena' were one aspect of the 'symptom-complex' of epilepsy[29]). In the interwar years, the three categories began to be differentiated but in many texts all three were still considered linked and terminology was applied in an erratic and arbitrary way.

A leading figure in the field of mental deficiency was Henry Goddard, an American psychologist and director of research at the Vineland Colony. In 1914, Goddard published his findings in 327 cases, mainly children with developmental disorders, resident in the Vineland Colony, of whom 79 had epilepsy.[30] Goddard's data and analyses were careless, and his science poor. His subjective biases were expressed as fact; yet, falling on freshly ploughed eugenical ground, they rapidly took root and his book had great traction with the public. He confirmed the prevailing opinion that mental defect was often the result of a diathesis inherited in a Mendelian fashion, 'transmitted as truly and accurately as colour of hair, stature or any other character' (p. 438), and in this category he

---

[27] A legal distinction was made in Britain only with the passage of the 1913 Mental Deficiency Act.

[28] Penrose, *Mental Defect*, p. 1. Lionel Sharples Penrose was Professor of Human Genetics at University College London, and a leading international figure in the field of intellectual disability. His major research project was the Colchester Survey of 1931–9, sponsored by the Medical Research Council (MRC), in which he examined 1,280 patients with mental defects and 6,629 siblings and parents in more than 400 families (Penrose, *Clinical and Genetic Study*).

[29] Turner, *Epilepsy*, p. 118.   [30] Goddard, *Feeble-Mindedness*.

included epilepsy. He subdivided the cases into three categories determined by IQ testing: morons (IQ 51–70), imbeciles (IQ 26–50) and idiots (IQ 25 or under). The most significant tribulations were encountered in the case of 'morons' (roughly equivalent to the English usage of 'feeble-minded'[31]), who Goddard found 'are often normal looking, with few or no obvious stigmata of degeneration ... yet they are persons who make for us social problems' (pp. 4–5). He listed pauperism, crime, prostitution, intemperance and truancy as examples of their moral defects – echoing late-nineteenth-century psychiatric theory. Over the next decade, Goddard's system of categorisation, based on IQ, became widely adopted, and patients with epilepsy were found in all three categories. As Stephen Jay Gould pointed out,[32] such measurement invoked two inherent fallacies: converting complex abstract concepts such as intelligence into single concrete entities, and ranking multiple complex variables into a single scale. However, at the time, the act of quantitation raised the profile of psychology to the level of a 'true science' and gave it legitimacy, despite the fact that the scheme was naïve and simplistic not to mention prejudicial.

To solve the problem of feeble-mindedness and epilepsy, Goddard turned to eugenics:

> The feeble-minded person is not desirable, he is a social encumbrance, often a burden to himself. In short it were better both for him and for society had he never been born ... It is perfectly clear that no feeble-minded person should ever be allowed to marry or to become a parent ...
> To this end there are two proposals: the first is colonization, the second is sterilization. (pp. 558, 565, 566)

To Goddard, epilepsy was the cause of feeble-mindedness in some cases, or part of the syndrome of inherited feeble-mindedness in others (p. 512). He did recognise that a minority of cases of epilepsy were not inherited, but most were, and for these cases he pressed for eugenic solutions.

According to Penrose, the hardening of attitudes towards the mentally ill in the second and third decades of the century reflected two fundamental and connected factors: first, the popularisation of ideas concerning heredity as a cause of illness; second, the growth of an agnostic materialistic outlook. He was surely correct. As a result, epilepsy and mental disorder changed in the interwar years, from being largely biological or medical problems to become what were essentially social and economic issues. As Penrose pointed out, a popular narrative arose that 'mental defectives' were

---

[31] In America, the term 'feeble-minded' was used to refer to all classes of mental deficiency ('morons, idiots and imbeciles').

[32] Gould, *Mismeasure*.

a class of vast and dangerous dimensions, and since it had already been shown that improvement on a large scale was not to be looked for, there was nothing to be done but to blame heredity and advocate methods of extinction … [T]he influence of the studies of Davenport and of Goddard both among medical men and among laymen has been such that they are largely responsible for the beliefs prevailing today.[33]

Two sociocultural factors contributed to widespread disparagement of those with mental disorders. First was the failure of the earlier, and over-optimistic, claims that training would provide a 'cure' (as suggested, for instance, by the progressive ideas of Maria Montessori and others).[34] In the 1910s, this view was increasingly challenged, especially by Alfred Binet and Theodore Simon, who maintained that the mentally defective had only limited educable potential.[35] The second was the widespread adoption of IQ testing as a scientific way of quantifying and categorising mental deficiency. Using these measures, to the alarm of the public, the number of individuals with low levels of intelligence was found to be much greater than previously thought. It was the burgeoning of the 'moron' class which caused particular concern, associated as it had become with the new concept of 'social incompetence'. The public became bewitched by numbers and rankings. This did serious harm to those at the lower end of the scales, and contributed to the prevailing trope that the defective was not so much an innocent deserving pity but more a 'menace' and an economic and social burden.

In 1908, Alfred Tredgold published what was probably the first significant twentieth-century theoretical text on mental deficiency. This was to become the standard book on the subject, going through eleven editions that reveal the evolution of thought in the interwar years.[36] To Tredgold, mental deficiency ('amentia') could be broadly divided into two categories: primary amentia, in which the amentia was due largely to an intrinsic inherited defect of germ plasm, and secondary amentia, in which external factors operated after birth and inhibited mental development. In the earlier editions of this book, Tredgold conceived the co-existence of epilepsy with amentia[37] in three different categories: (1) primary

---

[33] Penrose, *Mental Defect*, pp. 6–7.

[34] Much of the early work on mental deficiency, including epilepsy, was concerned with education. In the nineteenth century, 'idiots' were considered educable by physicians using techniques of sensationalism – an approach in which sensation or sense perception were considered the basis of knowledge, and the idea that the mind was a 'tabula rasa'. This was most clearly stated in the work of Édouard Séguin, *Traitement Moral*.

[35] Binet and Simon, *Mentally Defective Children*; Binet, *Intelligence of the Feeble-Minded*.

[36] Tredgold, *Mental Deficiency (Amentia)*. Tredgold was based at University College Hospital London and a leading authority on mental handicap. His book had a remarkable publishing history. The first eight editions were published during his lifetime: 1908, 1914, 1920, 1922, 1929, 1937, 1947 and 1952. Another three editions were published posthumously by his son in 1956, 1963 and 1970. Strangely, the dedication of the books was 'to all those persons of sound mind'.

[37] The term 'amentia' was coined by Theodore Meynert in 1890 and was also used by Freud. Meynert, Freud and Tredgold each used the term with entirely different meanings.

amentia, in which epilepsy occurs as a complication of the inherited impaired processes of development; (2) idiopathic epilepsy, in which the occurrence of epilepsy causes the amentia– a theory now recognised as false; and (3) gross cerebral lesions which causes both epilepsy and amentia (1908, pp. 196–7).

Primary amentia (category (1)) today would include what we know as specific inborn errors of metabolism and other congenital and genetic defects, most of which were not recognised at the time. Epilepsy was, in Tredgold's view, the commonest 'complication' of primary amentia (occurring in 11% of the feeble-minded, 42% of imbeciles and 56% of 'idiots'), and that it also contributed to mental decline in the same way as it might do in all patients, depending on the frequency and severity of the attacks. When seizures were frequent and severe, the patient would rapidly lose 'even his limited acquirements'; if slight or infrequent, no deterioration would occur (p. 191).[38]

It was category (2) which Tredgold considered true 'epileptic' amentia. In these cases he noted only slight evidence of the stigmata of degeneration. As he put it in the first edition of his book in 1908, the person with idiopathic epilepsy could be distinguished from the 'primary ament by being well developed and well grown, and by his comely and prepossessing appearance' (p. 194). Tredgold believed, completely wrongly, that as was 'common knowledge[,] frequently repeated severe convulsions ... occurring in a person of mature cerebral development may give rise to dementia' (p. 197). This result, however, 'is not invariable' (p. 211). In epileptic amentia, the seizures start in the first few years of life and impair mental development. The degree of mental deficiency varied, and in mild cases, not much headway was made at school and then manual employment was possible. 'But the persistence of the fits gradually strips these persons of any acquirements they may have possessed, and in the majority of cases dementia is but a question of time' (p. 199). All this was, of course, nonsense, but by the fifth edition of his book (1929), he still felt that the chronic idiopathic epilepsy led to dementia, especially if early onset,[39] but conceded that few of his patients (around 1%) were in this category.

Tredgold was also utterly mistaken in a second fundamental way – in his acceptance of the concept of the neuropathic diathesis ('the neurological trait') in a form largely unchanged since the late nineteenth century. He did not agree that the germinal impairment was atavistic or had ape-like characteristics, as claimed by Cesare Lombroso and reiterated by Davenport, so progress on this front at least had been made.[40] However, even in the later editions of his book, he still maintained

[38] This belief in the deleterious effects of seizures has been an orthodox view since at least Gower's time, but nowadays has been largely rejected.

[39] Tredgold cited, and agreed with, the statement of George Savage that 'epilepsy occurring before *seven* years of age is certain to leave the patient weak-minded' (Tredgold, 1908, p. 198).

[40] In fact, by 1915 Lombroso's theories were largely rejected, although his broad conception of the biological basis of behaviour was widely accepted.

that the neuropathic trait was at the core of the genetic inheritance.[41] In his Galton
Lecture of 1927 and the 1937 edition of his slightly retitled book,[42] he opined that
although not a mutation of any specific gene (or combination of genes), the trait
was 'a general impairment of the vitality and developmental potentiality of those
genes which are responsible for the growth of the brain' (p. 34), causing development to proceed in a certain particular direction and only up to a certain limit. He
accepted that the nature of the germ plasm defect was 'conjectural' for by then
attempts to show that mental defect was transmitted by Mendelian laws had
completely failed and Davenport's simplistic genetic theories of epilepsy were no
longer accepted. Tredgold also realised that eugenic measures against sufferers
would not reduce the number of carriers of poor genes. Nevertheless, in all editions
of his book, he favoured limiting procreation. Initially he focused on segregation,
but by 1937 his approach had hardened and he leaned toward voluntary
sterilisation.[43] One senses in his writings, over time, an increasing lack of compassion. For instance, regarding 'profound idiocy', he opined in 1929: 'The depth of
their degeneration is such that existence − for it can hardly be called life − is on a
lower plane than even the beasts of the field' (1929, p. 159). This noticeable shift
was perhaps a consequence of the propaganda of the eugenics lobby, which was
especially intense in the United States[44].

Tredgold also introduced the concept of moral deficiency, which was later
called psychopathy.[45] This became enshrined in Britain in the mental deficiency acts of 1913 and 1927, and in the latter was defined as a property of those
in whom 'there exists mental defectiveness coupled with strongly vicious or
criminal propensities'.[46] Moral deficiency was thought initially to be commoner in the mental defective population, and especially in those with epilepsy, but later studies showed this not to be the case. J. E. Wallace Wallin

---

[41] Tredgold did accept that environmental influences were important, and he believed that the germ
plasm could be weakened by external influences (disregarding 'Weismann's barrier'). An example
was stress in the precipitation of shell shock, but he nevertheless considered that the 'real cause of
breakdown [in shell shock] was constitutional rather than environmental' (p. 3).

[42] Tredgold, *Text-Book* (1937).

[43] Tredgold, *Text-Book*, p. 519. The British Mental Deficiency Act did not endorse sterilisation,
as Tredgold wrote, 'owing to a parliamentary outburst of hysterical sentiment' (p. 519). He
also noted that, by comparing the findings of the Royal Commission in 1908 with those of the
report of the Board of Education and Board of Control in 1929, the total number of 'aments'
in England and Wales had nearly doubled in the twenty-year interval, and the topic was
therefore one of great demographic importance.

[44] In the 1920s and 1930s, eugenic thought permeated many aspects of American art, literature,
film, social debate and social mores. The extraordinary profusion of eugenic ideas outside the
field of genetics was a remarkable phenomenon; see Currell and Cogdell, *Popular Eugenics*.

[45] The term 'psychopathie' was introduced by the German psychiatrist Julius Koch in *Die
psychopathischen Minderwertigkeiten* (1891–93), initially to encompass a wide range of mental
disorders. Its meaning changed progressively over the twentieth century.

[46] The term 'moral defective' was so defined in section 21 (1) of the 1927 act, replacing the term
'moral imbecile' of the 1913 act. See discussion in *Report of the Mental Deficiency Committee*, pp.
17–22.

summed up what was probably the prevalent view by the late 1940s: that this was a concept so vaguely defined as to have little value either in medicine or in legislation.[47]

By the 1920s and 1930s, medical concepts advanced in two further ways which were to render Tredgold's ideas of epilepsy obsolete. First, it was recognised that mental defect with epilepsy had a variety of biological causes and was not a unitary condition – and certainly not a condition inherited as a Mendelian recessive, as Davenport and Goddard had maintained. This, more than anything else, resulted in rejection of the theory of the neuropathic diathesis. A key figure was Archibald Garrod, then a physician at St Bartholomew's Hospital and the Hospital for Sick Children in London and later to become Regius Professor of Medicine in Oxford. He coined the expression 'inborn errors of metabolism' in his 1908 Croonian Lecture at the Royal College of Physicians.[48] Based on studies of alkaptonuria and three other conditions, Garrod considered that disease might be due to inherited enzyme defects in a metabolic pathway, and in 1909 he published his ideas in a book (a landmark in the field) titled *Inborn Errors of Metabolism*.[49] The idea that mental deficiency was not a homogeneous disease but could be the result of various distinct inherited biochemical defects in what Garrod called 'chemical physiology' was a paradigm shift.[50] Later, many more conditions would be added, and the discovery of phenylketonuria in 1934 by Ivar Asbjørn Følling[51] led to the first neonatal screening as a means of preventing mental deficiency and, as about half of sufferers have seizures, epilepsy.

The second advance from the point of view of epilepsy was the belated recognition both that the majority of persons with idiopathic epilepsy did not suffer from mental deficiency, and also that repeated seizures did not usually lead to mental deterioration. These conceptual shifts became self-evident when it was realised that findings from asylum-based studies could not be extrapolated to

---

[47] Wallin, *Mental and Physical Handicaps*. The concept of moral deficiency had a direct lineage from Lombroso. It was widely held that criminality was strongly associated with mental deficiency. Goddard, for instance, had estimated the frequency of mental defect among delinquents to be between 25% and 90% (see Woodward, 'Low intelligence in delinquency').

[48] Garrod, 'Croonian Lectures'.   [49] Garrod, *Inborn Errors of Metabolism*.

[50] As well as launching a new discipline within the field of medical genetics, Garrod's work provided an entirely new view of people's biochemical individuality and of the complex interaction between nature and nurture that underlies human disease. According to David Weatherall, 'there have been few fundamentally new concepts in the field of human genetics since his time … [T]he ideas that he set out in *Inborn factors* [in] *disease* are almost identical to those that led to current genome searches for genetic variation that underlies susceptibility or resistance to common diseases … [A]s well as opening up a completely new field of biological thinking they emphasised the critical importance of the role of physician–scientists, with their unique opportunity to take questions from the bedside into the laboratory' (Weatherall, 'Garrod's Croonian lectures').

[51] Følling, 'Über Ausscheidung von Phenylbrenztraubensäure'. Phenylkenonuria is also known as Følling's disease. Følling held the Chair in Biochemistry at Oslo University and was Physician-in-Chief at Oslo University Hospital.

persons with epilepsy in the community, as articulated clearly and precisely by Douglas Thom[52] in 1922 whose opinion still stands largely unchanged today:

> Until recently practically all of our observations on the subject of epilepsy have been considered from the institutional point of view. That is, our clinical observations, our pathological investigations, and, to a very large extent, our experimental therapy, have been confined to patients whose symptoms have been of such severity and long duration that they have necessitated their institutional supervision. This group not only represents less than 3 per cent of all individuals suffering from chronic convulsive disorders but as a group they appear to be quite different in their physical and mental symptomatology ... These cases stand out in marked contrast to the great majority of patients that one sees in our outpatient clinics and in private practice ... The general practitioner and the neuropsychiatrist in private practice find that but a relatively small per cent of their epileptic patients are deteriorated intellectually; psychotic symptoms are infrequent and neurological signs indicating organic disease are the exception. It is true that we do see the feeble-minded child who is having convulsions, but the convulsions are probably part and parcel of the same pathogenic condition which produced the feeble-mindedness. We are all familiar with those personality changes which so commonly are associated with epilepsy or any chronic disease of long standing; irritability, hypochondriacal ideas, depressions, self-centeredness, are certainly not confined to the epileptic, and we find many individuals who have suffered from epilepsy for years quite free from the so-called 'epileptic personality' ... A large part of this non-institutionalized group are carrying on either in school, the store, shop, factory, office or whatever their vocation may be. Inquiry has revealed that several large industries have had epileptics in their employ over a long period of time, and the occupational history of those individuals coming to our outpatient dispensaries or our clinics, indicates that they are in a very large measure industrially efficient. (pp. 626–9)

This was well said – and reflected the sea change in theory that was occurring in advanced neuropsychiatry in the 1920s.[53] It seems surprising today that the bias of studies restricted to asylums took so long to be appreciated (in 1923, there were said to be 24,018 epileptic patients in the US state mental institutions,

---

[52] Thom, 'Rational extra-institutional treatment'. Douglas Armour Thom was a psychiatrist whose work deserves to be better known. He did much to bring neuropsychiatry on a scientific basis. While he worked at the Monson colony in Massachusetts he investigated and concluded that epilepsy was seldom inherited. He was involved in work on shell shock in England during the First World War. He was best known as the pioneer of the Habit Clinic for Child Guidance, and for relating neurological and psychological disturbances to maladjustment in early childhood (see 'Obituary').

[53] In a similar vein, Lennox in 1931 wrote 'Much of the present-day misconception concerning epilepsy arises from the fact that although only approximately 1 in 20 of the persons subject to recurring seizures are in institutions, information concerning these piled-together, driftwood human beings has been easily assembled and when published has been accepted as representing all persons afflicted with seizures' (Lennox, 'Epilepsy').

with, it was estimated, 700,000 epilepsy cases in the population).[54] But Thom's conclusions did fly in the face of previously orthodox opinion, at a time when 'sane epileptics' hardly featured in any medical texts and were largely ignored by the medical profession, at a time when most patients in the community kept very quiet about their epilepsy and consulted doctors infrequently. Whatever the reasons, the contrast between the views of Thom and the earlier pronouncements of Spratling, Davenport, Godard or Tredgold could hardly be greater.

A leading theorist of the late interwar years was Lionel Penrose. His book *Mental Defect* (1933) and its successor, *The Biology of Mental Defect* (1949), were widely recognised as definitive works. They clarified much of the confusion surrounding the genetics of mental deficiency and showed how concepts had changed. In *Mental Defect*, Penrose derided Tredgold's view 'that all mental disease was essentially the same and due to neuropathic constitution' as a 'type of generalization too wide to be of much service in scientific investigation' (p. 137). He pointed out that epilepsy was 'a symptom and not a disease', and that it could be produced in 'a great variety of ways' (p. 138). He cited the different examples of mongolism, birth injury, post-encephalitic cases, those with cranial deformities, microcephaly, cretinism, pituitary dystrophy, epiloia (tuberose sclerosis), neurofibromatosis and so on. By 1949, after a decade of further genetic discovery, Penrose was able to differentiate heredity cases by their mode of inheritance – that is, dominantly inherited conditions such as epiloia and neurofibromatosis; recessive conditions such as phenylketonuria, Wilson's disease, cretinism, galactosaemia and amaurotic idiocy (Tay-Sachs disease); X-linked conditions; and 'defects of obscure origin', which included mongolism.[55]

Penrose also developed what became the modern view of idiopathic epilepsy. He considered idiopathic epilepsy to have genetic causes which lowered the inherited 'epileptic threshold' to a level at which spontaneous seizures occurred. He recognised that there was an increased rate of epilepsy in the families of subjects with idiopathic epilepsy, but that this increase was slight as the genetic influence on the threshold was not an all-or-nothing phenomenon; rather, it was a matter of degree. He noted, too, the important fact that genetic carriers would be unaffected. He considered (rightly, as it turns out) that these

[54] 'Most persons are surprised to know that there are as many epileptic persons in this country as there are diabetic and tuberculous persons ... Others find it hard to be believe that 700,000 epileptics can live in the United States without it being known to everyone .:. The "epileptic personality" has been shown to be derived from a small segment of the epileptic population. Mental deterioration has been shown to be caused by lesions or disease processes other than the mechanisms related to seizures' (Price, Kogan and Tompkins, 'Extramural epilepsy', p. 48). In 1948, the best estimate of prevalence of epilepsy in the USA was 6/1,000 (Malzberg, 'Intramural epilepsy', pp. 42–7).

[55] Penrose, *Biology of Mental Defect*, p. 175. (By 1963, in the further revised edition of the book, the karyotype abnormality was also recognised as the cause of Down syndrome.)

genes might act by making slight structural or chemical changes in the nervous system. He also recognised that intelligence could be normal or even exceptional and furthermore that there was no evidence that seizures resulted in deterioration. Perhaps most important of all was the stand Penrose took against public hostility to mental handicap. His humane view was very different from the punitive disgust which seemed to be the norm in the works of the leading US and German alienists.[56] In 1933 he wrote:

> Since those days there has been an extraordinary change of attitude amongst members of the general public and the medical profession towards the unfortunate idiots ... [T]he attitude implied is quite typical of views which are widely held at the present time, the word 'idiot' having become associated with ideas of sterilization and the lethal chamber.[57]

J. B. S. Haldane[58] would write in the preface to the first edition of Penrose's *Biology of Mental Defect* in 1949 that he hoped the book would not be used merely as a textbook by specialists but would be recognised as a contribution to thought and to humanism. In 1945, when Penrose was appointed to the chair in eugenics at University College London's Galton Laboratory, he shuddered at the title and eventually (though only in 1961) managed to persuade the university authorities to change it to 'Galton Professor of Human Genetics'. He hated the concept of eugenics and fought against it. But, as the 1930s progressed, as we shall see eugenic solutions to epilepsy were to take a new and ominous course.

Psychoanalytic Theory and Epilepsy

Another psychological theory impacting on epilepsy in the interwar years was psychoanalysis. In the nineteenth century David Ferrier, Hughlings Jackson and Victor Horsley had demonstrated that the anatomical location of epileptic fits was the grey matter of the brain. This, perhaps more than anything else,

---

[56] Penrose had a particular fondness for those with Down syndrome, admiring their 'secret source of joy'. He enjoyed playing with them in the kindergarten of the Galton Laboratory, and penned the doggerel: 'See the happy Mongol / He doesn't care a damn, / I wish I were a Mongol, / My God, perhaps I am.'

[57] Penrose, *Mental Defect*, pp. 3–4.

[58] Haldane, a highly original figure, held the positons of Fullerian Professor of Physiology at the Royal Institution, and Professor of Genetics and then the first Weldon Professor of biometry at University College London. He wrote of Penrose in the preface: 'Professor Penrose genuinely loves fools. When I presented him with certain calculations he accepted them with every mark of interest and pleasure. Soon afterwards I saw him examining the drawings of a defective, and expressing he same emotions. He was right. It is perhaps more remarkable that a boy who can hardly speak should be capable of excellent drawing than that one professor should be capable of helping another to analyse his data' (p. vii).

dispelled theories of possession and confirmed the physiological and organic nature of epilepsy. However, little progress had been made in establishing the cause or pathogenesis. It was into this knowledge vacuum that various erroneous theories flooded, including the aforementioned examples of autointoxication, reflex and contagion. Psychoanalysis, a term coined in 1896[59] by Sigmund Freud and developed progressively by Freud and his circle and successors, was to prove a particularly extravagant example.

Before the First World War, psychoanalysis attracted little attention in mainstream medicine, and most practitioners were fairly scathing about this seemingly outlandish theory. Rather typical was the exasperated outburst of a correspondent in the *British Medical Journal*:

> Surely the time has at last come when all psychologists, psychiatrics, and medical societies [should cease] to regard this modern and alien jargon about the 'unconscious' as matter for serious consideration, and follow the better course of killing the abounding nonsense of the Freudian 'Philosophy' by ridicule, or by letting it perish, at least in this country, from neglect of cultivation. At present it plays the part of a virulent pathogenic microbe in the wells whence psychiatrists drink.[60]

However, the large number of cases of battle neurosis in the Great War had shaken the medical profession and public, and both became interested in psychological mechanisms; the genie was out of the bottle. In an analysis of 1,043,654 British army casualties in the Somme, it was estimated that neurosis was the cause of around 35,000 cases (around 3% of the total, and up to 40% of those evacuated home). By 1918, a study of 160,000 pensioners found that around 20% were pensioned because of functional nervous and mental disease.[61] The curious theories of Freud and his associates then began to chime with the public mood. Psychoanalysis became an important element of popular culture, not only as an explanation of individual's personality defects but even for such issues as the progressive degradation of civilised life. Freud himself had taken the view that civilisation and repression were interlinked; the more civilised the behaviour, the more suppressed it was and thus neurotic. Psychoanalysis, like eugenics, offered a 'scientific' way forward. As *The Listener* put it:

[59] Freud, 'L'hérédité et l'étiologie'.
[60] H. B. D., 'Popular Freudism'. This letter was published in response to a review of Freud's *Psychopathology of Everyday Life*. Psychoanalysis was also strongly criticised by one of London's most colourful doctors, the forensic psychiatrist Charles Mercier. He (anonymously) wrote an amusingly sarcastic polemic in which he also poked fun at, amongst others, the neurologists at the National Hospital, Queen Square for their lack of treatment and hypocrisy. In other works, he also denounced Haldane and Bertrand Russell as traitors, attacked vegetarianism and published a satire on spiritualism.
[61] Wittkower and Spillane, 'Neurosis in war', p. 8.

Freud's work received little attention at first. When it began to be known, in the decade before the War, it met with bitter opposition on all sides. It was not till the twenties that complexes and repressions, transference and sublimation invaded the drawing-rooms of the English-speaking world. Freud's theories (half understood and loosely applied) served a convenient excuse for all sorts of public discussion and private behaviour.[62]

It was in this cultural context that psychoanalytic theories of epilepsy, amongst other conditions, became mainstream topics. Perhaps surprisingly, psychoanalytical theory also attracted some neurologists, particularly in the United States, including leading figures in the neurology of epilepsy, such as James Jackson Putnam, L. Pierce Clark, Charles Dana, Morton Prince and Smith Ely Jelliffe. All inclined towards this new explanation of mental processes.[63]

Psychoanalysis provided a novel explanation of epilepsy. As its theories matured, the view grew that essential epilepsy was the result of inhibited psychological development caused by inherited traits which prevented normal psychic development and were manifest both by epileptic seizures and abnormalities of personality. The Hungarian Sándor Ferenczi,[64] a leading early psychoanalyst. had the most to say about the condition. He had been a registrar at Szent Rókas Kórház (the 'Budapest Salpêtrière'), where he claimed to have observed hundreds of epileptic fits and wrote in 1916:

> Although I fully admit that in the question of epilepsy the physiological is difficult to separate from the psychological, I may call attention to the fact that epileptics are known to be uncommonly 'sensitive' beings, behind whose submissiveness[,] frightful rage and domineeringness can appear on the least occasion. This characteristic has up to the present usually been interpreted as a secondary degeneration, as the consequence of repeated attacks. One should, however, think of another possibility, namely whether the epileptic attacks are not to be considered as regressions to the infantile period of *wish-fulfilment by means of uncoordinated movements*. Epileptics would then be persons with whom the disagreeable affects get heaped up and are periodically abreacted in paroxysms.[65]

---

[62] *The Listener*, 14 (1935) p. 508.

[63] See Putnam, *Addresses on Psycho-Analysis*; Dana, 'Future of neurology'; Prince, 'American neurology'; Jelliffe, 'Fifty years'. Putnam was Professor of Diseases of the Nervous system at Harvard, founder member and president of the American Neurological Association, and later of president of the American Psychoanalytical Association. Dana was professor of nervous and mental disease at Cornell Medical College. His *Text-book of Nervous Diseases for the Use of Students and Practitioners of Medicine* went through ten editions between 1892 and 1925. Prince founded the American Psychopathological Association. Jelliffe was clinical professor of mental diseases at Fordham University, president of the New York Psychiatric Society, the New York Neurological Society, the American Psychopathological Association and editor-in-chief of the *Journal of Nervous and Mental Disease*.

[64] Ferenczi was one-time president of the International Psychoanalytical Association. He was an important theorist of the psychoanalytical movement and a member of Freud's inner circle.

[65] Ferenczi, 'Sense of reality'.

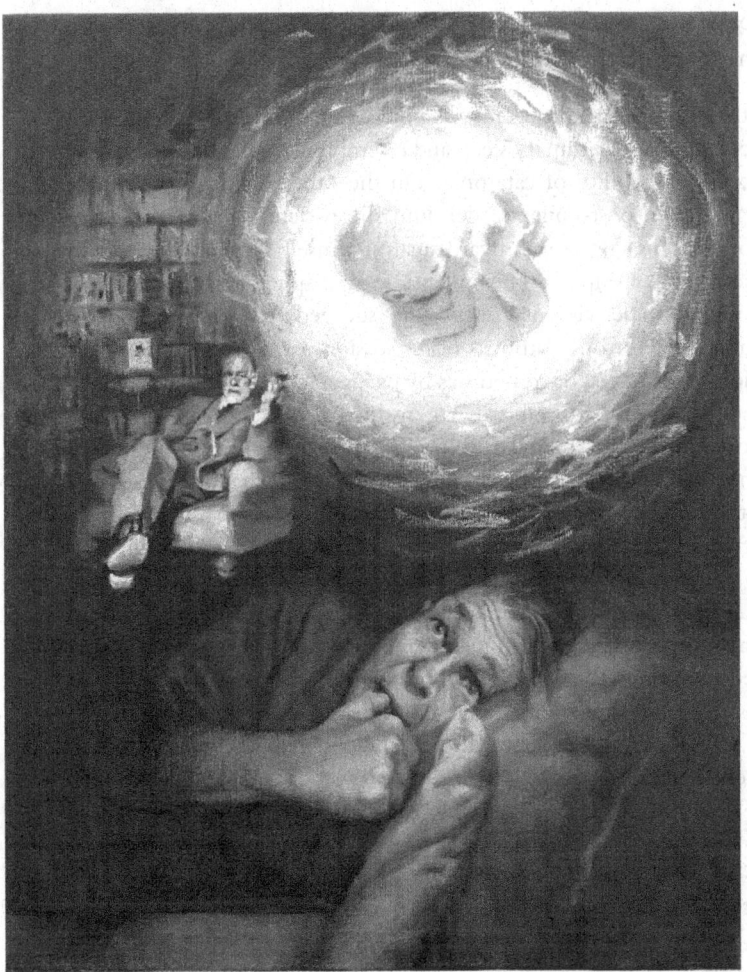

14. Infantile regression as the cause of epilepsy (A painting by David Cobley, 2021)

In his paper of around 1921,[66] Ferenzci offered a number of further observations and reflections which, although not sewn together into a coherent theory, do give a flavour of the psychoanalytical approach to epilepsy: '[Seizures are] a regression to an extremely primitive level of organization in which all inner excitations are discharged by the shortest motor pathway and all susceptibility to external stimuli is lost' (p. 197), or 'a regression to infantile omnipotence' (p. 198) and later a 'regression to an intra-uterine situation'. An epileptic seizure was similar to sleep, which psychoanalysis regarded as a state of regression to the antenatal state, with epilepsy being 'a state of exceptionally deep sleep'. Convulsions were reminiscent of the uncoordinated expressions of unpleasure

[66] Ferenczi, 'Epileptic fits'.

by a newborn, and during the later stupor the 'epileptic's attitude certainly resembles the foetus in the womb':

> When the fit is at its height we may assume a state of narcissistic regression far exceeding that of ordinary sleep and resembling cataleptic rigidity and the wax-like flexibility of catatonia. On the other hand, in the motor discharge and in post-epileptic delirium the patient rages at the outer world or turns his aggression inwards against himself; he thus clings fast to his 'object-relationship' ... The epileptic would appear to be a person of strong instincts and violent affects who succeeds for long periods in protecting himself from outbursts of his passions by extremely powerful repression of his urges, or sometimes by exaggerated humility and religiosity; but at appropriate intervals his instinctual drives break loose and rage, sometimes with bestial ruthlessness, not only against his whole environment but against his own person, which has become alien and hostile to him. This discharge of affect then brings about, often only for a few very brief moments, a sleep-like stage of rest, the pattern of which is that of the unborn child in the womb, or alternatively death ... The importance of the place occupied by sexuality among the instincts to which an epileptic fit gives rein is shown by the exceptional frequency of so-called sex criminals among epileptics, and the numerous sexual perversions, often in quite remarkable combinations, to be found among them ... In a number of cases, the fit appears to be actually a 'coitus equivalent'. (pp. 201–3)

To Freud, the symptoms of an epileptic fit expressed the frenzy of a tendency to self-destruction that is almost free from the inhibitions of the wish to live. Ferenczi agreed, and in accord with his experience in charge of a war hospital where one of his duties was to decide upon the fitness of many epileptics for service, he observed in genuine seizures life-threatening cessation of respiration and the risk of asphyxiation.[67]

Leon Pierce Clark was a leading figure in American neurology and psychiatry with a special interest in epilepsy, and, as we have seen, published definitive clinical and pathological studies of status epilepticus; he was also a convert to the theories of psychoanalysis. He considered the fit to be a regression, a flight from undue stress and a protective mechanism which withdraws or reduces the attachment and adjustment to reality, and in 1915, in a lengthy article in the *New York Medical Journal* on the nature and pathogenesis of epilepsy, argued:

> [that] the fit is a striving for expression of the libidinous energies in the unconscious; that the fit is therefore a libidinous outlet of the primal sexual energies and should be considered essentially as a pathological functioning of the unconscious; that this state is due to a condition of

[67] Ferenczi, 'Unwelcome child'.

mental infantilism caused by or coincident with a libidinous fixation in the earlier stages of psychosexual development.[68]

In an article in *Brain* in 1920 he stated that '[the fit] dispels an intolerable demand and the epileptic retreats to a state of harmony and peace'.[69] Muscular convulsions were comparable to the impulsive movements of the infant:

> We do not know just how the impulsive movements are incited further than to surmise that, being of the first, simplest and ontogenetic type of activities of the developing organism, their inciter is from motor centres of the lower order. In these latter structures are stored up a certain quantity of potential energy which is transformed into actual energy by the blood and lymph stream. With the increasing tissue growth and tension engendered thereby this energy finds its outlet in the random movements of the foetus and the infant, and their exaggerated distorted presence is seen in the major convulsion of epileptics. (p. 45)

As to the 'inciters' of the impulsive movements,

> deep sleep reduces them to the minimum. Satiation by food greatly curtails them. On the other hand, a duplication of the intra-uterine state by the use of the warm bath encourages them. The movements are then usually slow and rather rhythmic and graceful. One may even see in them the beginning of an expression of pleasure. The face may join in the picture of contentment with slow asymmetric contortions, which semblance has an odd mixture of pleasure with more than a hint of displeasure. The greater part of the impulsions, however, are purposeless, senseless and asymmetric and are found over the entire body from the first day of birth. Writhing and twisting of the body are also frequent accompaniments to the movements of the face and extremities. Just as the infant sinks into deep sleep these impulsive movements slow down and the body usually comes to a state of rest in the foetal position. (p. 46)

In his 1915 paper on the pathogenesis of epilepsy, Clark had noted that:

> neither the present accepted pathological anatomy of marginocortical gliosis nor its postulated pathogenesis, a still earlier chemicotoxic state, is really sufficiently constant in variation and extent to account for essential epilepsy … It must be admitted that the microscope has not solved the riddle of the nature and pathogenesis of epilepsy. All the careful and detailed work of Nissl and his school concerning the changes in the ganglion cell which result from fatigue and poisons has added little to our knowledge of the real pathogenesis of the disorder. There is not even a constant histological pathology of this affection. The marginocortical gliosis, whether primary or secondary (Alzheimer), occurs in about half of cases … There is no known tenable theory to connect such a lesion to the disorder of consciousness which is seen in the epileptic seizure.[70]

[68] Clark, 'Nature and pathogenesis' p. 386.   [69] Clark, 'Psychological interpretation'.
[70] Clark, 'Nature and pathogenesis', p. 386.

Clark also considered periods of lethargy and depression often to be symptoms of petit mal (and in his book on Napoleon ascribes the less-than-decisive Victory at Borodino to Napoleon's lethargy due to ongoing petit mal).[71]

To Clark, it was therefore in psychological theories of function that the cause and pathogenesis of epileptic seizures were to be sought, and in his view psychoanalytical concepts provided entirely plausible explanations for his clinical observations. Today such views are rightly ridiculed, but it was recognised then, and now, that psychological and physiological explanations are not mutually exclusive. Both probably do play a role in the pathogenesis of seizures, and as the pendulum of history swings, the former is now perhaps too neglected.

The Epileptic Personality

Most persons with epilepsy were, at the time, thought to have abnormal personalities. This was considered universal in those with mental deficiency, and as Tredgold stated in the first edition of his textbook (and repeated in many of the later editions), 'Epileptic aments are often exceedingly stubborn and difficult to manage; they are prone to sudden outbursts of temper and violence, and they are in fact, probably the most untrustworthy of all the varieties of mental deficiency, with the exception of moral imbeciles.'[72]

One might have expected psychoanalysis, with its emphasis on the individual, to have countered these absurd perceptions, but in fact the reverse was the case and psychoanalytic theorising strengthened stigmatising beliefs about epilepsy and linked them to sexual dysfunction and infantilism. Writing in 1910,[73] Freud's close colleague and biographer, Ernest Jones,[74] summarised orthodox psychoanalytical views of the mental state in chronic epilepsy:

> Perhaps the most important, practically, is the gradual reduction of intellectual capacity, which may progress to feeble-mindedness or even to profound dementia. Early evidences of this are the tardiness of general psychical reactions, a certain heaviness in thinking, a difficulty in seizing new ideas, a slowness in following the thoughts of others ... and a resulting conservative adherence to established and rigid opinions ... This narrowing differs from that of most dementing processes, particularly from that of dementia praecox, in being a concentric one, the patient becoming more and more confined to the interests and knowledge of his immediate environment. (pp. 223–4)

---

[71] Clark, *Napoleon, self destroyed*, p160.   [72] Tredgold, *Mental Deficiency*, p. 199.
[73] Jones, 'Mental characteristics of epileptics'.
[74] Jones was instrumental in arranging Freud's escape from Vienna in 1938. His personality and life are the topic of Maddox, *Freud's Wizard: The Enigma of Ernest Jones*.

Defects in memory and in rapport are common in epilepsy, Jones noted, and patients are very egocentric: their thoughts and interests centre on their own personality, resulting in high levels of personal vanity. He then moved on to

> the sexual activities of epileptics. It is notorious that these are often of a turbulent or even violent nature, and, further, that perverse acts of different kinds are especially common ... The sexual desires of epileptics ... overflow the normal channels of outlet, and are manifested not only in the normal manner, but in all kinds of perverse activities; there is no kind of perversion that may not commonly be met with in epilepsy. In this latter respect the sexual activities resemble those of normal young children. (pp. 226–7)

Jones cited Freud's description of the infant's sexual life as 'polymorph pervers' and the work of Alphonse Maeder, who characterised the sexual life of epileptics as 'polyvalent' and auto-erotic.[75] Jones also noted that algolagnia (the desire for sexual gratification through pain) is one of the best-known aberrant sexual tendencies of epileptics and is responsible for cruelty and violence.

Similar strange and prejudicial opinions were shared worldwide. An interesting example is a study of 89 patients with epilepsy from an asylum in the Punjab published in 1914 by Owen Berkeley-Hill, doyen of Indian psychiatry. He noted the same gradual reduction of intellectual capacity, impairment of speech and memory and abnormal behaviour, and 'polyvalent' sexuality of an infantile type. Moreover, epilepsy was associated with 'sexual perversion', and indeed 'sexual offences are committed with greater frequency by epileptics than by sufferers from any other mental disorder'.[76] Berkeley-Hill's case notes reported a tendency to exhibitionism and sadism, as well as extravagant and pathological religiosity. Sándor Ferenczi viewed the epileptic 'as a special human type, characterized by the piling up of unpleasure and by the infantile manner of its periodic motor discharge ... They take refuge in a completely self-contained and self-sufficient way of life as it was lived in the womb, that is to say, before the painful cleavage between the self and the outer world took place.'[77]

For Clark, disturbed evolution of the libido was the basis of the emotional defects seen in epilepsy. The epileptic had an 'essential polyvalent infantilism of the epileptic libido',[78] and memory defects seen in epilepsy might be 'directly due to the narrow range of the association of ideas which is born of a too

---

[75] Maeder, *Die Sexualität der Epileptiker*, p. 227. Maeder was assistant to Eugen Bleuler and Carl Jung.

[76] Berkeley-Hill, 'Short analysis'. This paper must be one of the first on psychoanalysis and epilepsy to come from a country outside Europe or North America. Berkeley-Hill was a major figure in Indian colonial psychiatry and a close friend of Ernest Jones. He held the post of superintendent of the European Asylum in Ranchi, was a founding member of the British Psycho-Analytical Society and later founded the Indian Psycho-Analytical Society.

[77] Ferenczi, 'Epileptic fits'.   [78] Clark, 'Nature and pathogenesis', p. 389.

attenuated and infantile emotional life'.[79] He wrote extensively about the psychology of essential epilepsy and made the important distinction, rarely noted at the time, that epilepsy can be a disorder of affect, independent from any disorder of intellect. The person with essential epilepsy had a personality structure (an epileptic constitution) that was invariably present, the nucleus of which was 'extreme hypersensitiveness and egotism'.[80] The seizure phenomenon was also 'the direct outcome of the inability of such persons to subordinate their individualistic tendencies to those of the so-called social demands and constitute a reaction away from the difficulties', which leads to the seizures – a personality full of infantile traits, characterised by sensitivity, lability of mood, lethargy, maladjustment, predisposition to rage and lack of good-fellowship, aloofness, and emotional and sexual underdevelopment. The epilepsy could be considered 'in the nature of a life-reaction, comparable to a state of rage or anger as seen in bad-tempered individuals, or excessive emotionalism in the supersensitive'.[81] In his view it was impossible to distinguish whether these traits are inherited or due to somatic structural anomalies which prevent proper emotional development.

In the sphere of forensic psychiatry, the 'epileptic character' was also firmly linked to criminality. A paper by John R. Harding, the resident physician in the psychological laboratory of the Elmira Reformatory, shows clearly the extent of the hostility experienced by persons with epilepsy in this period:[82]

> The epileptic is chronically nervous. The keynote to his character is emotional irritability. His varying moods change most unexpectedly, and he is actuated by quick, unreasoning impulse in much that he does. The epileptic shows a woeful disregard for consequences. He lacks foresight and planning ability, and pursues his irregular activities openly and boldly. He also has a violent, uncontrollable temper, and is usually jealous, suspicious and fault-finding in his dealings with others. Often he develops hatred, and assumes a persecutory attitude towards those with whom he is associated. In some cases fear is a prominent symptom, especially just preceding the attack. Some are cunning and treacherous, and inclined to trump up false charges against innocent people. These ideas against family and friends may temporarily pass into real delusions and thus lead to criminal acts … All epileptics are egotistic and self-centered. Sometimes this takes the form of self-pity and of a wholesale

---

[79] Clark, 'Nature and pathogenesis' p. 515. To Clark, essential epilepsy occurred in 'an apparently sound individual having epileptic attacks of apparent idiopathic or unknown origin' ('Psychological interpretation'). His book contains an extensive study of the individual's makeup and the stresses that result in epilepsy.

[80] Clark, *Clinical Studies in Epilepsy*, p. 2.   [81] Clark, 'Psychological interpretation'.

[82] Harding, 'Penal institution'. The Elmira Reformatory was an American penal Institution in New York. Although celebrated for its reforming approach, this is not evident from Harding's description, which owes much to Lombroso, and demonstrates the hostility epilepsy engendered in this period.

distrust of others, and thus leads to the 'shut-in' personality; these are the moody and melancholy cases which keep themselves in the background, and try to cover their symptoms. Other egocentrics are of a selfish, unethical type, who perpetually ignore and trample on the rights and feelings of others ... The volitional sphere of epileptics often suffers radical changes. While obstinate and uncompromising towards others, they are often strangely weak-willed and suggestible. Morally these individuals are apt to be spineless or perverted. They lack inhibitory force, and are frequently given to gluttony and debauchery. Many of them are oversexed, especially during the heat of emotional stress just preceding an attack. In general, as the higher mental attributes become dulled or effaced the animal instincts rise to the ascendency ... The epileptic psyche is always a restless and changeable entity. While the character defects just enumerated are usually intensified for varying periods immediately before or after the seizure, an unstable temperament is always in evidence. These individuals are essentially degenerate, and unable to adapt themselves to the requirements of a normal, social life. The defect is primal and in a broad sense due to a perversion of the varying attributes of the psyche itself, and is not to be confounded with the arrests of intellectual development found in the feeble-minded, or with the deterioration due to the destructive influence of the attack itself. (pp. 263–4)

To the public, psychoanalytic theories of disease were intellectually stimulating and attractive. However, and perhaps not surprisingly, they divided the medical profession, and psychoanalysis was viewed with great disdain by many, especially amongst the more physiologically inclined neurologists. As James Taylor wrote in a leading article in the *British Medical Journal* in 1921: '[I am] not a little disappointed and surprised at the tendency which has lately become obvious towards an attempt to approach [the] explanation [of epilepsy] on other grounds than that of physical disturbance.'[83] Taylor also disagreed with the view that patients with epilepsy had particular defects of their psychological make-up and that deterioration of mentation was an inevitable consequence of epilepsy, even if seizures were chronic or persistent. He attacked Clark's views and noted that these reflected his experience in asylum practice rather than private practice:

Does he not think that the so-called 'trained clinician' in an epileptic colony is much more likely to be biased in his views than is a man who is at least equally well trained, and much more widely experienced in varied forms of disease? He even claims that the colony physician has a much broader view of the whole problem, which, of course, is absurd, seeing that he is dealing with advanced and apparently incurable cases, and no experience (or ignores it) of patients subject to occasional attacks who are able to get about, to do good work, and of whose tendency to occasional attacks

---

[83] Taylor, 'Epilepsy as a symptom'.

everyone, except their immediate relations and their physician, is in complete ignorance. The colony physician surely has a narrow and restricted view of these phenomena because his patients are of a class only suitable for institutional treatment – for, as the author confesses, the institutional physician 'receives the most badly deteriorated patients'. (p. 4)

He followed this with examples from his own private (i.e. outpatient) practice at the National Hospital concluding that seizures were best explained physiologically not psychologically, and are: 'the result of changes occurring locally in the brain giving rise to signs of irritation in the peripheral structures, motor or sensory, related to the unstable brain area' and that the cause of the irritability – '[which] may, of course, be various' – does not determine the symptomatology (here carefully echoing Hughlings Jackson) (p. 5).

Indeed, it was psychoanalysis that deepened the divide between the disciplines of neurology and psychiatry, which diverged in this period, taking many decades to come together again. The psychoanalytic view of epilepsy then began to recede, at least in neurological circles. In 1940, in the standard neurological textbook of the period by S. A. Kinnier Wilson, who was isympathetic to psychiatry, there is no mention at all of psychoanalytic theories of causation or mechanism in epilepsy, and he ridiculed the idea of a typical epileptic personality:[84]

> On the *epileptic temperament,* inordinate stress has been laid. It is alleged that some form of mental obliquity distinguishes most epileptics, who are egocentric and volatile, of irritable temper and feeble judgment, suspicious or credulous, dreamy or impulsive, hesitant or hasty, timorous or fanatic – the 'character' of the epileptic can be made to comprise almost anything ... No doubt the neurologist, as a rule, sees early or uncomplicated cases, yet did the temperament pre-exist it would have been much more manifest in personal experience than it has proved. (p. 1508)

Wilson also considered that much depended on the 'class of the material studied'. As far as he was concerned, by 1948, when cultural attitudes to the disabled and to epilepsy had become far less prejudicial (not least as the abuses perpetrated by German medicine and psychiatry in the Second World War became known), the psychoanalytical school had generally conceded that the 'epileptic personality' applied only to a minority of cases. Nevertheless, Bela Mittleman, a leading American physician and psychoanalyst, could still in 1947 consider 'hostile, aggressive and self-centering, self-magnifying attitudes' to be typical of the epileptic character, and that seizures stimulated 'submissive and masochistic strivings, together with guilt, dependency, and expiation'. He also felt that seizures 'may represent to the patient ... escape from an unbearable

---

[84] Wilson and Bruce, *Neurology,* vol. 1.

situation, ... forbidden sexual activity, ... a threat, ... an aggressive act, ... suicide, ... destruction and rebirth'.[85]

It is difficult today to understand how the psychoanalytical theories around epilepsy, which now seem largely to be nonsense, could have held such sway amongst doctors and public alike, nor how such seemingly ridiculous theories could have been so extensively explored. Nothing illustrates better the relativity and culture-bound nature of science, a warning from history always to be heeded.

HEREDITY, EUGENICS AND EPILEPSY

Although the mechanisms of its inheritance were still almost completely obscure, as we saw in the previous chapter it was almost universally assumed that idiopathic (genuine) epilepsy was caused by inherited degenerative germ plasm, and this placed it at the forefront of the eugenic agenda. Furthermore, idiopathic epilepsy was the catch-all term for the wide spectrum of epilepsies in which no gross cerebral lesion was detected, and within which were institutionalised patients with mental deficiency and psychological disturbance as well as otherwise normal persons in the community; all were thought to have the same inherited condition.

Heredity was an area where science was shipped in to construct social policy, and perhaps the first full-scale example of this trend which has strengthened throughout the twentieth century. A discipline of 'scientific racism' grew up. Politicians, the press and the public spoke casually in scientific terms, using data from science in their pronouncements and writing without understanding the limitations and methodologies.[86] It was the erroneous theorising of science which fashioned the racist and hostile culture of the times that proved so detrimental to the handicapped and to those with epilepsy.

Very simplistic views around heredity were expressed. Warnings were made in scientific and political circles that the reproduction of those carrying genes of degeneration, including defectives and epileptics, would produce an ever-increasing number of similarly affected persons.[87] Calculations were published of the dire social impact of this rising tide, which would sap the genetic vigour

---

[85] Mittelmann, 'Psychopathology of epilepsy', p. 147. The same book featured descriptions of the use of the Rorschach test to identify the epileptic personality (Piotrowski, 'Personality of the epileptic'). This test, too, became a popular drawing-room game.

[86] As I write this, similar tendencies were notable in the press and governmental reaction to the Covid pandemic.

[87] Very similar predictions were made at the time about other groups, particularly in relation to race or immigrants to the United States from least desirable countries (see Grant, *The Passing of the Great Race*), and the 'demographic threat' proved a powerful propaganda weapon which struck seemingly at the heart of public disquiet. The same tool was used by the Nazis two decades later.

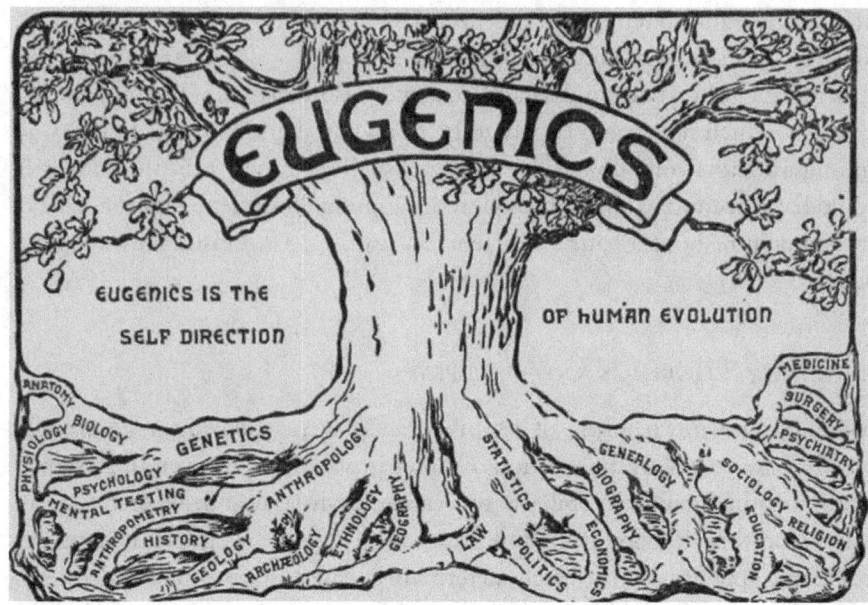

15. **'Eugenics is the self direction of human evolution'.** Poster of the Second International Eugenics Congress, held at the American Museum of Natural History in New York, on 25–27 September 1921.

of the population and pose an unbearable economic burden. Based on these demographic predictions, an impending social crisis was seen to be imminent. It became widely accepted that eugenic action offered the only way out and that without eugenic measures 'humanity will gradually destroy itself from within, will decay in its very core and essence'.[88]

Although this view was reinforced by many leading physicians and academics, including well-regarded figures in the interwar science community,[89] those with a clearer understanding of genetic mechanisms voiced dissent. An early example was an excoriating attack on Davenport's work by David Heron of the UCL Galton Laboratory in London. After a forensic analysis lambasting Davenport's poor methodology and science, Heron noted: 'Nothing is more astonishing than the amount of approval that this cacogenic doctrine has received in this country.'[90] A similar point was made by Abraham Myerson[91] in his landmark book of 1925. In a

---

[88] The blunt opinion of Julian Huxley, 'Eugenics and society'. Huxley was the grandson of Thomas Huxley and brother of Aldous Huxley. He and his student Charles Blacker led a call for eugenic sterilization that was never permitted in Britain. See Overy, *Morbid Age*, pp. 120–3).

[89] For instance, Julian Huxley and Cyril Burt.

[90] Heron, *Problem of Mental Defect*, p. 8. Heron was president of the Royal Statistical Society in the 1940s.

[91] Myerson specialised in the heredity of psychiatric and neurological disease and was a strong opponent not only of eugenics but also psychoanalytic theory. He was a remarkable man and a first-rate academic. He was one of the last to specialize both in neurology and psychiatry,

chapter on epilepsy, he derided the older theories of the neuropathic diathesis, and in regard to the papers of Davenport and Weeks he wrote: 'It seems to me that Davenport and his followers have been dogmatic offenders against logic and science – they have collected data in a thoroughly unscientific way, they have unified utterly diverse conditions into one "neuropathic effect due to lack of a unit determiner" which last is an arbitrary conclusion decided upon, apparently, beforehand.'[92] The doyen of British neurology, Russell (later Lord) Brain agreed:

> Davenport and Weeks have attempted to show that epilepsy is due to the absence from the inherited germinal material of a unit character which behaves according to Mendelian laws. These authors have been fully dealt with by Myerson and the greater part of his refreshingly outspoken criticism appears to be entirely justified. It is difficult to take seriously conclusions which are based on the indiscriminate inclusion in the concept 'neuropathic taint' of chorea, paralysis, neurosis, alcoholism, epilepsy, feeble-mindedness, prostitution, and migraine, which here again exercises its usual fascination for the statistician of psychopathology.[93]

Although carrying weight in the scientific community, such criticism was largely ignored in the populist public debate. In fact, partly as a result of Davenport's urging, programmes of involuntary sterilisation of persons with 'degenerate' germ plasm were initiated and legalised in United States,[94] Canada, Scandinavia, Switzerland and in Germany, where 375,000 surgical sterilisations were carried out, 14% of which were for hereditary epilepsy.[95] In Britain, sterilisation was never performed, despite pressure to do so from many, including some leading clinicians.[96]

It was in the United States that eugenic ideas regarding epilepsy initially gained most traction. Davenport's focus on epilepsy ensured that this condition was ensnared in the eugenic debates. The public were impressed by the visual impact of pedigree charts (family tree diagrams) purporting to show the

---

holding both the Professorship of Clinical Psychiatry at Harvard Medical School and the Professorship of Neurology at Tufts Medical School. A contemporary of William Lennox, he took a very different stance on eugenics.

[92] Myerson, *Inheritance of Mental Diseases*, p. 67.   [93] Brain, 'Inheritance of epilepsy'.

[94] This was not the first time such measures had been taken. In some American penal institutions in the 1890s, castration had been tried to control masturbation and sexual appetite.

[95] Weindling, *Health, Race*. Interestingly, abortion of those carrying degenerate germ plasm was not permitted. See also Bumke, *Richtlinien*, pp. 125–30.

[96] For instance, in his *Bradshaw Lecture on Some Points in Heredity* (1912; the lecture was delivered in December 1911), R. Clement Lucas considered that the political maxim 'liberty of the individual' had by then been replaced by the principle 'that the minority must yield in everything to the will of the majority'. He drew the startling conclusion that 'the germinal organs (testes and ovaries) do not actually belong to the individual, but to the next generation' (p. 19).

widespread presence of epilepsy, crime, pauperism, immorality and feeble-mindedness in these extended families, and accepted the dogma that unless the procreation of epileptics and the feeble-minded was restricted, it would drag down the entire population. This prediction seemed alarmingly imminent when studies using the Stanford–Binet test claimed to show that a significant proportion of the population was already afflicted with mild feeble-mindedness.[97] In 1907, when sterilisation of inmates in asylums began to be practised, numbers were initially small. But the medical authorities continued to press for greater activity, often on grounds of demography and economics. The 'rights' of individuals with epilepsy or mental disturbance were hardly considered.

In the epilepsy colony at Gallipolis, for instance, a socio-medical investigation was carried out using Davenport's methods in which it was concluded:

> At the Ohio Hospital for Epileptics the number of patients has been increasing at the rate of a hundred each year. The cost of segregation places such a burden upon the tax-payer that this method of negative-eugenics [i.e. segregation] is extremely unsatisfactory. It is necessary that some method be adopted which will materially lessen the number of epileptic individuals, and it is probable that sterilization would prove immeasurably valuable in this regard.[98]

The question of balancing the rights of the individual and the society was settled in America in the famous case of *Buck* v. *Bell*. Carrie Buck may or may not have had epilepsy (evidence is divided on this point). She was an inmate of the Virginia State Epileptic Colony and was to become the first person forcibly sterilised against her will under Virginia's Eugenical Sterilization Act of 1924. Her case was challenged in the Virginia Supreme Court of Appeals and later before the US Supreme Court. There, in his ruling, Chief Justice Oliver Wendell Holmes made the now infamous declaration that 'it is better for all the world if, instead of waiting to execute degenerate offspring for crime or to let them starve for their imbecility, society can prevent those who are manifestly unfit from continuing their kind ... Three generations of imbeciles are enough.'[99] Expert evidence relied on depositions by Harry Loughlin from the

---

[97] It was then that IQ measures began to be used in American legislation and in legal proceedings. Goddard's *The Criminal Imbecile* (1915) describes in detail the three (non-epileptic) cases in which the Binet–Simon tests were admitted in evidence and in which the mental status of the accused was determined by this method.

[98] Brown, 'Relatives of epileptics'. To the credit of the state of Ohio, laws permitting sterilisation of epileptics failed to pass through the state legislature despite repeated attempts between 1915 and 1965.

[99] *Buck* v. *Bell*, p. 274. See also Lombardo, *Three Generations, No Imbeciles*. In 1979 Carrie's sister, Doris Buck Figgins, discovered that she, too, had been involuntarily sterilised in 1928 at the age of sixteen, when she was taken to an operating room where 'they told me that the operation was for an appendix and rupture' (Boodman and Frankel, 'Over 7,500 sterilized').

Eugenics Record Office, who had not actually interviewed the family yet opined that they were members of 'the shiftless, ignorant, and worthless class of anti-social whites of the South'.[100] In fact, later evidence showed that Carrie and her siblings were not imbeciles nor, indeed, intellectually impaired. The effect of the ruling, however, was to legitimise eugenic sterilisation, and laws were subsequently passed in many states.[101] Eugenic solutions had become respectable and thereafter became widely accepted in popular culture.[102] As a consequence, by 1945, more than 65,000 compulsory sterilisations were said to have been carried out in the United States.

In Britain, an overriding concern for the liberty of the individual, as well as a general dislike of centralised coercion, prevented any such legislation despite the powerful lobby of the Eugenics Education Society. At the society's annual dinner in 1927, Arthur Tredgold delivered the Galton Lecture,[103] in which he reflected the widely held attitudes of British eugenicists of the time. One to two per cent of the population, he said, were affected by mental deficiency or lunacy, and an even larger number suffered from conditions such as epilepsy and 'states bordering upon Insanity and Mental Defect … [I]f the mating of neuropaths was rigidly restricted … the disease would eventually work out its own elimination' (pp. 7–8). The 'danger to the race [lay] in the contamination of [sound and healthy] stocks by those who are predisposed to the disease' (p. 9), and the mating not only of those with the diseases but also of carriers needed urgently to be prevented. This could be achieved by 'an educational campaign … [for] developing throughout the

---

Interestingly, Wendell Holmes' judgement has similarities to that reported in the seventeenth century by Robert Burton in his *Anatomy of Melancholy*: 'Heretofore in Scotland, (saith Hect. Boëthius) if any were visited with the falling sickness, madness, gout, leprosie, or any such dangerous disease, which was likely to be propagated from the father to the son, he was instantly gelded; a woman kept from all company of men: and if by chance, having some such disease, she were found to be with child, she with her brood were buried alive: and this was done for the common good, lest the whole nation should be injured or corrupted. A severe doom, you will say, and not to be used amongst Christians … [I]t comes to pass that our generation is corrupt; we have many weak persons, both in body and mind, many feral diseases raging amongst us, crazed families, *parentes peremptores*; our fathers bad; and we are like to be worse' (pp. 214–5).

[100] *Buck* v. *Bell*, pp. 40–2.

[101] In 1907 Indiana became the first state to legalise eugenic sterilisation. By 1909, laws had been introduced in California, Washington State and Connecticut. By 1936, legislation existed in 27 states (Myerson et al., *Eugenical Sterilization*). In the end, more than 65,000 individuals were sterilised in 33 states under state compulsory sterilisation programs (Kevles, *Name of Eugenics*). As an example, between 1924 and 1972, the state of Virginia sterilised more than 7,500 people confined in six mental institutions but mostly from the Virginia Colony for Epileptics and the Feebleminded in Lynchburg.

[102] One example of this was the movie *The Black Stork* (see pp.167). The film is the subject of a well-documented and thoughtful book that provides a balanced view of contemporary popular sentiment: Martin Pernick, *The Black Stork* (1966).

[103] Tredgold, 'Galton Lecture'.

nation the Eugenic ideal', by which he meant 'not merely the intellectual recognition of the desirability of producing sound and healthy offspring, ... but a feeling, or an emotion, ... the Eugenic sentiment, or if we prefer so to call it, conscience' (p. 11).

Eugenics had another consequence. It was a mechanism by which psychiatrists could shake off their 'alienist' reputations,[104] and many sought to advance their status by supporting eugenics and taking a more active role in public health and hygiene.[105] In America, a well-documented example is provided by G. Alder Blumer.[106] The power to sterilise, introduced in the United States and in Germany, elevated the psychiatrist's professional authority, but also steered psychiatry into new and dangerous waters.

It was Nazi Germany, though, in the 1930s that most keenly adopted eugenic solutions. Eugenics already had a strong foothold there. In 1924, Fritz Lenz outlining the development of eugenics in Germany, opened his remarks with a call for the 'eugenic cooperation of all nations of European race and civilization ... [As t]he existence of the best racial elements of all these nations is already more or less directly threatened'. He claimed that his views were 'in complete agreement with those of Anglo-Saxon eugenics', but regretted that, in contrast to the situation in the United States, neither sterilisation nor termination of pregnancy on eugenic grounds was permitted. Noting that there was much to be done on the legislative side, he added an ominous prediction:

> The Germans are more disposed toward scientific investigation than toward practical statesmanship. It is, then, perhaps no loss that the Anglo-Saxons have an advantage in the field of eugenic legislation. Too hasty legislation in this matter may also provoke disastrous reactions. The

[104] Psychiatry had become attractive as a profession in the nineteenth century for various reasons, not least because it was the first of the 'specialties' to be differentiated from medicine, there was an oversupply of medical doctors and a competition for fees, there were no effective therapies in medicine and the directorship of asylums provided a guaranteed income. Particularly on the continent, asylums for the uber-rich were generally well-appointed mansions in the countryside (see, for instance, Thomas Mann's descriptions of the 'International Sanatorium Berghof' at Davos-Platz in *The Magic Mountain*). However, as time passed and general medicine became more effective and powerful, the attractions of alienist medicine diminished. Eugenics provided an attractive option to pursue as it could be seen as 'preventative medicine'. Henry Maudsley had a strong influence at the time. In his view, psychiatric disease was incurable and had the potential to bring down civilisation and humanity and so supported eugenic ideas. But it was the 'medicalisation' of psychiatry in the 1950s which had the greatest impact in raising the reputation of the profession.

[105] A theme fully explored in Ian Dowbiggin's *Keeping America Sane* (1997).

[106] Blumer was at one time president of the American Psychiatric Association. Initially an avid supporter of eugenics, he later modified his opinions to avoid alienating himself from the families of his more patrician patients who were alarmed by his belief in the inherited neuropathic taint. (See Dowbiggin, *Keeping America Sane*).

main thing is that the eugenic education of the nation goes ahead; and it is going. Once public sentiment is won over to eugenics, the legislation will come of itself.[107]

Earlier, in 1916, Kraepelin and others in the German Society for Racial Hygiene had shifted the emphasis of the origins of mental disease away from social or environmental causes towards a purely biological explanation affecting the whole population (the 'folk body'). Kraepelin's younger colleagues, Alfred Hoche and Ernst Rüdin, gladly took up the baton. In 1920 Hoche published *Release and Destruction of Lives Not Worth Living* (co-authored by Rudolf Binding, a law professor), which argued that 'those who are not capable of human feeling – those "ballast lives" and "empty human husks" that fill our psychiatric institutions – can have no sense of value of life. Theirs is not a life worth living; hence their destruction is not only tolerable but humane.'[108] As Michael Burleigh points out, this text

> was essentially a search for a post-Christian, utilitarian ethic, [which] deliberately conflated the issue of voluntary 'euthanasia' with non-consensual killing of 'idiots' and the mentally ill; stressed the historical relativity of such notions as the 'sanctity of human life'; highlighted the objective futility of such emotions as 'pity'; ... and emphasised the emotional and economic burden allegedly represented by 'entirely unproductive persons'.

Moreover, 'it argued that in emergency wartime circumstances, where the healthy were making enormous sacrifices, one could justify "the sacrifice" of "not merely absolutely valueless, but negatively valued existences"'.[109]

Rüdin became a very influential figure in German psychiatry. He, and Kraepelin, considered the German race to be too 'domesticated', and this kindled Rüdin's interest in the genetics of psychiatric disease. He was the brother-in-law of Ploetz, and their friendship was one factor in linking psychiatric disorder to racial hygiene. In 1917 Kraepelin appointed Rüdin director of the Department of Genealogical and Demographic Studies at the Max Planck Institute of Psychiatry in Munich, the first unit in the world to specialise in psychiatric genetics. In 1931 Rüdin was made director of the entire institute, and subsequently president of both the International Federation of Eugenics Organizations and the Society of German Neurologists and Psychiatrists. The

---

[107] Lenz, 'Eugenics in Germany'. Lenz considered Alfred Ploetz (who in 1904 established the Archive for Racial and Social Biology and coined the term *Rassenhygiene*) and Wilhelm Schallmayer to be the German founders of eugenics. It is interesting to note that Schallmayer's 1903 essay 'Heredity and selection in the life-process of nations' was stimulated by the offer of a prize by the steel magnate F. A. Krupp, for a work on the topic 'What can we learn from the theory of evolution, for the internal political development and legislation of nations?' – in other words, for sociopolitical rather than biological or medical reasons. The essay won the prize and was widely discussed in German intellectual circles.

[108] Cited in Proctor, *Racial Hygiene*, p. 178.

[109] Burleigh, *Ethics and Extermination*, pp. 114–15.

Rockefeller Foundation funded much research at the institute, and Rüdin became the international face of German eugenics during these years. When Hitler came to power, Rüdin considered it a 'duty of honour' to assist him, and in 1934 he quoted the words of the Führer: 'Whoever is not physically or mentally fit must not pass on his defects to his children. The state must take care that only the fit produce children.' In 1939 Hitler personally awarded Rüdin the Goethe Medal for Art and Science.[110]

In the same year, under the influence of Lenz and Rüdin, the German Eugenics Society adopted a policy which resulted in a programme in Germany in which university chairs were created and mechanisms put in place for eugenic and race-hygiene measures against Jews, Roma other non-Nordic peoples, as well as those with feeble-mindedness. epilepsy and other disorders. In 1933 the first 'racial hygiene' law was passed for the 'prevention of genetically diseased progeny'.[111] Rüdin, who was then director of the Kaiser Wilhelm Institute for Genealogy in Munich, played a leading role in drafting the law, which was partly based on the Californian example. It permitted the compulsory sterilisation by surgery or by X-rays, based on 'eugenic indications', of persons suffering from inherited medical conditions, including imbecility, schizophrenia, Huntington's chorea, muscular dystrophy and epilepsy (and other conditions, including severe alcoholism). Patients with epilepsy were to be sterilised unless it could be shown that there was a symptomatic cause.[112] More than 200 genetic health courts were set up, whose proceedings were kept secret and which between 1933 and 1949 sanctioned the sterilisation of 320,000–350,000 persons with mental handicap and genetic disorders.[113] In three different studies, it was shown that between 8.1% and 24.6% were sterilised on the grounds of hereditary epilepsy. This massive sterilisation programme changed the nature of German medicine. In many ways, every doctor had to become 'a genetic doctor', and new training and courses in racial hygiene proliferated. This, linked to the theories of inherited personality defects of those with epilepsy, contributed to the striking lack of compassion evident in the medical writings of the time.

The selection of patients was based largely in asylums, and asylum directors enthusiastically embraced the task.[114] The finger of blame should not necessarily be

[110] Tucker, *Racial Research*, p. 121. Rüdin escaped censure after the war and continued his work. For a review of his life, see Welzel, 'Ernst Rüdin', and Weber, 'Ernst Rüdin'.

[111] Gesetz zur Verhütung erbkranken Nachwuchses was enacted on 14 July 1933, permitting the compulsory sterilisation of any citizen judged by the *Erbgesundheitsgericht* ('genetic health court') to suffer from any one of a list of eight genetic disorders, including epilepsy.

[112] Schou, 'Epileptics in Scandinavia'.

[113] See Proctor, *Racial Hygiene*, from which details are taken. This figure is probably derived from all Nazi euthanasia projects and Actions.

[114] An example was Otto Heinrich Moritz Hebold (son of the alienist Otto Karl Moritz Hebold, a founder of the ILAE), who was physician in charge of Eberswalde asylum in 1936, where he was involved in the implementation of forced sterilisation. He was then recruited by the

pointed *only* at the doctors, as they were in a sense just technicians. German society as a whole had adopted increasingly extreme and brutal attitudes, and as Lenz had predicted this allowed 'legislation to come of itself'. Conditions in asylums had deteriorated seriously. Care became increasingly pared down on grounds of cost, contributing to the idea that the inmates were subhuman. In 1935 the law was amended to include eugenic abortion up to the sixth month of pregnancy. Relentless Nazi propaganda churned out films showing a nation menaced by hordes of feeble-minded persons. Much was made of the cost of institutional care, which could be more usefully spent on housing the racially pure poor. Asylums were toured by the SS (*Schutzstaffel*) to reinforce the uselessness of the inmates, and mercy killing (*Gnadentod*) was increasing discussed. Compassion and pity were replaced by disgust as majority public opinion turned against the handicapped.

The sterilisation programme introduced in 1933 was largely ended in 1939. Less than 5% of the total number of procedures were carried out after this point, mainly it seems because sterilisation was superceded by an even more radical step. Hitler first mentioned ending the life of the handicapped at a Nazi Party rally in 1929, and from 1935 he was encouraged by a powerful medical lobby that pressed for the introduction of 'euthanasia'. A law was drafted but not implemented as there was significant opposition – not least from the families of targeted children. The killings were consequently hidden from sight. Initially, parents were informed that their children were being transferred to special clinics to receive up-to-date treatment; instead, they were taken to facilities where they were murdered by starvation or lethal injection. More than 6,000 were disposed of in this way, and the age range was subsequently extended to adolescents and adults. Schemes became increasingly ambitious, culminating in 1939 with the initiation of much larger-scale programmes of euthanasia, following Hitler's announcement that the average annual removal of 700,000–800,000 of the weakest babies in Germany would increase the power of the nation. A series of programmes were enacted, some informal but others more organised, such as the child euthanasia (*Kinder-Euthanasie*); Aktion 14f13 (the so-called *Sonderbehandlung* or 'special treatment'), which culled those in concentration camps; and, most notoriously (and the most studied), Action T4. It has been estimated that about 200,000–300,000 persons in total with hereditary diseases, including epilepsy, were killed in these various programmes.

Action T4 was a programme of extermination of those with incurable inherited diseases, focused on those with mental handicap and epilepsy. The programme started with children and was extended to adult cases. War provided a convenient backdrop. If healthy persons could sacrifice themselves during war, argued Hoche and Binding, why should the mentally handicapped not do the same? The psychiatrist Hermann Pfannmüller, one of the assessors in

Reichsarbeitsgemeinschaft für Heil und Pflegeenstalten and led the T4 selection process, was involved in gassing at two killing centres and also participated in Action 14f13 in the Sachsenhausen concentration camp. He was jailed in 1965 for these and other crimes.

Action T4, wrote: 'It is unbearable to me that the best, the flower of our youth must lose its life at the front in order that feeble-minded and asocial elements can have a secure existence in the asylum.'[115] Action T4 was overseen by the Reich Committee for the Scientific Registration of Serious Hereditary and Congenital Diseases. As no law sanctioned the killings, the programme operated under the radar and was considered a private matter between doctors and patients. A typically efficient apparatus was put in place that involved many highly educated but morally corrupt doctors and other individuals. A procedure for selecting and registering patients was established, and six killing centres were set up. Doctors in all hospitals and nursing homes were required to fill in a report form on any patient who had been institutionalised for five years or more and who had one of the specified conditions, which included epilepsy. About half of those killed were taken from church-run asylums, often with the approval of their Protestant or Catholic authorities. Some individual churchmen protested, and the Catholic Church hierarchy tried (and failed) to negotiate an opt-out clause for Catholic asylum staff. Only two questions related to epilepsy were asked: 'Was there an abnormal personality?' and 'What was the average seizure frequency?' Copies of the reporting forms were dispatched to one of a selection of 'expert physicians' and then to the central office, where one of three senior experts (*Obergutachter*) had the final word.[116] If the doctors filled out the empty box on the lower left of the form with a red '+', the patient was killed. If they chose to mark it with a blue '−', the patient would be allowed to live.[117] The killings were often carried out by SS officers to avoid any sudden change of mind, initially by lethal injection but later by gassing, which was considered far more efficient. In some settings, patients were transferred from their institutions to the killing centres in buses marked 'Community Patient Transport Services' and operated by teams of SS wearing white coats to give a professional appearance. The selected were usually killed within 24 hours of arrival at the centre, entering the gas chamber naked, with towel and toothbrush. A false death certificate was sent to the family along with an urn of random ashes, citing pneumonia or influenza or some other acute illness. Cremation was carried out in view of the risk of infection. More than 70,000

---

[115] Cited in Lifton, *Nazi Doctors*, p. 63.

[116] One of these doctors was Werner Heyde, Professor of Neurology and Psychiatry at the University of Würzburg. His whereabouts were identified in 1947 but he escaped and was recaptured twelve years later, having been working as a physician under a different name. He was charged with manslaughter in 1964 and committed suicide in his prison cell in 1964. Among the three experts for children was Werner Catel (1894–1961), who held the Professorial Chair of Paediatrics at Leipzig University and who, it is said, approved the killing of more than 5,000 children. Catel was never convicted. His career continued undisturbed until his retirement from the Chair of Paediatrics at Christian-Albrecht University Kiel (Germany) in 1960.

[117] This process was accurately portrayed in the film *Werk ohne Autor* (*Never Look Away*, 2018).

people were killed in Action T4, amongst whom were sometimes perfectly 'sane' epileptics although the exact number of those with epilepsy who perished through Action T4 or the other schemes is unknown.

Tissue from the victims of the killing centres was also used in experimental medicine. Julius Hallervorden,[118] head of the histopathology department and deputy director of the Kaiser Wilhelm Institute, and Hugo Spatz, the institute's director, were both members of the Nazi Party, and both willingly received many brains of those killed in concentration camps and from the T4 programme. (Hallervorden, though, noted that he did not bother with the brains of those with epilepsy, as he felt they showed nothing of interest.[119])

Despite its secrecy, the nature of the fate of the unfortunate people taken away in the buses became quite widely known, and voices began to be raised against the programme both by families and particularly by individual clerics who protested publicly.[120] The programme was then halted, although perhaps this was not so much because of public unease but because attention had turned to extermination of the Jews. To neutralise professional dissent, the psychiatrists in charge of Action T4, such as Paul Nitsche and Carl Schneider,[121] suggested the money saved could be used to provide better care for acute cases.

The Nazi authorities tried to institute similar policies in occupied countries, but there was more opposition. In Holland, for instance, the director of Meer and Bosch, Ch de Ledeboer, engineered a daring scheme for protecting the inmates.[122] In 1935, he had admitted a German patient from Bethel who, diagnosed as a hereditary case and facing compulsory sterilisation, fled to Holland and in Meer and Bosch had surgery for a cortical scar and became seizure free. What this demonstrated to Ledeboer was that the Nazis would deal similarly (or worse) with his patients. And so, when the occupying forces seemed likely to take over the running of Meer and Borsch, and its sister

[118] Neither Spatz nor Hallervorden showed remorse about the source of the pathological material and Hallervorden was indeed present at some of the killings in order to collect the brains. In the Nuremburg trials he informed his interrogator, Major Leo Alexander: 'you are going to kill all these people, at least take the brains out so that the material could be utilized … They asked me, "How many can you examine?" and so I told them an unlimited number – the more the better. I gave them the fixatives, jars and boxes, and instructions for removing and fixing the brains' (*Nuremberg Trial Proceedings*, vol. 7, p. 96). This testimony notwithstanding, Hallervorden and Spatz both managed to escape trial and punishment and continued to lead their respective institutes after the war as if nothing untoward had happened. In the event, and in what is surely an indictment of the process, only twenty physicians were prosecuted in the doctors' trial at Nuremberg despite the widespread collaboration of German doctors with the Nazi eugenic programme.

[119] 'Notice and review'.

[120] A well-known dissenter was Bishop von Galen, whom Hitler promised to deal with after the war.

[121] Nitsche headed the medical office of Action T4.

[122] Ds. J. C. van Dijk et al., 'Het verzet'.

colony Bethesda Sarepta, Ledeboer and his religious-based board members arranged to discharge the 600 patients to their homes, as far as was possible, in the company of staff members. When the Germans did take over the clinic in 1942, there were no patients and few staff. Other asylums were less fortunate, and in 1943 the approximately 1,100 patients of the institution and 50 staff from the Jewish mentally ill 'Het Apeldoornse Bos' asylum in Apeldoorn (including a number of non-Jewish inmates) were taken by train to Auschwitz; immediately upon arrival, all were murdered.

All in all, it is remarkable how little opposition there seems to have been from the German medical profession, which, like others in society, had become morally dulled and brutalised[123]. The whole programme carried out by doctors represents one of the worst ethical transgressions in the history of medicine. Eugenicists were prominent amongst the doctors prosecuted at the Nuremberg trials, but the usual defence was that German eugenics differed little from that in the United States. Certainly, many escaped punishment on the basis of this argument. Others defended the killings as being natural, or on the grounds that they were never illegal. The aftermath of this episode is also a salutary lesson. Most of those involved were not tried in court, and many who were tried emerged unscathed. Many of even the leading figures in the racial hygiene movement were able to continue their careers in 'human genetics' and to publish their research. Quite a few gained national and international reputations after the war.

Although eugenics had developed prominently first in the United States, it did not progress there as it had done in Germany. In fact, in leading neurological and psychiatric circles, the tide had begun to turn before the war. In 1936, Abraham Myerson and a five-man committee of the American Neurological Association, which included Tracy Putnam, produced a landmark report concerning sterilisation that marked an immensely important change of direction.[124]

Myerson's committee was highly critical of the eugenicist position, pointing out the fallacies in the demographic predictions, the Mendelian assumptions and that the institutionalisation probably costs much the same as having the person in the community. It also reminded their readers that those with the most severe forms of mental handicap will die before they can reproduce, and that the inheritance of crime is so complicated by environmental factors that eugenic explanations are fruitless. In the committee's view, sterilisation should be selective and voluntary (citing the opinion in Britain, and also amongst the

---

[123] The bases of the attitude of the German medical profession is explored in Kater, 'Doctors under Hitler.'

[124] Myerson, Eugenical Sterilization. This work further developed the views of Myerson expressed in Inheritance of Mental Diseases (1925).

vast majority of American members of the American Association for the Study of the Feebleminded). The report critically reviewed the laws in different states and different countries, and came to the conclusion that sterilisation should be not only voluntary, but also carefully overseen, carried out only after very careful selection and restricted to a small number of conditions – of which epilepsy in certain circumstances was one, but on mainly social not genetic grounds.

In regard to epilepsy, the committee laid out a view which held sway for the next fifty years:

> [Epilepsy is a term that] has been dropped by many workers, who now speak of the convulsive disorders. The term epilepsy denotes an entity which no more exists than does 'insanity'. We retain its use in this report merely because the heredity studies in the literature bear this name ... in many cases, there are clear exogenous or environmental, exciting or precipitating causes ... One of the most pretentious pieces of work is that done by Davenport and his group. Elsewhere one of us [Myerson himself] has criticized the work of Davenport, who comes to the conclusion that epilepsy is a hereditary Mendelian character, although in later writings, he directly modified his opinion. What is called Mendelism in Davenport's work is merely polymorphism of the widest type. (p. 136)

The report criticised earlier writers, especially Spratling and Binswanger, noting that the latter considered epilepsy to be due to degeneration of the germ plasm from a wide variety of causes, such that '[i]t is easy to see that such a widespread net might also make normality a degenerative disease due to defect in the ancestors' (p. 137).

The committee then cited what they considered to be the two most important pieces of recent work: Russell Brain's 'Inheritance of epilepsy' (1926) and Calvert Stein's 'Hereditary factors in epilepsy' (1933). According to Brain, epilepsy was not a Mendelian condition and heredity contributed a 'predisposition' to epilepsy in about 30% of cases. Stein maintained that 'the higher incidence of neuropsychiatric disorders in the families of epileptics [than in controls] may well be explained on the basis of an existing potential or latent germplasm defect', but, the committee concluded that his studies '[did] not justify the conclusion the symptom–complex known as epilepsy, either *per se* or as migraine, or as any other neuropsychiatric disorder, is an inherited [i.e. Mendelian] condition' (p. 143), and that epilepsy had a multifactorial character, and no single recessive Mendelian character was present. Even invoking multiple Mendelian characteristics would have little practical validity. Consequently, '[i]t is probable that the best efforts of science at the present time, insofar as the epilepsy problem is concerned, will be expended in the study of the pathology, chemistry, and general physical constitution of the individual patient himself in the hope of discovering both a pathogenesis and a cure' (p. 144).

The report strongly attacks – in fact ridicules – the idea of the neuropathic trait, which 'up to this day ... governs in most of the studies made of the heredity of mental disease and appears under a new guise in the Mendelian work'. In the committee's view,

> [a] great deal of the work which has been done is entirely invalid and has only historical significance. This applies quite decidedly to such work as is exemplified by the study of the publicized feebleminded families, the Nams, the Kallikaks, the Jukes, and such types. It invalidates, we believe, the earlier work which came from Davenport, Rosanoff, and the American Eugenic school with its headquarters at Cold Spring Harbor, New York. We may fairly state that the eugenic studies of Lombroso, Morel, Esquirol, and others, should now be relegated to the history of psychiatry rather than to its actively utilizable material. (p. 88)

Myerson later wrote interestingly about the committee conclusion in the *Yale Law Journal*.[125] About diseases whose cause was unknown, he wrote, 'All cats look gray in the dark' – and therein was a temptation to postulate heredity as a unifying mechanism (p. 619). He perceptively observed that

> certain groups of people tend to become strict hereditarians and thus to view failure in life and the occurrence of disease as evidence of congenital inferiority. Conservative groups, as a rule, take this point of view. On the whole, these people are well satisfied with the status quo. They do not like the idea that their success and the failure of others may be accidental and environmental. The arrogant and the proud tend to be hereditarians and to neglect the environment entirely. Thus a leading feature of Nazi ideology is the importance of blood, and all the studies which emanate from Germany have emphasized racial superiority, stock superiority and eugenics. (p. 624)

Conversely, the opponents of eugenics were 'a curious conglomeration of bedfellows' (p. 624): the Roman Catholic Church, which viewed sterilisation as an infringement of the sacred theology; the Bolsheviks, who felt that adopting communism would end much mental disease; and the liberals, who defended freedom of the individual. Myerson strongly rebuffed the suggestion that the numbers of the mentally ill were increasing, arguing that the public had simply become more aware of the illnesses. He was dismissive of the efforts of William Lennox:

> Recent work has tended to show that there may be more of an hereditary basis than was assumed to be the case, particularly the study of the brain waves by a notable Boston group of workers – Lennox, Gibbs and Gibbs. I do not believe, however, that the study of brain waves has reached the

---

[125] Myerson, *Eugenic Sterilization*.

precision and reliability which these workers assume it has. Nor do I agree that the kind of brain wave they describe is limited to epilepsy, so that their studies showing abnormal brain waves in the parents, collaterals and siblings of epileptics as proof of the hereditary basis of epilepsy are perhaps not as well founded as might be believed the case at first glance. Epilepsy, or, more precisely, the convulsive states, appears to be producible in all forms of life beyond the most primitive, can be brought about in any human being by drugs, electricity, and brain damage, and thus differs radically from schizophrenia and manic-depressive psychosis. The most that as yet can be said as to its relationship to heredity is that some individuals and familial groups are more liable to it. (pp. 630–1)

Myerson's work was wise and forward looking, He attacked the dogmatic nature of eugenics, pleaded for more neutral science and emphasised the need for law to be based on this and to face up to the task of 'manipulating a prejudiced society' (p. 633) to protect the individual, even if doing so seemed to retard reform. Myerson's position was shared, for instance, by Penrose, and indeed by then, by many academic geneticists in the United States and in Britain.

The report seems to have ended any enthusiasm for eugenics in America, but it did not disappear altogether. Lennox, the leading American epileptologist of the period, had written before the war that society should eliminate congenital 'idiots and monsters ... The selection of the congenitally and hopelessly mindless for elimination would offer no more difficulties than their selection for lifelong incarceration. A court-appointed medical committee would be sufficient.'[126] He stuck to his convictions after the war, writing in 1950, for instance: '[W]e unmercifully prolong the lives of imbeciles (clock cases without works whose only relief is death).'[127]

NEUROLOGY OF EPILEPSY

In the first decades of the twentieth century clinical neurology lost its emphasis on epilepsy, which previously had been at the centre of neurological thought and theory. Quite why this happened is not entirely clear. Disease is subject to fashion as much as any other human endeavour, and the lack of clinical progress, the retreat from the earlier and exaggerated advantages of surgery and from discredited conceptual theories may be partly to blame. Nor did epilepsy suit the style of practice that was developing amongst neurologists, who were more interested in rare diseases and subtle clinical signs, and tended to value the intellectual challenge of diagnosis and nosology more than the

[126] Lennox, 'Should they live?'. The idea echoed the German genetic health courts and is a chilling reminder that leaving decisions to medical examiners without oversight is fraught with risk.

[127] In an address given in 1950 titled 'Epilepsy then, now and a century hence', cited in Offen, 'Dealing with "defectives"'.

mundane aspects of epilepsy. Also, increasingly in the interwar years, neurologists wanted to distance themselves from psychiatry and asylum practice.

However, by the late 1930s neurology was itself under pressure. The perception had arisen that it was a diagnostic discipline, sandwiched between the more advanced specialties of psychiatry and neurosurgery. Neurology was seen as old-fashioned, backward-looking and elitist. It was a specialty with a reputation for obtuse diagnosis and a complete lack of, and disinterest in, any therapy. Neurologists were portrayed as working in an essentially primary care role with a practice dominated by neurotic conditions. This was all in marked contrast to psychiatry, which had reinvented itself, shedding its alienist image, boosted by the sciences of eugenics and psychoanalysis, both of which had popular support, and then by the rise of pharmacological and physical therapies. Psychiatry became perceived as forward-looking and therapeutically minded in tune with the times – the exact opposite of neurology. Similarly, neurosurgery emerged in the 1930s from a low position as a dismal cousin of general surgery into a fully fledged speciality of its own. New techniques and new operations gave it a glittering and innovative reputation. And, buttressed by the necessities of war, the number of neurosurgical units was rapidly expanding. In the United Kingdom, for example, only three neurosurgical departments existed in the early 1930s, but by 1961 there were at least twenty-five.[128] In every country, psychiatrists greatly outnumbered neurologists, and where specialists were involved in epilepsy, most were psychiatrists.[129] In 1951, in his paper on the past, present and future of neurology, Pearce Bailey, the doyen of American neurologists wrote: 'the neuropsychiatric movement in the United States did more to set neurology back in its bid for professional autonomy than any other single development in its history. This movement split neurologically trained physicians into two camps, neurologists and neuropsychiatrists, which tended to deplete them as a group.' Furthermore,

> the already budding specialty of neurologic surgery burst into full bloom under the astute and progressive leadership of Harvey Cushing. The new, young, spirited and closely knit group of neurosurgeons graduated way above the level of surgical technicians. They entered aggressively the field of neurologic research, especially along neurophysiologic lines, which had been neglected by the clinical neurologists; they were therapeutically minded in contrast to the traditional neurologist who began to assume a reactionary tinge; and in some instances, the neurosurgeons challenged the neurologist's specialized talent in neurologic diagnosis … Consequently, at the end of World War II, the clinical neurologist found himself out of harmony with the trend of the times, and was confused by the glare of a scintillating psychologic age … [I]t appeared

---

[128] Pennybacker, Unpublished memoirs.   [129] Weisz, *Divide and Conquer.*

that neurology, particularly clinical neurology, had reached its lowest ebb.[130]

In Germany, too, up until the 1930s, most neurologists worked in the community in private practice, and by 1930 there were vociferous complaints about the parlous state of their specialty, with only a minority of hospitals having special departments and only in the large teaching hospitals.

But fashions change, and so did the fortunes of neurology. In the years after World War II, diagnostic techniques and new treatments transformed the speciality. Indeed, over the subsequent few decades it again rose to a position at the pinnacle of medicine and, as it did so, separated entirely from psychiatry. Epilepsy played its full part in these developments.

Clinical Research and Medical Training

One other reason for neurology's post-war rise was its emphasis on research, and the seeds of this were planted in the 1930s, backed by the Rockefeller Foundation and, to a lesser extent, other funding sources. Clinical research began to flourish in several fields of medicine in the late interwar years, and one of these was epilepsy. Prior to the World War 1, scientific research was rare amongst medical practitioners, and when individual clinicians did carry out research (Horsley and Gowers being prime examples) this was a part-time and amateur activity.[131] It was only in Germany that full-time academic university positions were appointed, and this became a structure widely regarded as responsible for German primacy in science. This in itself had begun to cause widespread concern in the anglophone world (although the Nazi government then decimated German university structures, with many of the best German scientists fleeing to other countries). In America, the influential Flexner report,[132] published in 1910, had painted a contrasting and gloomy picture of contemporary American medical education and research, considering there to be only five institutions in the country which were centres of medical research. Urging the adoption of the German university-based model, the report had recommended the establishment of academic units in which training in laboratory investigation was a prelude to clinical training, in which the scientific investigation of disease was

---

[130] Bailey, 'Past, present and future'. It was in response to this crisis that Abe B. Baker, Chair of Neurology and Psychiatry at the University of Minnesota, and a cohort of about fifty 'young Turks' founded the American Academy of Neurology (AAN) in 1948. In contrast to the ANA (the American Neurological Association), which had a limited membership dominated by older members, the AAN became the forum for younger and more progressive neurologists and grew into a prominent and successful organisation.

[131] A PhD was a rare degree in clinical practise in those days; indeed, when Michael Foster was appointed to the first Chair of Physiology in Cambridge in 1883 he made it a stipulation that future holders should be barred from practising medicine.

[132] Flexner, *Medical Education in the United States and Canada*.

promoted, in which all physicians had a responsibility to create new scientific knowledge and in which medical schools and universities were to work closely together. Academic units were to be led by medical professors – full-time academics freed from any major responsibilities for patient care so that they could focus on research and teaching. The report also recommended the closure of so-called for-profit proprietary medical schools, responsible for the pall of mediocrity over American medicine. Its findings were taken to heart and although many criticised Flexner's vision for producing doctors who were too narrow in outlook and too over-specialised,[133] the report was a turning point. Stimulated by large donations from the Rockefeller and Carnegie Foundations, by the mid-1920s twenty or so academic institutions had been established. The reorganisation of the National Institutes of Health (NIH) in 1948 further boosted research, and this particularly had an electrifying effect on epilepsy research, as we shall see in the next chapter. In Britain, the Haldane Commission of 1913[134] came to similar conclusions and recommended that academic units, led by full-time professors on the newly proposed American model, be established; that medical professors should be of the same standard as their university counterparts and dedicated to teaching and research and not the pursuance of large private practices; and that training should be of the same standards as in the non-clinical sciences. The commission's recommendations though went largely unheeded as the powerful lobby of senior clinicians protested violently about what they considered an assault on the traditional apprenticeship model of medical education and their own self-interest; indeed, it was only in 1962 that the first established professorship of neurology was created in Britain, and that was in the face of staunch opposition from clinical colleagues.[135]

Radiology

The discovery of the clinical potential for X-ray in 1895 was a medical landmark, for which Wilhelm Röntgen was awarded the first Nobel Prize in Physics in 1901. But although X-ray revolutionised the investigation of patients in many branches of medicine, brain diseases (including epilepsy) were not much assisted.

---

[133] Sir William Osler warned that medicine would change as 'teacher and student chased each other down the fascinating road of research, forgetful of those wider interests to which a hospital must minister' (cited in Duffy, 'The Flexner Report'). As Duffy put it in 2011, absolutely correctly, 'the trust and respect that were extended to the profession 50 years ago have been substantially eroded. There has been a fall from grace of our vaunted profession. Physicians have lost their authenticity as trusted healers. We have become derelict in many realms' (p. 273).

[134] *Report of the Royal Commission on University Education in London.*

[135] See Shorvon and Compston, *Queen Square*, pp. 444—60, for the machinations around the establishment of the Chair of Neurology.

Plain X-ray cannot distinguish between grey and white matter or brain tissue and cerebrospinal fluid (CSF) – all are largely invisible (i.e. the difference in contrast-[136] between these substances was too small to be visualised) – and in this sense the brain proved a dark and unexplored continent. Bone and calcification, on the other hand, have very different contrast and can be clearly imaged. That meant that abnormalities of the skull and the calcified cysts of neurocysticercosis were detectable, but these are rare causes of epilepsy and the common important structural abnormalities underlying epilepsy remained imperceptible. Then, in 1918, Walter Dandy[137] introduced ventriculography, a technique in which a substance with markedly different contrast was injected into the ventricles of the brain rendering visible to X-Ray their shape and position.[138] His first experiments were on infants with gross hydrocephalus, then adults, with air introduced through holes ('burr holes') drilled in the skull. In 1919 he started to inject air via a lumber puncture and invented what came to be known as pneumoencephalography (or air encephalography).[139] Subsequently, in France Jan Sicard discovered that the opaque lipid lipiodol could be used instead of air, and lipiodol[140] ventriculography was born. Both methods became widely used as diagnostic tools in neurology. They enabled detection of abnormalities by looking for distortions of ventricular shape, which would prove useful in detecting tumours and other structural brain changes. Dandy's landmark chapter in Dean Lewis's *Practice of Surgery* of 1932 listed seventeen different pathologies causing epilepsy which could be visualised using ventriculography (Table 2.1). These technologies were an enormous boost to neurosurgery[141] and contributed to its growth in influence. As the techniques were performed by neurosurgeons, they also proved useful ammunition in neurosurgery's turf war with neurology.

[136] Contrast is the image density of a structure and is a function of the number of X-ray photons transmitted when an X-ray beam is directed through an object.

[137] Along with Horsley and Cushing, Dandy was considered one of the founding fathers of neurosurgery. He was a pioneer of air encephalography and ventriculography. Working at Johns Hopkins, at the peak of his career was said to have operated on more than 1,000 patients per year. He devised the hemispherectomy for epilepsy, but it is not clear whether he had any interest in other forms of epilepsy surgery.

[138] In 1917, a remarkable case was published in the English medical literature of a women with headache and a feeling that 'her brain was splashing'. She consulted a London Hospital physician, Dr Gilbert Scott, who carried out an X-ray which showed air inside her head, due presumably to an opening following previous surgery on a skull tumour. The air allowed the outline of the woman's brain and the ventricles to be visualised. Whether Dandy read this report is not known, but it was, in effect, the first ventriculogram, albeit produced by accident.

[139] In this procedure, air is injected into the CSF in the lower back. The patient is then turned upside down, gravity pulls the air into the head and an X-ray picture is taken. For an early description, see Sicard and Forestier, 'Méthode radiographique'.

[140] Lipiodol is an ethiodised oil composed of iodine and the ethyl esters of fatty acids of poppy seed oil.

[141] In this way, very similar to the effects of computed tomography and magnetic resonance imaging later in the century.

TABLE 2.1 *Walter Dandy's seventeen categories of brain lesions causing epilepsy which could be visualised by ventriculography*

Congenital malformation and maldevelopment, either general or focal
Tumors
Abscesses
Tubercles
Gummata
Aneurysms
Syphilis with or without demonstrable gummata or vascular occlusions
Areas of cerebral degeneration and calcification
Depressed fractures
Hamartomata
Foreign bodies
Injuries from trauma at birth or subsequently (focal or general)
Connective tissue formation after trauma
Atrophy of the brain after trauma
Thrombosis and embolism
Cerebral arteriosclerosis
Sequelae of obscure inflammatory processes including encephalitis

As Dandy wrote: 'Current opinion is … veering round to the view that all epilepsies are symptomatic, inclusive of the variety [idiopathic epilepsy] whose basis still elude search … the cause will eventually be revealed.' This is a curious list to modern eyes
(Dandy, 'Brain', p. 330)

In 1927, António Egas Moniz introduced cerebral angiography.[142] He had the novel idea that imaging the position of blood vessels in the brain could identify the presence of brain lesions with greater sensitivity than ventriculography. The key was to find the best substance (a 'contrast medium') to use – one which was sufficiently opaque to X-ray in the short time that it circulated around the blood vessels of the head but also safe to use. Moniz experimented with a variety of different opaque substances and concentrations, killing a number of patients in the process. Finally, he alighted on 25% sodium iodide as a suitable contrast medium and at the time of injection temporarily ligated the carotid artery to slow down the speed of blood flow. By 1928 he was able to diagnose the presence of a pituitary tumour using this method, and by 1931 had published a celebrated book describing 180 cases of sodium iodine cerebral angiography.[143] Nonetheless, it remained a hazardous technique, with significant mortality and morbidity, and few scrupulous surgeons were prepared to use it. In 1931, the introduction of thorium dioxide (Thorotrast), a radioactive compound, as a contrast medium produced greatly superior opacification without carotid ligation, and was safer. Cerebral angiography was then adopted

---

[142] In addition to angiography, Moniz devised the prefrontal leucotomy, for which he shared the Nobel Prize in Medicine for 1949.
[143] Moniz, *Diagnostic des tumeurs cérébrales*, p. 931.

worldwide.[144] A strikingly hostile debate between neurosurgeons ensued over whether angiography or pneumoencephalography was the superior technique. But, over the next three decades, it was appreciated that both methods were complementary, and they were used together with plain radiology.[145]

At the time, these new technologies were said to be able to identify causal brain lesions in 17–30% of cases of epilepsy,[146] which was almost certainly an overestimate. Dandy himself was not shy in wildly overstating the value of these new medical developments:

> Epilepsy is always regarded as an idiopathic disease. The theories of its causation are indeed so numerous as to reflect seriously upon any exclusive stand concerning its etiology or pathology. However, the writer is confident that there is now assembled from experimental, pathologic, clinical and surgical studies a sufficient number of unquestioned facts to place epilepsy unequivocally upon a pathologic instead of idiopathic basis … [T]he fundamental conception that in every case of epilepsy there is a lesion of the brain can no longer admit of doubt … The lesions causing epilepsy are most varied. Although superficially of such dissimilar character, fundamentally they act in the same way, i.e., each represents a defect in the nervous paths of the cerebral hemispheres.[147]

In fact, it was the later introduction of EEG, not the enhanced radiological techniques, which were to have the greatest impact on epilepsy. Nevertheless, by demonstrating the relevance of structural changes in the brain, radiology did contribute to the rising interest in symptomatic epilepsy. No longer was idiopathic epilepsy considered the only form of 'genuine epilepsy', and the idea that epilepsy was, in the vast majority of cases, an inherited condition had been seriously challenged if not entirely discredited. This represented a paradigm shift in the concept of the condition.

Kinnier Wilson and Non-Hereditarian Theories of Epilepsy

A key figure in the switch of focus from hereditarian to symptomatic causes was Samuel Kinnier Wilson.[148] Seen in the late interwar years as the European neurologist with the greatest intellectual grasp of epilepsy (although actually born in America), and brought up in the older neurological tradition, he was

---

[144] Thorotrast is insoluble in water and permanently retained in some tissues, and concern about the safety of its radioactivity began to be expressed in 1937. However, it was thirty years later when was it finally recognised to be the cause of the subsequent development of malignant tumours. As late as 1995, lawsuits were being pursued in the United States by sufferers given Thorotrast in these earlier years.

[145] Bull, 'History of neuroradiology'.   [146] Shorvon, 'Neuroimaging in epilepsy'.

[147] Dandy, 'Brain', pp. 324, 329.

[148] Samuel Alexander Kinnier Wilson was appointed neurologist to the the National Hospital, Queen Square and Kings College Hospital London.

very much a link between the vintage period of Jackson, Horsley and Gowers and the new generation of the 1920s and 1930s. Wilson's style was traditional and old-fashioned – aloof, elitist, narcissistic and obsessive – and he viewed his specialty as a clinical topic of a higher intellectual standard than other medical specialties.[149] He was trained in classics; studied with Joseph Babinski and Pierre Marie in Paris, as well as the physicians at Queen Square in London; was a fluent linguist; and had a rich understanding of French, German and English culture. He strongly rejected eugenics. Although deeply interested in psychiatry, he vehemently opposed the concept of the epileptic personality and psychoanalytic views of epilepsy. His masterpiece was his 1,838-page three-volume textbook of neurology, published posthumously in 1940.[150]

In relation to the aetiology of epilepsy, Wilson spoke for many when he wrote in 1929: 'The hereditary factor is persistently overrated ... It is time protest should be unitedly voiced by neurologists against the portentous ascription of a sinister prognosis to every case of epilepsy because of a supposed inheritance and consequent incurability.'[151]

Epilepsy, he believed, was the result of organic cerebral pathology (Table 2.2), often but not always structural in nature; in idiopathic epilepsy this pathology existed, but it had not yet been identified. Furthermore, all epileptic seizures could be considered as symptoms of an 'epilepsy', regardless of aetiology, and the idea that only idiopathic epilepsy was genuine epilepsy was outmoded. The widespread introduction of new investigatory techniques such as air encephalography, ventriculography and angiography had advanced the study of epilepsy particularly by detecting brain trauma and tumours. However, the shift in emphasis from the belief in heredity and degeneration was not only the result of advanced radiology. Epilepsy had also become a more widely treatable condition, which meant that its management moved away from

---

[149] Macdonald Critchley, Wilson's friend and colleague, once asked him about a British Medical Association lecture Wilson had given in Leeds, and the story is a vivid illustration of his style: '"I hate the North of England", said Wilson, "and if there is one city I particularly loathe it is Leeds ... I got there in the afternoon. It wasn't until nearly seven o'clock that I was offered a sweet glass of sherry. Then at dinner I was seated next to a woman who never stopped talking. Her sole topic was Bernard Shaw, and if there is one person I detest it's George Bernard Shaw. ... What about the lecture? ... My subject was epilepsy, and as you know the sort of material that intrigues me. What is the biological meaning, if any, of the convulsive seizure? What does it represent? An abrupt release of inhibition? an excitatory phenomenon? neurogenic? or chemically initiated? I hadn't been talking more than 10 minutes when a voice shouted out from the back, 'Speak up' ... I stopped and turned to the Chairman. 'Mr Chairman', I said, 'I have been lecturing for 25 years, and never before have I been told that my voice does not carry'. At the end of the talk the Chairman invited questions. There was a long silence, and then someone said 'I would like to ask the specialist from London what dose of the bromides he recommends'. My dear Critchley, I ask you!'" (M. Critchley, 'Remembering Kinnier Wilson').

[150] Wilson died prematurely in 1937 at the age of fifty-eight. His neurology textbook was virtually complete at his death, and the final editing was done by his brother-in-law, Ninian Bruce.

[151] Wilson, 'Problem of the epilepsies'.

TABLE 2.2 *Causes of epilepsy mentioned by Kinnier Wilson*

Exciting/ predisposing causes	Heredity, fever, sleep, menstruation, menopause, pregnancy, acute renal inflammation with albuminuria, psychical states
Humoral and vascular cerebral states	1. Diseases of cerebral blood vessels: occlusion, embolism, haemorrhage, arteriosclerosis, endarteritis obliterans, endarteritis calcificans 2. Disorders of cerebral circulation: morbus cordis, heart block, anaemia, asphyxia, interference with carotid and vertebral streams, anomalies of venous sinuses. Any condition causing venous obstruction or delay 3. Disorders of cerebrospinal fluid regulation and flow: hydrocephalus internal or external, fluid stasis, cerebral oedema, rise in fluid pressure, etc.
Cerebral disease conditions	1. Cerebral tumours 2. Infections and toxi-infections' encephalitis, syphilis, tuberculous abscess; toxins of many specific fevers and exanthema, of meningitic affections, etc 3. Toxi-degenerations and sclerosis, polysclerosis, tuberose sclerosis, diffuse sclerosis, Pick's cortical atrophy, Alzheimer disease, plumbism, alcoholism, cysticercosis, puncture of the pleura ('pleural epilepsy') 4. Cerebral trauma 5. Some forms of congenital and heredo-familial disease

(Derived from Wilson, *The Epilepsies* (1935) and *Neurology* (1940)).

institutions into routine outpatient practice. In this new setting it also became clear that most patients did not suffer mental deterioration and that the many eugenic assumptions about epilepsy, and the stigma under which patients thus laboured, were unwarranted and unjustified.

Perhaps the most definitive work on epilepsy in this period was Wilson's imperious 87-page chapter in the *Handbuch der Neurologie* of 1935,[152] which was longer and more detailed than the epilepsy section in his textbook, although both contain similar material. This volume firmly pointed the way towards the modern concept of epilepsy. He attacked 'the traditional view' that there is 'a disease called epilepsy' and that

> [t]his 'disease' is alleged to be progressive, rather intractable, and prone to result in mental deterioration. Its cause being unknown, it is labelled 'idiopathic' … But the epithet is obsolete, serving merely to cloud the issue. It is curious that the patently symptomatic nature of so many epilepsies has not yet sufficed to convince everyone of the untenable character of the hypothesis constituting this 'idiopathic' variety a self-contained and circumscribed entity. No less confusion has been engendered by resort to such terms as 'genuine' or 'essential' to characterise the

---

[152] Wilson, 'Epilepsies'.

'disease', as though fits of a symptomatic kind were merely casual or in some way 'false'. The best present-day opinion declines to accept the implication underlying the 'idiopathic' doctrine, viz. that of 'epilepsia sine materie', affirming on the contrary that all epilepsy is symptomatic, whether its basis is discoverable or not. (p. 1)

Wilson also pointed out that some patients have very occasional seizures and that infantile seizures often do not 'authorise a diagnosis of epilepsy' (p. 2). In view of its variability, and multiple causation, he wondered whether the term 'epilepsy' should be replaced by 'the epilepsies' or, better, by 'paroxysmal disorders' or 'convulsive states' (although he acknowledged the difficulties of such terminologies). He considered that the criteria for a classification of seizures could include clinical form (i.e. seizure type), aetiology (disengaging the 'exciting causes' from the underlying 'morbid conditions', p. 6), age of life and pathology. He was of course writing before EEG provided visual evidence of the physiological basis of seizures, and more is the pity that he died at about the time that the technique was being introduced into medicine, as his assessment of the technology would have been most instructive.

Interestingly, Wilson observed that the pathological tissue is itself not responsible for the liberation of energy and the positive symptoms which constitute the epileptic fit required the presence of 'normal cells … Thus, the various diseased states in whose presence fits have been remarked do not properly constitute the specific pathology of epilepsy, though their analytic study aids in penetrating the mystery of pathogenesis' (p. 6).

In dismissing heredity, he also noted: 'Were inheritance of much import as a determinant, out-patient practice should have brought me numerous instances of the condition among siblings, yet in point of fact this is distinctly rare.'[153] Based on his own experience, he concluded that 'at most, what can be thus handed on from one generation to the next is an obscure cellular tendency to excessive reaction demonstrable only if circumstances calculated to evoke it should arise' (p. 63). This is a notably modern view, made at a time when the mechanisms of heredity were unknown, and perhaps vindicated only in the past ten years.

By 1937, even William Lennox admitted that 'the hereditary factor in epilepsy is much less than imagined. It is smaller than for other non-infectious nervous and mental diseases and is about the same as for diabetes.'[154] Muskens ventured that 'the view was at one time very generally accepted that epilepsy was almost always hereditary, but it has long since been realised that this is not so'.[155] Similarly, at the International Congress of Neurology in London in

---

[153] In his 1940 textbook, Wilson wrote that heredity was operative in only about one-fifth of his cases (p. 1524)
[154] Lennox, 'Epilepsy'.   [155] Muskens, *Epilepsy*, p. 408.

1935, Jean Abadie[156] lectured on the general aetiology of common epilepsy and followed Wilson in making the point that epilepsy was not a true disease, but a lesional manifestation: 'The old idea of an epilepsy called idiopathic, as opposed to symptomatic epilepsy, had been completely given up ... Epilepsy is not a neurosis; it is due to organic injury of the nervous centers. Epilepsy is not a hereditary disease; it is an acquired affection.'[157] In 1938, H. P. Stubbe Teglbjaerg, a leading Danish epilepsy specialist, quoted Wilson and then remarked: 'The distinction between genuine and symptomatic epilepsy is not tenable any longer, and the distinction between cryptogenic and symptomatic epilepsy can only be considered a working hypothesis, which is maintained for practical reasons for the time being owing to defective diagnostics.'[158]

In addition to the new focus on structural causes of epilepsy, there was also interest in the chemical factors precipitating seizures. In the 1920s and 1930s, no doubt in part the result of the renaissance of academic medicine stimulated by the Flexner report in America, the science of clinical chemistry had developed in tandem with improvements in measuring technologies.[159] Much of the chemical research in epilepsy was led from Boston by Lennox and Stanley Cobb, the apogee of this work being their book titled *Epilepsy, from the Standpoint of Physiology and Treatment*.[160] It is an extended summary of their researches (supported by an exhaustive list of more than 600 references to the contemporary literature which covers almost all of the work in this area). Of the 193 pages, 120 are devoted to the 'the factors involved in convulsions' (and only 3 pages on treatment), where the known physiochemical changes in epilepsy are detailed. The authors described 'the so-called irritation, release, short circuit and explosive theories' of epilepsy (p. 225).

Other theories of causation had been rejected by the time Kinnier Wilson's book was published, including two mentioned in the previous chapter. Reflex theories of epilepsy had previously been widely promulgated, but

---

[156] Abadie was chair of neurology and psychiatry in Bordeaux, and one of the few neurologists in France at the time who had a specific interest in epilepsy.

[157] 'International Neurological Congress in London'.

[158] Stubbe Teglbjaerg, 'Modern hospitals for epileptics'. Between 1949 and 1957 Stubbe Teglbjaerg served as vice-president and then treasurer of the ILAE.

[159] Chemical analysis in epilepsy had a long tradition. In 1906, at the Craig Colony, Munson had a chemistry laboratory, and both Spratling and Turner gave lengthy descriptions of chemical changes in epilepsy.

[160] Lennox and Cobb, *Physiology and Treatment*. This was an early work by Lennox but had all the hallmarks of his later writings. It was perhaps also the first example of one of his typical diagrams – in which he divided the 'factors' involved in the production of a convulsion as brain factors (functional and structural) and factors 'outside the brain tissue' (sympathetic nervous system, gastrointestinal factor, etc.) (p. 130). The book was based on a series of seventeen papers in the *Archives of Neurology and Psychiatry* titled 'Clinical Studies of Epilepsy', which contributed to Lennox's reputation as the leading researcher of his time. The series included studies of sugar metabolism, bicarbonate, fibrin, basal metabolism, fasting, cerebral circulation and respiratory quotient.

Wilson hardly mentions them in his text.[161] Nevertheless, a few rare triggers were then, and have continued to be, recognised as reflex in origin, and seizures reliably induced by these factors retain the name 'reflex epilepsy', of which musicogenic epilepsy[162] is one the best known. One particular variant of reflex theory was elaborately worked on by Muskens, who experimented on hundreds of cats with seizures induced by monobromide of camphor. Muskens concluded that myoclonic fits in idiopathic epilepsy were a special form of reflex after-discharge (following Sherrington, who was Muskens' mentor, and whose amanuensis Muskens liked to consider himself), which in his view helped render toxins inactive. In this sense the seizure, like shivering and fever, was a healthy adaptation. Muskens also seems to have considered that the pons and medulla were the main generators within the nervous axis of a myoclonic seizure. One fears the cats died in vain. He was, however, correct in recognising that myoclonus was a common feature of idiopathic epilepsy, and also a most common form of epilepsy. His book *Epilepsy* (1924) provides a detailed description of his experimental studies and clinical observations, including a dissertation on what today would be categorised as juvenile myoclonic epilepsy.[163]

Another theory which by 1939 had withered due to lack of evidence was that seizures were caused by an internal toxin (the 'autointoxication' hypothesis). In earlier decades this theory had strong support. For instance, in 1924, the Queen Square physician (and colleague of Wilson) James Collier gave a paper on the causes of epilepsy, expressing the rather curious view that in the majority of cases, and possibly all cases, epilepsy was not a true disease of the brain but, citing Hermann Oppenheim, a 'toxicopathic condition with cerebral manifestations'. External toxins such as lead, bismuth and absinthe and internal toxins such as are produced in fever, metabolic dyscrasias, renal and hepatic disease, eclampsia and thyroid and pituitary disease were, he claimed, 'capable of producing manifest-ations in every way indistinguishable from those of epilepsy'. Once triggered by a toxin, the epilepsy could continue in the absence of the toxic precipitant.[164] This theory turned out to be a path leading nowhere, but reflected the fashions of an age obsessed with toxin theories of many diseases.

How marked the changing views on aetiology were in this period is dem-onstrated in the chapter on epilepsy by Kinnier Wilson in his 1940 textbook,

---

[161] The concept of reflex epilepsy underwent somewhat of a revival in the 1980s.

[162] Critchley, 'Musicogenic epilepsy'.

[163] This was a form of epilepsy already well described by Gowers, who called the myoclonic seizures 'starts'. Others described these using such names as: impulsions, secousses, commo-tions épileptiques (Herpin, 1867); petit mal moteur (Delasiauve, 1854; Féré, 1890); myo-clonies épileptiques (Rabot, 1899); intermittierende Myoclonusepilepsie (Lundborg, 1903); jerks (Turner, 1907); myoclonic petit mal (Penfield and Jasper, 1954); and impulsiv-petit mal (Janz, 1955).

[164] Collier, 'Nature and treatment'.

where he again attacked the idea that epilepsy is a unitary condition and an inherited degeneration.[165] He also dismissed the importance of 'bad teeth, septic tonsils, nasal polypi, refractive errors, phimosis, intestinal worm, and what not' (p. 1527). Amongst the symptomatic causes, he mentioned seizures during anaesthesia ('ether convulsions'), pleural epilepsy (today we would consider this vaso-vagal) and cysticercosis (an imperial disease, as he noted that 'although infestation may occur in England, the majority contracted the disease in Egypt, India, or the Malay States'; p. 1528). He also described precipitating factors such as cosmic influences (which he dismissed), sleep, menstrual epilepsy and pregnancy (including eclampsia) and psychical states.

Wilson listed the factors causing epilepsy in 'pathological states' (p. 1514), which he divided into two categories and eight subdivisions (Table 2.2). The two categories were neural (cerebral), and humoral and vascular. The five subdivisions of cerebral causes were tumours; infections and toxins; cerebral toxi-degenerations or scleroses; trauma; and some forms of congenital and heredo-familial diseases. The three categories of humoral and vascular states were diseases or disorders of blood vessels; disorders of cerebral circulation; and disorders of CSF regulation. He also considered the provocation of epileptic seizures in three further categories: mechanical (due to increased intracranial pressure, increased permeability of tissues, alteration of water balance, pressure on or ligation of carotids and vertebrals); exogenous (convulsants, insulin hypoglycaemia, foreign proteins, anoxaemia, alteration of acid-base equilibrium and alkalosis); and endogenous (endocrine disorders of parathyroid, thyroid, pituitary, ovary, etc.). He discussed the mechanisms by which seizures could be produced. Finally, he addressed the effect of intercurrent infections and pyrexia on seizures. To Wilson, epilepsy could be caused by almost any disease of the cerebral cortex. By 1940 this seems to have become the predominant view. For perhaps the first time, a modern and comprehensive list of causes of epilepsy had been produced; this laid the foundation for all subsequent views of causation, and finally put to rest the theories of inherited degeneration.

William Lennox and Boston Epileptology

The geography of epilepsy was changing. The two world wars decimated Europe, and the previously thriving research and clinical centres of Eastern

---

[165] Wilson and Bruce, *Neurology*, vol. 2. Wilson's colleague Francis Walshe expressed similar sentiments in his own textbook: '[Epilepsy] has always been regarded as a heritable condition, though it obeys no known laws of inheritance, and it is probable that what is inherited – if anything be – is an instability of function in the cells of the cerebral cortex ... [N]othing is known of what these exciting [causes of idiopathic epilepsy] may be ... [C]ertainly the heritable causes of epilepsy have been greatly exaggerated in the past, and in consequence severe restrictions upon the liberty of conduct of the epileptic have been imposed in the guise of medical advice' (Walshe, *Nervous System*, p. 115).

Europe shrank into insignificance. Basic science continued in Western Europe in a limited fashion, but the transition of clinical leadership in neurology to America, which had begun in the early interwar years, stimulated by Flexner and funded by Rockefeller and Carnegie, was greatly hastened by the Second World War. The output of epilepsy research from the leading European institutes in London (National Hospital, Queen Square), Paris (Salpêtrière) and Germany (Charité) dwindled, and was replaced by that from Boston, Chicago, New York and Philadelphia. Key figures in this growth of American epilepsy included Stanley Cobb, William Lennox, Herbert Jasper, Frederic and Erna Gibbs, and Tracy Putnam. The reasons are complex, but the energy, confidence and modernity of the American medical structures, especially with the backing of philanthropic money, were in sharp contrast to those in an exhausted and time-worn Europe.

William Lennox[166] is a name which has already appeared and which will appear time and again in this book. Lennox was born in 1884 in Colorado Springs, where his father was a pioneer settler who made a good living from his livery business and prospecting. Lennox's mother was from a long line of Quakers, and the boy was brought up in a devout, god-fearing family. From a young age, he seemed destined for service to the church. Yet when he applied for a place at Boston University Divinity School, his application was turned down because of his weakness in Latin and Greek. At college, Lennox's greatest influence was Edward Christian Schneider,[167] a physiologist and professor of biology. It was Schneider who persuaded Lennox to take up medicine as a way of furthering his faith. Lennox entered Harvard Medical School and, after obtaining his qualifications, spent the next four years in China as a medical missionary at Union Medical College. He lived frugally in China with his wife and two baby daughters, and Frederic Gibbs relates that he would have devoted his life to missionary work had his daughters not become repeatedly ill.[168] After four years Lennox returned to Boston and entered 'a new ministry, medical research'.[169] He did return to China once, in 1928, for a year, and there compiled a book titled *The Health and Turnover of Missionaries*.[170] In Boston, Lennox was employed as assistant to Stanley Cobb in 1922 (who in 1925 was appointed Professor of Neuropathology) at Harvard Medical School to investigate the ketogenic diet being proposed as a treatment for epilepsy.

---

[166] Details here are taken from Gibbs, 'William Gordon Lennox'; Millichap, 'William Lennox'; 'William Lennox, physician'; and Shorvon and Weiss, 'International League Against Epilepsy.'

[167] Schneider had a remarkable career, not least as a member of the extraordinary 1911 Anglo-American Expedition to Pikes Peak with J. S. Haldane, C. Gordon Douglas and Yandell Henderson; see West, *High Life*, and Schneider, *Burnet – Ferguson – Schneider*. Schneider not only persuaded Lennox to take up medicine but also taught Alan Gregg, later of the Rockefeller Foundation. Both were greatly to influence the course of epilepsy.

[168] Gibbs, 'William Gordon Lennox'.   [169] Gibbs, 'William Gordon Lennox'.

[170] Lennox, *Turnover of Missionaries*.

His interest in epilepsy is said to have dated from his time in China. Different sources state that his own daughter, or the eight-year-old daughter of a friend, was afflicted with the condition thus focusing his attention on the condition, and in *Epilepsy and Related Disorders*, published in 1960, Lennox also mentions the history of Ann, a cousin, with epilepsy.[171] There is no doubt that Lennox's daughter, Margaret, had epilepsy, as she mentioned it later, and it is interesting that Lennox himself never admitted this publicly despite his championship of better public acceptance. It was surely with a degree of hypocrisy that, in 1960 in *Epilepsy and Related Disorders*, he wrote about the 'canker of secrecy', which he considered the 'epileptic's most serious and implacable handicap' (p. 919).

His work, whilst under the tutelage of Cobb, and with Erna Leonhardt as research assistant, was published in a series of seventeen papers all bearing the title 'Studies in Epilepsy' in the *Archives of Neurology and Psychiatry*, and in the aforementioned book co-written with Cobb entitled *Epilepsy, from the Standpoint of Physiology and Treatment*.[172] These papers and the book describe well-conducted physiological and neurochemical studies. They were in many ways models of experimental method and equipped Lennox with a deep understanding of clinical research and investigation in his field. However, his neurochemical and physiological findings, although correct, were to prove to be culs-de-sac in the history of epilepsy. Neurochemistry was seen as a promising new field in the 1920s, and the discovery of chemical factors had led to experiments with a range of diets in epilepsy, but apart from the success of the ketogenic diet, these proved very disappointing. Lennox looked at other biochemical changes, including studies, in blood and CSF, of urea, sugar, fibrin, chloride and calcium, oxidation and carbon dioxide, but none were fruitful. The entire corpus of physiological and chemical work remains little more than a footnote, albeit an honourable one, in the history of epilepsy – as Lennox put it, 'blind tunnels off the main shaft of a deepening gold mine'[173] – and neither Cobb nor Lennox pursued this field after 1935. The last paper (number XVII) in *Studies in Epilepsy*, published in 1935,[174] however, was not concerned with chemistry and was of more profound importance – opening, as we shall see, the floodgates of EEG in epilepsy.

In 1930 Cobb was appointed director of the Harvard Neurological Unit at the Boston City Hospital. In 1934, when he moved to Massachusetts General Hospital as professor of psychiatry, Derek Denny-Brown[175] took over as director of the neurological unit. Thereafter, Lennox and his colleagues

---

[171] Lennox, *Epilepsy and Related Disorders*, vol. 1, pp. 79–80.
[172] Lennox and Cobb, *Physiology and Treatment*. [173] Lennox, *Epilepsy*, vol. 2, p. 739.
[174] Gibbs, Davis and Lennox, *The Electroencephalogram in Epilepsy*.
[175] Derek Ernest Denny-Brown, A New Zealander who became an American Citizen, had worked in London, Oxford. His work included studies of myoclonus much of which he considered of subcortical origin.

Frederic and Erna Gibbs[176] (Erna Leonhardt married Frederic Gibbs in 1930 and continued her work as Erna Gibbs) left the unit in turn to work at the Boston Psychopathic Hospital under the superintendentship of Harry Solomon.

In 1935, just at the time when Lennox's work on the brain physiology and chemistry of seizures was hitting the buffers, the Gibbses had visited Hans Berger in Jena.[177] They had already begun research on EEG, and Gibbs and Lennox then launched into the electroencephalographic clinical research programme that was to occupy them for several decades. Lennox was in the right place at the right time, and this research had a massive impact.

He presented the first results of his work on the respiratory quotient and on EEG at the International Medical Congress in London in 1935.[178] The event made his international reputation. On the same visit to London, Lennox was fortuitously elected president of the ILAE. In this position, he combined his interests in epilepsy and in writing as editor of the journal *Epilepsia* from 1941. With the coming of the Second World War, and as his European colleagues were subsumed in the processes of war, the centre of gravity of epilepsy moved unequivocally to Boston, with Lennox as its leading light.

In 1938, Houston Merritt and Tracy Putnam started their work on phenytoin in Boston, and Lennox also became deeply involved in this and the new wave of drugs for epilepsy that followed. This activity resulted in a series of further important papers by Lennox on the therapies of epilepsy.

Lennox moved to the Boston Children's Hospital in 1944 and there established the famous 'Seizure Unit', which was the first epilepsy unit of its time. As the unit director, Lennox trained many future epileptologists, all of whom were said to be devoted to him. Investigation was the mainstay of his practice, and although a conservative and paternalistic person, he unfailingly took a research-oriented view to the problem of epilepsy. As he wrote in 1937: 'In the US there are some 500,000 persons subject to epilepsy ... They are numerous, and are available to the research staff of the general hospital; they can usually give intelligent cooperation; they are pathetically anxious to be experimented upon; they have abrupt and unmistakable changes from normal to abnormal states.'[179]

---

[176] The Gibbses were integral to the success of Lennox's EEG work. Erna Gibbs was born in Germany and migrated to the USA in 1928. She found a post with William Lennox initially as a biochemistry technician and then took up electroencephalography with her future husband, Dr Frederick Gibbs. Frederic Andrews Gibbs graduated from Yale and Johns Hopkins. He was later appointed as Professor of Neurology at the University of Illinois.

[177] They had attended the International Congress of Physiologists in Leningrad and Moscow in 1935 and then visited not only Berger, but also Tönnies in Berlin and Adrian in Cambridge.

[178] Reported in 'International Neurological Congress in London'.

[179] Lennox, 'Problem of epilepsy'.

Lennox's work in relation to the two major clinical discoveries of the time – EEG and the novel medicament phenytoin – were examples of his intelligent application of research into clinical practice. J. Gordon Millichap provides a vivid picture of the unit at that time: 'Almost all his patients would form part of a study: a trial of a new drug, an electroencephalographic study of twins or relatives, biochemical and blood-flow studies, and the investigation of psychological factors. All aspects of epilepsy were studied, and a team of secretaries was at hand to aid with the many publications produced in his Seizure Unit.'[180]

Lennox was also a tireless campaigner for the alleviation of the social problems of epilepsy. He was deeply involved in founding the Layman's League Against Epilepsy,[181] the American Epilepsy League, the National Epilepsy League, the Epilepsy Federation, the United Epilepsy Society and the Epilepsy Information Center, and he wrote extensively on the education and social problems of patients with epilepsy and on fighting the prejudice that surrounded the condition. He worked closely with Merle McBride in the Layman's League and then with Gertrude Potter[182] to found the American Epilepsy League. He understood the patient's perspective in a way few others did at the time, and he was sensitive to and respectful of the societal as well as medical aspects of epilepsy. On May 24/25 1945, he appeared before US government hearings, informing the congressmen that 'Of all the handicaps which you and your committee are studying, epilepsy without doubt is the least understood by both the medical and general public and is the most neglected. Like the lepers of ancient times, epileptics still 'dwell without the city' of public understanding and philanthropy.' In 1949, the *National Epilepsy Act* was passed, 'to provide for research and investigation as to the cause, prevention, treatment and possible cure of epilepsy', and Lennox gave a powerful statement to the congressional committee looking into the issues.[183] In 1950, the National

---

[180] Millichap, 'William Lennox'. Gordon Millichap trained in medicine at St Bartholomew's Hospital in London before moving to Boston, and was later appointed Professor of Neurology at Northwestern University. He was a founding member of the Child Neurology Society in America.

[181] The Layman's League Against Epilepsy changed its name to the American Epilepsy League and later to the National Epilepsy League, for reasons which are not clear but which no doubt involved Lennox.

[182] Gertrude Brooks was appointed the first President of the American Epilepsy League.

[183] In part of this, Lennox stated: 'I speak for the half-million sick who dare not speak for themselves. Discovery of their illness would bring not helpful sympathy, but social ostracism … The epileptic must hide his condition or else be denied education and employment; therefore, the public does not know that epileptics outnumber persons who are crippled by polio or those with active tuberculosis or diabetes. Half the hospital beds in this country are taken by persons with nervous or mental disease, a tenth of these beds are for epileptics, yet 9 epileptics our of 10 are in the community … The big reasons for aiding the epileptic are two: first, pity; and second, economy. Pity to the point of nausea would be roused by a visit to some of the 50,000 epileptics now confined in our mental institutions. These, for the most part, are behold restoration. This is especially true of children irreparably defective at birth – their numbers constantly increasing because the mercy of death from infections is denied to

Institute for Neurological Disease and Blindness (NINDB) was established, and he was a key advocate to the congressional committee of NINDB and of the National Institutes of Health (NIH), providing evidence which ensured a rich trawl of public funding for epilepsy.

The jostling for positions of the lay and professional organisations in the arena of post-war American epilepsy has been an interesting example of the complexity of human behaviour, and are worth a short diversion. In the pre–World War I era, a single national professional and lay organisation represented epilepsy in America: the National Association for the Care and Treatment of the Epileptics (NACTE), based in New York and in existence from 1899 to 1914. In 1909 the ILAE was formed, and the NACTE affiliated itself with this new organisation – stimulating much American activity in epilepsy. The advent of war crushed both organisations, and nothing further transpired until the resuscitation of the ILAE in 1937. Lennox, elected ILAE President, worked hard to form a parallel lay organisation. This began a tangled and complicated story of mergers and demergers, with organisations and charities coming and going,due largely to geographical competition and professional jealously, resulting, finally, in 1967 in the emergence of the Epilepsy Foundation of America (EFA) and the American Epilepsy Society (AES) as the twin lay and professional representatives of American epilepsy – and both continue to this day.[184]

them by the use of inoculations and sulpha drugs. We cannot relieve society of this wreckage, but we can prevent many others from becoming a public charge. We should be most concerned with the thousands of useful lives and the millions of dollars that might be saved in the future by better care of epileptics in the community.' Lennox continued that 'key works in this saving' were prevention, early medical treatment and social therapy; and he believed that a saving of $6,000,000,000 in 30 years would be achieved by 'modern medical and social means of prevention and treatment' (*National Epilepsy Act*, pp. 6–7).

[184] The 1940–67 manoeuvrings can be summarised as follows: The Layman's League Against Epilepsy (Boston, 1940–4) was formed in April 1940 (some sources claim its date of origin to be 1939) with 370 members. In 1944/5, it changed its name to the American Epilepsy League (AEL; Boston, HQ, 1944–9) and Mrs Brooks Potter succeeded as president. The AEL opened chapters in Chicago (1946–9), Boston (1946–7) and New York (1946). The New York chapter split off immediately, objecting to paying part of its income to the parent organisation and changed its name to the National Association to Control Epilepsy (NACE; New York, 1944–9). In 1945, a second New York organisation was founded: the Epilepsy Association of New York. Then, in 1949, the National Epilepsy League (NEL) was formed from a merger of the AEL and the NACE. In the same year, three groups in New York – the Variety Club to Control Epilepsy, the Committee for Public Understanding of Epilepsy and the Epilepsy Association of New York (1945–54) – united under the name United Epilepsy Association (UEA). In parallel, in 1954, a new organisation, the Federal Association for Epilepsy, was incorporated in Virginia and this changed its name in 1956 to The Epilepsy Foundation (TEF). There was then intense negotiation involving the professional organisation, the American League Against Epilepsy, and in order to maximise fund-raising a 'committee of nine' was elected to form guidelines and by-laws for a national epilepsy organisation. As a result, the American Epilepsy Federation (AEF) was formed in 1957, headed by Ellen Grass, the main goal of which was the 'unity of all societies now concerned in the common cause of epilepsy' (and to support this effort, Lennox donated all the royalties

Paradoxically, given his public support of patients with epilepsy, Lennox was also an unapologetic eugenicist, and he apparently saw no contradiction in this position. He was a leading figure in the eugenics and euthanasia movements in the United States from the 1930s until his retirement. In 1938 he gave a lecture, which has since become notorious, to the Harvard Phi Beta Kappa chapter. In the lecture he stated: 'The principle of limiting certain races through limitation of offspring might be applied *intra*nationally as well as *inter*nationally. Germany in time might have solved her Jewish problems in this way. We zealously exclude certain aliens from our shores but both on the mainland and in overseas territories their entrance by birth is free and unlimited.'[185] He recommended both sterilisation and euthanasia for 'the congenitally mindless and for the incurable sick who wish to die' (p. 466). Lennox was an economic hawk, and one stated reason for his view on eugenics was that the mentally handicapped were an unacceptable drain on societal resources. Perhaps another was his desire to emphasise the normality of most sufferers, including his own daughter. Other aspects of Lennox's medical eugenics are covered in a recent article by M. Louis Offen[186] and make uncomfortable reading. In 1943, Lennox joined the advisory council of the Euthanasia Society of America. In 1949 he wrote an article entitled 'The moral issue', calling for the mercy killing of 'children with undeveloped or misformed brains' as a way of opening up space in 'our hopelessly clogged institutions'.[187]

Lennox was a gifted organiser and deeply involved in the international epilepsy movement. He almost single-handedly kept the ILAE in existence during the war, founded the AES, and later served as president of this society. He organised numerous conferences, including the first post-war congress of the ILAE in New York in 1949. He was a prolific author, with nearly 100 papers and 4 books to his credit.

Epilepsy and Related Disorders (see pp. 309–312) was published posthumously in two volumes in 1960, the year of his death, with the collaboration of Margaret Lennox. It is a central text in the history of epilepsy, possibly the best twentieth century book on the topic of epilepsy and a fitting culmination to his career.[188]

of his 1960s textbook to the AEF). In 1965, after protracted meetings and discussion, three major organisations – the AEF, the NEL and the UEA – agreed to merge into a new organisation named the Epilepsy Association of America (EAA), with headquarters in New York. Then in 1967, the TEF agreed to merge with the EAA to form a revised organisation named the Epilepsy Foundation of America (EFA). President Lyndon B. Johnson praised this development as a 'milestone in a major health field' and pledged sustained interest and cooperation. The NEL branch in Chicago withdrew from the plan, though, and budded off on its own (and continues today as the Epilepsy Foundation of Greater Chicago). (See 'Hearings', 'Epilepsy across the spectrum').

[185] Lennox, 'Should they live?'.   [186] Offen, 'Dealing with "defectives"'.
[187] Lennox, 'Moral issue'.
[188] Sadly, in recent years his reputation has been blemished by the eugenics connection. In 2018, the American Epilepsy Society changed the name of their lifetime achievement award from

Neuropathology and Neurochemistry

These were two areas in epilepsy on which experimental work was focused in the early and mid-interwar years. At the time, neuropathology was concerned mostly with histopathology and pathological (morbid) anatomy and was developing strongly because of new staining procedures and technical improvements in microscopy.

Much pathological interest was focused on Ammon's horn sclerosis (also called mesial temporal sclerosis, incisural sclerosis or hippocampal sclerosis), which was recognised to be a common finding in epilepsy. At the time, the lesion was considered by most authorities to be the result, not the cause of epilepsy, and hence there was no contradiction to including it as a common finding in cases of genuine (or idiopathic) epilepsy. The leading pathologist of the period was Walther Spielmeyer, who in 1925 supposed the lesion to be the result of ischaemic damage, analogous to the pattern of pathologies seen in global ischaemia.[189] In an influential monograph published in 1951,[190] Willibald Scholz would similarly emphasise the 'anoxic' nature of the damage and attributed this to the 'consumptive hypoxia' that occurs in a seizure where the energy requirement is high and cannot be met. The characteristic pattern of damage to the CA1 portion of the hippocampus and the relative resistance to damage of the CA2 portion (the 'resistant' sector), well recognised since the 1880s, was the subject of an important 1925 paper by Oskar Vogt,[191] who proposed that the different tissue had different vulnerabilities and attributed this pattern to paraclisis. Spielmeyer disagreed and argued that the difference in vulnerability was simply the result of the pattern of vascular supply. Although it is now known that the pyramidal neurons of these regions do indeed differ significantly, not least in respect of the high density of the excitatory glutamate receptor N-methyl-d-aspartate (NMDA). It was Spielmeyer's student Karl-Heinz Stauder who, on the basis of Spielmeyer's autopsy material, found that a proportion of patients with symptoms he ascribed to temporal lobe epilepsy had Ammon's horn sclerosis, making the link between this pathology and the seizure symptoms for the first time. In 1935 Stauder speculated that the lesion was due to contusional damage during falls,[192] but it was only in the 1950s and 1960s, with the advent of EEG and temporal lobe surgery, that the causal nature of the lesion became fully appreciated.

As noted earlier, neurochemistry was a fashionable field of study in the 1920s, although none of the findings of this period proved important or

---

the 'Lennox Award' to the 'Founders Award' – in my view a short-sighted 'wokish' decision that lacks historical perspective.
[189] Spielmeyer, *Zur Pathogenese.*   [190] Scholz, *Die Krampfschädigungen des Gehirns.*
[191] Vogt, 'Der Begriff der Pathoklise'.   [192] Stauder, 'Epilepsie und schläfenlappen'.

significant in the field of epilepsy. Early work was focused on endogenous compounds such as urea, uric acid, ammonium carbonate and phosphates, as well as glandular causes such as hypothyroidism, and intestinal causes. In early experiments, Gyula Donáth had tested various compounds by injecting chemicals into dogs, and this was taken to support the totally erroneous theory of autointoxication. By the 1930s, most interest was focused on acetylcholine, oxygenation and cerebral acid-base balance.[193] Gibbs and Lennox showed there was no anoxaemia before a seizure, challenging the contemporary orthodoxy that seizures were due to cerebral anaemia. They also noted marked anoxaemia after a seizure and correctly attributed it to the high oxygen utilisation during the event. They found that blood carbon dioxide concentrations were low prior to petit mal seizures but rose in the days before a grand mal seizure. Consequently, it was postulated that changes in acid-base balance might be the mechanism of seizure precipitation, either directly in the cortex in petit mal seizures or by release of cortical control of subcortical structures in grand mal seizures. Kinnier Wilson summarised Lennox and Cobbs' theory of humoral pathogenesis as follows:

> Contraction of cerebral vessels will cause deficiency of oxygen supply to brain tissues, and the anoxaemia will dilate capillaries, with outward passage of fluid through their walls. Lowered oxygen tension, oedema, or rise of intracranial pressure, singly or together, may then so interfere with neuronic function as to precipitate a fit. This will lead to accumulation of carbon dioxide and to relative acidosis; hence oxygen will be utilized by the tissues, fluid will pass back into capillaries and normal intracranial circulation be restored.[194]

He noted, though, that the initial vasoconstriction remained unexplained.

Support for the central role of acetylcholine metabolism was also demonstrated by seizures that occurred in low metabolic states and by the stimulating effects of camphor, metrazol and electrical shock.[195] Other studies had shown that hyperpyrexia precipitated seizures and was the explanation for the increased rate of seizures after a hot bath, assumed to be due to raised intracranial pressure.

The mechanism of action of antiepileptic drugs was also beginning to be studied in the 1940s. The predominant theory was that the anticonvulsant effect of drugs was exerted through cholinergic mechanisms, and various attempts were made to modify epilepsy by manipulating acetylcholine metabolism.[196] Animal screening tests for antiepileptic drug action were also

---

[193] Lennox, Gibbs and Gibbs, 'Relationship in man'; Himwich, *Brain Metabolism*; Page, *Chemistry of the Brain*.
[194] Wilson and Bruce, *Neurology*, vol. 2, p. 1519.
[195] Pope et al., 'Histochemical and action potential'.
[196] Williams, 'Cholin-like substances'; Toman, 'Neuropharmacology of antiepileptics'.

explored, following the success of Merritt and Putnam's method in the discovery of phenytoin. James Toman and Louis Goodman showed that no single test was sufficient in Sprague–Dawley rats, but a combination of four tests would be useful in differentiating specific anticonvulsant properties: the normal electroshock threshold, the hydration threshold, the metrazol test and the supramaximal electroshock test.[197]

The idea that epileptic seizures might be caused by a chemical change stimulated Penfield to establish a neurochemical laboratory in Montreal and to hire the Cambridge graduate Alan Elliott after the Second World War. Elliott and Penfield took samples of brain tissue during surgery in a search for 'X-substance', the existence of which they postulated might be the chemical trigger of epileptic seizures. Disappointingly, no such trigger was identified – neither then nor since.

EPILEPSY AS A CEREBRAL DYSRHYTHMIA: THE AGE OF ELECTROENCEPHALOGRAPHY

It was however neither the science of neuropathology nor that of neurochemistry which was to have the greatest impact on epilepsy by the 1940s; that honour was to go to neurophysiology, and particularly to the technique of electroencephalography (EEG).

At the opening of the twentieth century, physiology was already a favoured science of the nervous system (surely reflected by the fact that the Nobel Prize awards, founded in 1901, were awarded for 'Physiology or Medicine'). The key early text was Sherrington's *Integrative Action of the Nervous System*, published in 1906, which spurred the development of much subsequent work.[198] In 1897 Sherrington had coined the word 'synapse' and demonstrated one-way transmission across synapses. He viewed neural action as in essence an interaction between reflexes, and recognised that there was a balance between excitatory and inhibitory effects. In direct lineage from David Ferrier, to whom the book was dedicated, Sherrington also provided a subtle and nuanced view of cortical localisation, and in the next two decades, using the framework created by Sherrington, studies of neural and synaptic function made great advances, Curiously, neither Sherrington nor any of the basic physiologists of the period made any mention of epilepsy, despite the fact that their work had clear implications for the condition and the obvious relevance of these processes to the mechanisms of seizures.[199]

[197] Toman and Goodman, 'Convulsions in animals'.   [198] Sherrington, *Nervous System*.
[199] In Britain, this was partly because, during that period, the Medical Research Council (MRC) focused strongly on curiosity-driven ('blue-sky') rather than applied research, and basic rather than clinical science. This was the deliberate policy of the MRC secretary, Walter Fletcher, himself a Cambridge Physiologist and Fellow of the Royal Society.

Physiology appealed to the personality of neurologists as it was a stringent science, unlike psychology (or even worse, psychiatry). In the early interwar years, the battle over cerebral localisation, the burning neurophysiological issue of the preceding decades, had been won. Clinical neurophysiology moved mainly into the fields of peripheral nerve and motor physiology, and, prior to electroencephalography, epilepsy was ignored. Muskens's work in cats on myoclonus (mentioned earlier) was perhaps the most extensive experimental epilepsy physiology of its time, but this too come to nothing. The landscape, though, was to change radically with the advent of EEG and suddenly epilepsy was again brought to the forefront of neurological research.

It was EEG which, unlike neuropathology and neurochemistry, utterly changed not only clinical practice in epilepsy but also its very conceptual basis. As Lennox put it, the introduction of EEG made it clear that the epileptic seizure was 'a paroxysmal cerebral dysrhythmia',[200] a visualisation of Jackson's 'excessive neuronal discharge'.

But EEG did not arise out of the blue. Its early history has been well rehearsed in several important texts, and these form much of the content of the following account.[201] Although Hughlings Jackson had referred to epileptic seizures as a 'discharge', he was not implying an electrical basis, and it was Richard Caton of Liverpool who first demonstrated that the grey matter of the brain possessed an intrinsic electrical current in 1885:

> In every brain examined [of monkeys and rabbits], the galvanometer has indicated the existence of electrical currents ... Feeble currents of varying direction pass through the multiplier when the electrodes are placed on two points of the external surface of the brain ... The electric currents of the grey matter appear to have a relation to its function. When any part of the grey matter is in a state of functional activity, its electric current usually exhibits negative variation.[202]

Measuring currents by reflecting a beam of light on the meniscus in his Thompson's galvanometer (the 'moving mirror' method) onto a wall, Caton noted their variation with light, sleep and with anaesthesia, and their disappearance at death. In 1876, the Austrian Ernst Fleischl von Marxow found that stimulating different sense organs caused small evoked potentials on the surface of the brain. For reasons which are quite unclear, he made the strange decision

[200] Gibbs, Gibbs and Lennox, 'Paroxysmal cerebral dysrhythmia'.

[201] Brazier, *Electrical Activity*; Brazier, 'Role of electricity'; Collura, 'Instruments and techniques'; Stone and Hughes, 'Early history'; Gloor, 'Hans Berger'.

[202] Caton, 'Electric currents', p. 278. Caton was Professor of Physiology at the University of Liverpool, Lord Mayor of Liverpool (1907/8) and later pro-vice-chancellor of the university. His discovery of cerebral electrical currents was lost until Berger acknowledged his precedence. See Haas, 'Hans Berger'. Caton used non-polarising electrodes to minimise artefacts and a moving mirror system for display. It was a remarkable technical achievement given the primitive nature of his equipment.

not to publish his results but instead to place them in a vault at the Kaiserliche Akademie der Wissenschaften in Vienna to be opened in 1883.[203] Caton's observations were then followed up by the Polish physiologist Adolf Beck, who in 1888 demonstrated the waxing and waning of the current when stimulated with light, sound or tactile or other stimuli.[204] All prior work had been conducted on the exposed brain or dura mater; then Vladimir Pravdich-Neminsky in Kiev, using the newly developed string galvanometer, recorded electrical signals from the intact skull of a dog and published his findings in 1913. He called the output an electrocerebrogram.[205] He also described a 12- to 14-Hz rhythm under normal conditions and marked slowing during asphyxia. In 1912, Pavel Kaufman from St Petersburg was the first to suggest that a seizure might be associated with abnormal electrical discharges. By stimulating the exposed cortex of a dog, he demonstrated such discharges during the tonic and clonic phase of the electrically induced seizure. However, he did not have a camera, and no illustrations of these recordings exist; it was to be Napoleon Cybulski,[206] Beck's mentor in Cracow, who recorded electrically induced epileptic seizures in a dog in 1914 and first published photographs of the resulting cortical potentials.

The first human studies were performed by Hans Berger,[207] who reported these from 1929 in a series of fourteen papers all titled *Über das Elektrenkephalogramm des Menschen.*[208] It was in fact in 1920 that he had made his first attempt to record through the intact skull, but this failed. He persisted,

---

[203] Ernst Fleischl-Marxow was Professor of Physiology in Vienna and a close friend of Freud. He had an amputated thumb which left him in chronic pain. He was treated with opiate and cocaine, which led to addiction and his premature death.

[204] Beck's claim to have been the first to record the effects of arousal is possibly incorrect, as work by the Russian Vasili Danilevsky may have predated him. Beck was Chair of Physiology at the University of Lemberg. He was nominated three times for a Nobel Prize. He was Jewish and, having been in hiding, in 1942 committed suicide before the Nazis came to transport him to the gas chambers. See Coenen, Fine and Zayachkivska, 'Forgotten pioneer'; Coenen and Zayachkivska, 'Adolf Beck'; https://www.youtube.com/watch?v=NZfHafgDAp8.

[205] Brazier, *Electrical Activity*, p. 112. Also: https://www.youtube.com/watch?v=CwgfB3JMTrc

[206] Cybulski was head of the department of physiology and, subsequently, rector of Jagiellonian University in Krakow.

[207] Having qualified in medicine, Berger became assistant to Binswanger, who appointed him *Oberarzt* in 1912. In 1919 Berger succeeded Binswanger as Chair of Psychiatry and Director of the University Clinic for Psychiatry at Jena. He was nominated for a Nobel Prize by Edgar Adrian, although the Nazi regime forbade him to proceed. His interest in psychic energy is described in Millett, 'Hans Berger', and seems to have developed from a near-death experience as a youth. In 1924 he wrote: 'Is it possible that I might fulfill the plan I have cherished for over 20 years and even still, to create a kind of brain mirror: the *Elektrenkephalogramm!*' (p. 535). In 1929 he achieved his dream, and that year recorded hundreds of EEGs.

[208] All, bar the second report, were published in the journal *Archiv für Psychiatrie und Nervenkrankheiten.* Pierre Gloor published English translations in 1969 and provided an excellent commentary. It is from Gloor's translation and editing of the fourteen papers into English with commentary that most of the information in this section is taken (Gloor, 'Hans Berger').

however, and it is probable that the first human EEG recording was made on 6 July 1924, when Berger observed 'tremulous movements' on his galvanometer due to brain currents in a patient with a skull defect.[209] This followed a twenty-year period during which Berger had worked on 'brain energy', starting by recording changes in blood flow during various tasks and psychological states, and then examining brain temperature as an indicator of energy consumption. Part of the aim of his studies was to identify the existence of 'psychic energy' – energy that generated mental actions – hypothesising bizarrely that such energy might even underpin the transmission of thoughts and emotions by telepathy from one individual to another. This line of thinking no doubt contributed to the view of his colleagues that Berger was a crank. W. Grey Walter[210] visited Berger and gave an interesting account of his personality. He found him a modest and dignified person, with one major weakness: 'He was completely ignorant of the technical and physical basis of his method [and] knew nothing about mechanics or electricity' (p. 54). He was a 'most unscientific scientist' (p. 52).[211] Berger initially tried to adapt electrocardiological methods but made little progress, instrument insensitivity being the major hurdle. Then, in 1927, he acquired a Siemens moving-coil string galvanometer, which was sufficiently sensitive to record cerebral potentials through the intact human skull. Doing some of the experiments on his own son, he studied the EEG in mental tasks, in different psychological and neurological states, in sleep (describing sleep spindles) and in disorders of consciousness. In his papers, he described his methodology and discussed his findings in relation to the psychological significance of different patterns, and the EEG in different conditions and states. He identified alpha waves that were correlated with mental activity ('physical concomitants of conscious phenomena'[212]) and beta waves, which he considered to reflect metabolic activity of cortical tissue.

Advances in clinical neurophysiology were to a very significant extent technology driven, not least because the electrical potential changes of human EEG are so small that their measurement outside the skull on the surface of the head (shaven or unshaven) requires considerable amplification. The string galvanometer was a technology introduced in 1903 (replacing the moving mirror technology), followed by the moving-coil galvanometer in the 1920s. Vacuum-tube amplifiers were introduced into neurophysiology in 1920

---

[209] Gloor, 'Hans Berger', p. 8.

[210] Walter was not only a physiologist but also an inventor, and created one of the earliest robots (see Holland, 'Exploration and high adventure').

[211] Walter, *Living Brain*. Walter was sent to meet Berger by Frederick Golla, who was his chief at the Maudsley Hospital and who was himself experimenting with brain potentials using a Matthews oscilloscope. Berger 'was not a physiologist', Walter concluded: '[H]is reports were vitiated by the vagueness and variety of his claims and the desultory nature of his technique' (p. 52).

[212] Millett, 'Hans Berger'.

and were used by Edgar Adrian, and then by Alan Hodgkin and Andrew Huxley in the later work that led to their Nobel prizes. The introduction of transistors in 1947[213] elevated amplification to another level. Equally important were advances in recording oscilloscopes, electrode types (with their different impedances), and methods of paper writing and storage. The potential of EEG expanded with each improvement.

In 1931 Berger obtained a specially constructed amplifier/oscillograph from Siemens which had an input impedance that allowed direct recording. In 1932 he became the first to record the EEG (in one or two channels) in various epileptic seizures – an event which turned out to be epoch changing. He noted that absence attacks were associated with high-voltage 3 Hz discharges (without spikes), but delayed publication of this finding for several years as he strove to exclude the possibility of artefacts.

He worked extensively on electrodes, trying out a variety of types and materials. As his equipment improved, Berger described high-voltage potential oscillations in the inter-ictal EEG of patients with frequent seizures, which he interpreted, correctly, as illustrating a predisposition to epilepsy.[214] He recorded changes in minor (partial) seizures.[215] He was disappointed not to be able to record a generalised convulsion because of muscle and movement artefact, although he did record the post-ictal state and noted the suppression of electrical activity and high-voltage slow activity.[216] He also demonstrated focal high-voltage sharp waves over the left central region in a patient with clonic jerking of the right hand in the aftermath of a 'severe epileptiform paralytic attack'.[217] He correctly interpreted this activity as a demonstration that the jerks originated from discharges in the contralateral central cortex. In his last report, in 1938, he graciously referred to the publications of Gibbs and colleagues, who had taken over the baton of the EEG in epilepsy from him.[218]

Perhaps because of Berger's lack of physiological method, and his intellectual isolation, initially these publications did not gain much international recognition. This situation was to change when, in 1934, Edgar (later Lord) Adrian – a physiologist with impeccable credentials – and his colleague Bryan Matthews – a gifted electrical engineer – published a landmark paper in *Brain*. Matthews designed their three-channel equipment, including a home-made vacuum-tube differential input amplifier and ink-writing oscilloscope that recorded on moving bromide paper. And with careful location of electrodes, they confirmed the existence of oscillating rhythms, including the alpha rhythm, which

---

[213] The 1956 Nobel Prize in Physics was awarded to the Bell Telephone Laboratories team of John Bardeen, Walter Brattain and William Shockley for this discovery.
[214] The 7th report: Gloor, 'Hans Berger', pp. 91–207.
[215] The 5th report: Gloor, 'Hans Berger', pp. 151–71.
[216] The 3rd, 4th and 14th reports: Gloor, 'Hans Berger', pp. 95–132, 133–50 and 299–320.
[217] Gloor, 'Hans Berger', pp. 191–207; citation, p. 197.
[218] Gloor, 'Hans Berger', pp. 299–320.

Adrian generously termed the 'Berger rhythm', the occipital origin of which they were able to demonstrate.[219] This was the publication which moved EEG into the mainstream (and at a memorable meeting of the Physiological Society in Cambridge in the summer of 1934, Matthews applied electrodes to Adrian's head and demonstrated his fortunately prominent alpha rhythm to all present). Berger instantly became an international celebrity. In 1937 he attended the International Congress of Psychology in Paris, where he was greatly feted. Nonetheless, in September 1938 he was removed from his chair in Jena by the Nazi authorities, and his laboratory was dismantled. His scientific work came to an abrupt end, and Berger fell into a deep depression. In 1941, he took his own life.

David Millett provides an interesting analysis of Berger's work, noting that it was his early thermodynamic approach to brain function that moved the debate forward from discussions of cerebral localisation.[220] Berger's work also disputed Hughlings Jackson's theory of concomitance of brain and mind by showing the physical neural underpinnings of mental activity: 'It is particularly interesting to note that the central question of Berger's early experimental work, namely, the relationship between cerebral blood flow, neural activity, and mental phenomena ... has become a cornerstone of modern brain imaging' (p. 540). This is correct, and in this sense Berger was a pioneer of much that was to follow. But his lack of understanding of electrical technologies, as identified by Walter, meant that Berger failed to recognise the full potential of his work. Perhaps the greatest missed opportunity was his failure to appreciate the value of EEG in epilepsy. The same could be said of Adrian, who continued to work on theoretical aspects of the EEG and basic physiology, and was less interested in disease. His work though was to be the stimulus for advances in epilepsy made by others. For instance, he had recorded action potentials from single pyramidal neurons of the cat after excessive chemical or electrical stimulation of the motor cortex, and during seizures initiated from other cortical regions. He found that the characteristic activity in a seizure consisted of bursts of impulses of unusually high frequency, commenting that these discharges represented the maximal degree of activity of neurones, an excessive responsiveness to an excessive stimulation, and were probably the cause of the spread of epileptic discharges.[221]

One noteworthy aspect of the history of EEG is that, right into the 1960s, all the early clinical electroencephalographers tended to design and make up their own equipment for their clinical practice (not a feature, for instance, of the introduction

---

[219] Adrian and Matthews, 'Interpretation of potential waves'; and Adrian and Matthews, 'Berger rhythm'. Adrian was a key figure in the early history of EEG. See Hodgkin, 'Edgar Douglas Adrian'.

[220] Millett (in *Hans Berger*) cites the criticisms voiced by Jan Tönnies (1933) that Berger 'never carried out his recordings with the question of localization in mind', but instead conceiving 'the bioelectrical effects of the cortex as a unity which he explains as a basic phenomenon of brain activity'.

[221] Adrian and Moruzzi, 'Pyramidal tract'.

of computed tomography or magnetic resonance imaging – technologies provided by commercial companies, essentially black boxes bought off the shelf), and most possessed deep technical understanding. Perhaps as a result, almost all the fundamental technical concepts and major clinical features of EEG were established within twenty years of the first clinical recording, and subsequent work was essentially incremental. The first American clinical electroencephalographer was Herbert Jasper, who had been funded in 1933 by the Rockefeller Foundation to establish an EEG laboratory at the Bradley Hospital in Providence, Rhode Island. Here he made his first human recordings in 1934, a year after the publication of the paper by Adrian and Matthews. In 1935 he travelled to Paris to defend his doctorate and, whilst in Europe, visited the Europeans who were pioneering EEG: Berger in Jena,[222] Tönnies in Berlin, Walter in London, and Matthews and Adrian in Cambridge. During the visit he studied the 'polyneurograph' machine designed by Tönnies[223] and Matthews's instruments and implemented similar technologies on his return to America. In 1939 Jasper opened an EEG laboratory in Montreal and that same year carried out around 1,000 EEGs in 500 epileptic patients. He worked on many aspects of instrumentation and electrodes, and proposed the 10–20 system for electrode placement[224] and pioneered the use of sphenoidal electrodes.

The second electroencephalographer to make human recordings was Alfred Loomis,[225] working in Tuxedo Park in New York. He, too, made a number of important innovations, especially in relation to sleep. Most significant to the history of epilepsy, however, were the developments in Boston. In December 1934, Hallowell Davis,[226] working with Frederic and Erna Gibbs and William Lennox, began recording human EEG. They employed a single-channel portable EEG system, incorporating a Western Union Morse Code ink-writing 'undulator', designed by the Harvard engineer E. Lovett Garceau.[227] In May 1935, with

---

[222] His memories of Berger are recorded in Jasper, 'Preface'. Herbert Henri Jasper was working at Brown University when he published the first American paper on EEG in 1935. He moved to the Montreal Neurological Institute and was appointed Professor of Experimental Neurology at McGill in 1946 and then Professor of Neurophysiology at the Université de Montréal in 1965. A detailed appreciation of Jasper's contribution is given in Andermann, 'In memoriam'.

[223] Tönnies worked at the Institute of Brain Research in Berlin where he designed the polyneurograph, the first ink-writing oscillograph. In 1932, Tönnies went to New York on a fellowship funded by the Rockefeller Foundation and there also developed a differential amplifier, similar to the one designed by Matthews in Cambridge.

[224] 'Report of the Committee on Methods of Clinical examination in electroencephalography'.

[225] See Alvarez, 'Alfred Lee Loomis'; also www.youtube.com/watchv=qBCK8rU8byw.

[226] Davis graduated from Harvard and trained as an electrophysiologist with Adrian in Cambridge. He played a pivotal scientific role in developing EEG, and is said to be the first subject to have his EEG recorded in Boston. He then turned his attention to the inner ear and pursued a distinguished career in audiology.

[227] Garceau was an engineer at Harvard Medical School and one of the first to apply electronic methods in neurology. He built the first cathode ray oscillograph at Harvard and the first EEG machine for Hallowell Davis. Garceau and Davis, 'Amplifier, recording system'; Garceau and Davis, 'Ink-writing electroencephalograph'.

funding from the Macy Foundation, Frederic Gibbs contracted Albert Grass to 'build three channels of EEG amplifiers' to incorporate into an EEG machine. By autumn, the 'Grass Model I' had been constructed, complete with a three-channel preamplifier and moving-coil galvanometers.[228] EEGs were recorded on rolls of paper using an ink-and-pen writer, and in 1937 a system of folded paper was introduced. The inter-ictal spike, as a hallmark of focal epilepsy, had been described in experiments by Max Fischer and Hans Löwenbach in Berlin in 1934,[229] and Gibbs, Davis and Lennox described inter-ictal spike and wave and the 3-second pattern of clinical absence seizures in 1935.[230] Events moved rapidly, for as early as 30 July 1935 Lennox made a remarkable announcement to the International Congress of Neurology in London:

> For what takes place in the brain when a seizure occurs we no longer have to depend on the evidence of sensation or muscle movement, as, through a door unexpectedly opened, we can discern what is happening within the brain. We can speak plainly of its electrical activity. We have obtained graphs of electrical potentials of patients during hundreds of seizures. The fundamental clinical feature of the epileptic seizure is disturbance of consciousness. The large waves represent a synchronization of many disparate activities. They mean that the customary harmony of the symphony orchestra has become a single note, that constitutional government has given place to the totalitarian state. Probably our hope of knowing the pathogenesis of epilepsy rests on finding the physico-chemical process involved in the electrical activity of the neurons. We who are here can hardly hope to arrive at a solution of this problem, which is linked up with heredity, in our lifetime, but we have our rewards, and it is better to travel hopefully than to arrive.[231]

[228] Zottoli, 'Grass foundation', p. 219. The rolls of paper were a technology which continued to be used for at least fifty years. I remember, in the 1990s, the relentless task of reviewing huge piles of paper EEGs. Model I was the beginning of the commercialisation of EEG, with sixty units produced. The Grass Model II appeared in 1939, with 4- and 6-channel capability and a newly developed system for folded paper which was widely used by the military during the war. Around 1,000 machines were produced. Then, in 1945, Grass and his wife Ellen founded the Grass Instrument Company and in 1946 introduced the Grass Model III, the first 8- and 16-channel machines, of which around 5,000 units were produced and shipped worldwide. It was an early example of a 'spin off' and the commercialization of medical discovery. Albert Grass, an engineering graduate from MIT, first built EEG machines for Lennox's unit in Boston for human and animal studies, which is where he met his wife Ellen Grass (née Robinson), who was working in Hallowell Davis' laboratory. Ellen later played an active role in lay and professional organisations and served as the first President of the IBE.

[229] Fischer and Löwenbach, 'Aktionsströme des zentralnervensystems'. In 1936, Gibbs and Jasper independently reiterated that this was the focal signature of epilepsy.

[230] Gibbs et al., 'Electroencephalogram in epilepsy'.

[231] 'International Neurological Congress in London'. This conference was a milestone in the field of epilepsy. It was dedicated to the memory of Hughlings Jackson, and epilepsy was a main topic with fifty papers. Interestingly, only two dealt with the question of heredity. Penfield's paper was published a year later (Penfield, 'Epilepsy and surgical therapy'). In it he

Lennox, Gibbs and Davis then went on to describe various aspects of clinical electroencephalography, including the electrographic changes of grand mal seizures and the normal EEG patterns of wakefulness and sleep.[232] In 1936, only two years after Adrian and Matthew's publication, the first clinical EEG unit was opened at Massachusetts General Hospital, directed by Robert Schwab, who remained there until his retirement in 1968.[233] The work in Boston in effect marked the beginning of clinical electrophysiology, with epilepsy at its centre, and Lennox opens his 1937 *Brain* paper in characteristic style:

> Diseases change their names with increase, not of age (like Chinese children), but with increase of medical knowledge ... However, some diseases never have outgrown their baby names. For example, ever since the days of Hippocrates, recurring and sudden loss of consciousness and of muscle control has been called 'the falling sickness' or (in Greek) a seizure, 'epilepsy'. Thanks to the pioneer work of Berger in developing the electroencephalograph, we can now make good the lack of thousands of years and adopt for this condition a name based on the underlying pathological physiology. We now know that epilepsy is due to the development of abnormal rhythms in the cerebral cortex; it is a *paroxysmal cerebral dysrhythmia*. This discovery places the study and understanding of epilepsy on a different and deeper level and requires a reorientation of our thinking.[234]

Lennox and his colleagues reported that by then they had performed EEG on 400 epileptic patients, of whom 120 had seizures whilst being recorded, and they outlined what they called 'seven new facts about epilepsy': (1) '[A] clinically observed seizure is but the outward manifestation of a disordered rhythm of brain potentials' (p. 378). These were seen in all but 2–3% of seizures. (2) In grand mal, petit mal and psychomotor seizures, the patterns were different (as Lennox later put it: 'The writhings of the electrographic pen name the sort of seizure the patient is having'[235]). (3) The fundamental basis of the disorder was not the abnormal rhythm but a defective control of rhythm. (4) There were inter-ictal changes (Lennox called these 'subclinical seizures' (p. 382)) taking the form of spike–wave or spike discharges. (5) EEG

---

ascribed temporal lobe symptoms, including epigastric sensations, to the posterior inferior medial portion of the frontal lobe – something he would later revise. His already well-developed critical approach is immediately evident from this paper.

[232] There were four landmark papers: Gibbs, Davis and Lennox, 'The electroencephalogram in epilepsy'; Gibbs and Davis, 'Loss of consciousness'; Gibbs, Lennox and Gibbs, 'Localization of epileptic seizures'; and Gibbs, Gibbs and Lennox, 'Paroxysmal cerebral dysrhythmia'.

[233] Grass, 'The electroencephalographic heritage'. Schwab was a key figure in American EEG. He trained in physiology at Cambridge University and then in medicine at Harvard. He served as president of the American EEG Society, vice president of the IFSECM, and managing editor of the *EEG Journal*.

[234] Gibbs, Gibbs and Lennox, 'Paroxysmal cerebral dysrhythmia'.

[235] Lennox, *Epilepsy and Related Disorders*, p. 33.

changes could predict when a grand mal seizure would occur. (6) 'The point of origin of an abnormal rhythm' can be in one area (now referred to as a focus) or occur 'simultaneously in all leads' (now referred to as generalised). The authors also noted that 'one patient with abnormal spikes confined to the frontal area has greatly improved following bilateral amputation of his frontal lobes' (pp. 384, 388). (7) The effects of treatment could be seen by the effect on the EEG, often after only a few hours of recording.[236]

These findings formed the basis of all future EEG work in epilepsy, and the understanding and conceptualisation of epilepsy – now as a *paroxysmal cerebral dysrhythmia* – had been utterly transformed. EEG demonstrated that the previously invisible excessive discharge postulated by Jackson was indeed the mechanism of the epileptic seizure. The impact was enormous. Moreover, its promise seemed limitless as physiologists, especially in Britain and the United States, turned their attention to its clinical applications, and the basic science discoveries were rapidly translated into the clinic.

Much of the early American work was heavily influenced by the British school of experimental physiology, and especially the work of Sherrington and of Adrian in Cambridge. Adrian had visited and lectured in Boston in the early 1930s, and there were many exchanges of students. Devoting his time to experimental work, Adrian did not pursue clinical EEG, and in Britain the first and unsuccessful attempts to record brain electrical activity had been earlier made by Frederick Golla at the Maudsley Hospital in the late 1920s. In 1935 Golla recruited W. Grey Walter, who had been a student of Adrian. Walter set up an EEG recording laboratory of his own design, and for a time basic EEG work in Britain matched that in Boston. Walter's focus was initially on clinical localisation. In 1936 he described the presence of focal slow activity (he coined the term 'delta activity') indicating the position of an underlying brain tumour, and proceeded to develop a technique for localising EEG activity in tumours and other pathologies. He also determined that in about 50% of persons with epilepsy, the inter-ictal EEG showed subtle abnormalities.[237] In 1939 Golla and Walter moved to the newly opened Burden unit in Bristol, where Walter made further important contributions to frequency analysis and contingent negative variation. An EEG Society in Britain was established in 1943, the first in the world (the American EEG

---

[236] In *Epilepsy and Related Disorders* (1960), Lennox posed the question 'Of what use is the EEG?' and answered it with a slightly different list, demonstrating what had changed and what had not over the previous two decades: 1. Diagnosis of the disease; 2. The EEG patterns help define the type of seizure; 3. To assist defining aetiology by differentiating between genetic and acquired epilepsy; 4. Show the focus of the abnormality; 5. Conceivably help in deciding on marriage; 6. Prognosis; 7. Treatment; 8. Future use in many forms of brain disease (pp. 773–9).

[237] Walter, 'Electro-encephalography'.

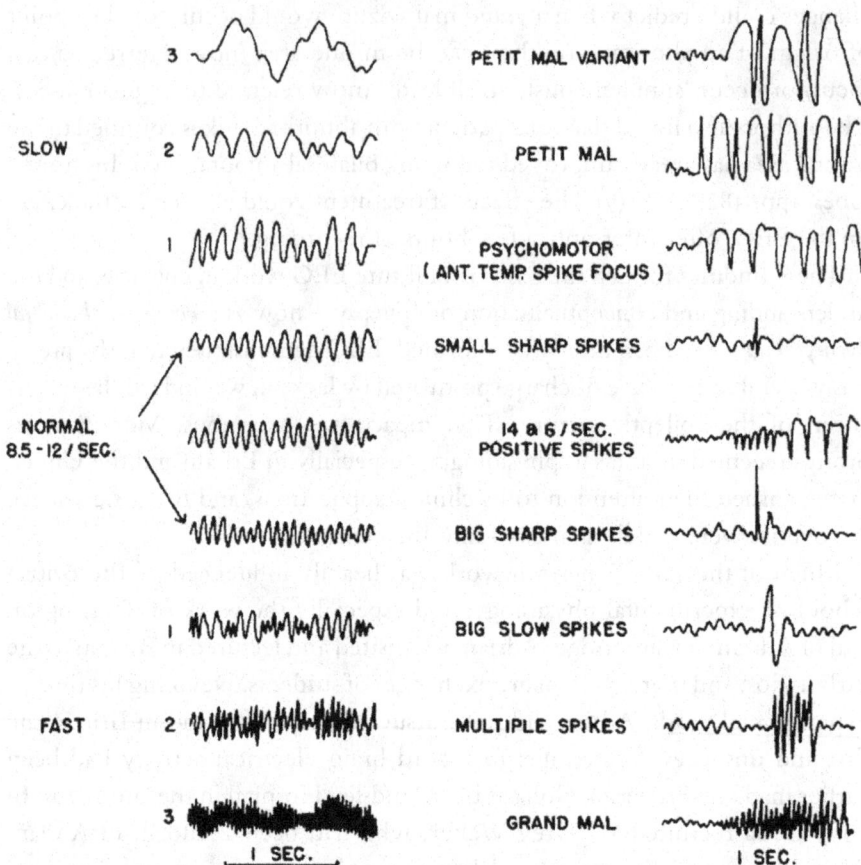

16. Early EEG. Within a few years of its introduction into clinical practice, Gibbs was able to catalogue many aspects of the normal and abnormal EEG.

Society was formed in 1947), and in 1947 the first international EEG congress was held in London, organised by Walter and chaired by Adrian.[238]

In some ways the meeting in 1947 proved a watershed, for by then the limitations of EEG were becoming apparent. As Adrian put it:

> Some of the dreams of the adolescent have been abandoned: the EEG is not the sure guide to the state of the brain that we may have hoped it would become, but we now know far better what it can show and what it cannot and the physician and surgeon have far better reason to trust the advice you can give them.[239]

Certainly, although its importance in epilepsy was apparent to all, its value in psychiatry, which had been exaggerated early on, was beginning to be doubted.

[238] This congress was notable, too, from another point of view. It was the first appearance of Henri Gastaut on the international stage, where he accompanied his mentor, W. Grey Walter. Walter recognised Gastaut's talent and was instrumental in introducing him to the then leading figures in the field.

[239] Adrian's opening address is reproduced in Nuwer and Lücking, 'History of the IFCN'.

In a typically caustic and pessimistic broadside, Francis Walshe, the leading British clinical neurologist of his generation, reflecting on his life in neurology and the future of the specialty in 1959,[240] noted that at the beginning of his career (in 1912) clinical neurology was the 'precise and complex study of phenomena' (p. 93) focused on description of diseases and classification. Thereafter, stimulated by Sherrington's work, attention turned to using the observed clinical phenomena to elucidate the nature of working of the nervous system, and many important contributions to the anatomy and physiology of the nervous system came from men who were primarily clinical observers ... So strong became this anatomical and physiological orientation of the clinical neurologist that the tradition was born that research into the anatomy and physiology of the nervous system was the most superior and important field of research for the neurologist (p. 94).

Then, he continued, the rise of 'electronic recording' and electrophysiology consumed resources and manpower but were abstractions which had contributed nothing to 'those age-old burning problems of the etiology, pathogenesis, and treatment of the many chronic, disabling, and killing affections of the nervous system'.[241] To Walshe the upsurge of interest in the electroencephalogram 'had got out of hand with its bloodless dance of action potentials'.[242] To Walshe, the future was neurochemistry.

Walshe's disparagement of EEG might well have been partly stimulated by his extreme dislike of Penfield[243] and was unfair, for EEG did contribute to pathogenesis and also to diagnosis. It had, however, been a curate's egg, and in many ways Walshe was correct: EEG has a narrow remit, and its place now in clinical practice is largely confined to investigating epilepsy and disorders of consciousness. The rapid dissemination of EEG units in psychiatric hospitals and the extravagant claims and widespread misuse of EEG in the 1950s and 1960s were a waste of resources. Few other areas of medicine produced charlatanism on such a wide scale (and it still does). However, EEG was to dominate the thinking and conceptualisation of epilepsy for the rest of century and, it could be argued, in some senses has held it back, and this is a point taken up in later chapters.

---

[240] Walshe, 'Present and future'.   [241] Walshe 'The present and future of neurology'.

[242] Rose, *History of British Neurology*, p. 197. See also Walshe, 'Mind and brain'.

[243] There exists a notorious correspondence between Walshe and Penfield, filled with animosity, revolving around the relative positions of neurology and neurosurgery. Penfield considered the former lacking in therapeutics, and Walshe the latter a lowly craft.

TREATING EPILEPSY

Healthcare for Epilepsy in the Interwar Period

Prior to the Second World War, healthcare services in most European countries were chaotic and uncoordinated. Funded largely by philanthropy, religious foundations or local authorities, healthcare was not considered a priority of central government. The principal reason may well have been that health was not then considered a right but a privilege, and there were great variations in access, distribution and quality.

In relation to epilepsy, Britain and Germany can be taken as examples, although situations were probably similar in most of the industrialised countries of the Western world. In both countries, healthcare in the first decades of the century was a patchwork of facilities, with access depending very much on the patient's class, geography and financial standing. The wealthy kept epilepsy out of sight and were treated privately at home or, if necessary, in private nursing homes or private asylums. The poor with severe epilepsy were treated without cost either in epilepsy colonies, workhouses (until these were closed in the years before the Second World War) or public asylums. Those with epilepsy from the middling classes mostly hid their condition from view and obtained care largely from local private practitioners. Many patients sought medical attention either on an occasional and sporadic basis or not at all. As time passed. with improvements in medicine and rising living standards, doctors were consulted more often and more formally. In large urban centres, physicians and surgeons provided their services free at the public hospitals and generally earned their living from their private practices, which for a fashionable physician or surgeon could be extremely lucrative; and grumbles about the 'doctor's fees' were commonplace.

As the twentieth century drew on, one of the most fundamental changes in medicine was the rise of the hospital as the principal locus of medical care. In Britain, in the early years of the century, at least in the large endowed teaching and general hospitals, although treatment was free to patients, hospital admission was considered by all a last resort (a place to die). Hospitals were seen as facilities for the poor, and no self-respecting citizen with even moderate resources would contemplate seeking hospital treatment. Furthermore, in these early years, in many hospitals patients with epilepsy were excluded from beds, which were reserved where possible for acute conditions. In London, for instance, it was initially only in the small voluntary hospitals that care for epilepsy was provided.[244] However, as the century drew on, medicine

---

[244] In 1914 in London, there were twelve large teaching hospitals in London (with 80% of the general hospital beds). Treatment for epilepsy, though, was only routinely available at the four London specialist hospitals ('voluntaries') devoted to neurological conditions with

became more effective, more scientific, more technological and more special-ised, and hospitals grew in importance and prestige. By 1920, the larger hospitals were attracting a more middle-class clientele, and were growing in size, number and influence in all Western countries.

Specialist-based hospital outpatient departments also developed. Prior to the First World War, outpatient facilities for persons with epilepsy were confined in Britain mainly to the specialist voluntary hospitals and in Germany to a few polyclinics. But because drugs such as bromide and phenobarbitone could be obtained without medical prescription, the lack of these services may not have greatly mattered to the majority of patients. However, in the first decades of the century, specialist departments began to develop. In Britain, the first neurology department in a large general hospital was established in 1907 (at St Mary's Hospital in London), and soon other large hospitals followed suit. In Germany developments were slower, due in part to the reluctance to disaggregate neurology from psychiatry, and even by 1930 there were still only a handful of neurology units.

Hospital care was also becoming more expensive, and by the 1920s these costs were increasingly unsustainable. General and voluntary hospitals reluctantly began to turn to the patients for payment, and in hospitals in Britain 'lady almoners' were appointed, whose role was to assess the finan-cial position of those seeking hospital care and to levy small charges on those who could afford it. In the economic crises of the 1920s and 1930s, many voluntary and local health facilities faced severe financial problems, and it was only then, to prevent wholesale hospital insolvency, that central governments across Europe and the United States reluctantly became involved.

Health insurance had its origins in the mid-nineteenth century when the first hospital insurance schemes were launched in France and Germany. The first statutory health insurance was created by Otto von Bismarck in Germany in the 1880s for low-income workers and some public employees (not out of any real concern for the sick, but to head off electoral threat from socialists). By 1907, 21% of the German population was covered. Around this time most other Western countries had some voluntary or statutory schemes, linked to employ-ment or to union membership. These were often available only to those in work, and most did not cover women or dependants. In the interwar years, government intervention grew. In Weimar Germany, state funding was seen as a way of motivating a population demoralised by defeat in war. Its constitution

outpatient departments and a few hundred beds: the National Hospital for the Paralysed and the Epileptic, in Queen Square; the Hospital for Epilepsy and Paralysis and Other Diseases of the Nervous System, in Maida Vale; the West End Hospital for Diseases of the Nervous System, Paralysis and Epilepsy, then in Welbeck St; and the Empire Hospital for Nervous Diseases, in Vincent Square.

of 1919 guaranteed comprehensive insurance, and by 1925 85% of dependants and by 1932 a third of the population had some sort of cover. In Britain the National Insurance Act 1911 protected 15 million persons, and by 1942 25 million persons were covered (over half of the population). Health insurance was introduced in Japan in 1928 based on the German model, and in France in 1928. In Holland the entire wage-earning population was covered. Charitable and private schemes also flourished, albeit in a patchy and haphazard fashion, in many countries – and in Britain were often run by trade unions or church-based organisations. In America, anti-communist feeling prevented any such developments, and even though a safety net was promised in the New Deal, the 1935 Social Security Act contained no provision for health insurance.[245] There, private, commercial and, increasingly, employment-based schemes were preferred. In many countries, as most schemes were related to employment, patients with epilepsy were often excluded from much of the health insurance cover, and for those unable to live independently in the community, mental asylums were the only option, despite the wide recognition that they were inappropriate, or, for the luckier few, epilepsy colonies.

In 1937, the newly resuscitated ILAE returned to its pre–First World War mission of procuring epilepsy statistics in different countries, and these provide a snapshot view of epilepsy care in the years 1937–9. By then, in the United States there were estimated to be half a million epilepsy sufferers, of whom 10% (40,000) were in public institutions (75% in state- or government-maintained psychiatric asylums and 25% in epilepsy colonies). The 19 epilepsy colonies housed a total of about 10,000 inmates, of which the Craig Colony was the largest with 2,083. There were just over 2,000 admissions each year to the colonies, and 500 discharges and 600 deaths. The anonymous author of the report from America noted that the American colonies were often very large and supported by the state, in contrast to those in Britain and continental Europe which tended to be smaller and run by philanthropic, often religious organisations. It was commented that 'whilst the class of "hopeless" epileptics can probably be given custodial care most cheaply in a large public institution, remedial treatment of incipient cases should be made available in small, well-staffed highly-motivated institutions such as exist at Lingfield in England and Filadelfia in Denmark'.[246]

In Britain, J. Tylor Fox reported that 'those epileptics certified as either insane or mentally defective' were housed in the county or borough mental hospitals for the insane (11,233 inmates). For sane patients with epilepsy there were 19 institutions (epilepsy hospitals, residential schools and colonies)

---

[245] Figures from Lawrence, 'Continuity in crisis', pp. 345–7.
[246] 'Institutional care of epileptics'.

containing 4,068 patients, the largest being the colony at Langho, which had 630 beds. Most were run by voluntary organisations, with patients receiving financial support from the public authorities. There were also patients living at home or admitted periodically to general hospitals, but the numbers were totally unknown. Tylor Fox also mentioned that epileptic inpatient and outpatients were common in the three specialised neurological hospitals in London.[247]

Schou reported on the situation in Scandinavia. Norway had one 70-bed epilepsy hospital; all other patients were either in institutions for the insane or mentally defective, or in private homes. Finland had one hospital equipped with 300 beds; Sweden had one hospital with 200 beds for male epileptics and 7 smaller nursing homes, amounting to a total of 300 beds; Denmark had one large hospital with 550 beds for adults and institutions for 150 children. In the Danish system, sane and insane cases were both found in these institutions, as were new cases who were housed separately and for whom modern investigatory facilities were available. Some chronic cases were distributed in private homes near the hospital. Schou cited the general opinion that about 10% of epilepsy cases required hospitalisation, but as there were only 1,500 beds, the provision was 50% less than that required. In his opinion, it was deplorable that epilepsy patients had to be treated in hospitals for the insane or feeble-minded; what was needed was real hospitals with neurologically trained physicians and facilities for investigation.[248]

Ledeboer, reporting in 1939, provided an upbeat assessment of the situation in Holland, where he deemed services to be the most comprehensive.[249] Most persons were treated in the community, with ten 'consultation offices for Epileptics'. In 1937 three associations were in existence, with four trained male nurses 'travelling by motorcar from place to place' following up patients who had been discharged and arranging admissions of others. A 'Christian charity' for engaging the public had also been formed, which boasted 1,000 branches around the country and 100,000 contributing members who were said to report cases of epilepsy in every town or village. There were also 2 hospitals for sane epileptics with facilities for modern investigation and 2 institutions for the insane (a total of 500 beds); others were admitted to the general psychiatric institutions. Elsewhere, Germany had 4 institutions; Czechoslovakia and Australia each had 1; and Belgium, Romania, South Africa and India had none. In all countries, other persons with epilepsy resided in 'lunatic asylums'. In India, it was reported that only 'insane epileptics' were admitted to lunatic asylums (there were said to be 734 patients with epilepsy in 19 mental hospitals in India), but in other countries the asylums still contained patients categorised as sane.

[247] Fox, 'Accommodation for epileptic patients'.   [248] Schou, 'Care of epileptics'.
[249] Ledeboer, 'Epileptics in Holland'. Ledeboer was medical director of the epilepsy colony in Heemstede.

In August 1939, at the 5th meeting of the ILAE held in Copenhagen on the brink of World War Two, the ILAE Secretary General, H. J. Schou, presented the results of an ILAE questionnaire summarising the situation of patients around the world.[250] He considered the hospital at Heemstede in Holland to be the best institution he had visited. It provided investigation, well-trained staff and excellent aftercare – and 'the importance of out-patients departments solely for epileptics and managed by the physicians of the hospital for epileptics can hardly be over-estimated'. In relation to the optimal arrangements, he divided patients into three categories.

First were the new ('fresh and acute') cases of epilepsy. He considered it an imperative that all patients be admitted to hospital and pass through a neurological service with specially trained staff and equipment: 'It is highly regrettable, and a sign of lack of civilization that in several countries it is impossible to send fresh cases of epilepsy to hospital for rational examination, and in still more countries the doctors have not yet discovered the importance of such examination'. It was only in Switzerland, Holland and Demark that all new patients could be admitted to special hospitals for epileptics, and in most other countries, admission was to neurological wards which were inadequate in size to cater for all patients. The second group comprised chronic epileptics who he considered should be treated in specialised epilepsy hospitals or nursing homes, which could be associated with other institutions such as 'nerve wards or nerve sanatoria' but unfortunately often ended up in mental hospitals. The last group were the 'insane epileptics' who should be admitted either to mental wards in epilepsy hospitals or to ordinary mental hospitals (the former being preferable). Some of the ILAE members were eugenicists, others directors of colonies, and some both, and in a separate article in the same year, Schou commented on

> sterilisation of epileptics, which to a great extent is performed in Germany. We have in Sweden and Denmark a moderate Act permitting the voluntary sterilisation of adult epileptics after petition to the Ministry of Justice. At our hospital we have used this act in about 10 cases with good results, and to the satisfaction of the patients. Compulsory sterilisation – as in Germany – in all cases where it cannot be proved that the epilepsy is symptomatic, seems to be a risk ... In Sweden marriage between epileptics is forbidden by law. In Denmark it is only permitted after information has been received from a doctor that the epilepsy was not severe and the inheritability was not marked ... The question is a very difficult one.[251]

It is notable that of the doctors writing in *Epilepsia* about epilepsy services, only Lennox emphasised that the majority of cases lived at home. The members of

---

[250] Published in 1940. Schou, 'Institutional care of epileptics'.
[251] Schou, 'Scandinavian Branch'.

the revived ILAE seemed most concerned with the provision of care in special epilepsy facilities – navel-gazing which perhaps reflected the isolation of epilepsy doctors, their small number and their lack of vision about the wider world of medicine.

Medicinal Therapies for Epilepsy: Phenobarbitone and Phenytoin

As described in the previous chapter, the antiepileptic properties of phenobarbitone had first been noted in 1912, but its use was initially confined mainly to German-speaking populations. It was only in the aftermath of the Great War that its value became more widely recognised and it percolated slowly into the practice of the leading American and European centres. In the United States, Julius Grinkler published his experience in 100 cases in 1920, and then in 200 cases in 1922, with impressive results.[252] In Britain, the first recorded use of phenobarbital was by Frederick Golla,[253] who wrote up his findings in the *British Medical Journal* in 1921.[254] At the National Hospital, Queen Square, Gordon Holmes and James Collier were also using the drug by then, as was Aldren Turner by 1922.

Its usage then spread rapidly, and over the next twenty years debate about the treatment of epilepsy was largely concerned with the relative effectiveness of phenobarbitone compared with bromide. Many considered the barbiturate to be a great improvement.[255] In 1928 Cobb and Lennox wrote that it was the

---

[252] Grinkler, 'Further experiences with phenobarbital'. Grinker, Professor of Nervous and Mental Diseases at Northwestern University, was the first American to try out phenobarbital, which he started to use in 1914.

[253] Golla was to become an important figure in the history of epilepsy, notably as the first director of the Burden Neurological Institute in Bristol.

[254] Golla, 'Luminal contrasted with bromide'.

[255] The archive of the Chalfont Centre for Epilepsy provides an interesting insight into the progress in the use of phenobarbital during that period. In 1922, Dr C. Brook, then resident medical officer at Chalfont, reported that treatment of 50 male patients left him with no doubt of the drug's effectiveness, particularly for 'cases of major convulsions (apart from group attacks), and where there is also mental deterioration'. By 1923 Brook considered phenobarbital to be superior to bromides. His successor, Dr. F. Haward, reported his own experience in 1928 in 124 patients who were naive to phenobarbital therapy. He observed that '46 showed a marked decrease in seizures, 58 some decrease and 20 no decrease'. He also noted that in the latter group, there had often been an initial period of from 4 to 6 weeks in which fits are much reduced and in some cases ceased, 'to be resumed in the old manner after this time'. The use of subcutaneous phenobarbital for cases of status epilepticus and severe fits was also described. In 1928, Haward issued treatment guidelines for newly admitted patients. Potassium bromide would be given as the treatment of first choice. If, after a time, there was no diminution of seizures, Luminal would be substituted. The patient would be monitored for 3 months and 'if at the end of this time there was little improvement, potassium bromide would be combined with the Luminal.' Luminal was given at a dose of one grain (65 g), night and morning, for adults and one-half a grain for children. The dose could be titrated upward according to clinical response, but should not exceed 6 grains a day in any case (Haward, *Report of the Medical Officer*). By 1934, very few of the colonists at Chalfont were taking bromides (see Sander, Barclay and Shorvon, 'Neurological founding fathers').

standard drug for controlling seizures and had replaced bromide in this role as it did not 'so greatly depress the mentality'.[256] Clearing the mentality was a property mentioned by many at the time, one presumes due mainly to the replacement of bromide rather than to any positive effects of phenobarbitone. However, not all authorities were as enthusiastic. In his 1940 textbook of neurology, Kinnier Wilson still considered phenobarbitone to be second-line, behind bromides (Table 2.3). He recorded its advantages, notably the 'absence of mental depression' and 'lowering of somatic function', but noted also that it was susceptible to tolerance, had a narrow therapeutic window and its withdrawal entailed a risk of status epilepticus. The drug was 'best in mild and moderate epilepsies, given alone; for the more severe or semi-chronic cases, its combination with bromide or other sedative' (for instance, borax) was recommended; it appeared 'to have least value in serial types recurring at longish intervals'.[257] In 1919 Alfred Hauptmann noted that phenobarbitone could be used in status epilepticus.[258]

Two books devoted to epilepsy in the pre-phenytoin era are also worth noting, providing as they do a snapshot of advanced therapy in the 1920s and 1930s. *The Treatment of Epilepsy* by Fritz Talbot was published in 1930.[259] Compiled by a well-known figure, but not an innovator, this book probably reflects mainstream paediatric practice. He considered prophylaxis to be possible by any measure which stops reproduction in families with 'a long history of mental deficiency'. As for treatment, the exhortation – 'The first endeavour should be to remove the cause' – is followed by a long section on the treatment of constipation by diet and drugs, for this, along with poor posture, 'lower[ed] the general resistance of the body' and facilitated seizures (pp. 82–6). However, Talbot dismissed both colectomy and the administration of bacillus acidophilus as ineffective. Rather, treatment should consist of physical hygiene, social and mental hygiene, diet and drugs. Physical hygiene meant regular exercise, sufficient sleep and a carefully regulated diet. Mental hygiene meant avoiding stress and 'nervous exercise' to develop 'nervous resistance' (pp. 102–10). Psychoanalysis was useful in some cases, but the value of hypnosis 'is questionable particularly for children'. It is clear from Talbot's book that he, too, viewed medication as having only a very limited role (in fact, drug therapy occupied only 5 pages of his 308-page book). Phenobarbitone was considered the standard drug, and then bromides. The use of other drugs is mentioned but 'without startling success', and these included borotartrate, zinc, asafoetida, nitroglycerine, ammonium chloride, iodide of mercury and calcium chloride. The second section of the book, over 130 pages in length, is devoted to dietary

[256] Cobb and Lennox, *Physiology and Treatment*, p. 254.
[257] Wilson and Bruce, *Neurology*, vol. 2, p. 1540.
[258] Hauptmann, 'Erfahrungen aus der Behandlung'; Wilson '*Neurology*', vol. 3, pp. 1534–44.
[259] Talbot, *Treatment of Epilepsy*. Several editions of this book appeared, beginning in 1930.

TABLE 2.3 *The drugs used in the treatment of epilepsy in the mid-1930s in America and Great Britain*

Lennox (USA)	Kinnear Wilson (Great Britain)
	Drugs of definite benefit
Bromides (various preparations and combinations, including gold and sodium tetrabromide)	Bromides – potassium, sodium, ammonium, lithium, calcium, calcium bromine galactogluconate Bromide combinations – bromocarpine (potassium bromide and pilocarpine), bromopin/brominol (bromide and sesame oil), bromalin (hexamin ethyl bromide), Gélineau's dragées (potassium bromide, antimony arsenate, picrotoxin), sedobrol (sodium bromide and sodium chloride), ozerine (potassium bromide and ammonium carbonate), Trench's remedy (potassium bromide, ammonium bromide), etc.
Phenytoin (first mentioned in 1937)	
Phenobarbitone	Phenobarbitone (Luminal)
Prominal	N-methylethyl-phenylmalonyl urea (Prominal) Borax, sodium biborate, double tartrate of borax and potassium
Ergotamine, ephedrine, prostigmine	Belladonna (with bromide, Luminal or caffeine)
Brilliant vital red, methyl blue	Nitroglycerine (as liquor trinitrini: with strychnine and sodium bromide) Dialacetin (allobarbital with allylparacetaminophenol)
Ketogenic diet, fluid restriction	Ketogenic diet
Anti-rabies vaccine	***Drugs of doubtful benefit*** Zinc, iron, digitalis, strophanthus, calcium, opiates and hypnotics,

Note

Lennox's list is derived from his annual review of epilepsy in America in 1937 and 1938 (see text), and reflects US practice in those years.

Kinnier Wilson's list is derived from his textbook (*Neurology*, 1940). It reflects British practice in the mid-1930s, before the introduction of phenytoin. He notes that bromide combinations 'were very much in vogue' and that there were 'many preparations ("secret" or otherwise) on the market' (p. 1540).

therapy, including a low-protein, low-salt diet and dehydration, but especially the ketogenic diet. Diet was, it seems in Talbot's opinion, the main thrust of therapy at that time, a conclusion he supported by comprehensive tables.

The second book, an important work in European epileptology of the 1920s, was the monograph on epilepsy by Louis Muskens.[260] Like Turner, Muskens[261] emphasised non-medicinal therapy in the prodromal phase (he was, it seems, somehow able to recognise 'unmistakable signs of epilepsy'

[260] Muskens, *Epilepsy*. Muskens's book was originally published in Dutch in 1924; the first English edition came out in 1928.
[261] See Eling and Keyser, 'Louis Muskens'.

even before seizures developed) and in the early stages, and considered this to be far more effective than in the later stages of the condition. Social hygiene was of primary importance, including attention to rest and graded exercises; the avoidance of extreme exercise or emotion; and the use of bathing, massage, good nutrition and appropriate work. Hydrotherapy was a popular form of therapy, with warm (or hot) baths, Turkish baths, douches and wet packs. Another important element was the removal of endogenous toxins by great attention to the bowels – and the avoidance of constipation by laxatives, enema and diet. Extreme measures such as colectomy were occasionally to be recommended. Muskens recognised the deleterious effects of alcohol on fits, which was the provoking cause of the epilepsy in 4.3% of his patients. Marriage between epileptics should be utterly discouraged ('such marriages seem absurd to the physician, but they do take place', p. 328), as should marriage of a person with epilepsy to anyone, though he commented 'curiously and fortunately epileptics as a class seem to be lethargic sexually' (p. 329; surprisingly, he did not seem to consider that this might have been due in part to the effect of bromide). His prescription for children in the prodromal stages of epilepsy was almost identical to that of Turner twenty years earlier: 'the form of a well-regulated system of life, with carefully regulated rest and nourishment. How difficult it is to get these two last factors in the life of the average woman of the poorer classes any doctor knows' (p. 332). His general advice included sleep, sunshine (illustrated by his treatment, the provision of a sunnier cage, of an epileptic ape in the zoo), open air, rest, regulated exercises, food given frequently and in small quantities, moderate brain work, proper functioning of the alimentary canal and psychical encouragement. Diet was also important, and he noted that various dietary measures were employed by different authorities, the most common being mixed diets with little meat, low salt and high milk content, the avoidance of fried food and alcohol, and an emphasis on moderation.

For the stage where 'patients ... have had a certain number of fits, but who have not reached the stage which could be classed as inveterate' (p. 340; how many seizures was not specified), Muskens recommended medicinal treatment with sodium or potassium bromide, borax and phenobarbital (these were the principal therapies), and with zinc, nitroglycerine, belladonna, veronal and Indian hemp (cannabis) as adjuncts. Bromides seem to have been his first choice, although he was lukewarm in their recommendation. Like Turner, he favoured the potassium or sodium salts and not the synthetic combinations. He also preferred low doses, and he recognised the need for tailored dosing and the deleterious effects of 2.5–3 g, which seems then to have been widely prescribed. He devoted only a page to

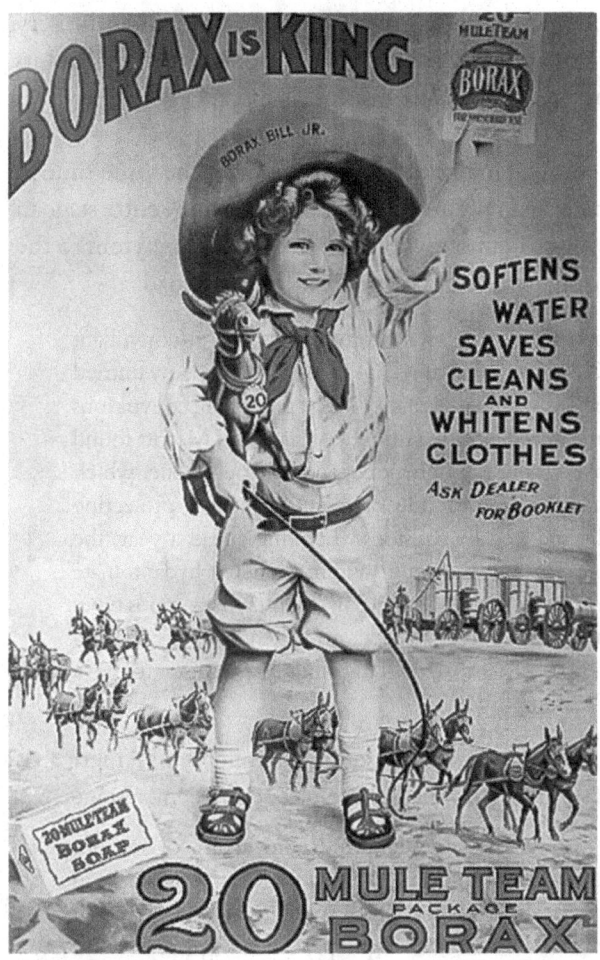

17. Borax is king. An advert for borax as a washing powder – 'softens water and whitens clothes'.

phenobarbitone, ranking it third after bromide and borax.[262] For inveterate cases, hygiene again was the primary measure, although mercury and drugs could be used. Iodide of mercury was a rather idiosyncratic recommendation of Muskens, and is a toxin which did not seem to catch on among other authorities. He also recognised, as many did at the time, that drug treatment was often ineffective and, furthermore, that it was suppressive not curative. 'What is achieved by drug treatment at its best', he wrote, 'is that the period between the fits is lengthened'.[263] Few would have disagreed.

Phenytoin made its first appearance around 1938, so its launch into practice coincided with the start of the Second World War. Because American epileptology was relatively unaffected by the hostilities, phenytoin was extensively

[262] Muskens, *Epilepsy*, p. 347.   [263] Muskens, *Epilepsy*, p. 341.

studied there, and multiple papers singing its praises were published in very short order. Phenytoin was seen as the paradigm of a modern therapy, and its impact was profound. The previously rather dismal landscape of epilepsy was suddenly brightened.

The drug had another consequence and, with its arrival at the same time as EEG, epilepsy suddenly once again hit the headlines and became centre stage in the theatre of neurology. It was Lennox who first introduced phenytoin to the epilepsy world in his *Epilepsia* review of progress for the year 1939:

> Not content with the generally complacent attitude towards anti-convulsant drugs, Putnam of Harvard determined to go broadside through many untried ones. To that end he devised a standardised method of producing convulsions in a cat by means of a measured electric current. Putnam and Merritt found three drugs, diphenyl hydantoin, acetophenone, and benzophenone, which were more effective than either bromide or phenobarbital in protecting animals from electrically induced convulsions. (Looking ahead a year, the authors have proved the value of the drug sodium diphenyl hydantoinate clinically. It is more effective than phenobarbital in stopping the various types of seizures, and is without the depressive effect on the mentality, but has a more marked toxic action on the skin. This finding promises to be a therapeutic advance of real importance.)[264]

By the time of his 1940 annual review (by now only of epilepsy in America, as Europe was steeped in war), phenytoin had come to occupy centre stage:

> The big news of the year is the discovery and clinical use of sodium diphenyl hydantoinate (Dilantin Sodium). Merritt and Putnam, working at the Neurological Unit of the Boston City Hospital, report the results of treating 200 non-institutionalised cases of epilepsy. Of 118 patients who received treatment from 2 to 11 months, grand mal attacks had been absent in 58%, and in an additional 27% they were greatly reduced ... results were relatively poor for petit mal ... Benefit ... was most dramatic in patients having psychomotor attacks. Besides being more effective than phenobarbital or bromides in controlling grand mal and psychomotor seizures, Dilantin has the great advantage of having only a weak hypnotic effect.[265]

The story of the discovery of phenytoin is well rehearsed by Anthony Glazko[266] and Walter Friedlander,[267] the latter being a model of historical detective work. As Friedlander points out, the development of phenytoin was a product of its times for two reasons. First was the growth in organic chemistry

---

[264] Lennox, 'Epilepsy in 1939'. From 1937 to 1946, Lennox published annual reviews of the literature in *Epilepsia*. These are important sources of information about trends during this period.

[265] Lennox, 'Epilepsy in 1940'.   [266] Glazko, 'Discovery of phenytoin'.

[267] Friedlander, 'Putnam, Merritt'. The details in this section borrow heavily from this account.

in the preceding thirty years. The chemical structure of drugs was well understood, as was the concept of manufacturing families of drugs that might have similar functions (e.g. the hydantoins and barbiturates). Indeed, phenytoin was not the first hydantoin to be synthesised that had known antiepileptic effects. Ethylphenylhydantoin (Nirvanol) was an important precursor with a hydantoin ring and the same attached radicals as phenobarbital. It was in general use as a hypnotic in the 1920s and 1930s and was known to be effective in epilepsy, but its toxicity limited its appeal. Mesantoin was the second antiepileptic drug (after phenytoin) to be introduced into wide practice and became very popular despite the fact that it is metabolised in vivo into ethylphenylhydantoin (i.e. Nirvanol). Had Nirvanol been more thoroughly assessed clinically in the 1930s, it is quite possible that it would have pre-empted phenytoin.

The second fact that made phenytoin a product of its times was Merritt and Putnam's use of an animal model as a screening test for antiepileptic drugs. This was not a new concept. In 1882 Pietro Albertoni had shown that bromide reduced convulsions in experimental animals. Then chemicals were assessed in electrically-induced convulsions in models devised by Viale in 1929, Krasnogorsky in Moscow in 1935 and Spiegel in Philadelphia in 1936. Chemical convulsants (thujone, camphor and metrazol) had been employed to induce seizures in experimental animals to assess potential antiepileptic drugs by both Lennox and Haddow Keith in the 1920s. What was new was Merritt and Putnam's systematic approach. They devised a model, based on that of Spiegel and Krasnogorsky,[268] using electrically induced convulsions in a cat and began their experiments between 1936 and 1937. Their method involved administering electric currents to cats via scalp and mouth electrodes, and seeing whether, and at what dose, a drug would prevent the seizure.[269] Each drug was rated by the amount of change in the convulsive threshold. According to Cobb and colleagues, who had used an animal model to test the antiepileptic potential for brilliant red, the idea of a systematic survey of potential drugs seems to have originated around 1935.[270] Putnam wrote that, having designed his screening methodology:

> I combed the Eastman Chemical Company's catalog, and other price lists, for suitable phenyl compounds that were not obviously poisonous. I also wrote to the major pharmaceutical firms … The only one of them that showed any interest was Parke-Davis and Company. They wrote back to

[268] Friedlander, 'Putnam, Merritt'.
[269] The relationship of Merritt and Putnam is itself an interesting story. When Merritt joined the Boston City Hospital in 1928, Tracy Putnam was already a Harvard professor. Although both published the seminal papers on phenytoin together, in 1945 Putnam claimed that the ideas were all his and that Merritt was the junior and not a full partner in the collaboration. This interpretation has since been challenged, and the truth may never be known.
[270] Cobb, Cohen and Ney, 'Brilliant Vital Red'.

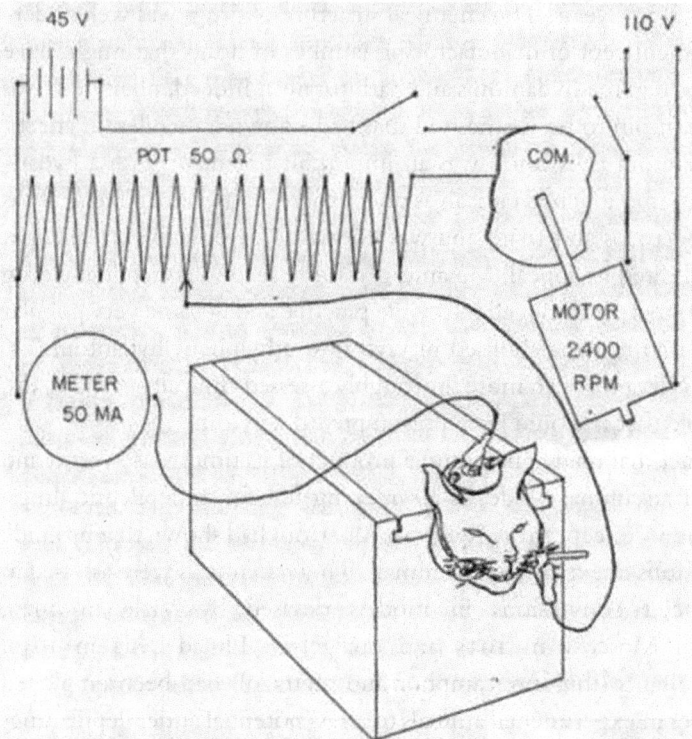

18. A diagram of the experimental model used by Merritt and Putnam to trial potential antiepileptic drugs. It was using this model, that the anticonvulsant action of phenytoin was identified. (From Putnam, T. and Merritt, H., Experimental determination of the anticonvulsant properties of some phenyl derivatives. *Science* 85: 525–6)

me that they had on hand samples of 19 different compounds analogous to phenobarbital and that I was welcome to them.[271]

These nineteen compounds had all been prepared by Arthur Dox of Parke-Davis, and phenytoin was first on the list. Putnam started to use the drug experimentally in 1936 and reported his findings in the 28 May issue of *Science* in 1937.[272] In fact, this cannot have been an entirely random choice of drug as knowing that other hydantoin drugs were antiepileptic must surely have contributed to the submission of phenytoin for testing. It was a drug originally synthesised in 1908 by Heinrich Biltz and again in 1923 by Dox and Adrian

[271] Putnam, 'Anticonvulsant action'.

[272] Putnam and Merritt, 'Experimental determination'. According to Lennox (*Epilepsy and Related Disorders*, vol. 2, p. 861), the 'versatile and popular' Tracy Putnam, head of Harvard neurological service at the Boston City Hospital, had a 'hunch' about phenytoin, and Hiram Merritt and his technician Dorothy Miller (later Mrs Robert Schwab) undertook the painstaking and 'laborious and unpleasant task of testing the ability of various drugs to prevent convulsions electrically induced in cats'.

Thomas in the Parke-Davis laboratories. They noted that hydantoins had a ring structure similar to barbituric acid and that, like barbiturates, aliphatic substitutions on the 5-position conferred hypnotic properties but not aromatic substitutions. They had tested diphenylhydantoin looking for a hypnotic effect, but found none and so ignored it.

At the time, it was widely accepted that an antiepileptic effect depended on the sedative properties of a drug (bromides and barbiturates were examples of drugs identified as sedatives), and this was an assumption that Putnam challenged, perhaps on the basis of earlier experience with the brilliant vital red dye which has no sedative action at all.

The first eight patients treated were reported to Parke-Davis in August 1937, and the results of the first clinical trials were presented in June 1938 at the annual meeting of the American Medical Association. Clinical observations in the first 200 patients were published in September 1938, but were not all that encouraging. Among the 200 patients, minor toxic symptoms were reported in 15% and more serious reactions in 5%. Merritt and Putnam reported that phenytoin was 'without doubt … considerably more toxic than bromides and the barbituric compounds … [and thus] … it is worth trying with proper precautions in patients who have not responded to less toxic modes of therapy … or the ketogenic diet'.[273] Others were also trialling the drug. O. P. Kimball[274] gave it to children and was the first to report gum hypertrophy. A year later, Merritt and Putnam made a more upbeat presentation to the American Psychiatric Association and published this four months later,[275] reporting 267 patients now treated in whom 74% with grand mal, 59% of petit mal and 85% of psychomotor seizures were controlled or greatly improved.

It was on this basis, after minimal testing by today's standards, that Dilantin Sodium was added to Parke-Davis's catalogue price list in June 1938, only a year after the first patient had received it and only two years after the first administration to a cat. A year later, in 1939, the American Medical Association Council on Pharmacy and Chemistry voted to include Dilantin for 'epileptic patients who are not benefitted by phenobarbital or bromides and in those in whom these drugs induced disagreeable side reactions'.[276] The first advertisements for phenytoin in *Epilepsia* appeared in 1943.

Within a few years the drug had become extremely popular, perhaps partly due to Lennox's enthusiastic and infectious support. Contemporary opinion was summarised in 1940 in a paper submitted to the American Psychopathological Association, wherein were distinguished three epochs in the history of drug

[273] Friedlander, 'Putnam, Merritt'.   [274] Kimball, 'Treatment of epilepsy'.
[275] Merritt and Putnam, 'Sodium diphenyl hydantoinate'.
[276] Friedlander, 'Putnam, Merritt'.

treatment in epilepsy: the first of bromide, the second of phenobarbital and the third era, 'very recent in origin and characterized by the introduction in 1938 of Dilantin Sodium'.[277]

Over the next few years, Merritt and Putnam continued to test other drugs using the same screening methods. By 1945 more than 700 compounds had been evaluated and the results of 618 compounds were published,[278] of which 76 were given a 4+ rating and grouped into 7 categories on the basis of their structure: barbiturates, benzoxazoles, hydantoins, ketones and phenylketones, oxazolidinediones, phenyl compounds with sulphur and phenyl glycol. Four of these drugs were selected for clinical trial (5-phenyl-5-isopropoxymethylhydantoin, ethyl-phenylsulphone, 5-methyl-5-phenylhydantoin and 5,5-diphenylenehydantoin) but none were shown to be more effective than phenytoin and were dropped.

It was the view of Merritt and Putnam that the drugs acted by acidifying the nerve cell milieu and in this sense were similar to carbon dioxide and the two ketones pyruvic acid and acetoacetic acid. It was to be many years before the real mechanism of the anticonvulsant action of phenytoin – inhibition of sodium channel conductance – was unravelled. Merritt and Putnam also recognised that the anticonvulsant action was entirely independent of any hypnotic activity, and suggested that the use of anticonvulsants in epilepsy 'may be regarded as a substitution therapy'.[279]

Mass animal screening has since become part of the developmental programme of all the major pharmaceutical companies and drug development programmes in epilepsy. Ironically, it is now known that Merritt and Putnam's method does not measure seizure threshold reliably, and one can wonder how many of the drugs rejected on the basis of this test might in fact have proved useful in epilepsy.

Other Therapies 1914–1945

Hygienic therapy did not disappear in this age of medicine, but its emphasis changed, with growing interest then paid to diet. In the 1920s and 1930s, much of the research into the treatment of epilepsy had focused on changing the internal chemical milieu of the body, and especially the acid-base balance, by restricting fluid or by dietary means. Dietary treatments of epilepsy were fashionable prior to the Second World War and persisted well past it. Even as

---

[277] Cohen, Showstack and Myerson, 'Treatment of institutional epilepsy'.
[278] Friedlander, 'Putnam, Merritt'.
[279] Friedlander, 'Putnam, Merritt'; Putnam and Merritt, 'Chemistry of anticonvulsant drugs'. This to an extent reflected the great interest at the time in Lennox's experiments which had shown that acid-base balance affected the frequency of attacks in petit mal epilepsy.

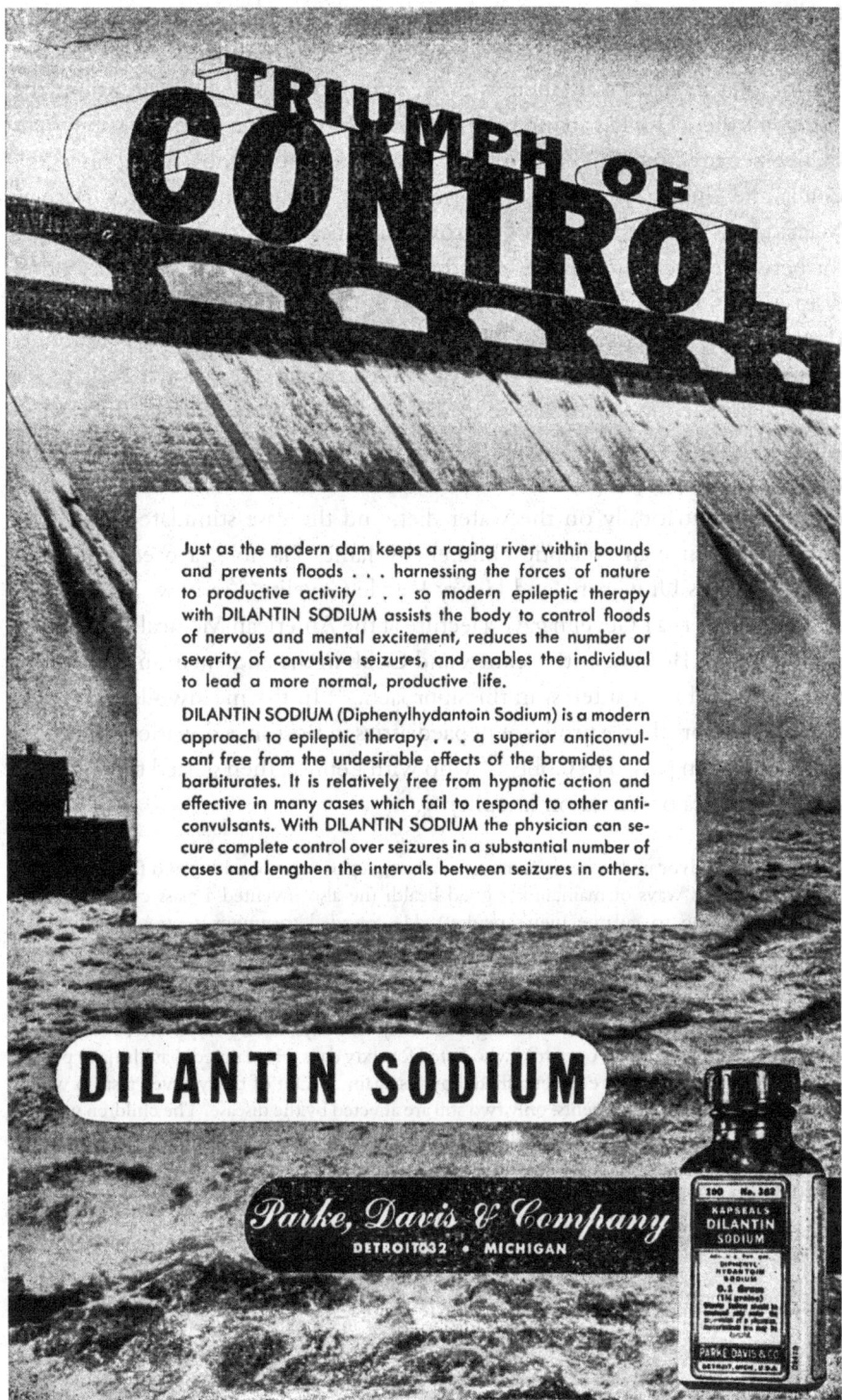

19. The first advertisement for phenytoin. A Speer-like dam holds back the seizure with a suitably fascist-era slogan.

late as 1960, Lennox reported a patient who had been given a typed list from his physician of 144 prohibited and 61 recommended foodstuffs.

One diet in particular, then as now, attracted considerable attention: the ketogenic diet. This has an interesting history. In 1911, starvation was shown to reduce seizure frequency (an observation made numerous times since) by Guillaume Guelpa and Auguste Marie in Paris. In the United States, Bernarr Macfadden,[280] a celebrated and controversial fitness fanatic, claimed that fasting for between three and twenty-one days could cure epilepsy and many other diseases. His assistant was Hugh Conklin, a physician from the little town of Battle Creek, Michigan.[281] Conklin began to treat epileptic patients routinely with fasting, which he called the 'water diet' (apparently on the basis of his belief that epileptic seizures were caused by a toxin secreted from the Peyer's patches in the intestines). A wealthy New York lawyer, Charles Howland, took his son, who had epilepsy, to see Conklin as a last resort. The child's seizures improved dramatically on the water diet, and the case stimulated studies of acid-base balance in epileptic children by James Gamble, a paediatrician at Johns Hopkins University, and Henry Rawle Geyelin,[282] a New York endocrinologist. In 1921 Geyelin gave a lecture at the American Medical Association convention in Boston, with Lennox and Cobb in the audience, and it was this that stimulated their interest in this approach.[283] In the meanwhile, Howland had given his brother, a professor of paediatrics in Boston, a donation of $5,000, which was then passed to Cobb [284] who with Lennox then started their famous series of studies of starvation in epilepsy.[285]

---

[280] Macfadden advocated extreme forms of exercise, vegetarianism, nudity and frequent sexual intercourse as ways of maintaining good health (he also invented a glass cylinder with a vacuum pump to enlarge men's penises). He founded treatment centres that awarded doctorates in 'physcultopathy' as well as a publishing empire of pulp fiction. He died a multimillionaire (see Ernst, *Weakness Is a Crime*).

[281] Bizarrely, Conklin believed that epilepsy was due to the improper functioning of certain glands in the bowels and that by fasting for twenty-two days, taking only water, a cure might be effected. He reported one child who fasted for sixty days. He claimed that "[m]any people ... fast thirty days and are never afflicted by fits again ... Out of thirty-seven tests in which children were used as patients, only two still are affected by the disease. The children were all under the age of 11 years, but we effect cures in older patients in from 50 to 60 per cent of the cases we undertake" ('Fasting as epilepsy cure'). Battle Creek, nicknamed 'Cereal City', was famous as being the site of the Sanatarium run by the arch eugenecist John Harvey Kellogg, whose brother invented Corn Flakes in 1894.

[282] Geyelin, a physician at the Presbyterian Hospital in New York, was best known for his work in diabetes.

[283] Lennox reported in *Epilepsy and Related Disorders* that Geyelin, whose results were never published, found long-term freedom from seizures in 15 of 79 children, but only 1 of 200 adults treated (vol. 2, p. 735).

[284] Wheless, 'Ketogenic diet'. On Geyelin, see Cecil, 'Henry Rawle Geyelin'.

[285] Lennox and Cobb showed that fasting between four and thirty-two days did have a dramatic effect. But it was only temporary, and seizure frequency returned to previous levels as soon as the fast was terminated. It was useful only as an emergency procedure. For good measure they also quoted Mark 9:24, where Jesus is presented with an unusually severe case of epilepsy

The effects of fasting also led Russell Morse Wilder at the Mayo Clinic[286] to suggest that a ketogenic diet was as effective as fasting in producing acidosis and could (obviously) be maintained for a far greater time. M. G. Peterman, a paediatrician at the Mayo Clinic, instituted the diet there with great success. In 1922, Wilder and Malcolm Winter[287] showed that ketosis occurred when the ratio of fatty acids to glucose was greater than 2:1 and recommended a diet with a 3:1 ratio, which became standard therapy. Temple Fay[288] subsequently suggested that by decreasing intracranial pressure, dehydration was a key factor, opening further avenues of work. In 1947 Peterman concluded that 'the new drugs [i.e. phenytoin et al.] … are no more effective than the ketogenic diet' and that 'the epileptic should not be given false hopes by articles in the popular literature to the effect that he may now be "cured" with a few pills or capsules'.[289] Lennox's annual review of the work in 1939 in *Epilepsia* reported that, at the Mayo Clinic, 267 children with idiopathic epilepsy had given the diet an adequate trial. Eighty-four (31%) had been rendered free of attacks for a year or more, and 73 of the 84 were reported currently to be back on a normal diet.[290] Water restriction was also advocated, especially by Fay.[291]

The ketogenic diet was taken up particularly at Johns Hopkins in Baltimore, where in 1972 the paediatrician Samuel Livingston reported more than 1,000 children treated with the diet, claiming that 52% had complete control of seizures and an additional 27% had improved. The previous year, in Chicago, Peter Huttenlocher had introduced a medium-chain triglyceride oil diet that allowed less restriction of other foods, improving tolerability. But despite Livingston's astonishing results, interest in the diet slowly receded – only to be stimulated again in the late 1990s.[292]

Other medicinal therapies employed in this period are now also largely forgotten, and almost all the contemporary leading physicians considered them to be inferior to bromide and phenobarbital. Borax remained the most widely used. Agents that were primarily simple chemicals or extracted from animals (rattlesnake venom was one exotic example) had largely disappeared in the first decades of the century, as had herbals, although some authorities continued to recommend the use of belladonna, valerian, zinc and cannabis.

and says: 'This kind (of evil spirit) goeth not out but by prayer and fasting' (Lennox and Cobb, 'Clinical effect of fasting').
[286] Wilder, 'Ketonemia', p. 307. [287] Wilder and Winter, 'Threshold of ketogenesis'.
[288] Fay was Professor and Head of the Neurosurgery department at Temple University School of Medicine.
[289] Peterman, 'Idiopathic epilepsy in childhood'. [290] Lennox, 'Epilepsy in 1939'.
[291] Fay, 'Dehydration of epileptic patients'.
[292] A key milestone was the Charlie Foundation, set up by the parents of a two-year-old boy who was treated with remarkable results. The foundation became the subject of a 1997 film titled *First Do No Harm*, starring Meryl Streep and directed by Charlie's father.

A curiosity of the period was the discovery that therapy with vital dyes – notably, but not exclusively, brilliant vital red – could stop seizures. The anticonvulsant potential of brilliant red was reported by Cobb following a paper presented to the Boston Society for Psychiatry and Neurology in 1936.[293] As has been often the case, the discovery of the anticonvulsant effects was the result of chance. Cobb and colleagues were trying to stain, in vivo, cerebral tissue subjected to anoxia, but the dyes would not take, and they attempted to increase uptake by chemically inducing convulsions. They observed that the convulsions were inhibited by the dyes, which they then systematically evaluated in camphor-induced seizures in rabbits and mice. Subsequently, ten children were treated with daily intravenous injections of a 1% solution of brilliant vital red until their skin turned bright pink. Five had a reduction in the number of seizures in the pink condition, and one remained seizure free. Two were then followed up on oral neoprontosil, a diazo-sulphonamide compound being used as an antibiotic and for ulcerative colitis, with marked diminution of attacks. In 1940 Lennox reported the results of several studies of brilliant vital red, including one of thirteen institutionalised boys with improvements in eight, and better results in petit mal rather than grand mal seizures (although some cases were worsened by the therapy). In another study, 2–20 ml of 1% methyl blue solution was administered in twenty-two cases of status with excellent results.[294] Robert B. Aird also reported positive results, postulating that the dye worked by rendering the blood–brain barrier impermeable to 'convulsive toxins' in the systemic circulation.[295] Further experimentation continued for some years, despite the obvious unpleasantness of this treatment – a colourful but futile interlude in the history of epilepsy therapy.

Calvert Stein, a senior physician at the Monson State Hospital in Massachusetts (mentioned earlier in relation to his work on heredity), wrote in 1934 on another topic of contemporary interest: the role of hormonal factors in the causation of epilepsy. Endocrine studies in dementia had been under way for some time, and endocrine replacement in deficiency diseases (for instance, thyroid extract in myxoedema and posterior pituitary extract in diabetes insipidus) had been found to be strikingly effective. Stein listed numerous available pharmaceutical preparations, comprising extracts of more than twelve 'glands' (including liver, prostate and testicles) for which over-embellished claims had been made. This was clearly a fashionable form of therapy for a variety of different diseases, despite an often dubious theoretical basis. The stage thus seemed to be set for studies in epilepsy. Among the more than 1,000 inmates of Monson, well over half had no obvious cause of epilepsy, which was assumed

[293] Cobb, Cohen and Ney, 'Anticonvulsive action'. Even by 2020, the cerebral effects of red dye in foodstuffs remain the subject of much controversy.
[294] Lennox, 'Epilepsy in America'.   [295] Aird, 'Mode of action'.

to be inherited (although few had near relatives with the disorder). It was on 68 such patients whose seizures were frequent and severe that Stein conducted his investigations. These studies were all the more notable for the inclusion of a control group of 70 non-epileptic nurses and attendants.[296] A variety of measurements were made, including pulse, blood pressure, weight (distribution of fat), peristalsis, menstruation and general well-being. Single-gland therapy was used in every case, namely extracts of whole pituitary, anterior and posterior pituitary, thyracoids, suprarenal tissue, corpus luteum, ovacoids, testacoids, ampacoids (prostate, testicle and ovary, respectively, for hypodermic use), panacoids and pancrobilin. If no clinical effect was noticed after two months, thyroid and whole pituitary extracts were added. No change in seizure frequency was observed with any of these therapies. Accordingly, Stein concluded that

> [E]ndocrine therapy should be but one part of the general therapeutic program; and does not deserve consideration to the exclusion of sedatives, dietary restrictions, gastro-intestinal regulation, psychotherapy, and the usual routine hygienic measures ... Patients who improved in general health while on treatment, and the majority of them did ... show a lessening of the post-convulsive debility, headache and weakness, and also a marked shortening of the post-convulsive period of convalescence. (pp. 757–8)

What is interesting about this paper is not so much the results, which were disappointing, but rather the systematic method used and the inclusion of a control group – one of the first epilepsy studies to do so (although Stein had also included controls in his studies of heredity published a year earlier in 1933, albeit with a choice of controls heavily criticised in the Myerson report).

Surgical Treatment of Epilepsy

This brings us to surgical therapy. Throughout the 1910s and 1920s, the idea that surgery could be primarily targeted at treating epilepsy faltered as the nascent specialty of neurosurgery focused on other topics, and was revived only in the 1940s.

In England, by the time of Horsley's death in 1915, epilepsy surgery had ceased almost completely. Indeed, the decline had begun probably a decade earlier (Horsley's last paper on epilepsy appeared in 1890, and his last epilepsy operation was said by one source to have been around 1897 – see footnote 285, p.129). What surgery there was focused on removing lesions, especially brain tumours, and operating on post-traumatic epilepsy.[297] Similarly, in France there was no interest at all. In the United States, although Cushing was

[296] Stein, 'Endocrine therapy in epilepsy'.
[297] Two such cases were described by Worster-Drought ('British Medical Association').

instrumental in reviving neurosurgery and in pushing the specialty forward, he too had given up epilepsy surgery in the early 1900s.[298]

Horsley's pupil Sir Percy Sargent[299] had become the leading neurosurgeon in London by the end of World War One. Sargent's contribution to epilepsy surgery was restricted largely to treating post-traumatic seizures, partly from his own very extensive wartime experience as the only specialist neurosurgeon in the British army. In 1922, he gave a paper[300] expounding his theory that post-traumatic scarring anchored the brain and meninges to the internal surface of the skull by adhesions, which caused traction on brain tissue and resulted in vascular constriction and post-traumatic seizures (this concept was then adopted by Otfrid Foerster and Wilder Penfield). In a series of more than 200 cases, Sargent found that separating the dura from the skull and inserting a piece of celluloid between them prevented traction and resolved the epilepsy in some cases. Results in other lesional focal epilepsies, however, were less good. Accordingly, it became his view that tumour surgery in epilepsy should be primarily directed at treating the tumour (p. 10) rather than the epilepsy, although he did concede that if the tumour was entirely removed, there was a reasonable chance that the epilepsy might resolve. In the absence of an obvious lesion, the results of 'exploratory surgery' were in his opinion wholly unpredictable (p. 11):

> 'Cynical friends have told me that operations upon the nervous system do but illustrate the truth that hope ever triumphs over experience. The surgeon must be an optimist, but his optimism need not be that of the ostrich. It should be based upon the expectation that inquiry into the causation of those diseases which he seeks to remedy will eventually furnish the clue to their successful treatment. The search may lead him into deep waters, and this must be my excuse for venturing so far out of my depth as to address a gathering of neurologists on such a subject as epilepsy. (p. 12)

Sargent was a brilliant surgeon, in the general surgical tradition, and had a significant influence on Penfield, who trained partly with him.[301] However, in this period orthodox opinion offered little hope for the surgery of epilepsy, and, as Sargent had intimated, neurosurgery was then widely thought of as a poor servant of neurology – a situation that was to be reversed within a few decades.

It was only in Germany, in two centres, that epilepsy surgery continued in any intellectual sense in these years, stimulated by the continuing work on

---

[298] In the 1910s and 1920s, neurosurgery flourished as a sub-specialty in America, not least because the oversupply of surgeons encouraged specialisation as a method of maintaining a good income. But in Europe neurosurgery remained largely the preserve of general surgeons.

[299] Sargent, like Horsley, practised at the National Hospital, Queen Square.

[300] Sargent, 'Observations on epilepsy'.

[301] Penfield's vascular hypothesis of seizures, a concept he maintained throughout his life, was based heavily on Sargent's ideas.

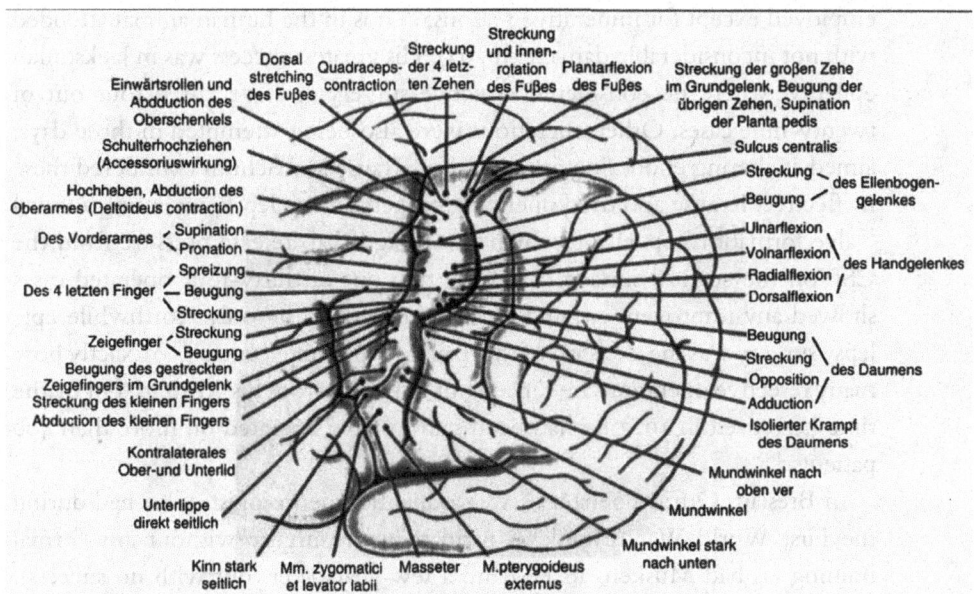

20. A map of responses to electrical stimulation of the motor cortex (from Fedor Krause, *Surgery of the Brain and Spinal Cord Based on Personal Experience*; 1912)

cerebral localisation. The theory was extended between 1901 and 1917 in Britain, notably by Sherrington and his brilliant associate Albert Grünbaum (who changed his name to A. S. F. Leyton in 1915), who together produced detailed motor maps of the brains of chimpanzees, gorillas and other apes. In Germany, in the same period, Oskar and Cécile Vogt produced cytoarchitectonic maps (maps based on the cellular composition of cortex) with the cortex divided into more than 100 zones. They worked on apes, transcribing their maps onto an outline of the human brain (their 'human homologue'). This was excellent work[302] and stimulated Fedor Krause and his co-worker, Heinrich Schum, to begin to practice resective surgery on the motor strip for Jacksonian epilepsy. Krause published a three-volume work on the surgery of the brain and spinal cord, the second volume of which (published in 1912) contained a chapter of more than 200 pages devoted to a detailed analysis of Krause's own operations on patients with epilepsy.[303] He developed maps of the human cortex based on cortical stimulation and used peroperative electrical stimulation to identify the 'primary spasm area' (p. 84; also called the primary convulsive area) but cautioning that: 'Electric stimulation of the brain should not be

---

[302] The culmination of their work, and a summary of their previous papers, was the massive paper published in 1919: Vogt and Vogt, 'Allgemeine Ergebnisse unserer Hirnforschung'.

[303] Krause, *Surgery of the Brain*, vol. 2. See also his later three-volume opus on brain surgery, Krause and Schum, *Die Spezielle chirurgie*. In volume 2, part 2, he refers to 446 operations for epilepsy, but it is not clear what their nature was; some might well have been simple trepanations (pp. 656–7).

employed except for imperative reasons, as it is in the human animal attended with not inconsiderable damage' (p. 93). His greatest success was in Jacksonian epilepsy, where he considered resective surgery to have cured four out of twenty-nine cases. Other operations were also being attempted in those days, aimed at altering endocrine function, but Krause and Schum considered these ineffective. Krause also tried operating on genuine epilepsy, inventing a novel 'valve formation' operation which was designed to release pressure from the CSF on the cortical surface. But only two out of thirty-four operated cases showed any improvement, and he concluded that the only worthwhile epilepsy surgery was the excision of the 'primary spasming centre'.[304] Exactly how many resective operations he carried out is unclear from his writings, but by the time he retired in 1923 he had been said to have operated on more than 400 patients.[305]

In Breslau, Otfrid Foerster[306] was a qualified neurologist, who had during the First World War turned his hand to neurosurgery without any formal training (as had Muskens in Holland a few years later, but with no success). In the 1920s he developed new techniques for epilepsy surgery, using awake craniotomy under local anaesthetic and intraoperative cortical stimulation to localise the area of epileptogenicity by observing the symptoms produced by stimulation.[307] Foerster was said to have operated on 100 patients with post-traumatic epilepsy. He presented a film of his human cerebral stimulation to a meeting in 1922, which may have triggered Berger's interest in the electrical currents of the brain.[308] He gained a reputation for this work, although the value of such surgery remained contentious. James Collier in London, for instance, claimed that he had never seen a case of post-traumatic epilepsy cured by surgery. But this was unfair. Foerster had a distinguished record but perhaps his greatest legacy was the fact that he interested Wilder Penfield in epilepsy surgery (Penfield had in 1928 spent six months with him learning his techniques. Percival Bailey and Paul Bucy were other influential American neurosurgeons who had periods of training in his clinic). Then, in 1930, Penfield and Foerster jointly published an influential paper on the surgical treatment of post-traumatic epilepsy, in which they ascribed the epilepsy to traction of the post-traumatic scar on the surrounding 'vaso-astral' framework

---

[304] Krause, *Surgery of the Brain*, vol. 2, pp. 389–90, 464–5.   [305] Horwitz, 'Fedor Krause'.

[306] See Zülch, 'Otfrid Foerster'; Kennard, Fulton and de Gutierrez-Mahoney, 'Otfrid Foerster'. Foerster studied medicine in Freiburg, Kiel and Breslau, and practised in Breslau. He was a renowned neurologist who treated Lenin after his stroke. In recognition of his work, he received the Hughlings Jackson Memorial Medal, and gave the Hughlings Jackson lecture, at the 1935 International Neurological Congress in London.

[307] Foerster, 'Zur operativen Behandlung der Epilepsie'.

[308] Foerster and Altenburger, 'Elektrobiologische Vorgänge'. Foerster's film was presented at the Gesellschaft Deutscher Nervenärzte in Halle in 1922.

of brain tissue. They used cortical stimulation under local anaesthesia, and wrote up seven of these cases in detail.[309]

In this surgery, they were guided by Vogt's cortical maps. But in 1935 the Vogts were dismissed from their posts by the Nazi government, and epilepsy surgery based on cortical localisation ceased in Germany, much as it had done in Britain. It was when Penfield returned to establish his unit in Montreal, adopting and developing Foerster's methods, that the baton of epilepsy surgery passed to North America.

In what was his first major international platform, Penfield spoke at the Second International Neurological Congress in London in July 1935, presenting the approach to epilepsy surgery that he had adopted, and which was not to change substantially in subsequent decades.[310] He first discussed the finding of what he called 'cerebral vasolability' (an 'irritability of cerebral blood vessels') and the lack of value of surgery in idiopathic epilepsy (as had Sargent and others), mentioning the failure of such procedures as cervicothoracic sympathetic ganglionectomy, carotid body removal, carotid sinus denervation, subtemporal decompression except in rare instances of chronic subdural fluid collection, and spinal insufflation of air (which he considered to be effective only in patients under sixteen years of age whose seizures had occurred for four years or less). He then described surgery in epilepsy due to subdural haematoma, birth injury and congenital abnormalities, tumour, cicatrix and cerebral atrophy, and the value of total resection, explorations without excision, ligature of the carotid arteries and evacuation of subdural fluid. He discussed functional anatomy and the use of peroperative electrical stimulation. This was a tour de force and established Penfield immediately in the first rank of academic neurosurgeons. Penfield considered resective surgery to have its most significant role in lesional epilepsy, and especially epilepsy due to scars (cicatrices) and atrophy (41–6% cure rate and 32% improvement rate). Penfield ended his London talk with a memorable quote from Hughlings Jackson: that there is only one physiologic cause of epilepsy, but many pathological causes.

In 1940 he extended his work, describing the features of epilepsy in a series of 703 cases of intracranial tumour, all but 6 of which were verified histologically.[311] This paper gave a clear description, hardly bettered today, of the features of tumoural epilepsy, including the higher incidence in slow-growing tumours, and he was also the first to show clearly that operative resection was more effective in encapsulated tumours than infiltrating tumours. Penfield considered the 'cure' rate of operative removal of an encapsulated tumour to be about the same as that from the resection of a focal post-traumatic scar (p. 315).

---

[309] Foerster and Penfield, 'Traumatic epilepsy'.
[310] His talk was published a year later: Penfield, 'Epilepsy and surgical therapy'.
[311] Penfield, Erickson and Tarlov, 'Intracranial tumors'.

THE EXPERIENCE OF HAVING EPILEPSY

The Dehumanisation of Epilepsy

Attitudes of individuals in any society will naturally greatly vary; however, the dominant *waltanschauung*, and the range of viewpoints, are to a large extent set by socio-political conventions and group norms. The attitudes towards epilepsy in this period were a case in point. Being influenced by medical theory and also by the public interest in such topics as eugenics, degeneration and psychoanalysis, epilepsy took on a life well beyond medicine. It became a victim of a tendency which might be called the dehumanisation of medicine, in which the medical focus moved away from the patient's best interest towards the societal and political aspects of the disease. It was in this period that, to an unprecedented degree, the balance between medicine's obligation to a patient and to society changed.

The process was facilitated by the accelerated value medicine began to place on scientific competence above all else and its active discouragement of any empathetic relationship with patients (an approach associated with quacks and charlatans). Neurologists particularly were renowned for their condescending and authoritarian stance towards their patients with epilepsy (and mental disorders), a reputation confirmed by the tenor of much of their writings. Many conversations must have taken the form 'I am the doctor. You are the patient, and you will do as I say.' Maintaining 'control' became a guiding principle of medical behaviour,[312] often mixed with the recognition that there was in fact not much that could be done for epilepsy.

Another aspect was the issue of consent. This hardly featured in public debate for it was assumed that the doctor would act in the patient's best interest. Although consent is a fundamental principle of medicine, the rising focus away from the patient led to an erosion of this core obligation.

In World War II, the process of dehumanisation reached its zenith in wartime Germany. There medical ethics, always relative and dependent on prevailing political mores, were massively coarsened. The concept of the sanctity of life, a fundamental pillar of medicine, was tossed away by large sections of the medical profession in policies which declared that the handicapped had 'lives which were not worth living' and that such individuals 'did not really fit into this world'. Similarly, consent of patients or families was completely ignored. Although originating from eugenic medicine and Nazi ideology, these policies became accepted by large swathes of the population as well as the medical profession. Although it was doctors who selected the cases for extermination, many others participated in the process of removal and killing – including nurses, hospital staff, drivers, railway workers, cleaners,

---

[312] See, for instance, *Report of the Royal Commission*, pp. 8–12, 392, 403.

administrators, officials and lawyers. The uninvolved general public also understood what was happening, but humanity was in short supply in the face of economic hardship and Nazi ferocity. Many in the community agreed or complied with the policies, some enthusiastically and some tacitly. What today are taken to be fundamental and inviolable principles of compassion and human rights seem singly to have been missing from the public responses and this must have made the experience of those with epilepsy particularly frightening. Those whose lives were discarded were not all severely handicapped or severely affected, and the position of ordinary epileptic persons in society must have felt very precarious.

Epilepsy in Early Movies and in Literature

Changing societal and medical attitudes were reflected in film and literature. The immediate impact of a visual image is greater than that of the written page, and for this reason the depiction of epilepsy in film, including films based on books, is particularly instructive. Film can be said to have emerged in 1895, when the Lumiere brothers patented cinematograph in France, coincidentally the same year as Freud published his first major work (*Studies in Hysteria*, with Josef Breuer); the two topics, cinema and psychoanalysis, advanced in parallel, and both were central to defining cultural thought throughout the twentieth century. Film was later to prove the medium best suited to conveying to non-sufferers, with great immediacy, what having epilepsy feels like, but in its early days this was far from the case. The earliest movies treated patients like exhibits in a circus. Epilepsy was a relatively rare theme, appearing probably for the first time in a motion picture in *Le Déshabillage impossible* (*Going to Bed Under Difficulties*, 1900) a film directed by Georges Méliès.[313] This short, primitive, comic sequence shows a man struggling to undress and then collapsing in what is called an epileptic seizure (although the end of the film is lost and what is left actually bears little relationship to a genuine seizure). It demonstrated epilepsy as a humiliation and hilarious, but not much else. Romeo Bosetti and Alice Guy directed the 1906 short *Le Matelas épileptique* (*The Epileptic Mattress*), which again made fun of convulsive movements. Following the pioneering work of Eadweard Muybridge and others, the motion picture industry developed in earnest in the first decade of the twentieth century, and in the late 1920s silent films began to be replaced by 'talkies'. It was then that epilepsy began to appear as a significant element in the plot. A very early example was 'To What Red Hell' (which in fact was first made as a silent film) in which the main character, Edwin Greenwood, is an alcoholic who strangles a prostitute in an epileptic seizure and ends up dying by suicide. A review in the *New York Times* in 1929 mentions

[313] A useful list of films featuring epilepsy is found in Kerson and Kerson, 'Truly enthralling'.

that 'Criticism has also been made of the theme in which a drunken epileptic plays one of the chief parts'.[314]

Amongst the first movies to address epilepsy seriously were those involved in eugenics. Many revolved around the theme of marriage, with one partner finding out the other has a history or family history of insanity or epilepsy. The revelation was portrayed as carrying a dire risk of degeneration in any offspring – and the plot was sometimes resolved by the discovery that in fact, due to adoption or some other circumstance, there was no such danger. *The Black Stork* (1917), written by and starring Chicago surgeon Dr Harry Haiselden, was a prominent eugenic film and emblematic of this genre. The story revolves around two couples. The spouse (Claude) of the first couple has inherited degenerative tendencies, the result of his grandfather's impregnation of a 'vile filthy' black slave. His doctor tries to dissuade the marriage by showing Claude and his sweetheart Anne a variety of deformed and mentally defective children. They ignore the advice and produce a defective son who needs an operation at birth to save his life. His mother has a vision of her son being saved by the operation but then being inevitably burdened by his deformities, condemned to a life of pauperism and crime and with his own defective offspring. In a fit of rage, the son kills the surgeon 'who condemned' him to life. Horrified by this premonition, Anne agrees to withholding treatment and the child leaps into the arms of a waiting Jesus. The female (Miriam) of the other couple believes that her mother had epilepsy, and because of this refuses to marry her suitor. She then discovers that her mother was in fact a 'stepmother', not a blood relative, and so proceeds to marry and has a beautiful and healthy baby. The film has other complex themes,[315] but it paints a terrible picture of epilepsy, with its links to insanity, crime, degeneration, dementia and physical as well as behavioural deformity. Interestingly, the same theme – that someone with epilepsy carries an inherited weakness and should not marry – occurred in movies right through to the 1940s and later. For instance, in *Dr Kildare's Crisis* (1940) the young doctor's imminent marriage to Mary, a pretty nurse, was about to be cancelled because Mary's brother is diagnosed by Kildare as having epilepsy. All was saved, however, when a clever colleague elicited a history of head injury which removed the danger of the hereditary taint.

The literature of the period dealt with epilepsy in a more subtle and nuanced manner, and retained their focus much more on the individual, than was the case in the early films. Nevertheless, many of the same tropes were in evidence and the experience of epilepsy in most of these novels was portrayed as negative and fear-laden. As in the nineteenth century, epilepsy interested a number of the important novelists and writers of the interwar years. Thomas Mann, who received the Nobel Prize for Literature in 1929, was fascinated by medicine and, in particular, by the social metaphors of disease. Amongst the illnesses that he wrote about was epilepsy,

---

[314] Marshall, 'London Film Notes'.   [315] Pernick, *Black Stork*.

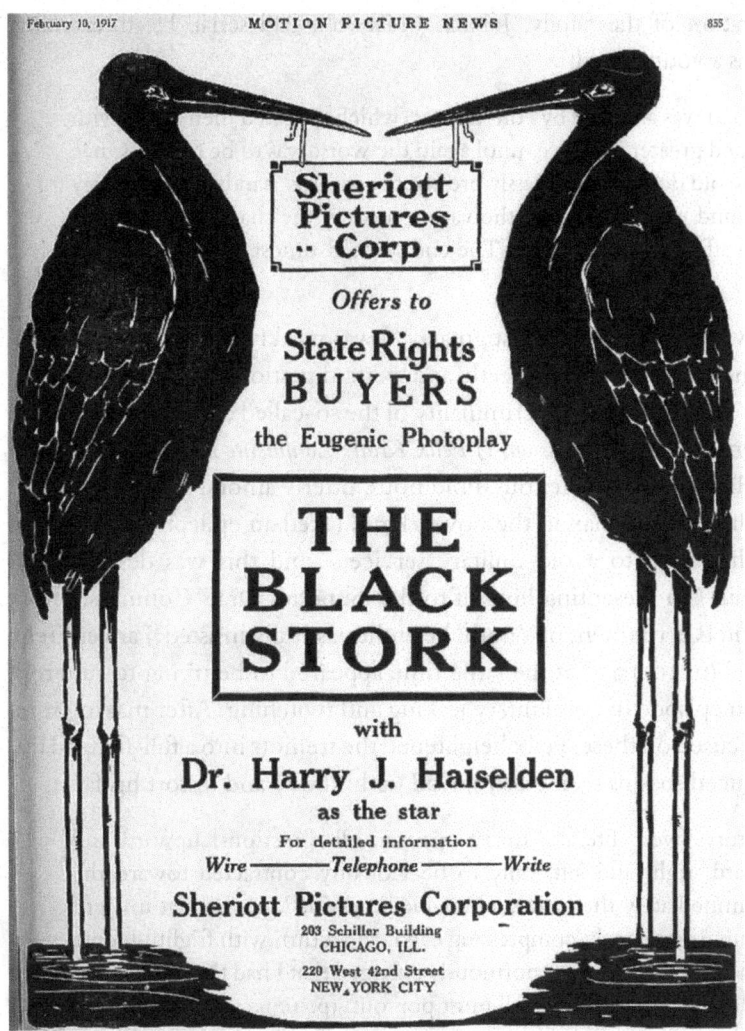

21. The poster for the movie *Black Stork*

which features in three of his novels. One recurring theme in Mann's writing (and evidence of the influence of Friedrich Nietzsche) is the relationship between epilepsy and creativity. As Mann wrote about Fyodor Dostoevsky's epilepsy, 'something comes out in illness that is more important and conducive to life and growth than any medically guaranteed health or sanity ... In other words: certain conquests made by the soul and the mind are impossible without disease, madness, crime of the spirit.'[316] Another theme of Mann's work was an interest in degeneration and the theories of progressivity (the worsening of degenerative manifestations over generations). This was the central theme of *Buddenbrooks: The Decline of a Family* (1901), written when Mann was only twenty-five.[317] The last born of the

---

[316] Mann, 'Dostoyevsky – within limits', p. 443.   [317] See Mann, *Buddenbrooks*, p. 485.

fourth generation of the family, Johann ('Hanno'), had serial, life-threatening convulsions as a young child:

> [T]he child was attacked by convulsions, which repeated themselves with greater and greater violence, until again the worst was to be feared. Once more the old doctor speechlessly pressed the parents' hands. The child lay in profound exhaustion, and the vacant look in the shadowy eyes indicated an affection of the brain. The end seemed almost to be wished for.
> (p. 445)

Hanno had various degenerative stigmata,[318] was weakly and sick, withdrawn and melancholic, with terrible teeth and poor digestion, until he died as a young man. The amorality and criminality of the so-called epileptic personality was in evidence in *The Confessions of Felix Krull, Confidence Man* (1922). Krull, the central character, is duplicitous, libidinous, utterly amoral and deceptive, a cheat and a liar. In a climax in the novel, Krull faked an epileptic seizure as a form of malingering to avoid military service – and this was described in accurate detail. On presenting himself to the 'Superior Draft Commission on the Fitness and Recruitment of Youth' he enthusiastically insisted 'I am entirely fit for service' (p. 101) and at the same time appeared to be trying to suppress and ignore an episode of involuntary jerking and twitching. After making sure the doctor focused on these, Felix heightened the tremors into a full-fledged fit. The self-induced spasms seemed to spread up his body and distort his face:

> My features were literally thrust apart in all directions, upward and downward, right and left, only to be violently contracted toward the centre immediately thereafter; a horrible, one-sided grin tore at my left, then at my right cheek, compressing each eye in turn with frightful force while the other became so enormously enlarged that I had the distinct and frightful feeling that the eyeball must pop out. (p. 109)

The commission members reacted with 'consternation, indignation and even disgust ... amazement ... I saw one who was holding both fists against his ears, and another had two fingers of his right hand pressed against his lips and was blinking his eyelids with extraordinary rapidity'. Despite Felix's apparent keenness to sign up, he is told with contempt 'You are rejected' (p. 113). Mann must have had personal knowledge of epilepsy, for his descriptions, like those of Agatha Christie (and unlike those of Raymond Chandler), are accurate and well described. Another accurate description of an epileptic convulsion occurs in *The Magic Mountain* (1924), when the teacher, Popov, collapses during lunch in the institution: '[O]ne day, while the meal was in full swing, the man was seized with a violent epileptic fit, and with that oft-described

---

[318] His condition has been ascribed to the 'hyper-E syndrome' (Fischer, 'Hanno Buddenbrook?'), but this is a banal explanation. Mann was really describing the stigmata and sign of inherited degeneration in the Lombrosian tradition.

demoniac unearthly shriek fell to the floor, where he lay beside his chair, striking about him with dreadfully distorted arms and legs.'[319] The other inmates are disturbed and appalled by the sight, and the doctor, Krokowski, gives a distorted and perverted psychoanalytic explanation of the epilepsy.

Epilepsy associated with visions and mysticism was another literary thread, well demonstrated by John Cowper Powys (nominated three times for the Nobel Prize in Literature), who had epilepsy himself.[320] In his novel *Wolf Solent* (1929), Solent describes a vision which is so convincing as to be based surely on personal knowledge:

> Once more the scent of pinks came quivering through his brain and he felt a nameless twirl of pleasure … [T]he voices of his companions became a vague humming in his ears, and all manner of queer detached memories floated in upon him. He felt himself to be walking alone along some high white road bordered by waving grasses and patches of yellow rock-rose. There was a town far below him, at the bottom of a green valley – a mass of huddled grey roofs among meadows and streams – round which the twilight was darkening. Along with all this he was conscious of the taste of a peculiar kind of baker's bread, such as used to be sold at a shop in Dorchester, where, as a child, they would take him for tea during summer jaunts from Weymouth. (pp. 463–4)

In his autobiography (1934), although Powys never directly refers to having epilepsy, he describes sudden falls, episodes of 'absent-minded foolishness' and also 'thrilling experience[s] … when an ecstasy of happiness came over [him] so intoxicating that it was as if [he] trod upon air'.[321] These episodes are not dissimilar to the ecstatic experiences of Dostoevsky. Both Powys's and Dostoevsky's symptoms seem to confirm my own clinical impression that the more creative a person is, the more complex are the phenomena of the focal (temporal lobe) seizures. Powys also wrote a book (*Dostoievsky*, 1946) and essays about the Russian author, holding that 'weakness and disease and suffering can become organs of vision',[322] much as was the view of Mann and Nietzsche. In *The Art of Growing Old* (1944), Powys wrote: 'I believe it is a peculiarity of this *sacred sickness* that it heightens, almost to a point of rapture, the smallest detail of the story of all persons and of all things that can possibly have a story.'[323] Seizures occur in other novels by Powys, including *Ducdame* (1925), *A Glastonbury Romance* (1932) and *Owen Glendower* (1941). Some of his characters seem to be able to induce seizures or feign at will, as part of what Robin Wood

[319] Mann, *Magic Mountain*, p. 298
[320] For two interesting articles about Powys and epilepsy, see Verbeek, 'John Cowper Powys', and Wood, 'Queer attacks and fits'.
[321] Powys, *Auto Biography*, pp. 408, 219.   [322] Powys, *Visions and Revisions*, p. 251.
[323] Powys, *Art of Growing Old*, p. 208.

has called 'a spiritual discipline … the ancient shamanic pathway to spiritual insight' and a 'doorway to heightened consciousness'.[324] Another theme in Powys' work, common in the writing of many at the time, including that of his Welsh compatriot, the artist Sir John Kiffin Williams, was social isolation because of epilepsy.[325]

Both Powys and the Austrian novelist Joseph Roth illustrate another aspect of epilepsy that of transformation (taken up later as a theme in pharmaceutical advertising of antiepileptic drugs). In Roth's novel (actually, more of a fairy tale) *Job* (1930), Menuchim, a misshapen, mentally retarded and epileptic child, miraculously turns into a beautiful, elegant, world-famous musician. The transformation does not happen during a seizure (as in the gothic novels), but it allows a happy ending to a life of misery. Roth may have suffered alcoholic seizures, as is implied in his correspondence with Stefan Zweig,[326] and perhaps this is what he hoped for as his life drifted into alcohol, debt, depression and misanthropy.

Mann, Powys and Roth are very much in the tradition of Dostoevsky, seeing epilepsy not only as a plague but also as a means to different planes of emotional and creative consciousness. There are echoes of Cesare Lombroso,[327] for whom epilepsy and genius were manifestations of the same cerebral irritation and linked by similar amorality. This has been a recurring theme in epilepsy studies, although not all agreed.[328]

Epilepsy appeared in a number of crime fictions in which there are obvious references to the post-Lombrosian folk-perception that criminality is part and parcel of the condition. In Agatha Christie's *The ABC Murders* (1936), the central character, Alexander Bonaparte Cust, has major

---

[324] Wood, 'Queer attacks and fits'.

[325] Because of his epilepsy, Williams avoided marriage, like Flaubert and Lear before him. The mood of his self-imposed isolation was described in his obituary in *The Guardian*, 4 Sept. 2006: 'The darkness implicit in so many of Kyffin's mountain landscapes was a facet of his own make-up. He recognised in it the Celtic tendency to melancholy, but believed it to be exacerbated by circumstance, instinctively feeling that a certain despair and gloom were the logical sequel to his grand mal seizures … [His complex personality] was reflected most tellingly in his turbulent seascapes and it was stormy weather, over land or sea, which fuelled the nervous excitement and apprehension that tormented him but, paradoxically, produced his greatest work'. (a very Lombrosian concept).

[326] Davidson, 'Letters of Joseph Roth'.   [327] Lombroso, *Man of Genius*.

[328] See the letter by a reader in the *British Medical Journal* disputing that idiopathic epilepsy could ever be associated with genius, and pointing out that '[o]ther seizures, such as those due to insolation, uraemia, or even the hysteria of fanaticism, have been in times past confused with true epilepsy'. The author viewed this as a reason for the 'neglect in hospital teaching of the tendency of epileptics to become insane, and on the frequency with which hysteria and other morbid mental phases are manifested in those epileptics who are not actually lunatics or dements' (F. G. C., 'Epilepsy and genius').

convulsions associated with periods of amnesia. Attempts are made to pin a series of murders on him. Cust himself is a timid person with no self-esteem and is tricked into believing that he did in fact carry out the crimes during periods of epileptic amnesia. He is saved from the gallows at the last minute by Hercule Poirot, who unravels the deception. Cust is a sympathetic but simple character (an innocent fool) and exhibits many of the stereotypes of epilepsy – rage attacks, criminality, loss of control, lack of self-confidence and naivety, all of which make an appearance in this novel. The descriptions of the seizures are so good that it is clear that Christie, like Mann, had first-hand knowledge of epilepsy. She included epilepsy in several other novels (*Murder on the Links*, 1923; *Nemesis*, 1971). In Raymond Chandler's *The Big Sleep* (1939), one of the central characters, Carmen Sternwood, has epilepsy and is painted as a childish, wild, promiscuous and violent women. She is saved from a murder charge but ends up being institutionalised. In these novels, amnesia and lack of control during a seizure are also used as devices to explain the plot and move the narrative along.

The negative aspects of the portrayal of epilepsy in this period were matched by the complete absence from the literature of any autobiography or memoirs in which epilepsy was disclosed. Surely this represented the then almost universal impulse of patients and their families to hide the condition or deny its existence. In the hostile environment of eugenics and medical disdain, the person with epilepsy inhabited a shadowy personal world, where being out of sight and mind were ways of remaining safe.

THE INTERNATIONAL LEAGUE AGAINST EPILEPSY

The fact that epilepsy could be differentiated early on as a sub-specialty of neurology and psychiatry was due partly to the opportunity provided by the large international conferences. There, friendships could be formed and contacts made across national boundaries. As described in Chapter 1, the ILAE itself was founded at the 16th International Medical Congress in Budapest in 1909, and its annual meetings continued to be held in conjunction with other international meetings until 1913. The First World War, however, ended these collaborations. The ILAE was disbanded, *Epilepsia* ceased publication and no further conferences, nor any other activity, took place until 1937.

The first evidence in the interwar years of a renewed interest in forming an international organisation was a visit to Europe in 1929 by a group of American epileptologists and psychiatrists accompanied by Kirby Collier and Arthur Shaw, president and secretary, respectively, of the National Association for the Study of Epilepsy.[329] The group set sail for Liverpool on the SS *Caronia*. In a letter to Adolf Meyer, dated 3 January 1928, Shaw had written, 'This is an attempt to revive the Internationale Liga contra l'Epilepsie.' During the month-long trip the group were to visit all the major European epilepsy centres and meet with previous ILAE members Louis Muskens, Alfred Ulrich, Henri Claude and Otto Wuth, among others (also promised were a 'glimpse of life on the Rhine', 'a day and a half in the capital city of the oldest republican government in Europe [Zurich] and a Saturday afternoon on the Parisian boulevards').[330] How the trip went is not recorded, but it led to no obvious immediate initiative, and the League remained dormant.

The next attempt seems to have been at the first International Congress of Neurology in 1931 in Berne, when representatives from six or seven countries were said to have met. Muskens remarked that, 'On that occasion our voice ceased to be a vox clamans in the desert' but having said that there were no further developments until 1935, perhaps due in part to Musken's own lack of political intelligence.[331]

At the Berne congress, epilepsy does not seem to have featured much on the congress programme. But this was certainly not the case at the 2nd International Congress of Neurology, held from 29 July to 2 August 1935 at University College London. The officers of the congress were Gordon Holmes (president), S. A. Kinnier Wilson (secretary general), and Macdonald Critchley[332] and E. A. Carmichael (assistant secretaries). All were physicians

[329] The association's letterhead carries the wording 'associated with l'Ligue [sic] Internationale Contre l'Epilepsie: object – to promote the scientific, therapeutic, pathologic, medico-legal and sociologic study of the epilepsies' (Arthur L. Shaw to Adolf Meyer, 3 January 1928, Adolf Meyer Collection).

[330] Shaw to Meyer, 3 January 1928. Adolf Meyer trained in medicine in Zurich, studied with Hughlings Jackson at the National Hospital in London and Charcot in Paris, and emigrated to the United States in 1892. He was appointed Professor of Psychiatry at Johns Hopkins in 1910 and introduced Kraepelin's classification systems and Freud's psychoanalytical ideas into American psychiatric practice. He developed 'Meyerian psychobiology'. He served on the advisory council of the American Eugenics Society between 1923–35.

[331] See Muskens, 'War and post-war time', and correspondence from Meyer to Collier which describes Muskens as badgering Ulrich 'to arrange an international meeting of those interested in epilepsy together with the 1931 Neurological Congress in Berne. Ulrich has not any great confidence in this scheme and would not like to work with Muskens.' But undated notes among Meyer's papers assert that 'the prime mover in the reorganisation is Dr Muskens. Unfortunately, he was showing the effects of cerebral arteriosclerosis and his thoughts were not always consecutive' (Adolf Meyer to Kirby Collier, 1 July 1929, Adolf Meyer Collection). In total, 890 people from 40 countries attended the congress in Berne, with Bernard Sachs as president. There was much discussion of the role of neurology, which was struggling to assert itself, in contrast to neurosurgery which was very much in the ascendency (see Kesselring, 'Early global-ization of neurology').

[332] Macdonald Critchley was a neurologist at the National Hospital, Queen Square, a debonair person, a brilliant raconteur and a master of written English. He published nineteen books, including a biography of Hughlings Jackson, written jointly with his wife, published posthumously in 1998. He was, at various times, president of numerous

at the National Hospital for the Paralysed and Epileptic, and all had a track record of publication in epilepsy, even if it was not their primary field of research. In fact, the congress turned into a showpiece for epilepsy, and the whole of the first day was devoted to the aetiology, pathogenesis, physico-chemical factors and treatment of the disorder. Epilepsy was also the commonest condition featured in the 'short talks' (40 out of 250 talks) presented in the afternoons.[333] Then, as noted in the *British Medical Journal*: '[t]hose interested in the social and institutional aspects of epilepsy spent a day at Lingfield Epileptic Colony, where 250 children and 200 adults were resident, and there an informal discussion took place on the types of institutional treatment in various countries'.[334]

The Lingfield Colony was located south of London in a rural setting, but the visit, held on 31 July 1935, had much greater significance than a simple day out in the country. As it transpired, it was during this visit that thirty-two doctors from fourteen countries unanimously decided that the International League Against Epilepsy should be reinstituted. The adjourned meeting then continued on 2 August, electing William Lennox as the new president, Hans Jacob Schou from Denmark as secretary and Joseph Tylor Fox from Lingfield as treasurer.[335] Lennox claimed later to have been attending the meeting as an 'innocent bystander' in place of Stanley Cobb, who had had to cancel his trip to London at the last minute. Muskens urged 'that the presidency of the newly formed ILAE should be an American uninvolved with the politics of Europe, which had proved so disastrous,' and the captaincy of the new ship was passed to Lennox.[336] Membership was set at 5 shillings a year or 15 shillings for the four-year period.[337]

organisations, including the World Federation of Neurology and the ILAE. He was the antithesis of a subspecialist, and was interested in epilepsy only in the context of general neurology. His main specific contributions to epilepsy were his papers on musicogenic epilepsy.

[333] Summaries of the epilepsy proceedings were reported in the *British Medical Journal*, 3 August (1935), pp. 223–6 and 10 August (1935), pp. 269–72; *The Lancet*, 3 August (1935), pp. 268–9 and 10 August (1935), pp. 332–6. In its report of 10 August, the *British Medical Journal* noted that the congress was distinctive for being 'predominantly German-speaking, but except in the business sessions there was no demand for interpretation, and apparently everybody understood everybody else. Even humour … managed to "get across"' (p. 269). There was an extraordinary international cast of speakers, many involved in epilepsy, including Otto Marburg, Ottorino Rossi, Joseph Abadie, Vito Buscaino, William Lennox, Ernest Spiegel, Felix Frisch, Mieczyslaw Minkowski, Miguel Prados y Such, Sixto Obrador, Philippe Pagniez, Alfred Ulrich, Max Sgalitzer, Louis Muskens, Wilder Penfield, Otfrid Foerster, H. Urban, Arthur Schüller, Hugh Cairns, Lewis Weed, Charles Sherrington and Ivan Pavlov.

[334] 'International Neurological Congress in London'.

[335] Schou was medical director of the Filadelfia colony in Dianalund; Fox was superintendent of the Lingfield colony.

[336] Shorvon, 'First 100 years'.

[337] The details were recorded in the first edition of the newly formed *Epilepsia* in February 1937.

It was also decided to revive publication of *Epilepsia*. The first issue of this 'second series' was produced in February 1937, with Schou as editor, 'in collaboration with Tylor Fox, Lennox and Muskens'. On the first page of the newly formed *Epilepsia*, Lennox provided the following raison d'être for the new ILAE, which should 'forward the fight against epilepsy' in the following ways:

1. By collecting and presenting detailed information concerning the extent of epilepsy and the institutional care available for epileptics in the various countries of the world.
2. By encouraging investigation and by facilitating the spread of new knowledge gained among both physicians and the public.
3. By personal acquaintance of those most interested in the problem through visitation and through attendance at the International gathering every four years.[338]

This vision was very similar to that of the ILAE founders in 1909, and like the then chair, Auguste Marie, Lennox presented his own version of a work plan for the League. The emphasis, though, was not on asylums (colonies) as before, but on research, publishing literature reviews and disseminating clinical information.

It is interesting to note that Schou had different ideas for *Epilepsia*, writing in his first editorial:

> In the course of the past 20 years (1915–1935) neurological and psychiatric periodicals have appeared in so great a number that all scientific works on epilepsy and its treatment can be published there. The first aim of the reorganised League must be the social care of epileptics and not so much scientific research into epilepsy. The new edition of *Epilepsia* must follow these lines. It must be the organ for our League.[339]

Tension between the societal and scientific strands, a recurring issue throughout the ILAE's history, seems to have been present from the beginning.

The League in its newly revived form consisted only of the American, British and Scandinavian chapters. The new journal, published once a year, largely contained reports from the three chapters, their membership lists and the programmes of their meetings. By the end of 1936 there were 248 members (195 of whom were anglophone, showing how different the new League was from its predecessor, the centre of gravity of which had been firmly in central Europe): 86 members in America; 102 in Britain; 31 from Scandinavia (Sweden, 11; Norway, 5; Denmark, 14; Finland, 1); and 29 members from countries without chapters. Some of the members were active eugenicists, others directors of colonies, and some both.

---

[338] Lennox, 'Message from the president'.   [339] Schou, 'Reorganisation'.

In the April 1939 issue of *Epilepsia*, Lennox published a paper titled 'The future of the International League Against Epilepsy', setting out his message.[340] He urged that branches be set up in as many countries as possible, for 'the ability of an organism to reach its destination depends on its legs and on its powers of coordination. In our organization the branches in various countries are the limbs, and the officers and "Epilepsia" provide for coordination' (p. 174). Size was no bar, and he cited the example of Czechoslovakia. He lamented the lack of interest in France, Germany and Italy. He ended his paper with a message typical of Lennox's style:

> The International League Against Epilepsy is an unselfish effort to assist an unfortunate group of the population … The officers of the League are determined to do their part in keeping the organization alive and growing no matter what may come. The world is desperately in need of people who will work together for the good of mankind. Therefore, in addition to scientific and humanitarian aspects our League plays a part in maintaining the stability of civilization. (p. 176)

Brave words, but events were to prove otherwise. The 1939 meeting of the ILAE took place in August in Copenhagen, at which time the League had nearly 300 members in 5 countries. At the congress, Karl-Heinz Stauder was appointed vice president of the new ILAE, which was a remarkable choice as Germany had no chapter and war was imminent.[341] As Lennox later wrote: 'In the midst of this Congress the German forces began their blitzkrieg. The banquet was a tragic affair. There were brave speeches for freedom but silence on the part of German colleagues. Delegates who were neighbours of Germany began leaving for whatever fate might meet them.'[342]

THE SECOND WORLD WAR AND EPILEPSY

As Europe descended into war, international activity ceased again, and the ILAE no longer met nor even communicated. The position of *Epilepsia* became precarious as Schou, based in Denmark, found it impossible to continue editing the journal. This task fell to Lennox in Boston, who almost single-handedly kept the journal going and became de facto editor (although Schou continued to be listed as editor on the title page until 1947). The American branch did meet, and had this not been the case, the League would certainly have been wound up (as Lennox put it, 'the American branch keeps

---

[340] Lennox, 'International League Against Epilepsy'.
[341] Karl-Heinz Stauder was the son of the physician Alfons Stauder. The younger Stauder was an opponent of Nazism and refused to join the party, thereby losing his prestigious position in the Munich clinic where he worked and his scientific career. He then gave up his epilepsy research and wrote novels and travel books under the pseudonym Thomas Regau.
[342] Lennox, *Epilepsy and Related Disorders*, vol. 2, p. 1034.

the flame burning').[343] Lennox wrote most of the copy in *Epilepsia*, including annual reports of the activities of the chapter, a few papers concerned with US epilepsy practice and an annual review of the published epilepsy literature (taken from the newly formed *Cumulative Index Medicus*). He later remembered 1939 to have been a 'good year' – on the face of it a seemingly strange sentiment, but it reflected the introduction of phenytoin and the growth of EEG. One topic strikingly absent from the pages of *Epilepsia* in these years was the eugenical killing of those with epilepsy by the Nazi government. This should have been of great concern, yet there was no mention of this, let alone protest, in the journal. The fact that the ILAE failed to speak out for its patients is a shameful subject still in need of full documentation.

Post-traumatic epilepsy returned to become the main focus of epilepsy research, as it had been in the Great War. A good summary of the issues concerning the rehabilitation of head-injured soldiers was provided in the book by Kurt Goldstein, Clinical Professor of Neurology at Tufts Medical School, who showed just how far psychometric testing and psychological therapy had advanced.[344] His book also reflected how psychoanalytical thought had permeated neurology – for instance, viewing the loss of consciousness in a seizure as a psychological mechanism for evading 'catastrophic situations, and the threat of catastrophe' (p. 73). Regarding the position of those with post-traumatic epilepsy in American employment practice, Goldstein wrote:

> The possibility of an epileptic fit is, of course, especially serious. Although epileptics sometimes do astonishingly good work even in big factories, the chance of an attack during working hours is a constant danger to other workers and to machines as well as to the patient himself. Thus it is understandable why employment bureaus are reluctant to take on men subject to such attacks. The question of insurance and compensation creates further complications. Only under special conditions are epileptics occupied in industry, even though they are good workers. (p. 210)

Goldstein considered that 50% of patients with penetrating wounds should be considered 'potential epileptics', that early and late seizures should be distinguished and that the results of both medical and surgical treatment were not very satisfactory.

In November 1945, a post-traumatic epilepsy centre for the US Army was set up at Cushing General Hospital in Framingham, Massachusetts, to establish

---

[343] Lennox, 'Epilepsy in 1939'.

[344] Goldstein, 'Aftereffects of Brain injuries in war'. In the First World War, Goldstein directed the Institut zur Erforschung der Folgeerscheinungen von Hirnverletzungen in Frankfurt, from where many of his ideas and procedures were formed; as he put it in the preface of his book, the Second World War allowed him to test 'their validity'.

best practice.[345] The next year, the clinical course and outcomes were described in 246 military patients with penetrating head wounds.[346] This paper is probably the earliest comprehensive modern account of post-traumatic epilepsy, showing what medical and surgical treatments were available. Epilepsy was thought to occur in the more severe injuries and in cases complicated by sepsis, and depended on the location of the injury (the parietal region being the most frequent site of injury causing seizures). The idea that heredity predisposed to post-traumatic epilepsy was roundly rejected. Focal features in seizures occurred in 76% of cases and were the only form of seizure in 13%. Although EEG had entered routine practice by then, it was found to be totally unhelpful in predicting which person with a severe head injury would develop epilepsy. As the first-line therapy in late epilepsy, large doses of phenytoin and phenobarbitone were used, and surgery was considered only when they were ineffective. Surgical principles were laid down which hardly differ from today's surgery, with the newly developed practice of corticography used to define the epileptogenic focus, scars and foreign bodies removed, debridement carefully performed, the dura closed and the bone flap replaced. Surgery was undertaken only after six months had elapsed after any wound infection, was avoided in those with extensive neurological or any mental disturbance, and was performed under sulphadiazine and penicillin cover. Where possible, surgery was also carried out under local anaesthetic so as not to affect the corticography. In a paper by A. Earl Walker and his colleagues, the approach pioneered by Penfield and Foerster was extended with detailed electrocorticographic studies in thirty-nine patients with post-traumatic epilepsy, using cortical stimulation demonstrating areas of hyperexcitability, in whom seizures were found to arise in locations adjacent to the scarred area.[347]

In some ways war had been 'good for medicine'. For epilepsy, the experience of the First World War led to improved neurosurgical technique and, by better understanding of neurosis, improved psychiatric practice. There were general improvements in healthcare provision and diet as well. The Second World War led to far better management of post-traumatic epilepsy and, importantly, also showed that central organisation of healthcare could be efficient and effective. The lessons learned led directly to the development of systems of universal care in peacetime, especially in Europe, and this greatly benefitted epilepsy. War also

---

[345] The hospital was established in Framingham in 1944 with 1,800 beds, and named after Harvey Cushing, who had died in 1939 (see Wallace, *Pushing for Cushing*).

[346] Quadfasel and Walker, 'Problems of posttraumatic epilepsy'. This is an interesting and important paper. A. Earl Walker was Chief of Neurology at Cushing General Hospital, where he developed an interest in epilepsy. In 1947 he was appointed Professor of Neurological Surgery at Johns Hopkins, and there made numerous contributions to the topic of epilepsy surgery. He was one of the leading epileptologists in America and served as ILAE president between 1953 and 1961.

[347] Walker, Marshall and Beresford, 'Electrocorticographic characteristics'.

promoted science and pharmaceuticals and, by accelerating the development of penicillin, changed for the better whole areas of medical practice. It also provided the stimulus for the rapid professionalisation and specialisation of neurology and neurosurgery, and the development of neurosurgical units.

On the other hand, there was an almost complete cessation of academic work on epilepsy in Europe, and it was war which moved the centre of gravity of epilepsy research to the United States, where advances in EEG, metabolic investigation and medicinal therapy were made despite rather than because of the conflict raging in the rest of the world. As Joanna Bourke pointed out, war also changed the relationship between doctor and patient. The primary focus of medicine in war shifted from the best interests of the patient to subservience to the goals of the military and to the return of men to the battlefield. The practices and rituals of medicine were altered by military structures, and medicine developed a punitive, coercing aspect – not only in epilepsy (and 'hystero-epilepsy') but also, for instance, in the treatment of venereal disease and malingering. As a result, doctors in the military were often resented by common soldiers.[348]

Zachary Cope,[349] the editor of two volumes of the official British medical history of World War Two, drew up a balance sheet and found that, overall, war was indeed a positive influence on medicine. The many bodies left in the Somme or in Hiroshima might have seen it differently, but it is true that, for epilepsy, benefits did ensue.

---

[348] The RAMC was said to be known in the ranks as standing for 'Rob All My Comrades' (Bourke, 'Wartime', p. 593).

[349] V. Z. Cope, 'The Medical Balance-sheet of War'.

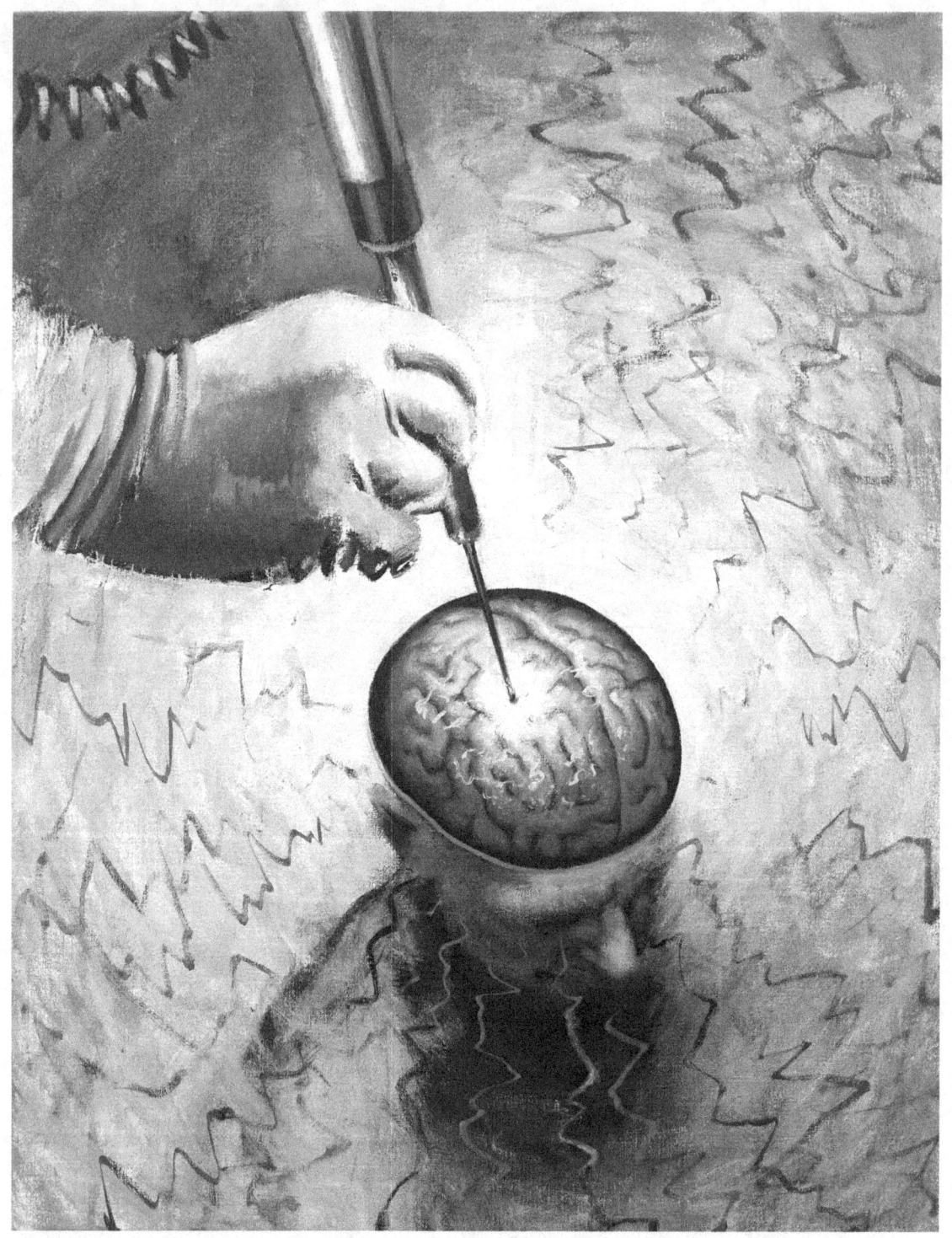

22. **'What can it be like to have electrical brain stimulation?'** (A painting by David Cobley, 2021)

THREE

1945–1970: EPILEPSY AND THE NEW WORLD ORDER

T HE WORLD WAS A DIFFERENT PLACE WHEN PEACE DESCENDED OVER the battlefields of the Second World War. Much of Europe was devastated, its empires evaporating and its Eastern territories were falling into Soviet control. As imperialism faded, the developing world, released from colonisation, was beginning its independent course. The hopes of Western democracy were led by America and it was America that set the pace. Vying with the Soviet Union for supremacy, America and its Western allies, and their world system based on globalised capitalism, eventually triumphed. The period also marked a process of rapid change in Western culture and society – 'the greatest and most dramatic, rapid and universal social transformation in human history' according to Hobsbawm.[1] Therein was a momentous opportunity for those with epilepsy. Hobsbawn considered the death of the peasantry to be the most far-reaching social change, but for those with epilepsy it was the impact of social democratic philosophies, the growth of capitalism and the rise of science which had the greater impact.

The rise of liberal democracy in Western cultures was in part a reaction against the horrors of the Nazi regime, which were fully exposed in the post-war period. International bodies were formed and, in December 1948, the Universal Declaration of Human Rights was proclaimed, which reset social

---

[1] Hobsbawm, *The Age of Extremes*, p. 288. His words were referring to the years 1945–90.

norms.[2] These ideals led to a slow transformation of societal attitudes towards disadvantage, illness and disability, allowing, for the first time, the voice of people with epilepsy to be given a sympathetic hearing. This was a process facilitated by the growth and establishment of lay organisations and aided by legislation. As rights were asserted and public attitudes changed, the dreaded stigma of epilepsy lessened. In the new liberal democracies, access to healthcare became possible for more persons with epilepsy than ever before, and new facilities were provided. Matching these societal changes was activity of unparalleled intensity in the medicine and science of epilepsy. Stimulated by new public and political support, research received an enormous boost by the award of lavish public funds. These fuelled its engines of growth. There were many developments – 'advances' is too strong a word, implying as it does inevitable progress or benefit, for although generally positive, some were regressive and detrimental. There was nevertheless an air of optimism as the medical problems of epilepsy seemed now potentially tractable. Basic neurophysiology and neurochemistry made enormous progress, and although not focused much on epilepsy, the discoveries of this period laid the foundations for much future basic epilepsy research. Much of the funding boost was predicated on the realisation that financing healthcare brought economic benefits on many fronts. Furthermore, the munificence was not without self-interest as markets and industry benefitted with more immediacy than did the sufferer. It was in America that most funds became available, and it was to America that most of the leadership in epilepsy moved. The establishment of an epilepsy section in National Institutes of Health (NIH) was an important stimulus, as was the rapid growth in power and influence of the pharmaceutical industry. A series of new drug treatments were marketed which banished older remedies to the outermost circles of the epilepsy firmament. The randomised controlled trial (RCT) improved the assessment of drug therapy, as did more stringent regulation. Clinically, the period was marked by the rise of neurology, which displaced psychiatry as the 'epilepsy specialty'. EEG was now seen as the fundamental investigation in clinical epilepsy, and increasingly complex intracranial EEG procedures and technologies were devised. Epilepsy was now conceptualised as an electrographic phenomenon – a cerebral dysrhythmia – and no longer as primarily a mental disorder. The ILAE too established itself as a leading authority on epilepsy, not least by cleverly producing an official classification of epileptic seizures, based largely on clinical and EEG criteria, and, with it, officially sanctioned terminologies. New forms of epilepsy were identified – most importantly, temporal lobe epilepsy – and, in parallel, temporal lobe epilepsy surgery was devised and widely promulgated. More significantly, though, than any medical advance for the person with epilepsy, this period

---

[2] See Greyling, *Towards the Light*.

marked the beginning of a slow climb out of the pit of heredity and mental defect and deficiency and into the brambles of organic disease. A long path lay ahead, but for those with epilepsy, optimism seemed justified.

HEALTHCARE

As Virginia Berridge has noted, all history is political, especially when it comes to health.[3] This assertion was never more evident than in the second half of the twentieth century, and the world of epilepsy was not left untouched. Its fortunes differed greatly depending on geography. As the Soviet Union and its new vassal states in Eastern Europe took up positions behind Churchill's 'iron curtain', the rich thread of scholarship on epilepsy from Russia and Eastern Europe, which had shaped the condition in the previous decades, was almost immediately severed. In the post-war period, almost nothing of note emerged from these countries in terms of epilepsy theory or practice. Similarly, communist theory and the Marxist interpretation of history paid little attention to the handicapped, and none at all to epilepsy. Whilst medical care was taken over by the state, and provided for all in most communist countries, little has been published about the quality of the lives of those afflicted by the condition.

In contrast, in America the course of epilepsy changed dramatically. In many ways, America had had a 'good' war. The country was spared desolation and destruction, and its gross national product increased by more than 60%. Indeed, at the war's end, US factories were responsible for two-thirds of the world's production, including their weapons of destruction. Without the period of austerity experienced in Europe, a new world economic order was created, led by the United States, and in the years between 1951 and 1973 capitalism entered what has been called its Golden Age.[4] Prosperity increased dramatically for the middle classes and there was no appetite for state intervention in healthcare, not least because the idea of 'socialised medicine' (or, indeed, anything with a whiff of communism) had become an anathema to American society. Indeed, only in 1965 was any health insurance provided at all, as part of Lyndon Johnson's Great Society project, in the form of Medicare to people over 60 and Medicaid for the poorest. But for the rest, there was no state support. As the centre of gravity of epilepsy research and development had moved to the United States, and in an entirely market-driven environment, both the pharmaceutical industry and the basic sciences of epilepsy flourished as never before. Both were to shape the course of epilepsy for much of this period.

The situation in Western Europe was rather different. The war had devastated much of the continent: thirty-six million Europeans had lost their lives in

---

[3] Berridge, *Health and Society*.   [4] For discussion, see Skidelsky, *Keynes*.

the conflagration, and millions more due to famine and disease in its aftermath.[5] The war's end initially brought in its wake extreme austerity, as rebuilding the shattered continent was the priority, but within a decade sustained economic growth began to take root (in fact, not only in the West but also in the Eastern bloc). It was on the crest of this economic upsurge, in 1957, that Harold MacMillan proclaimed to the British people that they had 'never had it so good'.[6] With regard to healthcare, the experience of war had also fundamentally changed the priorities of the citizens of Western Europe. In marked contrast to the situation after the Great War, there was no desire to return to the pre-war social order. The ruling class, in whose name the populations had sacrificed much, gave considerable ground, and the curtain was raised on a new era of social reform. European governments, some more than others, adopted the concept of the welfare state: 'a vast conglomerate of nationwide, compulsory and collective arrangements to remedy and control the external effects of adversity and deficiency', and between 1945 and 1964 this greatly extended governmental responsibility for healthcare. [7] In Britain, for example, in 1948 the government took control of the whole creaking and hitherto fragmented healthcare system by creating the National Health Service (NHS), funded entirely and centrally from taxation. It was the most wide-ranging scheme of its time. The voluntary hospitals (including the National Hospital, Queen Square) were taken into the state system, and all hospital doctors and other staff became salaried by the state. In the majority of countries (possibly all), doctors' organisations were opposed to 'state socialism' in healthcare. They resisted government efforts to centralise insurance on the basis that this restricted choice, endangered clinical freedoms, damaged income and might transform an elite medical professional into a lowly civil servant. Despite the opposition of the medical profession, the NHS was vastly popular amongst the general public. Even the grandees of the ruling class, such as Winston Churchill, were strong supporters.[8] Crucially, for the first time, access to

[5] The situation in Europe is well described in Judt, *Postwar*. Amongst the statistics quoted are: the destruction of 1,700 towns and 70,000 villages in the Soviet Union, with 25 million persons made homeless; 20 million made homeless in Germany; the death of 1 in 5 amongst the Polish pre-war population, 1 in 8 in Yugoslavia and 1 in 11 in Russia. Everywhere, millions of children were orphaned, and rationing and food shortages caused starvation and sickness (in England rationing continued up to July 1954).

[6] A speech at a political rally in Bedford on 20 July 1957. Economically speaking, he was right, and the same applied to all countries in Western Europe and North America.

[7] De Swaan, *In Care of the State*, p. 218. The view that there was a political or societal consensus in favour of establishing welfare and healthcare has recently been challenged (see Berridge, *Health and Society*). What is not in doubt, however, is that attitudes towards, and the landscape of, healthcare changed completely after the war.

[8] In a speech to the Royal College of Physicians on 2 March 1944, Churchill announced: 'The discoveries of healing science must be the inheritance of all. That is clear. Disease must be attacked, whether it occurs in the poorest or the richest man or woman . . . Our policy is to create a national health service in order to ensure that everybody in the country, irrespective

adequate treatment was a *right* not a *privilege*. A social contract was in effect formed between the government and the governed, promising healthcare 'free for all'[9] and available to all. Other European countries developed different systems with similar aims, but in all these systems the person with epilepsy was placed on an equal footing with all others for the first time in history. This was profoundly liberating. The person with epilepsy could now throw off the cloak of heredity and degeneration and have a place in the waiting-room queue like anyone else. This was a step change, occurring at a time when new options for medical and surgical treatment were being introduced, and it is difficult to overstate the ontological importance of this development. In practice, much prejudice remained; but establishing such a right for those with epilepsy constituted a fundamental change.

Other countries took different paths. In China, where healthcare had been developing along Western lines prior to the war, the Communist Party take-over in 1949 had profound effects. To compensate for the very small numbers of trained doctors, emphasis was placed on local 'barefoot doctor' schemes, on blending traditional Chinese medicine with Western allopathic medicine, and on a system of regional hospitals and clinics based on the Soviet model. How epilepsy fared is not recorded. Asia, and particularly Japan, copied the American model. Australasia and Canada followed Britain's state welfare model. But much of the Third World[10] remained mired in poverty at a time when population growth was explosive, and there healthcare remained the privilege of the few.

The cost of healthcare rose in all Western bloc countries, and faster than general inflation. The proportion of care that was publicly funded varied to different degrees in different countries and at different times (Table 3.1). but in this 'Golden Age of Welfare' between 1945 and 1975, there was an inexorable expansion of all governmental healthcare provision. By the mid-1970s, 4.9% of GDP was being spent on healthcare in the OEDC (Organisation for Economic Co-operation and Development) group of industrialised countries – a level of spending perceived increasingly to be a noose around the necks of government. As it turned out, the amount was only a fraction of what it would be in subsequent decades.

of means, age, sex, or occupation, shall have equal opportunities to benefit from the best and most up-to-date medical and allied services available. The plan that we have put forward is a very large-scale plan, and in ordinary times of peace would rivet and dominate the attention of the whole country; but even during this war it deserves the close study and thought of all who can spare themselves from other duties for that purpose' (Hodgson and Shorvon, *Physicians and War*, p. 91). For a detailed discussion of the attitude of doctors, see Webster, *Welfare State*.

9 'State take over doctors'. 10 A term coined in this cold-war period

TABLE 3.1 *Medical expenditure per capita (in US dollars) in four countries, and the percentage of this which was funded publicly (in brackets)*

	1890	1910	1930	1950	1970
USA	$8.4 (0.9%)	$14.3 (6%)	$25.2 (9%)	$43.3 (18%)	$119.4 (31%)
France	$5.6 (7.1%)	$4.4 (17%)	$3.6 (36%)	$14.4 (54%)	$51.9 (64%)
Great Britain	$8.3 (6.0%)	$8.4 (11%)	$9.6 (16%)	$28.2 (82%)	$56.8 (86%)
Sweden	$1.5 (21%)	$3.9 (25%)	$7.6 (29%)	$17.4 (52%)	$69.7 (57%)

NB: Dollar expressed in purchasing power parity
(From Webster, 'Medicine and the welfare state 1930–1970', p. 127)

SCIENCE AND MEDICINE

A central theme, enormous and overwhelming as the century progressed, was the impact of science on society and on its citizens. Scientific discovery not only influenced the course of events directly but also changed the way society and its citizens perceived the world. Scientific progress was seemingly inexorable and mesmeric. The interaction was not all one-way, for the path science took was itself heavily dictated by social, political and economic thinking and practice.

Medicine had had a good war. The discovery of penicillin (and other early antibiotics) had contributed greatly to both national survival and morale. Governments were impressed, and over the next twenty years it suddenly seemed possible that whole disease areas might be conquered, such as infections by antibiotics, inflammation by corticosteroids, and psychiatric diseases by psychoactive drugs and physical treatments. Epilepsy was imbued with similar optimistic tropes, and from its becalmed state during the early interwar period, clinical and scientific work blossomed as never before, especially on the east coast of the United States. These successes led to the further medicalisation of society, a phenomenon born of the interwar years and one which was to become one of the great social recensions of the time. The doctor's reputation rose, the number of doctors and health professionals rapidly increased, new medical facilities were built, and medicine pervaded popular culture. New research and care structures arose, and the world of medicine massively enlarged. In 1999, James Le Fanu[11] has listed what he calls '12 definitive moments' in post-1940 medicine, of which nine are clustered in that first remarkable quarter-century: 1941, penicillin; 1949, cortisone; 1950, streptomycin; 1950, smoking and Bradford Hill;[12] 1952, chlorpromazine and the revolution in psychiatry; 1952, the Copenhagen polio epidemic and the birth

---

[11] Le Fanu, *Modern Medicine*.

[12] The inclusion in this list of James Bradford Hill was for his work, with Richard Doll, demonstrating the connection between cigarette smoking and lung cancer. From the point of view of epilepsy, however, Bradford Hill's critical importance was his development of the

of intensive care; 1953, open-heart surgery; 1961, hip replacement; 1963, kidney transplant; and 1964, stroke prevention. Le Fanu did not include the discovery of the genetic code and structure of deoxyribonucleic acid (DNA), the divination of chemical transmission, the introduction of electroencephalography (EEG), the evolution of the operating microscope or the clutch of new antiepileptic drugs, all of which were to have a positive and pervading impact on epilepsy. Others might have chosen a different set of developments; there were a lot to choose from.

No one could doubt that a scientific revolution was underway, and it attracted public debate. C. P. Snow delivered his celebrated Rede Lecture in 1959, claiming that advancing science had resulted in a culture quite distinct from that of traditional intellectuals and that the 'two cultures' failed to understand the other: 'The great edifice of modern physics goes up, and the majority of the cleverest people in the western world have about as much insight into it as their Neolithic ancestors would have had.'[13] Snow can be fairly criticised for vagueness, but he had addressed an issue which still resonates today. The ascent of science was to dictate much of *Epilepsy's* direction of travel in the second half of the century, not least because of the claim that science differed from other forms of intellectual activity by virtue of the rational nature of the scientific method. This idea though was an illusion debunked by the many who realised that whilst it was true that science had an inner logic which did distinguish it from other activities, actual scientific behaviour is far more intuitive and random.[14] The methodology, the choice of topic, the facilities available, the personalities of scientists and co-workers, and the environment and system within which science was conducted all depend on political and social influences. This was particularly the case in medicine and in the field of epilepsy, where personality and politics played a major role.[15]

Snow's contemporary, Michael Polanyi, had another important message: that science depends on the liberty of the individual to pursue truth as an end in itself, that knowledge arises from personal judgement and that scientific discovery is a function of the scientist's personal choices. These points were taken

randomised controlled clinical trial and the 'Bradford Hill' criteria for determining a causal association.

[13] Snow's Rede Lecture of 1959 was published in Snow, *Two Cultures*, pp. 15–16. The lecture caused ferocious arguments, not least after the celebrated broadsides of F. R. Leavis: 'The intellectual nullity is what constitutes any difficulty there may be in dealing with Snow's panoptic pseudo-cogencies, his parade of a thesis: a mind to be argued with – that is not there' (cited in Otolano, *Two Cultures Controversy*, p. 3).

[14] Polanyi, *Science, Faith and Society*.

[15] It has also been said, with some justification, that most arguments and contention in academic epilepsy circles are due to personality clashes and professional jealousies (as the saying goes: 'Do not turn your back on a medical academic').

to heart in the post-war years in the United States, where funding was surprisingly free of conditions and remarkably productive. But balance was needed. The free market approach has been considered to have most benefitted a 'microcausal' approach to disease – attributing epilepsy, for instance, to brain abnormalities or genetics – as opposed to a 'macrocausal' approach, which paid more attention to the social and economic factors.[16] Such niceties notwithstanding, in this post-war period the march of science was dramatic and would become more so. Medicine had turned a corner, and scientific medicine in epilepsy was not going to retreat.

The Rise of Basic Research and the Funding of Science

Prior to 1920, most medical research was financed privately by individual doctors, universities or philanthropy. Research in fields such as epilepsy was a relatively amateur affair, conducted by clinicians, and was characterised by a general focus on clinical description augmented by physiology. As noted, almost no laboratory science was directed at epilepsy in the first decades of the century, and only in the 1930s did the idea arise that basic science might turn its attention, in any specific manner, to epilepsy. For the first time, pure scientists began routinely to collaborate with clinicians, a trend in epilepsy especially in America. As basic and laboratory research became more complex, previous funding models became increasingly unsustainable. Following the Wall Street Crash of 1929, President Herbert Hoover appointed a national committee to study 'recent social trends'.[17] The committee's report painted a sorry picture of confused and ineffective financing and urged more involvement of central government – a message heeded as thereafter allocation of funds became centralised under the top-down control of the Committee on Medical Research, part of the National Defense Research Committee. Grants were awarded for post-traumatic epilepsy and surgery, and never before had so much centralised research money been made available.[18]

---

[16] Hollingsworth, *Political Economy of Medicine*, pp. 95, 31.

[17] Mitchell, *President's Research Committee*, p. xi. In some ways the conclusions were a parallel of those of the Flexner Committee in relation to medical education.

[18] Shryock, *American Medical Research*, p. 289. This book is a detailed study of research funding to 1946, and much of the detail in this chapter is taken from it. The belief in pouring money into research funding was a legacy of Roosevelt's New Deal policies. It marked an enormous shift from the 1920s view that government should be as small as possible. In these expansionist years, the high levels of funding signalled the new confidence in the power of science and the promise of new drugs.

TABLE 3.2 *Rise in expenditure on medical research in the USA between 1947 and 1966, and the proportion of which was federal and NIH expenditure*

	1947	1966
National expenditure on medical research	$87 million	$2.05 billion
Federal expenditure (and percentage of total national expenditure)	$27 million (31%)	$1.4 billion (68%)
NIH expenditure (and percentage of total national expenditure)	$8.3 million (10%)	$800 million (40%)

(From Shannon, 'The Advancement of medical research', p. 97).

In 1946, President Franklin D. Roosevelt asked Vannevar Bush (later president of the Massachusetts Institute of Technology) how to proceed in the 'war of science against disease'.[19] Bush responded with a report titled *Science: The Endless Frontier* (1945). A powerful expression of the mood of the time, the report expressed the belief that basic science was an 'essential key' to security, to better health, to employment and a higher standard of living, and to cultural progress (p. vi). Bush's wartime experiences had shown him how scientific innovation had contributed to America's world hegemony, and he urged his government to extend financial support to basic medical research partly as a way of cementing its economic benefits. Bush's recommendation was timely, as science was increasingly expensive, and endowment income and private donations – the traditional sources of funds – were proving insufficient. Science, he maintained, was 'a proper concern of Government' (p. 11).

A key step in the rising profile of medical research in epilepsy was the founding in 1950 of the National Institutes of Health (NIH), which provided a mechanism for channelling central funding via its intramural and extramural programmes. Between 1947 and 1966, even after applying the gross national product deflation factor, there was a fifteen-fold rise in expenditure on medical research. James Shannon (NIH Director from 1955–1968) noted that by 1966, federal monies accounted for the majority of funds provided for science, much of which was channeled through the NIH.[20] (Table 3.2) Between 1945 and 1975, 41 American scientists who had received substantial NIH grants were awarded Nobel Prizes. By 1970 the NIH was supporting more than 67,000 senior research investigators and was providing more than 35,000 individuals with funding for training in the basic and clinical sciences. Stimulated by these funding mechanisms, basic science became embedded in American medical schools, as much as in other parts of the universities, and the medical schools greatly expanded their research activities. Prior to the war, research in universities

[19] Bush, *Endless Frontier*, p. 3.   [20] Shannon, 'Advancement of medical research'.

was a 'relatively minor adjunct of the higher educational process'.[21] Twenty years later it had become the dominant feature of the major institutions. In the United States, the abundance of grants resulted in a threefold growth of the faculties of medical school between 1962 and 1976; and by 1970 more than half of the faculty were salaried through grant funding. One-third of US PhDs in the biological sciences were awarded to physicians and scientists in medical school graduate programmes. This reliance on research funding resulted in another development, the rapid expansion of specialisation and subspecialisation, a trend led by the emergence of epileptology, but one which some thought had a detrimental effect both on patient care and on training.[22] Nevertheless, it seemed that Flexner's earlier proposals were at last being fully implemented, large scientific teams were formed, and research was no longer the lonely self-taught existence it had previously often been.[23] 'For the first time in its history', Shannon wrote,

> the government reached out directly in a time of peace to affect the social and economic security of the people of the nation in a massive way ... Building upon a foundation of European basic effort, American biomedical scientists made key contributions to microbiology, biochemistry, and physiology ... The impetus of war-related problems brought this [research] capability to impressive potential. As a consequence, the end of World War II found American bioscience ripe for major expansion. (pp. 98–9)

This transformation was due to the 'promise of science':

> The awesome detonation over Hiroshima imbued us all with a sense of what technology, built upon the results of basic science, could accomplish through massive effort. In like manner the nation was impressed with the emergence of penicillin and other war-accelerated 'wonder drugs'. These generated high expectations of science as a major instrument for the solution of national problems. Thus, the nation emerged from the war disposed toward generous support of science and its institutions. (p. 99)

Although government funding began to dominate the research arena, private philanthropy did continue to play an important role. Of all the non-governmental organisations which had an impact on epilepsy in this period, none was more directly beneficial to epilepsy than the Rockefeller Foundation. The funds

---

[21] Shannon, 'Advancement of medical research'.

[22] Hollingsworth, in *Political Economy of Medicine*, quotes R. H. Ebert, professor of medicine at Harvard, as saying that 'bootlegging the support of education from research dollars has been one of the most destructive by-products of NIH policy' (p. 228), and also Paul Beeson, a leading American medical academic, who wrote in 1975: '[T]he rapid progress made in the last 30 years has brought its own kind of medical pollution' (p. 231). According to Beeson, medical training in 1970 was inferior to that twenty-five years earlier in America, and to that in Britain.

[23] One interesting sign of this was the appearance of multiple authorship on medical papers, previously rather uncommon but by 1960 increasingly the norm.

dispensed by the Foundation[24] for medical research were about $3 million in 1913, $182 million in 1927 and $323 million in 1940. By 1938, more than 3,000 fellows from other countries had been brought to the United States for training and research, and 1,383 Americans had been sent abroad. Epilepsy profited immensely from these programmes; and indeed, it is remarkable how many of the major epilepsy figures of the period were beneficiaries of Rockefeller funding at one time or another. A key figure in the promotion of research into epilepsy was Alan Gregg, through his backing of individual scientists and clinicians.[25] Other philanthropists followed suit. By 1974, the total funding for medical research in the United States had reached $4.4 billion, a prodigality which reflected the public's optimistic belief that throwing money at science will inevitably result in cure. The new interest in basic science was also accompanied by an even bigger rise in spending by pharmaceutical companies on their own in-house research. By 1945, US-based pharmaceutical companies were estimated to be expending nearly twice as much on research as all the universities, foundations and research institutes put together.

In Europe the story was rather different. In the early interwar years, Germany had had the largest and best scientific medical research establishment. Medical research had been supported by the university system and research establishments such as the Kaiser Wilhelm Institutes to a greater extent than elsewhere in Europe. This system was ruined in the Nazi era. Many scientists either fled or immigrated, largely to the United States, and political interference, with a focus on racial hygiene and 'folksy' medicine, left German medical science foundering.[26]

Britain had the second largest scientific infrastructure in Europe, and although relatively modest compared to America's, it tended to follow the same general model. Money from the government was channelled through the Medical Research Council (MRC). Founded in 1913 as the Medical Research Committee and initially intended for research on tuberculosis, the group's

---

[24] The well-known story is that John D. Rockefeller was persuaded by his pastor, the Rev. Frederick T. Gates of Montclair, New Jersey, to fund medical research after Gates had read Osler's *Principles and Practice of Medicine*. Gates convinced him that he could have the greatest impact by reforming medical education, sponsoring curative research and eradicating diseases (such as hookworm), which reduced national efficiency.

[25] This is a history not yet fully explored but deserves to be so. Gregg trained in medicine at Harvard, and then worked in the Rockefeller Foundation, where he ultimately assumed the office of vice president. Under his influence, the munificence of the foundation in funding neurology and psychiatry and supporting talented individuals was key to the development of epilepsy from the 1920s onward.

[26] The dire effect of Nazi scientific policy is well described in part five of Watson, *German Genius*. The vital importance of immigration to American and British science is evident from the fact that of the 47 Nobel Prizes for Medicine or Physiology awarded between 1950 and 1970, 70% went to work conducted in America and 33% of the laureates were immigrants; 11% went to work in Britain and 40% of the laureates were immigrants.

remit rapidly broadened to encompass an agenda shaped largely by Cambridge physiologists.[27] The MRC was also concerned that most of the medical schools in Britain considered research to be 'a private hobby',[28] a way of thinking that the MRC was determined to change.[29] In the post-war period, most MRC grants went to basic research and were modelled on US examples.[30] As Robert Platt stated in his 1967 Harveian Lecture, this was a deliberate policy: 'The phenomenal success of modern medical treatment seems to have depended almost wholly on non-clinical, often non-medical scientists, frequently working in, or in close collaboration with, the pharmaceutical industry.'[31] The chief medical officer, George Godber, noted in *The Lancet* in 1964 that '[m]edicine will never again be self-sufficient. It has not only a large group of professions supplementary to medicine but also a great and increasing need for the aid of other scientists from disciplines only occasionally concerned with the care of patients or with health.'[32] The 1950s and 1960s were indeed notable for the growth of non-clinical scientists and fairly quickly, as the NIH and MRC had predicted, the real advances that were to benefit medicine were taking place outside the clinical settings; research in medicine was increasingly to be reliant on discoveries made in other fields. This was especially true of epilepsy medicine which became a largely applied or translational science.

Of the 180 MRC units and groups formed by 1972, only 13 were related to neurology. And, in contrast to the situation in America, no grants explicitly supported clinical studies of epilepsy. This was left to non-governmental agencies. The main source of private funding in Britain was the Wellcome Trust, founded in 1936 with a philanthropic vision similar to that of the Rockefeller Foundation: 'The acceptance of the trust could only be regarded as a public duty – a duty not only to the past, to carry out the wishes of the testator of a philanthropic vision, but also to the future, to the various work with unimagined possibilities which may be started as a result of this inheritance.'[33] Initially slow to grow, the trust's charitable donations reached £1.2 million by 1956, and rapidly increased thereafter. Fast-forwarding to 1986, the foundation's assets amounted to £1 billion, with £26 million spent each year on medical research grants. By 2000 the fund had grown to £15 billion, with £650 million spent annually on medical research by 2007 and epilepsy was well represented.

---

[27] Thomson, *Medical Research*.   [28] *Fourth Annual Report*, 1918.

[29] The exception was the University College Hospital medical school in London, which received considerable sums from the Rockefeller Foundation in order to transform it into a university health centre along the lines of Johns Hopkins Hospital. The National Hospital at Queen Square also benefitted from Rockefeller munificence in the 1930s to develop neurosurgery in the Cushing mode. This was part of the Rockefeller Foundation's interest in supporting Hugh Cairns in Britain, which also resulted in the £2 million grant to the Oxford medical school in 1936 – something the Rockefeller trustees congratulated themselves on (Fisher, 'Rockefeller Foundation').

[30] Timmermann, 'Research in postwar Britain'.   [31] Platt, 'Master or servant?'.

[32] Godber, 'Measurement and mechanisation'.   [33] 'Wellcome Trust' (1937).

Epilepsy and the National Institute of Neurological Diseases and Blindness

As we have seen, it was in 1950 that the NIH established a division for neuroscience: the National Institute of Neurological Diseases and Blindness (NINDB).[34] This was to be of the utmost importance to epilepsy. Indeed, the NINDB completely transformed the research landscape for epilepsy as well as for other neurological conditions. As the renowned American neurologist Robert Daroff put it in 2001: 'The epicentre of neurological research, which in the 1950's was Cambridge, England, has since shifted to Bethesda, Maryland.'[35] It is difficult to overemphasise the impact this had on epilepsy.

The NINDB had its origins in the mid-1940s as pressure began to build in Congress to enhance medical research. Individual philanthropists and citizen groups for various neurological conditions, including epilepsy, began to lobby for the establishment of a government research–funded institute with the help of leading AAN members – especially Merritt, Putnam, Hans Reece and Lennox, who testified on their behalf before Congress. The priority given to research rather than clinical services would not have happened in any previous period, but was justified by the argument that it was through research that clinical services in neurology would improve – and so it turned out. At the same time, a campaign to promote neurology as a specific specialty was prosecuted, with Pearce Bailey[36] and Lennox being particularly persuasive advocates. As a model of what might be achieved, all had in mind the National Cancer Institute, set up in 1937. Although initially the various lay groups desired individual institutes for each of the common neurological diseases, a bill to establish the NINDB covering all of these diseases (the Omnibus Medical Research Act) was proposed in 1949 and signed into law in 1950.

Pearce Bailey was appointed the first director of NINDB. Bailey appointed G. Milton Shy as director of the intramural programme. Shy, in turn, put neurosurgeon Maitland Baldwin in charge of NINDB intramural epilepsy research in 1953 and also brought in Cosimo Ajmone-Marsan to head up the EEG laboratory. All were interested in epilepsy which thereby re-found its place at the high table.[37] By 1956 the intramural budget for clinical epilepsy was $820,000; for extramural grants it was $608,000. By the late 1950s, as funding of neurological

---

[34] The NINDB was subjected to a merry-go-round of name changes: to the National Institute for Neurological Disease and Stroke (NINDS) in 1968, the National Institute of Neurological and Communicative Disorders and Stroke (NINCDS) in 1975 and the National Institute for Neurological Diseases (NINDS) in 1980. The history of the institute is well told in two books, from which much of the detail here is taken: Farreras, Hannaway and Harden, *Mind, Brain, Body*; and Rowland, *NINDS at 50*.

[35] Daroff, 'NINDS at 50'.

[36] Bailey was the first director of the NINDB. He is credited with raising the status of the field of neurology within the United States (see Burkholder, 'Pearce Bailey: The "Fifth Horseman"').

[37] This may partly be because so many of the new faculty had spent time at the Montreal Neurological Institute. Indeed, there were said to be more MNI alumni at NINDB than anywhere outside Montreal, a tribute to Penfield and one which placed epilepsy in the forefront of NINDB research.

disease programmes became a priority, the NIH's budgets continued rapidly to expand, from $81.1 million (including $7.6 million to NINDS) in 1955 to $1,076.4 million (including $128.6 million to NINDS) in 1968. Bailey was succeeded by Richard Masland in 1959, who in 1964, recruited J. Preston Robb to survey epilepsy research facilities in the United States and Canada. The findings were published as a 69-page book,[38] which proved to be a template for further research funding. In 1966, epilepsy research was to enter a transformative stage, with Masland's appointment of J. Kiffin Penry as head of the newly formed Epilepsy Section (later named the Epilepsy Branch).[39]

Penry was born of humble origins in Denton North Carolina in 1929 and qualified in medicine from the Bowman Gray School of Medicine in 1955. His exceptional talents were immediately evident to his teachers. In turn, Penry appreciated their influence, naming his sons after three of them: Martin Netsky, Richard Masland and Derek Denny-Brown. It was from these three, respectively, that he gained an appreciation of high-quality clinical work, administration and experimental neurophysiology. On his recruitment to the Epilepsy Branch at NIH, he began his phenomenally productive thirteen years at NIH. His major work focused on stimulating antiepileptic drug development and treatment and is described later. But there was no area of epilepsy in which he was not involved, and it is no exaggeration to say that he dictated the direction of American and, by extension, world epileptology for the next twenty years. His organisational genius was evident in his success in getting academic centres all over America to form a network of collaborators co-ordinating studies of both new antiepileptic drugs and basic research. He was involved in a number of massive publishing ventures and in 1968 also organised a computer program to provide abstracts specifically on the topic of epilepsy ('*Epilepsy Abstracts*') when the National Library of Medicine,[40] founded in 1836, was incorporated into NIH. His work with ILAE, as its Secretary-general and then President, is described in the next chapter.

[38] Preston, *Epilepsy: A Review*. This publication provided a succinct guide to the then current knowledge of epidemiology, aetiology, classification, diagnosis, pathology, treatment and prognosis (and was excellent value at only 45 cents). James Preston Robb studied medicine at McGill and succeeded Francis McNaughton as Professor of Neurology and Neurologist-in-Chief at the Montreal Neurological Hospital from 1968 to 1976.

[39] In 1965, a Departmental Committee on Epilepsy was established and, after several reorganisations, was restructured as the Epilepsy Advisory Committee, headed by Penry. Three subcommittees were subsequently formed: on epidemiology, basic research and anticonvulsant drug therapy. Each was highly successful.

[40] The National Library of Medicine initiated *Index Medicus*, a massive annual publication which indexed and abstracted all articles published in selected medical journals, including much of the international and non-English language literature. It was a very valuable service. At its start, it weighed in at around 2 kg each year, but at the end of the 1970s, 14 kg. It was computerised in 1964 as *MEDLARS*, then put online in a limited fashion in 1971 as *Medline*, and in 1996 made publicly and freely available via the Internet as *Pubmed*. By 2000 it was adding 400,000 articles each year.

In 1979 Penry left NIH and returned to Bowman Gray. There, he turned his attention to training, creating a series of 'epilepsy mini-fellowships' that consisted of week-long seminars for epilepsy fellows, residents and clinicians. By 1996, 2,200 'mini-fellows' had attended these courses and spread the Penry vision of epilepsy worldwide. Sadly, in his retirement, he became increasingly afflicted by diabetes and diabetic neuropathy, and was also profoundly affected by the tragic death in 1981 of one of his beloved sons.

The Pharmaceutical Industry

Difficult as it might be to believe now, the origins of the pharmaceutical industry were rather modest. Early stirrings were apparent in France in the first part of the nineteenth century, where methods to extract the active ingredients of plants (botanicals) were developed in local family businesses. By 1850 most of the active botanicals used in medicine had been largely identified and isolated. For epilepsy these included valerian and belladonna, amongst numerous other herbals and chemicals of more doubtful efficacy. Subsequently, especially in Germany, companies involved in dyestuffs and chemicals began to take an interest in drugs, which proved a rich vein to mine. Synthetic dyes, alkaloids and coal-tar products were found to have biological activity. A key step in the development of the industry was the discovery of the benzene ring by German chemist Friedrich August Kekulé in 1865. Drugs from botanicals or chemicals were initially sold wholesale to local pharmacies and dispensaries, and, in turn, pharmacies and dispensaries prepared the compounds for retail sale – bromides were the prime example in epilepsy. By the later nineteenth century, many (often small) companies had begun manufacturing pharmaceuticals. In the early twentieth century, a thriving but still relatively small industry existed in Germany (Bayer, Hoechst, Boehringer Ingelheim), which was the world leader, and in Switzerland (Ciba, Roche, Geigy, Sandoz), Britain (Burroughs Wellcome & Company) and America (H. K. Mulford, which merged with Sharp & Dohme in 1929, and Eli Lilly).

The industry grew slowly at first, but then more rapidly, not least by turning to the distribution of drugs, as well as their manufacture – in doing so usurping a time-honoured role of pharmacists and pharmacies. The most important product in epilepsy was phenobarbitone, produced by Bayer in 1912 and sold as Luminal. By 1914, methods for large-scale mass production and distribution were being introduced, along with modern techniques of management. Germany was still the powerhouse, but German leadership had been damaged by the First World War, not least by the confiscation of the American branches of German companies by the US state and the infringement of their patent rights. American industry flourished, and by 1928 America boasted 19,000 industrial laboratory researchers, a figure which had trebled by 1940. In

America, too, industry funded university research, and this was also to pay dividends in epilepsy.

The Second World War, and specifically the discovery and manufacture of penicillin in the later period, provided the greatest boost to the industry. Other antibiotics preceded and followed penicillin, as well as a long line of other useful drugs, including antipyretics, steroids, analgesics, vitamins and hormones. Scientific discovery was only partly responsible for the success of the pharmaceutical industry; the maturing of global capitalism and societal demand for better health services played a role. American companies again, as in the first war, overrode German patents, justified as the spoils of war. Companies saw opportunities for profit that previously did not exist, and it was around this time that the commercialisation of epilepsy medicine began in earnest.

Before the Second World War, the world market for pharmaceuticals was valued at $600 million; this figure rose to $4,000 million in 1960, $180,000 million in 1990 and around 1,000 billion dollars by 2020. As companies' balance sheets grew, their activities became progressively more controversial. Governments struggled to regulate and control abuses. In few other industries did the public gaze become so intense and the public so suspicious. Nonetheless, it was also clear that pharmaceuticals had become central to the success of medicine, and in future decades they would rule over the epilepsy agenda to an unprecedented extent.

A number of post-war legislative changes were the spur to a further rise of the American industry. Key amongst these were amendments to patent law. Previously, in most countries patents could only be issued for processes, not products. But in 1946 the US rules changed, overturning precedence and allowing the patenting of 'naturally occurring substances'. This event proved a turning point, giving the edge to American industry, not least as product protection was delayed in most European countries and Japan for many years. For one thing, academic leaders in Britain such as Henry Dale, Nobel Prize winner and president of the Royal Society, and Edward Mellanby, the post-war secretary of the MRC, believed that patenting life-saving drugs was unethical. Nonetheless, the experience of penicillin – discovered in Britain, patented in the United States and then licensed back at huge cost to British pharmaceutical companies – showed that in the post-war environment commercial interests could trump ethical concerns. According to Judy Slinn,[41] in no other industry did patents play as important a role as in pharmaceuticals. With patent protection, companies began investing heavily in their own research and manufacturing plants, and instead of licensing out their rights to other companies, tended to retain them, thereby gaining a monopoly on supply. Large research and development (R&D) facilities were created, along

[41] Slinn, 'Patents'.

with sophisticated legal, marketing and commercial practices. The R&D-to-sales ratio in US companies increased from 3.7% in 1951 to 15–20% in the 1980s.[42]

The Federal Food, Drug, and Cosmetic (FDC) Act of 1938 had brought about another important change in US regulation which strongly influenced the structure of the industry. This act made most drugs available to the public only through a doctor's prescription (a regulation further tightened in the1951 Durham–Humphrey Amendment).[43] At a stroke, elasticity of demand was greatly reduced, drugs became less price sensitive, and industry marketing switched massively towards doctors who were in effect acting as purchasing managers for their patients. Whereas previous advertising activity was directed at patients in a relatively low-key manner, companies began to target doctors with intensive and sophisticated marketing methods. Armies of representatives ('detail men', as they were known in the United States) were employed to deliver ever more skilfully crafted marketing under the guise of medical advice.[44] In 1958, 24% of the income of the largest American pharmaceutical companies was spent on advertising and promotion; by 1970, that share had risen to 40%. The profit margins of the big companies also increased, with typical annual rates of return after taxes at around 21–22% in the 1960s and 1970s.

In the field of epilepsy, a large number of drugs were investigated and licensed between 1940 and 1960,[45] in marked contrast to the poverty of new compounds in previous decades. It is not difficult to see commercial potential as the main driver.

In these years, two companies dominated epilepsy. The story of both is an instructive illustration of the then lack of control or regulation, and the consequences that ensnarled the industry in controversy. The first example is Abbott, which started life in 1888 when, in his own kitchen, Wallace Calvin Abbott began to produce small 'dosimetric' granules of several psychoactive drugs which previously were available only as liquids; by skilful and hyperbolic advertising, the company flourished. By 1900 the enterprise was incorporated as the Abbott Alkaloidal Company, and within five years it was generating sales of $200,000. In 1915 the company changed its name to Abbott Laboratories. By

---

[42] Malerba and Orsenigo, 'Pharmaceutical industry'. The number of new drugs (so-called new molecular entities) increased from 25 in the 1940s to 154 in the 1950s, 171 in the 1960s and 264 in the 1970s.

[43] Prior to 1938, in America, non-narcotic drugs could be purchased across the counter. In 1929, less than a third of all drugs taken in the United States were prescribed by a doctor, a figure which had risen to around 80% in 1969.

[44] The growth continued and by 2000 it was noted that there was one representative for every eight general practitioners and that $7,000 dollars per physician was spent on advertising.

[45] Merritt and Putnam reported that 700 compounds had been investigated using their cat model between 1937 and 1945 (Merritt and Putnam, 'Anticonvulsive activity'; Merritt, Putnam and Bywater, 'Sulfoxides and sulfones').

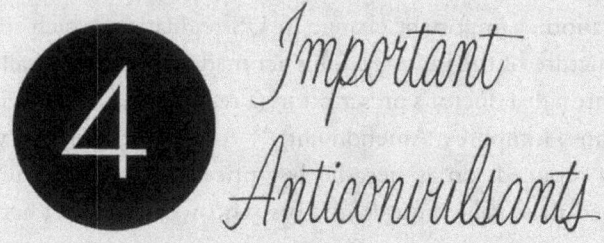

Do you have all the facts on these

4 *Important Anticonvulsants*

TRIDIONE®
(Trimethadione, Abbott)

First successful synthetic agent—now agent of choice—for the symptomatic control of *petit mal*, myoclonic jerks and akinetic seizures.

PARADIONE®
(Paramethadione, Abbott)

Homologue to TRIDIONE. An alternate preparation which is often effective in cases refractory to TRIDIONE therapy. For treatment of the *petit mal* triad.

GEMONIL®
(Metharbital, Abbott)

A new drug of low toxicity for *grand mal*, *petit mal*, myoclonic and mixed seizures. Effective in conditions symptomatic of organic brain damage.

PHENURONE®
(Phenacemide, Abbott)

A potent anticonvulsant for psychomotor epilepsy, *grand mal*, *petit mal*, and mixed seizures. Often successful where all other forms of therapy have failed.

These are names to remember. Each, in turn, has signaled a dramatic advance in the field of antiepileptic medicine. Used properly, discreetly, these four drugs will add inestimably to the scope and progress of your treatment of various epileptic disorders. Write us today for literature on any or all of these important anticonvulsants. Abbott Laboratories, North Chicago, Illinois. *Abbott*

23. An early advertisement. Abbott was the 'epilepsy company' manufacturing four drugs widely used in the 1950s

1950 Abbott had entered the epilepsy market, manufacturing and distributing a range of antiepileptics that included Tridione (trimethadione), Paradione (paramethadione), Phenurone (phenacemide), Gemonil (metharbital) and Peganone (ethotoin). These drugs were heavily advertised, along with exaggerated claims, but their lack of safety soon became an issue. Amongst 1,562 patients treated with

Phenurone, 6 were reported to have died from blood dyscrasia or hepatic failure. The drug also severely affected behaviour, yet it remained on the formulary and was widely touted. Tridione and Paradione were advertised by Abbott as 'two vessels of hope in the petit mal triad', along with a cartoon of two happy boys playing with a toy boat. But within two years of Tridione's licensing, in 1946, fatal renal failure, nephrotic syndrome, skin reactions and blood dyscrasias were reported. In 1948, the jury in a coroner's court in London opined that the drug should be scheduled as a poison; however, it continued to be widely marketed and used. Only in 1970 was it acknowledged that 30–50% of foetuses born to mothers taking Tridione were afflicted with severe congenital deformities and mental retardation and that the foetal loss rate was up to 87%. Despite this appalling record, no legal proceedings seem to have been launched concerning the drug's teratogenicity, reflecting perhaps the then subservient position of the patient. By 2000, Abbott reported sales of $13.75 billion and an R&D budget of $1 billion, and the company remains active in the field of epilepsy in many countries.[46]

The other dominant company in the field of epilepsy was Parke-Davis,[47] to whom fate was less benevolent. The company was founded in Detroit in 1871 and incorporated in 1875. It produced mercurial ointments and herbal laxatives. By 1900 it was marketing epinephrine, over which it was involved in a patent lawsuit, and cocaine, a drug which it advertised to 'supply the place of food, make the coward brave, the silent eloquent, and ... render the sufferer insensitive to pain'.[48] In 1946 the company synthesised chloromycetin. Within three years the product had yielded $120 million, and Parke-Davis became the largest pharmaceutical company in the United States. Its epilepsy products included Dilantin (phenytoin sodium), which became the most widely used drug in epilepsy, Celontin (methsuximide) and Milontin (phensuximide). Parke-Davis and Abbott had by then became known as the 'epilepsy companies'. However, by 1952, reports of hypoplastic anaemia due to chloromycetin appeared, and by 1960 the company was mired in bad publicity, not least from the apparent advice it gave to its representatives to stay focused on sales and to ignore good practice: 'Look, without sales there is no Parke-Davis. We all have to sell on some level ... Just don't leave anything behind. Above all, don't put anything in writing.'[49] In 1968 its vaccine Quadrigen was withdrawn from the market after a series of lawsuits, in one of which the judge ruled that although government regulations had been met, these 'standards were minimal' and that

---

[46] (www.fundinguniverse.com/company-histories/abbottlaboratories-history/, accessed 21 January 2020). In 1969 Abbott's sales amounted to around $180 million, but the company continued to be embroiled in controversy: in 1966 over the accusation that it had sold two million doses of methamphetamine in powder form to a criminal ring, and in 1970 over carcinogenic effects and bacterial contamination of cyclamate.

[47] Hoefle, 'Parke-Davis and Company'.   [48] Bourke, 'Enjoying the high life'.

[49] Critser, Generation RX, p. 103.

the company had failed to warn customers of the known risks or to exercise reasonable care. Following heavy fines, Parke-Davis was then purchased first by Warner Lambert in 1974, and then by Pfizer in 2000. In 2002 the company was again trouble, and in court proceedings admitted illegally marketing its new antiepilepsy drug Neurontin. In 2007 its research facilities were closed down.

Regulation of the Pharmaceutical Industry

In the nineteenth century, as industrialisation proceeded, regulation of the industry was largely restricted to addressing issues around the adulteration and labelling of drugs. Indeed, the market was crammed with 'patent medicines' – that is, those with a secret composition. Slowly regulation was tightened but at a glacial pace. The examples of Britain and the United States are cited here, but elsewhere there were similar political pressures and the passage of similar laws. In 1860, in the face of public concern, Britain passed the Adulteration Act, essentially the first regulation related to the manufacture and sale of drugs. This was amended in 1872 and then strengthened in 1875 into the Sale of Food and Drugs Act, which became the model for all subsequent legislation worldwide. The act sought to prevent the adulteration of an article with any 'mix, colour, stain or powder . . . any material . . . so as to render the article injurious to health',[50] and analysts were appointed by the state to police this law. A fine of £50 could be levied on offenders. Minor amendments were made over the years, leading finally to the Food and Drugs Act of 1938, which mandated clear and precise labelling and prohibited false advertising. In the United States, from 1902 factories began to be inspected and manufacturers licensed, and in 1906 the Pure Food and Drug Act, the regulation that led to the founding of the Food and Drug Administration (FDA), was passed into law. In the laissez-faire spirit of the day, government interference in business was discouraged, and there was no requirement to demonstrate either the effectiveness of any compound or its safely other than in very broad terms. Because drug effects were generally mild, their regulation was drafted alongside that of foodstuffs, which at the time were considered a greater risk to health. As a prototypic law of the Progressive Era, the Pure Food and Drug Act was also intended to ensure that fair value was received by the consumer. For seventeen drugs, it was mandated that the quantity should be stated; bromide was included in this list, along with atropine and strophanthin, which were still occasionally used in epilepsy.

In Britain, the first committee to advise on what drugs should be allowable for prescription under a national insurance scheme was established in 1929. However, in the face of opposition from the pharmaceutical industry, and because of the

---

[50] Sale of Food and Drugs Act 1875, chapter 63.

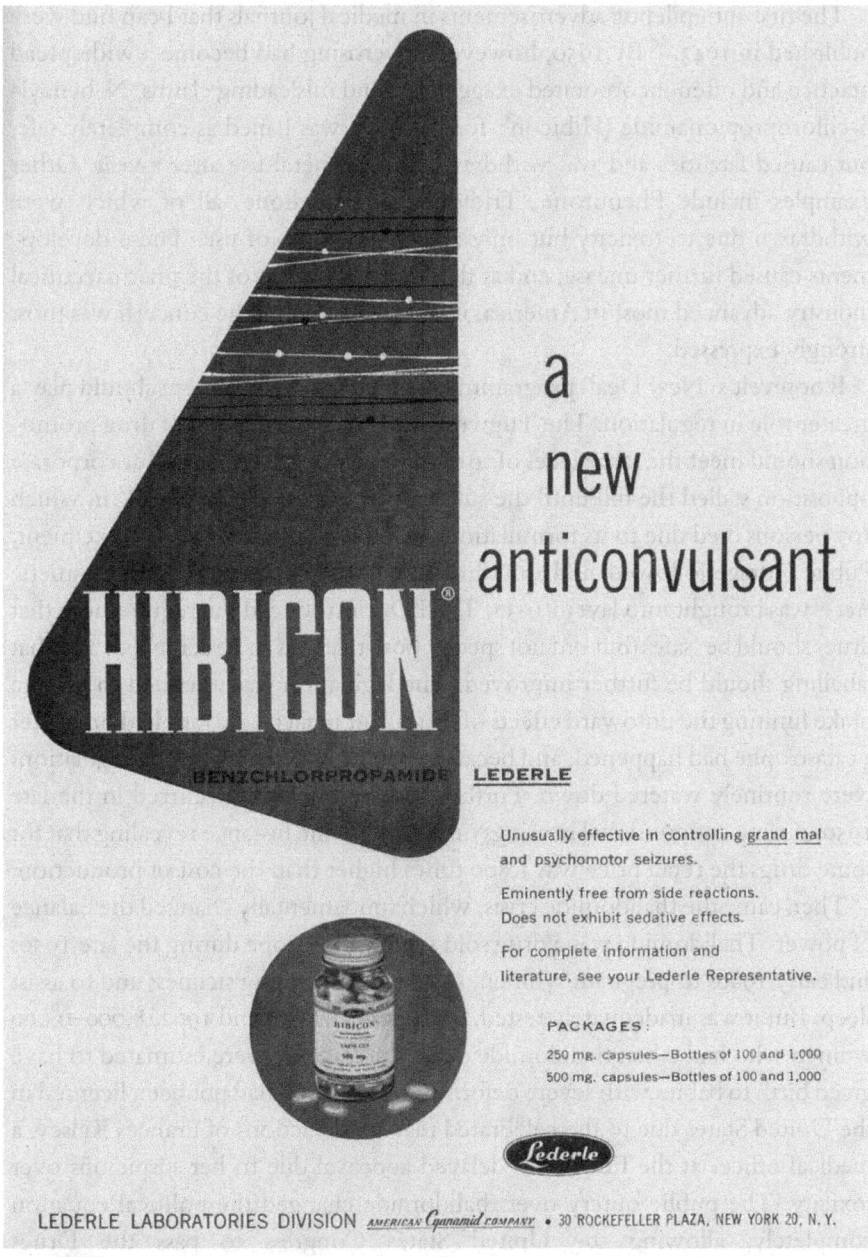

a new anticonvulsant

HIBICON

BENZCHLORPROPAMIDE   **LEDERLE**

Unusually effective in controlling grand mal and psychomotor seizures.

Eminently free from side reactions. Does not exhibit sedative effects.

For complete information and literature, see your Lederle Representative.

PACKAGES:

250 mg. capsules—Bottles of 100 and 1,000
500 mg. capsules—Bottles of 100 and 1,000

Lederle

LEDERLE LABORATORIES DIVISION *AMERICAN Cyanamid COMPANY* • 30 ROCKEFELLER PLAZA, NEW YORK 20, N. Y.

24. Hibicon advert. It is proclaimed that Hibicon was 'eminently free from side reactions'. The drug was withdrawn soon afterwards because of fatal blood dyscrasia.

value of that sector to the national economy, restriction was minimised. Drugs were licensed with sparse preclinical testing and with human studies confined to uncontrolled observations on only a few hundred patients, or less, often treated for a matter of weeks or a few months. Many of the drugs licensed then were subsequently shown to be ineffective or toxic.

The first antiepileptic advertisements in medical journals that I can find were published in 1943.[51] By 1950, however, advertising had become a widespread practice and often incorporated exaggerated and misleading claims. N-benzyl-β-chloropropionamide (Hibicon), for instance, was hailed as completely safe, but caused fatalities and was withdrawn from general use after a year. Other examples include Phenurone, Tridione and Paradione, all of which were withdrawn due to toxicity but only after many years of use. These developments caused further unease; and as the industrialisation of the pharmaceutical industry advanced most in America, it was there that public concern was most strongly expressed.

Roosevelt's 'New Deal' programme deemed that government should play a greater role in regulation. The Tugwell Bill of 1933 required that drug promotion should meet the same level of truthfulness as drug labelling. But corporate opposition stalled the bill until the sulphanilamide scandal of 1937,[52] in which 107 persons died due to its formulation with the inclusion of a toxic excipient. Public outrage followed, and a modified bill – the Food, Drug, and Cosmetic Act – was brought into law in 1938. The FDA introduced the requirement that drugs should be 'safe' (but did not specify how that was to be achieved) and that labelling should be further improved. The legislation was intended to act as a brake limiting the untoward effects of drugs, but in fact it was applied only after a catastrophe had happened, and because of industry's strong lobby, regulations were routinely watered down. Further adverse publicity occurred in the late 1950s during congressional hearings on prices, in one instance revealing that for some drugs the retail price was 1,800 times higher than the cost of production.

Then came the thalidomide crisis, which fundamentally changed the balance of power. Thalidomide was a drug sold widely in Europe during the late 1950s and early 1960s to pregnant women, to alleviate morning sickness and to assist sleep. But it was inadequately tested, and between 1956 and 1962, 8,000–9,000 women who had taken thalidomide during pregnancy were estimated to have given birth to babies with severe deformities. The drug had not been licensed in the United States due to the celebrated rear-guard actions of Frances Kelsey, a medical officer at the FDA who delayed approval due to her suspicions over toxicity. The public outcry over thalidomide changed the political equation completely, allowing the United States Congress to pass the Drugs Amendment Act (the Kefauver–Harris Amendment) in 1962.

---

[51] The advert for Dilantin (Figure 19).

[52] In 1937, the chief chemist at S. E. Massengill Company, a small pharmaceutical firm in Tennessee, decided to dissolve sulphanilamide in diethylene glycol (DEG) along with a raspberry flavouring. This was done without any consideration of the toxicology of DEG, which was used in industry largely for keeping products such as glue moist. Within a very short time, 107 patients died of renal failure and other toxic effects of the solvent after ingesting the elixir (www.fda.gov/files/about%20fda/published/The-Sulfanilamide-Disaster .pdf, accessed 10 May 2021).

This amendment was a milestone in the history of epilepsy. It required evidence of both efficacy and safety, not only of new medicines but also a retrospective evaluation of the efficacy of antiepileptic drugs introduced between 1938 and 1962. It further required drug advertising to disclose accurate information about the side effects and efficacy of treatment, and it obligated the FDA to establish guidelines for testing all classes of drugs, including antiepileptics. Rules about disclosure of information and the keeping of side-effect records by companies were put in place. Safety testing was made far more stringent. A new system of licensing was devised over the next few years that required each company to obtain an IND (Investigational New Drug application) before it was permitted to use the drug in human subjects. Complete chemical and manufacturing information, preclinical screening and animal investigation, including toxicology, teratogenicity and safety, had to be submitted to the FDA before the IND was granted, and in 1979 the NIH tightened regulations further, requiring further minimum standards before any license was awarded. Once an IND was granted, clinical testing could begin: this was divided into Phase 1 (healthy volunteers); Phase 2 (small-scale controlled studies to identify dose and other matters); and Phase 3 (broad and varied clinical studies). The FDA was given powers to withdraw existing drugs from the market if it deemed evidence of efficacy to be insufficient.[53] Similar regulations followed in some European countries and elsewhere, and this bill, more than any other, reset the balance between industry and government worldwide. And, in broad terms, the provisions, philosophy and procedures of the act continue to apply, changed only in detail, to this day.

In other countries, regulation varied, as governments struggled to balance public alarm with the need to stimulate industrial growth. In the communist bloc, the pharmaceutical industries were nationalised and regulation was widely extended. In developing countries, though, regulation remained largely absent, and corruption, fraud and malpractice were commonplace.[54]

Although the new regulations undoubtedly introduced a new level of protection for the public from dangerous compounds, there were significant negative consequences in epilepsy (and other branches of medicine). The cost of developing antiepileptic drugs rose steeply as a result of the very large increase in the number of animals and experimental procedures needed in preclinical testing, the complexity and scope of testing, and the requirement for large controlled clinical trials in human subjects. Gone were the days when a few short open studies were sufficient – as was the case, for instance, in the licensing of phenytoin and ethosuximide (bromide and phenobarbitone were

---

[53] This led to very public clashes between the industry and the agency, which had benefitted from large donations from the industry, and political interference from the Nixon government.

[54] See Silverman, Lee and Lydecker, *Prescriptions for Death*.

introduced without the need for any testing). Consequently, a number of companies, especially in the United States, withdrew from the field of epilepsy. The number of licences for antiepileptic drugs came to a sudden halt. There was a similar fall-off in the number of new drugs in other fields of medicine as well and, in Colin Dollery's words in 1978, it was the 'end of an age of optimism' in pharmaceutical development[55] – although, as we shall see, this was over-pessimistic, and in subsequent decades the industry continued to make huge profits.

THE BASIC SCIENCE OF EPILEPSY

Between 1900 and 1970, tremendous progress was made in understanding the chemistry and physiology of neuronal function. Although much of this early work focused on the nature and mechanism of transmission in the neuronal axon and at the synapse, epilepsy rarely featured.

Neurochemistry and neurophysiology were both products of Sherrington's discoveries of the synapse and of excitatory and inhibitory transmission. A central research question occupied this early neuroscience, namely, whether the transmission of impulses between cells and at the synapse was chemical or electrical. By the 1950s the debate had been resolved, and chemical transmission was recognised unanimously to be the predominant method in the 1950s. This revelation opened the door to new scientific research on chemical (i.e. drug) treatments of disease.

Neurochemical receptors were central to the idea of chemical transmission. Their existence was first posited in 1900 by Paul Ehrlich, who noted that '[c]hemical substances are only able to exercise an action on the tissue elements with which they are able to establish an intimate chemical relationship . . . [This relationship] must be specific. [The chemical] groups must be adapted to one another . . . as lock and key.'[56] In Ehrlich's time, nothing was known of the mechanism of this process, but knowledge slowly advanced. Landmarks in the field of neurotransmitters and neurochemical receptors are listed in Table 3.3, and these led to the new discipline of neuropharmacology. In the central nervous system, attention was focused first on transmission by dopamine, noradrenalin and acetylcholine, which were to have little impact on epilepsy, and later on GABA and glutamate. In the later decades of the century, it was to be these two brain chemicals that put epilepsy at the centre of neurochemical research and in receipt of massive investment of time and money in a search for new anticonvulsant drugs.

In the 1940s and 1950s, neurochemical interest in epilepsy was concerned mainly with cerebral energy metabolism and on acetylcholine metabolism

---

[55] Dollery, *End of an Age*.   [56] Ehrlich, 'On immunity'.

TABLE 3.3 *Timeline of some of the key advances in understanding the chemical and physiological basis of neurotransmission between 1900–1970*

1897–1906	Sir Charles Sherrington	In 1897, he coined the term 'synapse', and in his book *The Integrative Action of the Nervous System* described inhibitory and inhibitory transmission in the CNS.
1900–6	John Newport Langley and Thomas Renton Elliott	Langley introduced the term 'autonomic nervous system', and in 1905 suggested that noradrenaline was a transmitter in sympathetic nerves. In 1906, he suggested that the chemicals act on 'receptor substances'. In 1904 Elliott, his student, had suggested that sympathetic nerve secrete adrenalin.
1900–7	Paul Ehrlich	Hypothesised that there must be 'chemoreceptors'.
1914	Sir Henry Dale	First experiments with acetylcholine on smooth muscle and the vagus nerve.
1920s	Otto Loewi	Discovered acetylcholine (Vagusstoff) conveyed signals from the vagus nerve to the heart. He identified this as acetylcholine in 1926. Introduced the concept of neurohumoral transmission.
1933	Alfred Joseph Clark	Refined the concept of receptor occupancy by neurotransmitters.
1933	Henry Hallett Dale	Confirmed acetylcholine as neurotransmitter in peripheral nerves of mammals.
1934	John Henry Gaddum	Suggested that each impulse causes the release of a small quantity of acetylcholine at the synapse.
1936	Edgar Douglas Adrian	Showed that repetitive stimulation induced 'self-sustaining' activity (later called kindling).
1940	Birdsey Renshaw	Identified inhibitory interneurons in the nervous system (Renshaw cells).
1940	Theodore Erickson	Postulated that epileptic discharge spread via the corpus callosum.
1946	Ulf Svante von Euler	Confirmation of noradrenaline as neurotransmitter in peripheral nerves.
1949	Alan Lloyd Hodgkin and Andrew Fielding Huxley	Defined the action potential and membrane permeability to sodium and potassium ions.
1951	John Carew Eccles	Described experiment which disproved the hypothesis that nervous transmission was electrical, of which he previously was a leading supporter, and accepted the chemical hypothesis.
1950	Jorge Awapara, Eugene Roberts and Samuel Frankel	Demonstrated conclusively the presence of GABA in CNS, and this was later found to be the chief inhibitory neurotransmitter in the CNS.
1953	John Welsh and Betty Twarog	Serotonin identified as a potential neurotransmitter in CNS.

(continued)

TABLE 3.3 *(continued)*

1953	John Carew Eccles	Showed how acetylcholine was an inhibitory transmitter in Renshaw interneurons in the spinal cord.
1954	Sanford Palay and George Palade; Eduardo de Robertis and Henry Bennett	Using the electron microscope, described the synapse and its structure and the synaptic space.
1954	Bernard Katz	Suggested that synaptic vesicles contain neurotransmitter.
1956	John Carew Eccles	Showed that acetylcholine was a neurotransmitter in CNS (spinal cord and Renshaw cells of cat).
1960	David Curtis and Jeffrey Watkins	Demonstrated the presence of glutamate in the brain as a potential neurotransmitter.
1960	Henry Gaddum	Defined a receptor as a 'chemical group in the tissue with which a single molecule of drug combines'. This paved the way for identifying many other receptor types such as dopamine, opioids, cannabinoids, etc.
1960s	Arvid Carlsson	Provided evidence for endogenous agonists and neurotransmission in the CNS.
1961	Julius Axelrod	Described reuptake of neurotransmitters with noradrenaline as his example.
1965	Bernard Katz	Modelled synaptic neurotransmitter release (of acetylcholine at the synapse) and the role of calcium.
1967	Graham Goddard	Demonstrated and coined the term 'kindling'.
1967	Krešimir Krnjevic and Susan Schwartz	Demonstrated that GABA was an inhibitory neurotransmitter in mammalian brain.

(Sherrington, Adrian, Loewi, Dale, von Euler, Eccles, Hodgkin, Huxley, Carlsson, Axelrod and Katz were awarded Nobel prizes).

(the 'acetylcholine wave').[57] A symposium held at the American League Against Epilepsy in Louisville in 1952 summarised contemporary knowledge.[58] Alfred Pope presented a paper on the biochemistry of neuronal discharges, focusing on energy metabolism via the Krebs cycle and glycolytic pathways, and acetylcholine and acetylcholinesterase. Donald Tower discussed the 'biochemical lesion present in epileptogenic cortex' and the central role of the acetylcholine system, believing that a defect in acetylcholine binding and the relationship of the 'acetylcholine system' with the 'glutamic-acid system' might

[57] As a sign of potential importance of neurochemistry in epilepsy, Penfield established the first neurochemical laboratory in a hospital, at the MNI, directly involved in clinical studies of epilepsy. This was headed by the Cambridge graduate Alan Elliott, whom Penfield invited into the operating theatre to take samples during open brain surgery in his fruitless search for the 'X-substance' (Eccles and Feindel, *Wilder Graves Penfield*, p. 485).

[58] The symposium, chaired by A. Earl Walker, consisted of four papers by Paul Yakovlev, Horace Magoun, Alfred Poe and Donald Tower.

TABLE 3.4 *What was known about the neurochemistry of seizures by 1958*

1. Pre-ictal
Rise in cerebral ammonia
Fluctuation in cerebral acetylcholine

2. Ictal
Increase in: cerebral blood flow, oxygen consumption, lactic acid production
Decrease in: cerebral acetylcholine, cerebral glutamic acid, high-energy phosphate
   compounds

3. Inter-ictal
Free acetylcholine in CSF
Decreased acetylcholine binding
Increased cholinesterase activity
Increased glutamic acid utilisation
Impaired maintenance of cellular potassium

(From Tower, 'Evidence for a neurochemical basis of seizures'. Based on brain slices from patients
undergoing temporal lobe surgery and blood/CSF studies in patients with epilepsy)

be involved in the production of seizures (Table 3.4). In his 1951 textbook of
brain chemistry, Henry Himwich concluded: 'Much work has been done on
the biology of epilepsy but the enzymatic approach to the national history has
not been sufficiently explored.'[59] Following the work of Lennox and others in
the 1930s (described in the previous chapter), it was by then generally agreed
that, during a seizure, the principle changes were increased cerebral blood flow,
oxygen consumption and cerebral lactic acid levels; decreased levels of cerebral
acetylcholine, glutamic acid and high-energy phosphate compounds; and
variable electrolyte shifts.[60] Himwich also noted, with evident excitement,
that drugs which influenced cholinesterase activity, such as prostigmine and
eserine, were said to modify the course of petit mal epilepsy. But by 1976 and
the second edition of his textbook, the focus on cholinesterase had faded
completely, for by then epilepsy neurochemistry had moved to studies of the
GABA and glutaminergic systems.

The fact that little of the neurochemical work in epilepsy of this period has
proved of enduring value illustrates four problems central to the study of
epilepsy neurochemistry. First, of the thousands of potential brain chemicals
which could be studied, technology provides access to only a few. As a result,
studies were often driven by technology and not hypothesis. Second, brain
chemicals are interconnected in complex pathways, which means that changing levels in one will change levels in others which are merely onlookers.
Third, it is difficult to identify the exact microscopic location of chemicals: for
instance, whether they were intra- or extracellular, in glial tissue or neurons, or
at the synapse or elsewhere. Finally, the chemical changes in seizures are

[59] Himwich, *Brain Metabolism*, p. 363.   [60] See also Tower, 'Neurochemical basis of seizures'.

transient, a fact noted as early as 1910 by Aldren Turner, and dissecting cause from effect was difficult and often impossible. These problems continue to plague neurochemical study today.

That brings us to experimental neurophysiology. As with neurochemistry, it was the work of Sherrington which opened the field, and the role of ionic movements became the focus of much research. Julius Berstein had suggested as early as 1912 that propagation of the nervous impulse was due to changes to the ionic permeability of the nerve cell membrane. In the 1920s, Birdsey Renshaw[61] and colleagues devised electrodes for single-cell recordings which became fundamental to studies of epilepsy physiology. But elucidation of the mechanisms of propagation had to await the technological advances of the post–Second World War period. In 1949 Bernard Katz and Alan Hodgkin suggested that the axonal membrane might have different permeabilities to different ions, and showed the crucial role of sodium permeability in creating the action potential. In turn, Hodgkin and Andrew Huxley applied the 'voltage clamp' technique, first described in 1947, to make single-cell recordings in the giant axons of the squid. This approach enabled the pair to determine membrane permeabilities to sodium and potassium ions, and in five landmark papers they described the mathematics, neurochemistry and physiology of the action potential. For this fundamental work they were awarded the Nobel Prize in Physiology or Medicine in 1963. In 1963 John Eccles's single-cell studies of synaptic function earned him a Nobel Prize, and in 1962 Bernard Katz modelled neurotransmitter release and showed that it occurred in quantal amounts, for which he won a Nobel Prize in 1970. Subsequently, neurotransmitters were found to be stored in synaptic vesicles and released into the synaptic cleft when the vesicles fuse with the presynaptic cell membrane at the synapse. It was recognised that an action potential in presynaptic neurons triggers this release of neurotransmitters, which then bind to post-synaptic receptors and thereby transmit the action potential from one neuron to the next. Technological improvements, including multi-array electrodes and microelectrodes using glass, iridium and platinum, were introduced in the late 1960s. These were golden years in neurophysiology and the discoveries of this period opened up the new field of molecular biology. However, as with neurochemistry, none of this basic work was specifically addressed to the problems of epilepsy – a situation that would change in subsequent decades.

Most physiological work on epilepsy in the 1950s was concerned with identifying the anatomical structures underpinning seizures and seizure spread.

---

[61] Birdsey Renshaw was a researcher at Harvard and the Rockefeller Institute, and then died from polio two months after being appointed as Associate Professor in Physiology at the University of Oregon.

At the 1952 symposium of the American League Against Epilepsy, Paul Yakovlev gave a paper emphasising the importance of cortical–subcortical circuits, and Horace Magoun spoke on the reticular activating system. Much of the work was influenced by the long shadow of Hughlings and his concept of three levels of epilepsy. By then all were agreed that the lowest order (seizures arising from the medulla or spinal cord) were so rare as to be non-existent. Most work was centred on 'second-order' motor seizures in an attempt to elucidate the relationship between cortex and subcortical centres in relation to such questions as the genesis of the tonic and clonic components of generalised convulsions, and the genesis of spike–wave discharges in petit mal epilepsy. The role of the corpus callosum, the pyramidal and extrapyr-amidal tracts, and deep subcortical nuclei was extensively studied. E.D. Adrian's studies between 1934 and 1939 of the 'deep response' induced by strong cortical stimulation established that a wave of changing electrical potentials spreads outwards from an area of stimulation due to lateral spread in the neurons of the deep layer of the cortex, accompanied by clonic movements. In 1940, Theodore Erickson in Montreal showed neurophysio-logical changes spreading from one side to the other via the corpus callosum. In 1940, Renshaw and colleagues used their novel microelectrode recording methods to show that inhibition in the spinal cord was due to inhibitory interneurons – named Renshaw cells in his honour – and attention then turned to single-cell recording in the hippocampus where inhibitory inter-neurons were also found. The anatomical and physiological basis of spike–wave and petit mal epilepsy was intensively studied, a key question being whether these had a cortical or diencephalic origin.[62]

Animal models of epilepsy were crucial to this work. The first experimen-tally produced seizures were observed as early as 1660 by Robert Boyle in birds, cats and mice exposed to low air pressure. From the mid-nineteenth century a number of researchers produced focal seizures in primates by cortical electrical stimulation, the application of strychnine or freezing portions of cortex. Lenore and Nicholas Kopeloff, working in New York,[63] carried out a systematic series of experiments over thirty years using the focal application of alumina cream and heavy metals (especially cobalt) to the sensorimotor cortex or the temporal lobe in various primate species. This resulted in a model of chronic focal epilepsy which could be used for testing antiepileptic drugs and exploring the pathology and physiology of focal epilepsy and which seemed to induce patho-logical, physiological and behavioural changes similar to those of human epilepsy;

---

[62] Despite sparse and conflicting evidence, the idea of a subcortical origin led to the vogue for stereotactic stimulation of subcortical structures in human epilepsy and also laid the founda-tion for Wilder Penfield's centrencephalic theories.

[63] Reviewed in Kopeloff et al., 'Epilepsy in animals', pp. 163–80.

for many years, this was the experimental model of choice.[64] Focal destruction of areas of cortex by freezing was another widely used method, first introduced in 1883, for inducing seizures in dogs, cats and rabbits. Using this model, Frank Morrell was the first to demonstrate mirror foci in dogs in 1960.[65]

Another model of great importance to epilepsy was electrical kindling. In 1936 Adrian had demonstrated that repetitive stimulation was capable of inducing 'self-sustained' activity (i.e. EEG activity extending beyond the period of actual stimulation). Subsequently, it was found that spontaneous epileptic seizures could be produced after a course of repeated stimulation.[66] This permanent lowering of the seizure threshold by repeated electrical stimulation became known as 'kindling', a term coined by Graham Goddard in Ontario in 1967.[67] Applied to rats, cats and other sub-primate laboratory species in the decades after 1970, kindling became a commonly used method of investigating various aspects of epilepsy. The relevance to humans, though, was and remains uncertain as it has proved difficult to induce kindling in primates.

The generalised epilepsies were studied experimentally, also notably by the application of chemicals to the cortex of monkeys or kittens (conjugated oestrogens, strychnine, pentylenetetrazol, alumina gel, cobalt and, later, penicillin were all used). Then, in 1966, the Senegalese baboon, *Papio papio*, was discovered to suffer spontaneous photic-induced seizures. This species was extensively studied by Robert Naquet[68] in France and Brian Meldrum in

---

[64] Other convulsant agents used in this period included: penicillin, tungsten acid, strychnine, amino acids, conjugated oestrogen, tetrazoles such as metrazol, bemegride, picrotoxin, camphor derivatives, fluoroacetates, methionine sulfoximine, compounds affecting pyridoxal-5-phosphate-dependent enzyme systems, inhibitors of cholinesterases (organophosphates), bicuculline and thujone. Animal models using hypoxia, hypoglycaemia and other metabolic disturbances were also employed.

[65] Morrell, 'Secondary epileptogenic lesions'. Frank Morrell was Professor of Neurological Sciences at Rush Medical College. He qualified from Columbia University, and trained in neurology at the Montefiore Hospital, the National Hospital, Queen Square, Montreal Neurological Institute. (See Cohen, 'In memoriam'; Engel, 'Legacy of Frank Morrell'.)

[66] Alonso-Deflorida and Delgado, 'EEG changes in cats'.

[67] Goddard described his work in seventy-seven rats, with electrodes implanted in various subcortical areas, noting the particular 'progressive sensitization' ('Development of epileptic seizures', p. 1021) of the amygdala. Goddard did acknowledge the precedence of Louis (Jack) Herberg who in 1966 had observed that 'daily electrical stimulation of certain sub-cortical areas of the rat brain will eventually cause convulsions even though the intensity of stimulation is relatively low and initially has no such effect' (Herberg and Watkins, 'Epileptiform seizures'). Adrian had also made a similar discovery. Graham Goddard obtained his PhD at McGill, worked at Dalhousie and Stanford, and was appointed Chair of Psychology at the University of Otago in New Zealand. He died prematurely by drowning in a storm-swollen river whilst hiking (see Morrell, 'Graham Goddard').

[68] Robert Naquet was a French experimental neurophysiologist who was 'to French experimental epilepsy what Henri Gastaut, his mentor and friend, was to French clinical epilepsy research' (Capeda et al., 'Naquet'). He first worked on the baboon model of photosensitive epilepsy with Keith Killam, and these studies were then taken further by Naquet and Meldrum.

England, and it proved an ideal model for investigating the pharmacological effects of drugs and the pathology of status epilepticus. Strains of mice, rats and rabbits were also discovered which exhibited seizures brought on by loud sounds and other stimuli.

Another experimentally produced phenomenon was 'spreading depression', a term used to describe the slowly propagating loss of cortical electrical activity triggered by focal electrical stimulation. It was first described by Aristides Leão from Harvard in 1944 in studies of rabbits in an attempt to understand the electrocorticogram in experimental epilepsy.[69] Although a fascinating phenomenon, its relevance to epilepsy still remains unclear despite numerous investigations in the post-war years.

The key discoveries made in the basic science of neuropharmacology were dependent on technical developments, of which most important were those of X-ray diffraction and crystallography. These enabled scientists to determine the three-dimensional structure of small molecules and then of large proteins.[70] Antiepileptic drugs and brain proteins were not initially studied and these basic discoveries had no early impact on epilepsy therapy. In subsequent decades, however, using similar techniques, the structure of thousands of proteins and pharmaceuticals was uncovered, and X-ray crystallography came to be routinely used to show how a drug binds to its target, with obvious consequence in the field of epilepsy.

PSYCHIATRY, MENTAL HANDICAP AND EPILEPSY

Psychiatry, Epilepsy and Society

Psychiatry has always been influenced by sociocultural as well as medical trends, and in the quarter-century after the war, as Western social structures and culture dramatically changed so did psychiatric theory and practice. Amongst the crucial societal changes, first was the growing public interest in 'human rights', and in parallel the rights of the disabled and the mentally ill. The *disability rights movement* gathered force especially after the 1960s, in part a reaction to the revelations of the abuses of psychiatry, the rejection of theories of racial hygiene and eugenics, and in part to the exposure of the dire conditions in asylums throughout the world. Also influential were the ending of post-war austerity, the rise of a youth culture (as post-war baby boomers

[69] Leão, 'Spreading depression of activity'.

[70] Dorothy Hodgkin described the structure of cholesterol in 1937, then penicillin (1946), vitamin B_{12} (1956) and insulin (1964) – for which work she received the Nobel Prize in Chemistry in 1969. The first of the complex proteins studied was myoglobin, the structure of which was worked out by John Kendrew and Max Perutz, who shared the Nobel Prize in Chemistry in 1962. Identifying the structure of DNA depended on x-ray diffraction which was, as described later, to change the science of epilepsy in a fundamental manner.

entered early adult life), the liberalisation of social and sexual behaviour and norms, the decline of religious authority, the rise of science, the pharmaceutical industry and materialism. All were accompanied by a parallel transformation of the discipline of psychiatry. This by and large had a positive impact those with epilepsy; four changes in particular are worthy of comment.

The first was the rise of biological psychiatry. Throughout the history of psychiatry, the question of whether major psychiatric disorders are the result of psychosocial stresses or an organic (neurochemical or neurobiological) disorder had been debated, and by 1950 the biomedical model was in the ascendency. Psychoanalysts despised what they considered a materialistic approach 'akin to explaining the music of a violin by the physical properties of the horse-hair scraping on cats' entrails'.[71] But their influence was on the wane. The physical treatments for psychosis – insulin coma, barbiturate coma, electroconvulsive therapy (ECT) and lobotomy – had come first but were followed in the 1950s by the introduction of medicaments, 'liquid coshes' such as chlorpromazine and the benzodiazepines, replacing hours on the couch with a few seconds of tablet taking.[72] The medications were perceived to be 'curative treatments' in a speciality where few medicinal cures previously existed, and they certainly alleviated some of the psychiatric comorbidity of epilepsy (such as anxiety, depression and psychosis). The drugs supeceded the use of insulin coma and lobotomy, when 'like a large shoal of fish [psychiatrists] simply switched direction to follow the lights of the more fashionable pharmacotherapy'.[73] For the first time in its history, the specialty could claim to be on the same level as general medicine, giving psychiatrists a sense of medical identity,[74] and this dramatically changed attitudes to epilepsy, which was also increasingly seen as a primarily medical not mental condition, and one with a unique set of pharmaceutical solutions.

A second, and linked, trend, and perhaps the most important for epilepsy, was that of deinstitutionalisation. Conditions in asylums, and all aspects of the

---

[71] Dicks, *Clinical Studies in Psychopathology*, p. 237. Dicks was later celebrated for his psychological examination of Rudolf Hess and his work on the Nazi mentality. Dicks also held the view that there was a gradation from hystero-epilepsy to true 'idiopathic epilepsy' and the nearer to 'the true epileptic attack the manifestations are, the more primitive aggression is present, so that idiopathic epilepsy may, after all be a regression to the massive tension-discharge of infantile rage' (*Clinical Studies in Psychopathology*, p. 101).

[72] Insulin coma therapy was a landmark in the medicalisation of psychiatry, although any suggestion of an organic medical mechanism was resisted by the psychoanalytic school. To Smith Ely Jelliffe, its success was in 'withdrawing the libido from the outside world and fusing it with the death impulse for the maintenance of the narcissistic ego' (cited in Shepherd, 'Neurolepsis').

[73] Shepherd, 'Neurolepsis'.

[74] The title 'physician in psychological medicine' and even 'behavioural neurologist' came to be assumed by those who previously would have been known as a 'psychiatrist'.

care of those with psychiatric illness and/or learning disability, became widely discussed in public. Gone were the earlier days when these topics were taboo in polite social discourse. In 1948 Albert Deutsch published a damning critique of conditions inside twelve mental institutions in the United States that housed people with mental handicap and epilepsy, where 'humans [were] herded like cattle' in filthy, barnlike wards without any vestige of human dignity or decency.[75] At the time, 51% of people admitted to hospitals in America were 'mental' patients, and, in Deutsch's view, mental illness had to be the number one health priority. Increasingly concerned about the numbers of handicapped persons and the rehabilitation of brain-injured veterans, the public seemed to agree: the book sparked outrage and became a bestseller. In 1972, ABC news included the epilepsy colony of Letchworth Village in its piece 'Willowbrook: The Last Great Disgrace'. Residents of Willowbrook and Letchworth Village were found to be living in awful conditions, with a lack of clothes, baths or attention to even basic needs. The facilities were extremely understaffed, and residents received little or no actual schooling, training or even access to simple activities – a far cry from Letchworth's original vision. In Britain and Europe, where facilities for the mentally handicapped had also been badly squeezed during the war as beds were diverted for military cases, conditions in the asylums were also severely criticised. Accounts surfaced of the devastating effects of mental illness and abuse of inmates.[76] Effective, well-supported public campaigns, such as that launched by the National Council for Civil Liberties, raised the temperature of the debate. With the demise of hereditarian and nativist theories, attention switched both to social influences on mental illness and to the nature of treatment. Similar trends occurred in many other European countries.

Russell Barton, a psychiatrist, coined the term 'institutional neurosis' for the passive and submissive condition that many such asylum patients developed.[77]. The asylums were increasingly seen as outdated relics and pressure grew to move patients into 'community care'. In Britain, the mood of the moment was

---

[75] Deutsch, *Shame of the States*, p. 42.

[76] See, for instance, Vincent, *Inside the Asylum*, the film *Snake Pit* (1948), and, perhaps most influential of all, Ken Kesey's book *One Flew over the Cuckoo's Nest*, which was turned into a play in 1953 and a film in 1975. In Britain, there were at least twenty highly publicised 'scandals', for instance at the asylums in Ely, Farleigh, Whittingham, Napsbury and South Ockendon, which were the subject of TV programmes (e.g. a *World in Action* programme in 1968 claiming that ECT was being given without anaesthetic or muscle relaxant) and books (e.g. Robb, *Sans Everything*). Similar events occurred in other countries.

[77] Barton, *Institutional Neurosis*. Barton framed this as a medical 'condition' (p. 12). The symptoms were apathy, lack of initiative, loss of interest (especially in things of an impersonal nature), submissiveness, apparent inability to plan for the future, lack of individuality and sometimes a characteristic posture and gait. The causes included loss of contact with the outside world, enforced idleness, loss of responsibility, bossiness of medical and nursing staff, drugs, ward atmosphere and loss of prospects. Similar behaviours were also observed in other non-mental institutions, such as prisons. The symptoms were, as Barton humorously noted, similar to 'Oblomovism' (p. 11). See Goncharov, *Oblomov*).

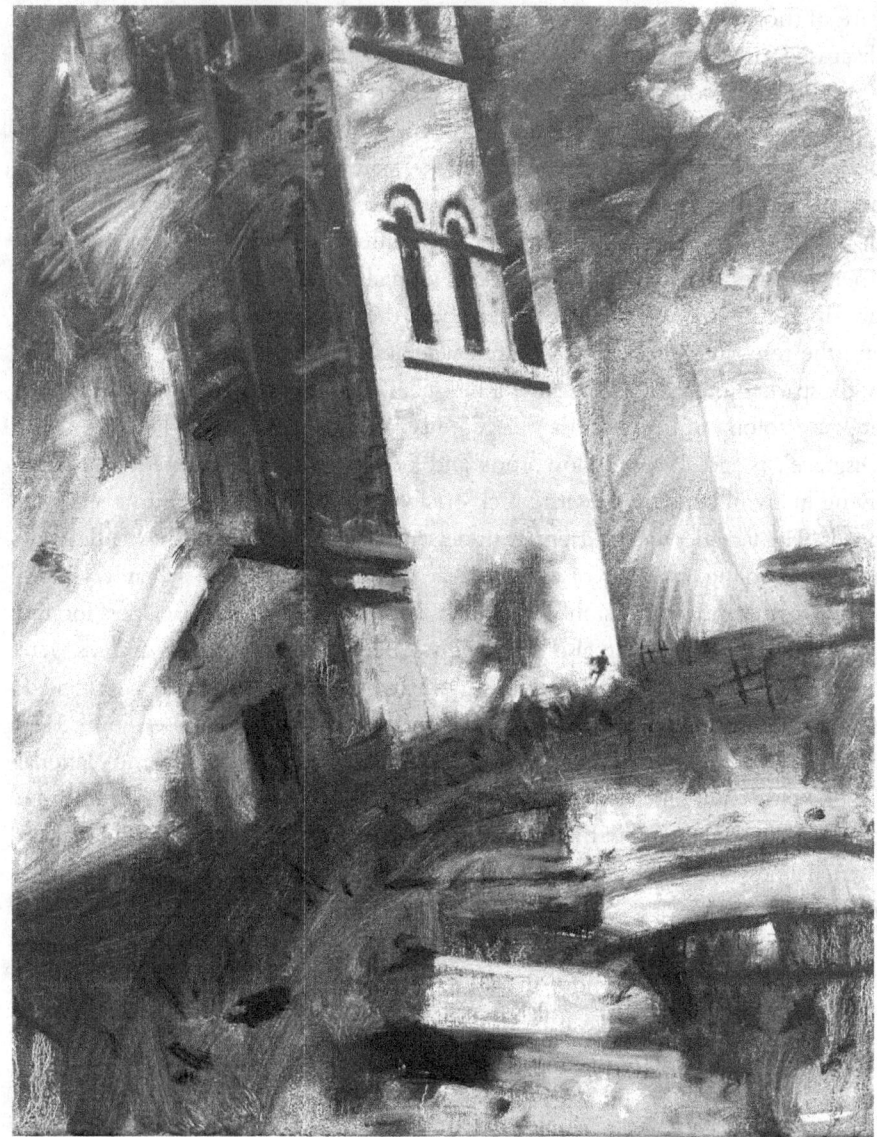

25. 'Fleeing the watertower'. (A painting by David Cobley, 2021)

reflected by Enoch Powell, then Minister of Health, in his notable 'water towers' speech about mental hospitals, delivered in 1961: 'There they stand, isolated, majestic, imperious, brooded over by the gigantic water-tower and chimney combined, rising unmistakable and daunting out of the countryside – the asylums which our forefathers built with such immense solidity to express the notions of their day.'[78] A converse, more understanding and more balanced picture of asylum care was provided by Richard Hunter and Ida Macalpine in

[78] Powell, *Address.*

their history of the Colney Hatch Asylum (later, the Friern Hospital) in North London which opened in 1851 as the largest asylum in Europe: 'Here society's impossibles, victim of the double misfortune of lunacy and pauperism, found asylum whatever the disease that made them so. Its riches were its patients, not its image'. They railed against determining care by the 'old vice of economy' (p.16) and the principle that there should be 'first class establishments for cure and second class for care' (p. 20). They urged for the retention of beds for those too vulnerable to thrive in the community. But theirs was a minority view.[79] Bed numbers rapidly fell in all countries and many large asylums in the Western world were closed down as psychiatry became a largely outpatient and community-based specialty. 'Community care' was the catchphrase, but it was never properly funded by any government. Many of those with epilepsy were transferred into the community, but whether their lives improved is arguable. The epilepsy colonies themselves, as we shall see, did to some extent buck this trend because their inmates with severe epilepsy were still considered to need constant supervision.

In the new philosophies of the 'welfare state', it became accepted that training 'higher-grade defectives' for life in the community was possible and desirable,[80] and in Britain The Disabled Persons (Employment) Act of 1944 obliged local authorities to provide occupation centres for rehabilitation and training. Large companies had to ensure that at least 3% of their workforce comprised disabled persons. The Education Act of 1944 extended special school placement to age sixteen, and in 1945 regulations replaced the term 'mental defective' with 'educationally subnormal' in an effort to lessen stigma. The National Insurance Act of 1946 provided money to assist parents in maintaining subnormal children at home, and the National Health Service Act, which came into effect in 1948, brought the management of mental institutions within the control of the regional health services, in part a well-meaning attempt to lessen stigma, although the success of this endeavour was arguable. Mathew Thomson,[81] for instance, felt that the changes simply strengthened the hand of centralised bureaucracies and of psychiatrists, and lessened that of pressure groups.

A third change was the rise of the anti-psychiatry movement, which gained traction partly in response to the wide application of pharmacological and physical therapies. In Britain, its leaders included R. D. Laing and David Cooper; in the United States, Erving Goffman and Thomas Szasz; and in

---

[79] Hunter was a psychiatrist at Friern Hospital and also at the National Hospital, Queen Square. He recognised the value of asylum care and his history of Colney Hatch ('Psychiatry for the poor') is a useful analysis of the benefits of asylum care. Friern Hospital was finally closed in 1993, and the transitioning from hospital to community care is well described by the historian Professor Barbara Taylor, who had been a patient at Friern ('The last asylum').

[80] O'Connor and Tizard, *The Social Problem*, p. 6.

[81] Thomson, *Problem of Mental Deficiency*, p. 262.

France, Michel Foucault.[82] In their different ways, each challenged the very concept of mental illness and thus the validity of psychiatric therapy. The movement was as much a public statement of liberation from the shackles of a medical model as a theory of mental illness. It was embedded in the growing counterculture movements in Western societies, left-wing politics, and other liberation movements and campaigns. It challenged the authority and power of psychiatrists and saw the physical and pharmacological therapies in psychiatry, and asylum care, as weapons of oppression and coercion. These developments impinged on epilepsy mainly at the margins, although Thomas Szasz (himself a psychiatrist) noted:

> In the initial decades of this century much was learned about epilepsy. As a result, physicians gained better control of the epileptic process (which sometimes results in seizures). The desire to control the disease, however, seems to go hand-in-hand with the desire to control the diseased person. Thus, epileptics were both helped and harmed: they were benefited in so far as their illness was more accurately diagnosed and better treated; they were injured in so far as they, as persons, were stigmatized and socially segregated. Was the placement of epileptics in 'colonies' in their best interests? Or their exclusion from jobs, from driving automobiles, and from entering the United States as immigrants? It has taken decades of work, much of it still unfinished, to undo some of the oppressive social effects of 'medical progress' in epilepsy, and to restore the epileptic to the social status he enjoyed before his disease became so well understood.[83]

Linked to these new directions was the fourth and very significant development for epilepsy in many countries: the rise in the lay patient movement. The establishment of the International Bureau Against Epilepsy (IBE; described later in this chapter) was a direct result of the changing public attitudes to medicine, psychiatry and mental handicap. In all fields of psychiatry, patient groups became more militant, better organised and highly influential – and they engaged in what was in essence a power struggle between the patient (the customer) and the doctor (the provider) in an increasingly consumerist society.[84] For the first time, medical practice in epilepsy was forced to take into account the perspective of patients as expressed by well-informed and well-structured associations.

---

[82] R. D. Laing (1927–89) was a British psychiatrist, whose books *The Divided Self* (1960) and *The Self and Others* (1961) were important tracts for the anti-psychiatry movement. The book *Folie et Déraison: histoire de la folie à l'âge classique* (1961; English translation, *Madness and Civilisation*, 1965) by Michel Foucault (1926–84) is a classic text in the understanding of the meaning of mental disease.

[83] Szasz (*Myth of Mental Illness*) considered mental illness to be a metaphor for human 'problems in living' (p. xi) and that much was feigned as a method of communicating distress (c.f. the concept of non-epileptic seizures today).

[84] In Britain, the National Association for Mental Health (which evolved into the mental health charity MIND in 1972) proved a powerful advocate, especially concerning issues of consent to treatment, patient rights and adequate funding. Two particularly influential figures in the 1970s were its director, Tony Smythe, and its legal director, Lawrence Gostin, who moved later to become Professor of Global Health Law at Georgetown University.

The Organic Psychiatry of Epilepsy

Stimulated by changes in public attitude, social policy and the medicalisation of psychiatric practice, a new specialty arose in the post-war years which came to be known as *neuropsychiatry*.[85] Epileptic psychosis and epileptic behavioural disturbance were central to the work of neuropsychiatrists,[86] and tended to focus around the psychosis and other psychiatric phenomena in temporal lobe epilepsy.

Thinking in this area had evolved from the 1920s. Previously, epilepsy itself was considered a psychosis, and the psychotic and behavioural symptomatology was considered to be intrinsic to the epilepsy spectrum and an integral part of the degenerative process. In the later interwar years, interest grew in the anatomical basis of the primary psychoses, initially focused on the hypothalamus, and then in the 1930s on anatomical systems such as the 'Papez circuit'[87] (proposed by James Papez) underlying emotional responses and a 'baso-lateral circuit' (proposed by Paul Yakovlev) modifying emotions. The combination of these two concepts gave rise to the notion of the limbic system, a term coined by Paul MacLean in 1949, as the 'emotional brain' – an anatomical network which included the mesial temporal lobe structures. Following the influential primate experiments of Heinrich Klüver and Paul Bucy in the late 1930s in which bilateral temporal lobe resections were made, it was soon proposed that 'limbic dysfunction' under-pinned aspects of the emotional disturbances of temporal lobe epilepsy.[88] Most then accepted that the psychosis was an organic physiological phenomenon and not degenerative. This too became a controversial topic. Some believed the

[85] Neuropsychiatry emphases organic and biological mechanisms in preference to psycho-dynamic and social models of disease and psychoanalytical treatment. Neuropsychiatrists take an altogether different approach to the management of mental health symptoms (see Lishman, 'What is neuropsychiatry?'). Francis Walshe, a neurologist who disliked psychiatry and who could always be relied on for a hostile remark, considered neuropsychiatry to be 'like the mule, [which] has neither pride of ancestry nor hope of progeny' (Shorvon and Compston, *Queen Square*, p. 236).

[86] Of course, the fact that epileptic patients could suffer psychotic symptoms had been well recognised long before the era of temporal lobe epilepsy (for reviews, see Gruhle, 'Über den Wahn'; and Slater and Beard, 'Psychosis of epilepsy').
See, for instance, Pond, 'Psychiatric aspects of epilepsy'; Gibbs et al, 'Psychomotor epilepsy'; Pond, 'Psychological disorders'; Hill et al. 'Temporal lobectomy for epilepsy'.

[87] James Papez was a neurologist at Cornell University. The 'Papez circuit' was similar to Broca's 'great limbic lobe', a fact not mentioned by Papez.

[88] Papez, 'Mechanism of emotion'; Yakovlev, 'Neural coordinates in behavior'; MacLean, 'Psychosomatic disease'; Klüver and Bucy, 'Psychic blindness' and 'Temporal lobes in monkeys'. Subsequent work has not led to any firm conclusion about the anatomical basis of epileptic psychosis, a field in which there are many unsubstantiated hypotheses. Paul Bucy qualified in the University of Iowa, did a period of training in Europe at the National Hospital, Queen Square with Gordon Holmes and in Breslau with Otfrid Foerster, and was appointed Professor of Neurosurgery at Northwestern University and then Bowman Gray School of Medicine. He served as president of the World Federation of Neurosurgical Societies between 1957 and 1961.

abnormal behaviours to be the direct consequence of altered physiological function in limbic areas, with others holding the contrary view that they were due to the social consequences of a chronic and highly stigmatised condition. Still others postulated that these problems applied to epilepsy generally, not just temporal lobe epilepsy (by then sometimes called limbic epilepsy).

In 1957, Desmond Pond suggested classifying psychotic symptoms in epilepsy into those associated with seizures (pre-ictal, ictal and post-ictal psychoses) and those with no clear time-locked association with seizures (inter-ictal psychoses).[89] Previous authors (right back to Jackson) had pointed to similar phenomena, but Pond's formulation was simple and clear. His terminology became widely accepted and has provided a useful framework for further investigation. Pre-ictal psychiatric changes were relatively rare and took the form of dysphoria, irritability, anxiety and hyperactivity. Ictal psychosis was characterised in studies which correlated the clinical signs with the concurrent EEG findings,[90] and showing this to be in effect a form of non-convulsive status epilepticus. Post-ictal psychosis − a phenomenon well known to all the nineteenth-century physicians, and sometimes called epileptic mania, furor epilepticus and epileptic delirium − was found to tend to occur after a severe convulsive seizure, or more often a series of convulsive seizures, usually after a 'lucid interval' of up to 24 hours.[91] This form of psychosis was florid, often with visual hallucinations, and associated with overactivity and excitement rather than retardation. It tended to die away after hours or days, and it too was postulated to be in some way related to deep-seated epileptic discharges.

The condition which attracted most interest was the inter-ictal psychosis of temporal lobe epilepsy, the salient features of which were established in the early 1960s, especially through the studies of Pond, Eliot Slater and A. W. Beard.[92] They found that it developed only after the epilepsy had been present for many years (a mean of fourteen years), and was often initially transient and

[89] Pond, 'Psychiatric aspects of epilepsy'. Sir Desmond Pond was a psychiatrist at the Maudsley Hospital in London and the first Professor of Psychiatry at the London Hospital.

[90] The ictal psychoses were clearly delineated in the decades after the introduction of EEG, although nomenclature and classification were confusing. Many cases previously described as 'epileptic twilight states' were now explained as episodes of non-convulsive status epilepticus.

[91] Temkin cites a case reported by the Paracelsian Martin Ruland, in 1580, of a sufferer who regained his strength but not his reason following a seizure and who 'fled to forests, fields, and other places in a state of madness, running this way and that, until his reason was restored and he returned home' (Temkin, *Falling Sickness*, p. 143). Ruland attributed this to witchcraft and others to possession.

[92] Slater and Beard, 'Psychosis of epilepsy'. Eliot Slater was the leading British academic psychiatrist of his time. He trained in London and was awarded a Rockefeller Foundation travelling fellowship to study genetics in Germany, where he did much to help Jewish psychiatrists escape from Nazi persecution. He married Lydia Pasternak, sister of Boris Pasternak, and returned to London to the Maudsley Hospital and the National Hospital, Queen Square.

usually related to bursts of seizures, before becoming permanent and not linked to seizure occurrence. They noted that the symptoms were similar to those of primary schizophrenia, although in the inter-ictal psychosis of epilepsy, cata-tonia was generally less common and loss of affective response less marked. Others erroneously proposed that the inter-ictal psychosis of left temporal lobe epilepsy was likely to be 'schizophreniform' and that of right temporal lobe epilepsy 'depressive'. Early investigators of the inter-ictal psychosis recom-mended temporal lobectomy in the hope that this would remove the psychotic symptoms.[93] However, the practice was soon abandoned when it became clear that the psychosis actually often worsened and that non-psychotic patients with temporal lobe epilepsy were sometimes rendered psychotic by the surgery.

Another, more controversial form of epileptic psychosis was the so-called forced normalisation, described by Hans Landolt in 1958. This was the devel-opment of a psychosis that seemed to occur when 'electroencephalography becomes more normal or entirely normal, as compared with previous and subsequent EEG findings'.[94] As originally described, it was an EEG phenom-enon, but the concept was then extended to the psychoses that occurred when seizures were brought under control. Whether this is a specific phenomenon is doubtful, but it generated a large literature.[95] The mechanisms were (and remain) unknown.

This period was a high point in deterministic neurobiology; and the physical basis of epileptic behavioural disorders attracted the interest of many neuro-psychiatrists. Violence in particular had been repeatedly attributed to epilepsy, an association which had its origins in cultural prejudices and that was, as we have seen, given especial prominence by early criminologists and eugenicists. As the anatomical concept of the limbic system became fashionable, so did the idea that limbic dysfunction caused violent behaviour. In the 1970s, Harvard neurosurgeons Vernon Mark and William Sweet, and the Harvard psychiatrist Frank Ervin set up a 'Violence Unit' at Boston City Hospital, partly in response to the 1967 Detroit riots. With chronically stereotactically implanted elec-trodes, sometimes in place for several months, they had demonstrated epilepti-form EEG changes, and also frank seizures, in the hippocampus or amygdala of epileptic subjects during violent episodes – noting too that recordings from the scalp and surface electrodes were often normal during these periods. They also found that, in both epileptic and non-epileptic individuals, violent behaviour ('loss of control') could be induced by stimulating the amygdala through depth

---

[93] The first 100 patients operated on in the Maudsley series included 12 with a history of psychosis. The acute post-ictal psychosis (two cases) did respond well to surgery if the seizures ceased. However, in only 50% of those with chronic paranoid or schizophrenic psychosis did the psychosis resolve post-operatively (Serafetinides and Falconer, 'Epileptic patients with psychosis').

[94] Landolt, 'Serial EEG investigations'.

[95] Including a book: Trimble and Schmitz, *Alternative Psychoses of Epilepsy*.

electrodes. In 1970, Mark and Ervin published a short book, at the core of which were four case reports claiming excellent effects in controlling violence by amygdalotomy.[96] Julia S was one of the cases. The daughter of a physician, she had developed temporal lobe epilepsy due to encephalitis at the age of 18 months, and was prone to cursive seizures and also rage attacks. She had a history of repeated serious and unprovoked assaults on acquaintances and strangers, and in one of these she stabbed to death a girl who had brushed passed her in a cinema washroom. Norman Geschwind referred her to Vernon Mark, who implanted depth EEG. This showed periods of intermittent epileptic activity in both amygdalae, similar to that at the onset of her seizures, and during such periods Julia tended to exhibit aggression and violent rage. Stimulation of the amygdala also produced the typical symptoms which occurred at the beginning of seizures, and on occasions resulted in her attacking a wall and violently smashing her guitar. A right amygdalotomy was performed and her violence was said to have improved. According to Mark, she became hyperphagic after the operation and lost her musical ability, but her behaviour was improved and she was able to leave the institution and live at home. The surgeons considered this operation a success; however, Julia's nurse reported that after the operation 'she began to deteriorate in front of my eyes … She stopped her wonderful guitar playing. She stopped wanting to engage in long intellectual discussions. She became more and more depressed. Suicidal.'[97] This notwithstanding, Mark's reports started a fashion, and both unilateral or bilateral amygdalotomy then became widely performed worldwide on violent persons with or without epilepsy.[98] The surgery, however, was from the onset highly controversial, and was, according to the state senator Chester Atkins, 'the equivalent of using a sledge hammer to tune a piano'.[99] Julia's experience became a cause célèbre and Mark was accused of turning her into a vegetable. There was then a concerted effort by the psychiatrist Peter Breggin and others to expose what they considered unethical and mutilating neurosurgery. This attracted mounting public concern

[96] Mark and Ervin, *Violence and the Brain*. William Sweet had been a Rhodes Scholar and developed an interest in stereotaxy in Oxford. He developed stereotactic methodology in Chicago and then in Boston, with Vernon Mark as his resident. A recorded discussion in 1989 between Vernon Mark and William Sweet goes into detail about their stereotactic work and their work on aggressive behaviour, and *inter alia* attacking Thomas Szasz and Peter Breggin. They describe the televised event at the Association for Research in Nervous and Mental Disease in the Roosevelt Hotel in 1972 when Vernon Mark was physical and verbally attacked, and also his subsequent law suit (www.youtube.com/watch?v=obWq7d95Mig).

[97] See Baird, 'Mindbending controversy'; Edson, 'A court of last resort'.

[98] An early series, which remained one of the largest, was from Japan (Narabayashi et al., 'Stereotaxic amygdalotomy'). It was said that patients with epilepsy responded better than those without, and Narabayashi also reported that the operation improved co-existing epileptic seizures as well as the behaviour. However, none of the surgeons assessed long-term outcome, and as time passed it became abundantly clear that these operations were often ineffective and sometimes extremely damaging – with some patients ending up institutionalised and totally dependent.

[99] Baird, 'Mindbending controversy'.

(with some student placards declaring 'stop pithing'), and within a decade amygdalotomy had largely fallen from favour.[100]

Stereotactic brain stimulation and recording were one aspect of the strong behaviourist movement in neuropsychiatric practice. Another extreme example was the work of José Delgado, who was appointed Professor of Physiology at Yale in 1950, in John Fulton's department.[101] Delgado devised the 'stimoceiver', a device consisting of depth electrodes which could record and stimulate in ambulant persons via radio waves. In some subjects, stimulation of different points in the amygdala produced dramatic changes in affect and behaviour. Delgado also created a 'chemitrode', which could release drugs into the deep brain structures via implanted electrodes. His experiments were carried out on schizophrenic and epileptic patients, and were highly controversial.[102] Even more so was the work of Robert Galbraith Heath, who in the 1950s carried out a programme of research with depth electrodes implanted into limbic structures of patients with schizophrenia, and some with epilepsy.[103] He found that episodes of violent behaviour coincided with electrical activity in these deep structures, in effect resurrecting the nineteenth-century concept of larval epilepsy.[104] He also undertook controversial experiments with self-stimulation in schizophrenic patients via implanted electrodes in the caudate, septal area, amygdala, thalamus and hypothalamus.[105] From the point of view of epilepsy, his work on the septal areas of the brain is of

---

[100] Frank Ervin and Vernon Mark were subject to malpractice proceedings in 1978/9 as the result of amygdalotomy on Mr Leonard Kille, one of the patients reported in their book, but they won their case. This was the first case involving psychosurgery. Interestingly, Michael Crichton had been a student of Ervin, and his book *The Terminal Man* contains many elements of Julia's case.

[101] Fulton was a highly regarded and widely respected physiologist, and later a medical historian. He studied medicine in Minnesota, and moved to Harvard and then to Oxford as a Rhodes Scholar. He then moved back to Harvard in 1927 and was appointed as the youngest Sterling Professor at Yale and Chair of Physiology in 1930, and Chair of the Yale Department of History and Medicine in 1951. His role in promoting leucotomy has been well described, but his promotion of other forms of physical treatments, including brain stimulation, is a story largely untold.

[102] See Delgado, *Psychocivilized Society*. Delgado contrasted his work with what he considered the illusion of the liberal idea of 'free will'. Delgado was appointed Professor of Psychiatry at Yale, and was singled out in Congress as 'the great apologist for Technological Totalitarianism' ('Statement of C. E. Gallagher', p. 5575). This topic spawned a number of novels, films and TV documentaries, and Delgado's eye for publicity reached its zenith when he was filmed using his stimoceiver to stop a bull charging him in a bull ring in Códoba. (www.discovermagazine.com/mind/the-man-who-fought-a-bull-with-mind-control)

[103] Heath, *Studies in Schizophrenia*. Robert Galbraith Heath founded and was the first Chairman of the Department of Psychiatry and Neurology at Tulane University. It was there that he engaged in his controversial researches. He used his method to 'treat' not only schizophrenia and epilepsy, but also other mental disorders and, notoriously, homosexuality. The ethical basis of Heath's entire oeuvre has been persistently challenged by various groups. See O'Neil et al., 'Dr. Robert G. Heath', and, for a defence of Heath's work, see Frank, *Pleasure Shock*).

[104] Heath, 'Psychosis and epilepsy'.

[105] Bishop, Elder and Heath, 'Intracranial self-stimulation'.

especial interest, and his idea that stimulation in this area can control seizures has been recently explored again.[106] His experimental subjects were drawn partly from black prisoners in Louisiana jails, for whom consent was inadequate, and when public concern over psychosurgery surfaced in the 1970s, this work became viewed as a particularly egregious example of coercive and unacceptable practices in psychiatry.

Fulton, Sweet, Mark and Ervin, Delgado, Heath and the behavioural determinists followed a long tradition in the field of epilepsy that considered the psychiatric symptoms of the condition to be 'biological' and 'organic' – that is, due to physical brain mechanisms relating somehow to the epileptic seizures or the brain damage causing or resulting from the epilepsy. The contrary argument – that the symptoms were the product of social factors such as parental overprotection, school environment, stigma and social rejection – was the position of other more liberal psychiatrists and psychologists. The differing stances reflected of the cultural and philosophical turmoil of the times.[107]

The conclusions of biological determinists raised further issues. If behavioural disturbances were organic, then should the sufferer be considered legally 'responsible'? Furthermore, if spontaneous electrical seizure activity in deep brain structures triggered behavioural changes, then it followed that the behavioural disturbances were as inherent and integral a feature of epilepsy as the seizures themselves. This was, in effect, a return to the late-nineteenth-century conceptualisation of epilepsy as an organic mental disorder. Although not mainstream views in medicine, such ideas continued to influence popular culture and public attitude.

The Psychiatric Effects of Temporal Lobe Surgery

As discussed later in the chapter, it was in this period that temporal lobectomy was pioneered for epilepsy, and, as we shall see, with often striking benefits on seizure reduction. In the general euphoria about this new treatment for seizures, the more perceptive surgical teams also noted changes in behaviour and mood. The early series from the Maudsley Hospital was a paradigmatic example. Their patients, selected as they were from a specialist psychiatric hospital, had a high rate of sometimes severe psychiatric disturbance, as well as epilepsy, prior to surgery. After surgery, despite the fact that no significant change in formal intelligence nor in the Rorschach responses were observed and that seizures were often improved, there were often striking changes in behaviour. Hill described the first 14 patients of Falconer's series. Prior to surgery: 'All but 2 had severe personality disorder showing excessive irritability and a liability to aggressive behaviour. 8 had been dangerously violent, 5 were

---

[106] Takeuchi, 'Stimulation of the medial septum'.
[107] The extreme behavioural determinists were particularly prominent in the United States.

paranoid, 7 had shown severe short-lived depressive episodes and 4 had fairly constant psychotic symptoms.' After surgery, there were improvements in general behaviour in most of the patients. Hill described, for instance: 'A girl of 14 who had been deemed beyond control, broken out of remand homes, smashed windows in hospitals and could only be nursed in the refractory wards of a mental hospital, has returned to live with her parents where she has been now for nine months, to their great satisfaction'. On the other hand, in other patients behaviour deteriorated. The husband of a 43-year-old women reported that

> Although the results of this operation from a physical point of view are a miracle in that she has not had any seizures and her memory for current events is much better than it was and she speaks more fluently, yet from the temperamental point of view I think her condition is poor. Whereas before [the operation] she had explosive periods, they were succeeded by periods of comparative calm and amiability, but now I am afraid her condition is evened out at a constant level of sullenness, depression, quarrelsomeness and abusiveness. She abuses her son on the slightest thing.

Another patient in clear consciousness began to expose himself and to masturbate in front of other patients and nursing staff, as frequently as twenty times a day, although Hill noted that in most of the patients the operation resulted in a reduction of libido. There was no doubt in his mind that temporal lobe surgery was a form of psychosurgery.

D. W. Liddle, the psychiatrist at the Runwell Asylum, found that a temporal lobe EEG focus was present in 50% of his epilepsy patients and that

> whatever their individual outlook on life, depending, of course, on their various personality traits, [they] have in common a restless aggressiveness. They never fully settle to any task, often wanting to start something new before they have completed the job on hand. They work hard but fitfully, are quick to take offence over trivial incidents, and at times are openly hostile for no adequate reason. Following lobectomy they become friendly, concentrate on the job in hand and are able to sit and enjoy life. As one patient remarks 'I feel satisfied and content now'. It is tempting to make a visceral comparison. Before operation they are hungry, restless, asocial, and have their fits, and afterwards they are replete, friendly, and cease to be explosive. In fact, they are changed from carnivora into herbivora.[108]

In this sense, temporal lobectomy was in effect a form of psychosurgery. Caution was needed, and many took the view that pre-existing psychiatric disturbance should be a contraindication to surgery due to the risk of

[108] D. Hill, 'Discussion'; D. W. Liddle, 'Discussion'.

deterioration, and also because of questions of consent. This is an approach still largely adhered to. However, in a paper presented to the American Epilepsy Society in 1972, Murray Falconer disagreed. He reported on more than 250 patients he had operated on using his en bloc technique, in which psychosis and aggression improved.[109] Furthermore, the psychiatrist in Falconer's team, David Taylor, believed that it was the successful control of epilepsy which, by providing a propitious milieu that allowed the individual to mature, was the key factor in resolving aggressive and other psychopathic traits.

During this time, there were various case reports of other psychiatric disturbances occurring after surgery, but none were then, or indeed have been since, subjected to rigorous study.

NEUROLOGY OF EPILEPSY

Specialisation in Medicine and the Rise of Neurology

One of the greatest metamorphoses in post-war medicine was the rapid growth in specialisms, including neurology. So dramatic was this that by 1970, in Western medical systems at least, the care of the majority of those with epilepsy, uncomplicated by behavioural disturbance or mental handicap, had been moved into neurological outpatient settings and out of the psychiatric arena. In part this shift was simply a matter of human resources, as the numbers of neurologists had greatly increased, but perhaps more important were the impact of EEG and the new antiepileptic medications, which placed epilepsy firmly in the camp of organic physicians, and the liberalised attitudes of Western populations who no longer viewed epilepsy as a mental disorder.

Specialisation was entirely predictable, and in many ways inevitable, given the increasingly scientific nature of epilepsy practice, its technologies and its treatment. The downside was the risk of isolation of the specialist from the rest of medicine – and the epileptologist from the rest of neurology. Indeed, as early as 1887, Hughlings Jackson had noted:

> As scientific medical research goes on, there is greater specialization of investigation, just as, in the development of society, there is that continually increasing specialization, called division of labour. This being so, all the more need is there that there should be greater integration, just as along with division of labour there is need for co-operation of labourers.[110]

---

[109] Falconer, 'Reversibility'. In fact, only 15% of Falconer's large series were considered mentally normal prior to surgery; 40% were diagnosed as having psychopathy and 40% had been institutionalised in a mental hospital or prison at some point in their lives.

[110] Cited in Brain, 'Neurology'.

The course of specialisation in neurology varied from country to country. In America, in the 1930s neurology was, as we have seen, in the doldrums, with its utility as a separate specialty doubted by some, but its fortunes were changed radically by the war. Public alarm was voiced at the number of individuals rejected from the draft on the basis of neuropsychiatric disorders: about 4% of all those called up, and about one-third of all those rejected.[111] Furthermore, during the war large numbers of traumatic neurological injuries were sustained by active troops, and better neurological rehabilitation was urgently needed. In the post-war years, neurologically disabled veterans accounted for about 25% of the patients in general hospitals and 10% in psychiatric hospitals. By 1946, 60% of the 74,000 Veterans Administration hospital beds were filled with neuro-psychiatric patients, costing at least $40,000 per bed per year.[112] Neurological services suddenly became an issue of American public policy. It was estimated that 1% of the US population had a disorder which would be appropriately treated by a neurologist, yet even as late as 1950, only 250 physicians in the country claimed to be neurologists. Some states (e.g. Connecticut) and some cities (e.g. Detroit) had no neurologist at all.

The fortunes of the specialty then began to turn around. The number of neurologists started to increase, especially in the medical schools and university hospitals, and a style of practice evolved which was firmly based within a research setting. Similar trends occurred in other medical disciplines, and within a few decades academic physicians in teaching hospitals displaced private practitioners as the most powerful force in the post-war American medical system. By 1966, 69% of all doctors were full-time specialists, compared to 24% in 1940. Medical empires – networks of hospitals, for instance in Chicago, Philadelphia and New York, formed, sucking in funds from the system and leaving rural and inner-city areas and state institutions behind. As Paul Starr observed: 'Gleaming palaces of modern science, replete with the most advanced specialty services, now stood next to neighbourhoods that had been medically abandoned, that had no doctors for everyday needs, and where the most elementary public health and preventive care was frequently unavailable.'[113] By the 1960s this disjunction was all too evident and caused public dissent; it is an inequality that remains to this day.

At the other extreme was Britain, with its strong traditions in general medicine. There, neurological units were much slower to be established, and neurology as a specialty trailed far behind neurosurgery in perceived priority and growth. By the 1960s, in marked contrast to the United States, 70% of British doctors were generalists, and only 30% were in specialty practice. In 1939 there were only 25 neurologists in Britain (19 of whom were in London),

[111] Pols and Oak, *War and Military Mental Health.*
[112] Farreras, 'Establishment of the National Institute'. [113] Starr, *Social Transformation*, p. 363.

a figure which had risen to 60 in 1945, and to only 90 by 1965. Up until this time, much of the burden of neurology was managed by general physicians 'with an interest in neurology', rather than by card-carrying neurologists, and the powerful generalist lobby in the Royal College of Physicians did what it could to inhibit neurology.[114] Before 1965, specialised epilepsy services (of which there were few) still tended to be run by psychiatrists or general physicians, with only a handful of neurologists professing a special interest or practice in epilepsy.

In other European countries, different levels of specialisation emerged. In Germany, for instance, with its tradition of combining the training of psychiatry and neurology into a single entity, most neurologists in the 1930s practised both disciplines, and in a community setting; pure neurology units existed only in the largest university hospitals, a subject of repeated complaint. The first neurological department in Austria was formed only in 1939, and many smaller countries had only a handful of neurologists.

As healthcare systems and medical practice varied from country to country, whether it was a generalist, a psychiatrist or a neurologist who treated epileptic patients in this period depended largely on the interplay between political priority, manpower, finance and lobbying by professional self-interest. It is not possible to fully appreciate how patients with epilepsy fared in different systems, as no comparative figures of outcomes are available.

Albeit slowly, as numbers of neurologists increased, subspecialisation within neurology began in Western countries. Epilepsy was the first to begin to split away to form its own sub-specialty. This was partly due to EEG and the complexity of the new drug therapies – for epilepsy was the first common condition within neurology to have effective specific drug treatments. At the time this development was celebrated, but the isolation that Hughlings Jackson articulated was later to become a pressing issue. Finding the correct balance of generalism, specialism and sub-specialism was then, and remains, one of the central challenges in medicine.

Leading Figures in Clinical Epilepsy

Three figures of this period deserve particular mention: William Lennox, Wilder Penfield and Henri Gastaut. All took epilepsy to new levels in the immediate post-war years, each by specialising almost entirely in epilepsy, exploiting the potential of EEG and, in the case of Lennox and Gastaut, advances in pharmaceutical medicine. If anything, their presence in twentieth-century epilepsy

---

[114] In his comparison of the American and British medical systems, Hollingsworth (in *Political Economy of Medicine*) noted that although the dominant medical paradigms were similar, what differed was the power and influence of pressure groups. This was certainly the case in relation to neurology.

could be considered a vindication not only of specialisation but also of Carlyle's 'great man theory' of history, and each had an enormous impact on the course of epilepsy history.

First to William Lennox, whose earlier biography was covered in the previous chapter. By 1945, Lennox was the undisputed world leader of epilepsy. Living as he did to the age of seventy-four, he helped to fashion many of the post-war theories and concepts of epilepsy. He epitomised the notion of 'can-do', a very American ideal of his time, and his self-confident demeanour must have been a tonic after the exhaustion of war. It was Lennox who, more than any other person, moved the centre of gravity of epilepsy from Europe to the East Coast of the United States. As described earlier, he carried out work on cerebral blood flow and vasculature and on the biochemistry of epilepsy, blind tunnels in the mining for epilepsy gold, and then in EEG, which proved a very rich seam. He also helped define the clinical role of phenytoin and Tridione and the new wave of drug therapies. At the same time, he turned his attention to clinical genetics and opened the field of twin studies in America (pioneered earlier by Rosanoff in America and Klaus Conrad in Germany).[115] Lennox was to some extent lucky, it seems: always in the right place at the right time and surrounded by intelligent and loyal co-workers. Nevertheless, his genius and his importance to epilepsy cannot be overstated, and his enthusiasm and drive rejuvenated the field after the war.

He died just before the publication of his two-volume work on epilepsy that was to be his crowning legacy. *Epilepsy and Related Disorders* (1960) was an extraordinary intellectual achievement and his *vale dictum*. Co-authored with his daughter Margaret,[116] but bearing all the hallmarks of having been written almost entirely by Lennox himself, this book stands as a glorious monument to his work. In my opinion at least, Lennox was the greatest clinical epileptologist of the twentieth century and his book the century's most important epilepsy text.

As an authoritative summary, in thirty chapters, of the contemporaneous knowledge of epilepsy from the medical perspective, *Epilepsy and Related Disorders* has absolutely no equal. Its influence will be apparent in many different aspects of epilepsy in the subsequent pages of this chapter. The title refers back to the book by Gowers of 1886; indeed, only someone with Lennox's self-confidence would compare themselves to Gowers. Lennox's book is perhaps less original, but it is equally comprehensive. In Lennox's words: 'The first volume is concerned with wide orientation, with history, the many manifestations of epilepsy, and its etiology, genetic and acquired. The second volume explores mentality, origin, means of diagnosis and treatment,

---

[115] Rosanoff was a keen eugenicist and Conrad a proponent of Nazi racial hygiene.

[116] Margaret also later confirmed that she should not have allowed her name to be included in the authorship of the book as she had nothing to do with its writing.

and the psychological and social problems involved' (vol. 1, p. x). The seventeen chapters of the first volume take a conventional form, as do the chapters on acquired epilepsy and treatment in the second volume. More unusual are chapters titled 'The doctor and his helpers', 'Epileptics of worth and fame', 'Social-emotional problems that impinge', 'Who cares for the epileptic?' and 'The altitude of things'. In all chapters, the published literature is combined with his rich personal experience, and the resulting text carries enormous authority. Not surprisingly, the book hinges on EEG, a technology which had matured over two decades and that permeated the conceptual structure of Lennox's view of epilepsy.

His clinical classification into five categories and nine subdivisions formed the basis for Henri Gastaut's later ILAE classification. Lennox had himself defined the EEG changes of petit mal, and the 108-page chapter on the 'petit mal triad' is a triumph of acute clinical observation, although it included conditions which nowadays would not be categorised strictly speaking as petit mal. He differentiated cases with 3 Hz spike and wave from those with the EEG signature of slower spike and wave, which he called the petit mal variant and which later became known as Lennox–Gastaut syndrome. Similarly, 95 pages on psychomotor epilepsy constitute a masterful summary of contemporary knowledge. The chapter titled 'Borderlands of epilepsy', covering conditions such as migraine, to which Lennox devoted twenty-five pages, is another concept borrowed from Gowers. The chapter on genetics summarises contemporary knowledge. The chapter on acquired (symptomatic) epilepsy includes most of the known causes of epilepsy and ends with a quote from J. Russell Reynolds to the effect that idiopathic epilepsy should be considered an entirely different entity from acquired and sympathetic epilepsy – a concept with which Lennox evidently agreed.

The chapter on 'The origin of epilepsy' is where Lennox's concepts of the mechanisms of epilepsy are most fully expounded. It is divided into four sections: neuroanatomy, neurophysiology, neurometabolism and neurochemistry. The section on neuroanatomy shows the extent to which electro-clinico-anatomical localisation had now permeated the topic, and there is an instructive table listing the cerebral localisation of seizure phenomena (interestingly, with a question mark as to the localisation of amnesia). The neurophysiology chapter emphasises the interdependent roles of cortical and subcortical structures and the concept of seizure spread. The section on neurometabolism includes a good summary of Lennox's own work on cerebral metabolism and on cerebral blood flow, cerebral metabolism and oxygenation in epilepsy.

Lennox was instrumental in popularising EEG, and perhaps initially overemphasised its potential. Within a decade, the clinical place of EEG in epilepsy had become more clearly understood and the earlier extravagant views of its benefits tempered. Lennox realised this, and in 1960 was able to answer the

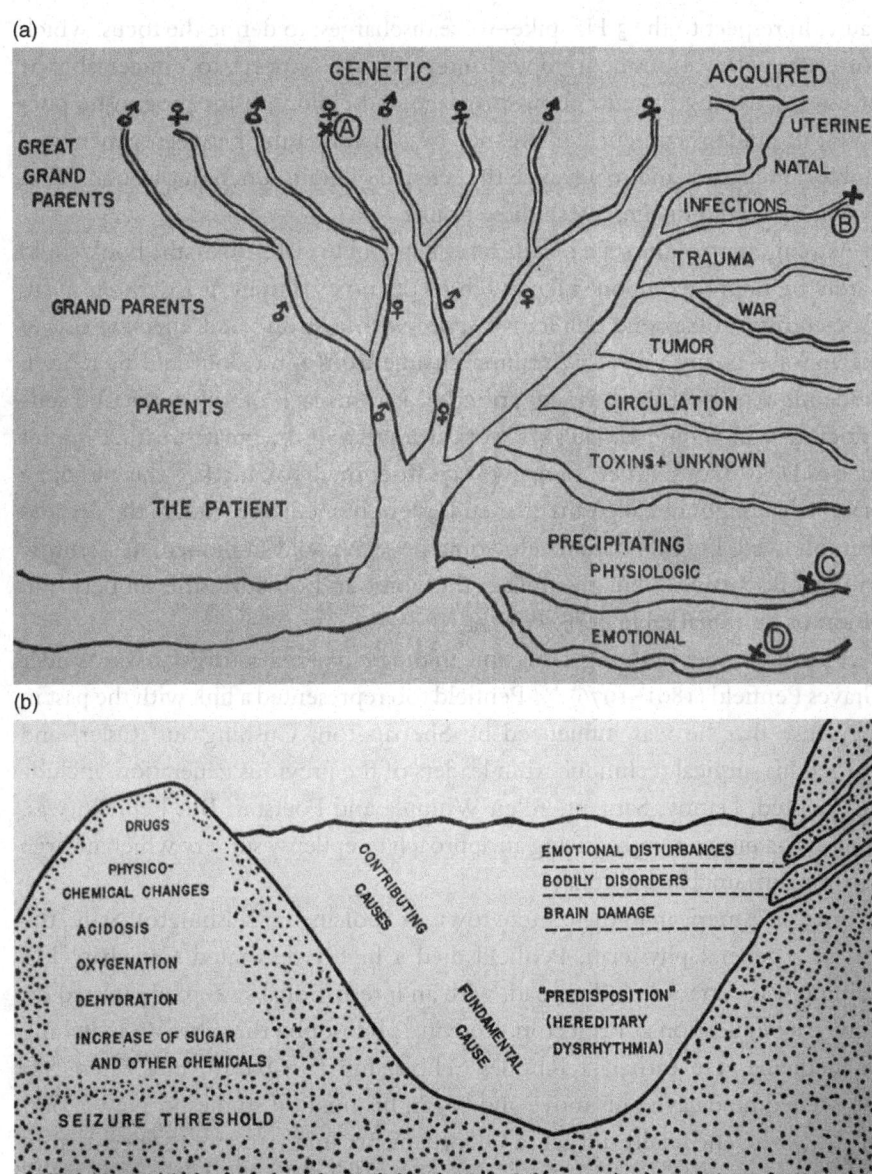

26. The analogy of the river, reservoir and dam. The first illustration conveys the idea of the multifactorial nature of epilepsy, with various streams filling the main 'river' of epilepsy; and the second that of the 'epileptic threshold' – the level at which water flows from the river to the reservoir and is held up by the dam. (From Lennox, *Epilepsy and Related Disorders*).

question 'Of what use is the EEG?' by stating eight ways in which it had clinical value (p.773–9): in diagnosis – he wrote that 75–80% of EEGs made routinely in epilepsy show abnormalities, compared with 15% in the normal population; to define the type of seizure, especially in absence epilepsy; to point to a genetic cause, in respect to the 3 Hz spike–wave discharges; to define the focus, which correlates with various neurological and psychiatric aspects; to 'conceivably be of use in advising patients about marriage and children'; for prognostic purposes; to guide treatment, for instance by differentiating between generalised and focal seizures; and to advance the science of brain function through EEG. Few now would disagree with these points.

As a summary of the state of clinical epilepsy in the late 1950s, the book could hardly be improved upon. Like much of Lennox's output, it is written in his characteristic folksy and alliterative style, with a strong and effective use of metaphor – in my view a refreshing change from most dour and ill-written academic works. If there is one criticism, it is his lack of self-doubt and self-criticism, which differentiates his work from that of the greatest earlier figures such as Jackson or Turner. In many ways, too, the book marked the end of an era of what might be called amateur endeavour in medicine, and, in the decades that followed, Lennox's approach would be seen as old-fashioned, unscientific and too discursive – but this misses the point and obscures the subtlety and vision of his remarkable book.

A second leader of the age, this time in the field of neurosurgery, was Wilder Graves Penfield (1891–1976).[117] Penfield too represented a link with the past in the sense that he was influenced by Sherrington, Cushing and Osler, and learned his surgical technique from leaders of the previous generation, including Halsted, Dandy, Sargent, Allen Whipple and Foerster. But Penfield was, above all, a pioneer, introducing an approach to epilepsy surgery which in large part remains unchanged today.

Born an American in the remote town of Spokane in Washington State, the son of a general physician, Penfield died a highly decorated Canadian. His training was extraordinarily broad, with an international sweep. He started his university education at Princeton, studying philosophy there before switching to medicine. He earned a Rhodes Scholarship to Oxford, but when war intervened he delayed his move and began his medical studies in New York. In 1915, when he finally did get to Oxford, he became a student of Sherrington, who introduced him to neurophysiology, and developed a close friendship with William Osler.[118] He obtained a BA in physiology from Oxford in 1916, and then returned to Johns Hopkins to finish his medical studies, graduating in

---

[117] Penfield's biographical details are well summarised in his own autobiography – *No Man Alone* (1977) – and in his various obituaries, especially that by John Eccles and William Feindel ('Wilder Graves Penfield'). The influences on Penfield's work are well described by Feindel, the third director of the Montreal Neurological Institute (MNI) (Feindel, 'Horsley, Cushing and Penfield'; Preul and Feindel, 'Penfield's surgical technique').

[118] His friendship with Osler had an interesting beginning. In 1916, en route to work at a Red Cross hospital in France, Penfield's ship was torpedoed in the English Channel. He was picked up, injured and clinging to wreckage, and transferred to Oxford, where he convalesced in Osler's house, starting a lifelong association.

1918. After a surgical internship at the Peter Bent Brigham Hospital in Boston, he returned to England on a Beit Fellowship and worked at the National Hospital, Queen Square under the tutelage of Gordon Holmes, J. Godwin Greenfield and Percy Sargent (he wrote his first paper with Sargent). In 1921, Penfield returned to New York and the Columbia-Presbyterian Hospital, where he continued his neurosurgical training, after which he spent six months in Madrid learning neurocytology from Pío del Río-Hortega. On his return to New York, he established a neurocytology laboratory with William Cone, supported by a grant from Mrs Percy Rockefeller. In 1928, Penfield accepted an invitation to move to Montreal to become the first specialist neurosurgeon in Canada. Before taking up the post, he spent a highly influential six-month period with Foerster in Breslau, learning the method of operating under local anaesthesia with electrical stimulation.[119]

Penfield and Cone then moved to Montreal[120] where, with the neurologist Colin Russel, they established a combined Department of Neurology and Neurosurgery at McGill.[121] Finally, after protracted negotiations with the Rockefeller Foundation, Penfield helped found the Montreal Neurological Institute (MNI), which opened its doors in 1934. The MNI was to prove immensely important in the history of epilepsy surgery, and Penfield was its first and greatest director. In 1967 he wrote about the origins of his vision for the 'Institute' and the germination of his ideas about epilepsy surgery and functional anatomy:

> I suppose it was after I realized that a man cannot make the approach to all the frontiers alone. As editor of the handbook [his 1932 cytology text], I saw what teamwork could do. At Oxford when I began to hope that I could made a basic physiological and pathological approach to the human brain, I did not dream how vast the task could be . . . Only a well-selected team of specialists can ever hope to carry out the plan . . . But that is not all . . . Something very exciting has developed. In itself, it deserves and needs a new establishment. Studying the experimental brain wounds, I could see how a surgeon might remove one or more convolutions of the brain cleanly and without producing another scar that would continue to cause epilepsy . . . I heard a rumor of successful work by Otfrid Foerster in Breslau Germany. He was a distinguished neurologist who had not published anything as yet about his surgery. According to the rumor, he admitted

---

[119] The idea of electrical stimulation to identify human brain areas was not new – and in fact was pioneered by Horsley and mentioned in his 1886 paper (see Horsley, 'Advances in the surgery'). In Germany, Fedor Krause introduced the technique later in the 1890s.

[120] And there completed his first major (and monumental) work: Penfield, *Pathology of the Nervous System*.

[121] Colin Russel trained at McGill and Queen Square and became the first neurologist at the Montreal Neurological Institute

epileptic patients to hospital, found the focus of discharge and removed the focus surgically although he had had little training as a surgeon. So in 1928, on the way from New York to Montreal, my wife and I moved our family to Breslau ... We stayed six months. Professor Foerster had operated on twelve patients who were sufferers from epilepsy. The fits were caused in some of the cases by war wounds to the brain. In others, the brain injury had been received at the time of a difficult birth. The patients were alive and grateful after operation. I studied the scars he had removed ... We published those cases together and I have continued such operations with new studies since coming to Montreal ... Foerster and I believe it will be possible, someday, to locate, in the case of more and more epileptics, the place in the brain in which the electric discharge originates, causing the fits ... But here is something else, something even more important: during such operations, which are carried out under local anesthesia, the opportunity presents itself to study the living brain of man as never before in history.[122]

In 1938 he was joined at the MNI by Herbert Jasper, who brought with him the then new technique of EEG. At the MNI, Penfield and his team – especially Jasper, Theodore Erikson[123] and Theodore Rasmussen – developed a new style of physiological epilepsy surgery, with the patient awake, using electrical stimulation and recordings to identify both eloquent areas of the brain and also the epileptic focus. And, at the same time, taking the opportunity of operating on the awake patient to record the clinical effects of cortical stimulation and thus derive maps of *functional anatomy*. This was, of course, an extension of the principle of mapping the human cortex pioneered by Horsley and Ferrier, but Penfield was the first to apply this systematically in an awake human subject and to extend the work to study the effects of stimulation on sensory and intellectual, and not just motor, functions.[124] His most intriguing discoveries were in relation to the temporal lobe, which soon became his main focus. Penfield demonstrated that stimulating the temporal lobe resulted in 'experiential responses', in which the patient reported memories – as of looking in on past experiences – and 'discover[ed] himself on the stage of the past as well as in the audience of the present' (pp. 524, 537). Illusions of déjà vu and familiarity were found when the first temporal convolution of the non-dominant hemisphere was stimulated, and of distance or sound with stimulation of either lobe. Illusions of taste and smell were evoked in the peri-insular regions, and abdominal sensations in the insula itself. Thus, Penfield not only established temporal lobe surgery for epilepsy but also demonstrated the role of the

---

[122] Penfield, *Epic of Alan Gregg*, pp. 248–9. Some criticised this research as being conducted without informed consent.

[123] Theodore Erickson trained in neurosurgery at the Montreal Neurological Institute and then moved to take up the inaugural Chair of Neurosurgery at the University of Wisconsin.

[124] Penfield, 'Temporal lobe seizures', p. 515.

temporal lobe in the mechanism of memory, perception and consciousness. His work was detailed in a series of books,[125] culminating in his landmark works *The Cerebral Cortex of Man*, co-authored with Rasmussen in 1950, and *Epilepsy and the Functional Anatomy of the Human Brain*, co-authored with Jasper in 1954. The former book, based on his Lane Medical Lectures of 1947, described his experience of, by then, around 400 craniotomies carried out under local anaesthetic. The book was concerned with the functional anatomy revealed on cortical stimulation (and resection), and described such aspects as somato-sensory and motor responses; head and eye movement; the autonomic system; vision, speech, hearing and balance; secondary sensory and motor representations; memory and dreams; and sensory perception. Also included were what may have been the first detailed descriptions of illusions, hallucinations and dreamlike conditions produced by temporal lobe stimulation; and therein can be found the origins of Penfield's later work on memory and perception. The age-old question of the site of consciousness was also debated, and he noted that under local anaesthetic, the anterior frontal lobe could be amputated in its entirety under local anaesthetic without the patient experiencing any symptoms nor impairment of consciousness or indeed seemingly without any symptoms at all (p. 226). Penfield and Rasmussen wrote about the subcortical and transcortical projections of the cortex, and they hypothesised about the anatomical basis of consciousness, which Penfield considered to lie in the diencephalon. Much of the book is in the form of case reports, with the anatomy marked out in diagrams and by photographs of numbered markers placed on the surface of the exposed brain – a method devised by Horsley.

Epilepsy and the Functional Anatomy of the Human Brain is perhaps the most important surgical epilepsy book of the twentieth century.[126] It was dedicated to Hughlings Jackson and Charles Sherrington, whose influence on Penfield's thought is clearly evident, and it represented the pinnacle of achievement of his method. The twofold aims of the book were, first, clinical, to provide detailed clinical descriptions of epileptic phenomena arising in different sites of the brain, and, second, scientific, to explore the anatomy and physiology of sensory, motor and psychological functions of the brain (i.e. its 'functional anatomy'). In both aims, the book brilliantly succeeded, and packed into its 896 pages was Penfield's experience of (by then) 750 patients with epilepsy operated

---

[125] Penfield and Erickson, *Epilepsy and Cerebral Localization*; Penfield and Kristiansen, *Epileptic Seizure Patterns*; Penfield and Jasper, *Human Brain*.

[126] The book is in effect a 'revised edition' of the earlier book *Epilepsy and Cerebral Localization* (1941), but significantly extended. The earlier book, 623 pages in length, was based on a smaller number of patients with less extended descriptions and a different joint authorship. The structure and approach, though, were very similar (as was the dedication to Hughlings Jackson and Sherrington). Included was an interesting and original chapter on 'ictus infra-tentorialis', seizures caused by interference with brain stem function, downplayed in the second book.

on under local anaesthesia. Most innovative was his work on the temporal lobe, but other original contributions included his discoveries of the functions of the supplementary motor area, four centres for speech (including two in the supplementary motor area), the second somatic sensory areas and 'suppressor strips' on the lateral aspects of the hemispheres. The immensely detailed descriptions of the anatomical basis of epileptic symptomatology, supplemented by fascinating photographs of different seizure phenomena, set the standard for all subsequent work. With these books, and Penfield's numerous other papers, books and articles,[127] Penfield and the MNI rose to international prominence.[128]

Penfield's interest in the functional anatomy of the temporal lobe initiated a programme of research on the anatomical basis of memory, which he conducted with the psychologist Brenda Milner, who had immigrated to Canada from England in 1944. She was educated at Oxford and recruited to the MNI by Penfield in 1950, where she began working on the memory defects of his patients with temporal lobe epilepsy, completing her PhD at McGill University entitled *The Intellectual Effects of Temporal-Lobe Damage in Man* in 1952. This was the start of their long collaboration.

Prior to their work, the functions of the temporal lobes were essentially unknown. Jackson, on the basis of the celebrated case of 'Dr Z', had surmised in 1888 that '[T]he particular variety of epilepsy' manifested by dreaminess, absence and cognitive symptoms had a temporal lobe origin. It was thereby a demonstration that the temporal lobe was involved in memory and, as Jackson put it:

> He who is faithfully analysing many different cases of epilepsy is doing far more than studying epilepsy. The highest centres ('organ of mind'), those concerned in such fits, represent all, literally all, parts of the body sensorily and motorily, in most complex ways, in most intricate combinations, &c. A careful study of many varieties of epileptic fits is one way of analysing this kind of representation by the 'organ of mind'.[129]

This was exactly what Penfield was engaged in. In the same year, 1888, another early and important investigation was reported by Sanger Brown and Edward Schäfer at University College London. They resected both temporal lobes in monkeys and demonstrated marked changes in behaviour, including loss of aggression, changes in feeding behaviour and loss of intellectual functioning (becoming 'like idiots').[130] Then, in 1900, Vladimir Bekhterev showed that a patient with a severe amnesic syndrome had bilateral mesial temporal lobe

---

[127] More than 300 papers and articles, and 12 other books, covering a wide variety of topics.

[128] There were only a few other surgeons interested in epilepsy at that time, including Bailey, Earl Walker and Green in the United States, and Falconer at the Maudsley Hospital in London.

[129] Jackson, 'On a particular variety'.

[130] Brown and Schäfer, 'Monkey's brain'. See also Vannemreddy and Stone, 'Bilateral temporal lobe ablations'.

destruction, but apart from these isolated examples, very little further work into the functions of the temporal lobe seems to have been carried out until, in the late 1930s, Klüver and Bucy essentially reproduced Brown and Schäfer's findings using more advanced methods of assessment. They showed that bilateral lesions of the medial temporal area in monkeys caused profound changes, including visual agnosia (what they termed 'psychic blindness'), changes to feeding behaviour, taming and loss of aggression, and hypersexual behaviour. This constellation of symptoms became known as Klüver–Bucy syndrome, and, furthermore, as mentioned earlier provided some support for Papez's theories of the anatomy and functions of the limbic system.[131] Following Klüver and Bucy's work, most surgeons – including, for instance, Falconer, Bailey and Penfield – were wary of resecting both temporal lobes.[132] But in the early 1950s, William Beecher Scoville, a neurosurgeon in Hartford, Connecticut, had few such inhibitions. He began to perform bilateral temporal lobe resections, including the removal of the mesial structures, on patients with schizophrenia and in his initial cases there was said to be little change in memory. Then, in 1953, he operated on a patient known as HM (now identified as Henry Molaison), a man of normal intelligence with refractory seizures. As a result of the operation, HM was left with a profound inability to lay down new memories. Milner seized the opportunity of this surgical disaster and extensively studied HM's memory functions. The case formed the basis of the theories of the anatomical basis of memory, which she and Penfield subsequently developed; and HM could be consoled by the recognition that he had become perhaps the most celebrated patient in the world at the time.[133]

Penfield was also an active nosologist, and proposed a classification of epileptic seizures based on clinico-anatomical, aetiological and chronological criteria – a classification which was perhaps superior to any others before his and, indeed, to the roughly contemporary ILAE classification.

---

[131] The Papez circuit comprised: the hippocampal formation connecting to the fornix, then to mammillary bodies, then to the mammillothalamic tract, then to the anterior thalamic nucleus, then to the cingulum, then to the entorhinal cortex and then back to the hippocampal formation.

[132] Penfield later reported one patient in whom he had carried out a unilateral left temporal lobectomy which resulted in profound memory disturbance. Autopsy revealed that the right hippocampus in this patient was also atrophic. In one of the cases reported by Green, Duisberg and McGrath ('Focal epilepsy'), a bilateral temporal lobectomy had been performed without appreciable change, 'except that there is now an increased "hypermetamorphic impulse to action", loss of social consciousness and increased sexual interest – a modification of the results following bilateral temporal lobectomies in monkeys ... His parents feel that the loss of viciousness compensates for the factors mentioned above' (p. 165). In 1957 Kendrick, who was Scoville's assistant in his operation on H. M., reported his results in 24 patients treated with bilateral temporal lobectomy and concluded (belatedly!) that 'Radical bilateral temporal lobectomy should not be performed' (Kendrick and Gibbs, 'Origin, spread and neurosurgical treatment').

[133] See a memoir by Scoville's grandson: Dittrick, *Patient H. M.*

He also had his failures. He had previously worked on cerebral circulation, especially the cerebral vasodilator nerves from the medulla, with Stanley Cobb and with Francis McNaughton. This work culminated in a symposium in New York in 1937, where Penfield hypothesised that an unidentified factor was involved in controlling the circulation in epilepsy.[134] He experimented with bilateral denervation of the autonomic nerves around the carotid arteries as a way of controlling seizures, but this approach proved disastrous and was abandoned. His view that the frontal lobe could be resected without any adverse sequalae, that memory is 'stored' in the temporal lobes, that the central reticular formation 'integrates' memories and cortical function, and his theories of the role of the speech centres and suppressor strips are now also discarded.

His most contentious theory was that of the existence of a centrencephalic system. Penfield defined this as 'that central system within the brain stem which has been, or may be in the future, demonstrated as responsible for integration of the function of the two hemispheres'.[135] In *Epilepsy and the Functional Anatomy of the Human Brain*, he saw this system as the anatomical mechanism linking his theories of consciousness and of 'highest level functions [which] cannot ... be strictly localized, but result from a dynamic interaction between centrencephalic mechanisms and those areas of cortex the function of which is momentarily being employed at a given time'.[136] In his view, the centrencephalic system helped explain the mechanism of consciousness, the impairment of consciousness during epileptic seizures and the amnesia caused by bilateral temporal lobectomy. He considered this to be the anatomical structure underpinning petit mal and grand mal seizures, and to explain loss of consciousness in secondary generalised seizures spreading from cortical foci in the anterior frontal regions. Penfield had earlier proposed that the centrencephalic system 'lies not in the new brain but in the old – that it lies below the cerebral cortex and above the midbrain'.[137] Later, he placed it in 'parts of diencephalon, midbrain and pons'.[138] As its function was to integrate higher mental functioning, it was in effect the seat of consciousness. According to Jasper, this notion was

> one of Wilder Penfield's most stimulating legacies to neurology and the neurological sciences. As a working hypothesis it has challenged leading clinical neurologists, neurosurgeons and many experimental neuroscientists throughout the world. It has also had an important impact on neuropsychology and neuropsychiatry, as well as on philosophic discussions of the nature of the mind. In the field of epilepsy the designation 'centrencephalic seizures' motivated research in leading laboratories throughout the world.[139]

[134] Cobb et al., *Brain and Spinal Cord*.   [135] Penfield, 'Epileptic automatism'.
[136] Penfield and Jasper, *Human Brain*, p. 482.
[137] Penfield, 'Cerebral cortex and consciousness'.
[138] Penfield, 'Mechanisms of voluntary movement'.
[139] Jasper, 'Centrencephalic system'.

This was over-laudatory, and the theory had numerous critics. Francis Walshe, who had by then become Penfield's implacable enemy, violently objected to the idea and scorned the lack of evidence evinced in its favour.[140] In a paper in *Brain* (a journal of which he had been the editor), he devoted twenty pages to demolishing the theory and concluded, '[A]s we read it we find ourselves back in the intellectual climate of mid-nineteenth century pre-Jacksonian imaginings'. Moreover, in relation to consciousness, '[t]he cerebral cortex, of course, could not be wholly ignored, but it is perhaps not unfair to say it has been stretched upon the Procrustean bed of a preconceived centrencephalic system, so that we scarce can recognize it'.[141] Walshe's authority damaged the theory's credibility, but it did not disappear. The pendulum of opinion then swung in favour of the cortex being responsible for consciousness, and there it has remained.

Penfield made another contribution, for which he is most publicly remembered. With the help of his student Edwin Boldrey, his coup was the construction of a visual diagram of the motor and sensory areas of the brain (with findings similar to those of many other investigators, including Horsley and Ferrier) which he displayed as a 'homunculus'.[142] This 'little man' caught the imagination of the public, the press and the profession alike, although the map frankly added only incrementally to others developed over the previous fifty years. What Penfield's homunculus did do was provide an intriguing image in which the size of the areas of cortical representation correlated well with the sensitivity and dexterity of that body part – for instance, with large areas involved with the tongue, mouth, fingers and genitalia. Many, not least Walshe, heavily criticised the device on grounds of inaccuracy, simplification and opportunism,[143] but the 'little man' has remained embedded in the public consciousness ever since.

---

[140] In a hostile exchange of letters with Penfield, Walshe wrote: '[The centrencephalic system] has never had a sure morphological foundation, and in effect you have dropped a unbodied hypothesis, like a cuckoo's egg, into Magoun's reticular activating nest – which is very hard upon his little family of ideas growing innocently therein, and not at all wanting this preposterous foundling foisted upon them' (Feindel and Leblanc, *Wounded Brain Healed*, p. 267).

[141] Walshe, 'Brain-stem'.

[142] Penfield and Boldrey, 'Electrical stimulation'. The homunculus was drawn by Mrs Hortense Cantlie (see Gandhoke et al., 'Edwin Boldrey'). Boldrey held a visiting residency with Penfield (1935–9).

[143] The most strident criticism came from Francis Walshe, whose vituperative attacks on Penfield exceeded the bounds of decency. About the homunculus he wrote, 'Of course, I have had many a laugh at your homunculi, anyone brought up on "Alice through the looking glass," and knowing his Jabberwocky, could not refrain from finding them funny, and still funnier when you try to explain away their defects – and yet keep and breed them. Are you really unable to see that they have an element of the ridiculous?' (Gandhoke et al., 'Edwin Boldrey').

The third leading epilepsy doctor in these post-war years was the French neurologist Henri Jean Pascal Gastaut, a remarkable figure who occupied a dominant place in the medical history of epilepsy for more than thirty years.[144] Born in Monaco to a family of modest means, Gastaut was an indifferent student who dabbled in banking and politics before embarking on medical studies in Marseille. A turning point in his life was the six months he spent in Bristol in 1946 studying with W. Grey Walter, whom he considered his lifelong mentor. He was fascinated by Walter's intelligence (as many were) and his originality. Walter, who had visited Hans Berger and had built his own EEG machine, taught Gastaut the basics of EEG and inspired his attachment to the technology. On his return to France, Gastaut grew a beard, said to be the result of a bet made with Antoine Rémond, traded his motorbike for a car and set up a small EEG laboratory at the Timone Hospital using a small, four-channel Grass machine. In 1949, he enjoyed a three-month sabbatical at the MNI with Penfield and Jasper, and was brought up to speed on the techniques of epilepsy surgery. With the aid of a Rockefeller Foundation grant, he began a research programme which culminated in 1961 in an INSERM unit in neuro-biology. In 1953, Gastaut became head of the Neurobiological Laboratories at the Marseille Hospital and created the Centre Saint-Paul to treat epileptic children. In 1967, he was elected dean of the medical school in Marseille, a post which involved dealing with the student unrest of 1968 (the epitome of countercultural power), and in 1971 was made president of the new University of Aix-Marseille. In 1984, he created the Institute of Neurological Research, co-sponsored by the World Health Organization (WHO). Gastaut won many awards and prizes, including corresponding membership of the Académie Française de Médecine, and election as Commandeur of the Ordre National du Mérite, as Commandeur of the Ordre des Palmes Académiques and as an officer of the Légion d'Honneur (he was promoted to Commandeur the day before he died).

Gastaut was a consummate 'fixer' who used his genius for organisation, politics and administration, and his unending energy, to promote the 'international epilepsy movement'. In the process, he also pretty well single-handedly resusci-tated French epileptology, which in the nineteenth century had had a distin-guished record but which in the first three decades of the twentieth century was largely dormant.[145] He was a founding member of the French EEG society in 1948, and played a major organising role in the second International Congress of EEG in Paris in 1949, at which the International Federation of Societies for

---

[144] For details from the various tributes by his students, see, for instance: Naquet, 'In memoriam Henri Gastaut'; Dravet and Roger, 'Henri Gastaut 1915–1995'; M. A. Lennox, 'Professor Gastaut's contribution'.

[145] One neurologist with a truly international reputation for his epilepsy work was Jean Abadie in Bordeaux.

Electroencephalography and Clinical Neurophysiology (IFSECN) was founded. Gastaut was appointed secretary (1949–61) of the IFSECN, and then president (1961–9). According to Charlotte Dravet and Joseph Roger, it was at the instigation of Lennox that he founded the French chapter of the ILAE in 1949.

Gastaut used the ILAE as a vehicle for his activities. In doing so, he elevated the profile of what was essentially then a small and insignificant organisation, and one in the shadow of the IFSECN, to a major force in international epilepsy. As organiser of the 1949 IFSECN conference held jointly with the fourth World Neurology Congress in Paris, he proposed that the ILAE should be a partner organisation and hold its quadrennial meeting at the same location just before or after the main meeting. He thus established a pattern of joint congresses with that organisation which continued until 1985, by which time the ILAE was financially strong enough to hold independent congresses. He was chair of the 1953 congress in Lisbon on temporal lobe epilepsy, and thereafter was appointed ILAE president-elect (at the young age of thirty-eight). However, as he was already president of the IFSECN, he took up the ILAE secretary-general position instead and became president in 1969. He was present at the 1957 ILAE meeting in Brussels, held in conjunction with the international societies of neurology, electroencephalography, neuropathology, neuroradiology and neurosurgery, and billed as the First Congrès International des Sciences Neurologiques (the word 'science' was said to have been added to appease the neurosurgeons, who felt marginalised). This was an exceptional meeting as it marked the centenary of the births of Sherrington, Horsley and Babinski.[146] A medal was struck in their honour. At this event, the World Federation of Neurology (WFN) and the World Federation of Neurosurgical Societies (WFNS) were founded and, due to Gastaut's astute manoeuvring, the ILAE was now supping at the top table. Earl Walker, then ILAE president, noted with satisfaction that 'the [ILAE] has been given a very favourable spot in the programme: It has been assigned the first morning (Sunday) for its symposium [on temporal lobe epilepsy] ... This will enable the League to hold a meeting without competition from any other society, and should promote considerable interest in its activities'.[147] Gastaut led the discussion on the

---

[146] For neurology, 1857 was indeed a vintage year.

[147] Walker, 'The president's report', p. 109. At the 1957 meeting, Walker gave a lecture on operations for extrapyramidal syndromes in the neurosurgical section, and Penfield and Walshe sparred over the centrencephalic system. The proceedings of the entire conference were published in a 704-page volume (van Bogaert and Radermecker, First International Congress). The anonymous review in Brain, though, was not favourable: 'This volume which contains papers given at the combined meeting with the Fourth International Congress of Electroencephalography and Clinical Neurophysiology, and the Eighth Meeting of the International League Against Epilepsy seems the ultimate condemnation of giant congresses. The editors have done their best, but the large volume contains a tedium of abstracts in several languages. Facts are buried in an expensive mass grave, their epitaphs the one minute index which occupies less than three of the 700 pages.' ('Shorter Notices').

anatomy of temporal lobe epilepsy; Macdonald Critchley on the classification
of the epilepsies; and Frederic Gibbs on the changes of EEG with age.

Between 1950 and 1980, Gastaut also organised 25 meetings, known universally as *Les Colloques de Marseille*. Each attracted 300–500 participants, and
the series established Marseille as an internationally important centre of epilepsy
work, elevating French epileptology. The 1958 colloquium took place in
Moscow, and there Gastaut launched the idea of the International Brain
Research Organization (IBRO), which at its foundation remained closely
associated with EEG and neurophysiology.[148]

Gastaut's major clinical contributions depended on EEG, and over forty years,
from 1947, he made a series of definitive clinical-EEG correlations that comprised the core of the 1969 ILAE classification of epileptic seizures. Although the
clinical features of generalised seizures were by then well known, he added the
ictal and inter-ictal EEG features and subdivided generalised seizures into tonic–
clonic seizures, tonic seizures, atonic seizures and atypical absence seizures. He
also described the syndrome of generalised epilepsy that now bears his name:
Lennox–Gastaut syndrome. He was one of the pioneers in clinically defining
subtypes of temporal lobe seizures and photosensitivity and startle epilepsy. He
coined the term 'hemiconvulsion-hemiplegia-epilepsy (HHE) syndrome' and
defined the features of benign partial epilepsy of childhood with occipital spikes
(a syndrome which also carries his name). He described mu rhythm, lambda
waves and posterior theta rhythms. He also studied the EEG of syncope, and
various non-epileptic behaviours of sleep, such as night terrors and sleepwalking,
as well as EEG findings in different personality types.

In April 1975, he worked on the first computed tomography (CT) scanner in
France, installed at the Timone Hospital; and this technology stimulated his
interest and passion in the same way that had EEG. He presented his first results
on 500 epilepsy patients in September 1975 at the 21st Colloque de Marseille.
This and the subsequent meeting were devoted to the topic. He was also one of
the first to explore the clinical uses of benzodiazepine drugs, especially in status
epilepticus. Over a nineteen-year period he tried out twenty-one different
benzodiazepine drugs, and in the latter years was an advocate for clobazam in
particular. The 16th colloquium (1968) was in part dedicated to the problem of
epilepsy in Africa, the first international conference devoted to epilepsy in
developing countries.

Gastaut had an infectious enthusiasm which led him to hog the limelight. This
tendency was sometimes interpreted as bullying, and, whatever anyone else
thought, he had a knack of always getting his own way. He had a quick temper

---

[148] See Marshall et al., 'Early history of IBRO'; Lichterman, 'The Moscow Colloquium'. The
Colloques de Marseille were one example of Gastaut's genius in the organising international
meetings and in influencing clinical science internationally.

and could be 'frank'. As Robert (Bobby) Naquet put it, he would have 'received more honors from his peers if his very Mediterranean and "unusual" personality had not frightened more than one person in the Capital'.[149] Nevertheless, he was a superb teacher and trained a whole generation of epileptologists, mainly French-, Italian- and Spanish-speaking, who were devoted to his memory. French epileptology rose into prominence due to his efforts, and many of his students subsequently came to occupy positions of importance nationally and internationally.[150] Whilst the epicentres of epilepsy remained in Boston and Montreal, by 1970 its main European outpost was Marseille, and justly so.

The ILAE Classifications of epileptic seizures and of the epilepsies[151]

The introduction of EEG into epilepsy practice had one further far-reaching effect – the renewal of the classification first of 'epileptic seizures' and then of 'the epilepsies'. Since the time of Jackson, classification in epilepsy had been based on the clinical appearance of seizures ('seizure type') and had not changed in any fundamental way for eighty years. EEG opened a Pandora's box and raised the possibility of introducing physiology into what was previously only a clinical classification.[152] This seemingly more scientific approach proved irresistible and stimulated considerable activity in the field of classification. Important contributions were made, incorporating EEG, by Charles Symonds (the leading British clinical neurologist of the time), Francis McNaughton (ILAE president from 1961 to 1965) (Table 3.5), Richard Masland (director of the NINDS from 1958 to 1968, President of the WFN from 1981 to 1989 and of the IBE), and jointly by Penfield and Jasper.[153]

Gastaut got into the act with his proposal to create 'an international classification', as he put it, to provide a uniform system and to standardise communications worldwide. The process he adopted was fascinating. He drafted a classification scheme himself and then gathered 120 leading figures to a meeting in Marseille on 1–2 April 1964. They debated his scheme intensively for two

---

[149] Naquet, 'In memoriam Henri Gastaut'.
[150] Robert Naquet recounted that when, as a young researcher, he told Gastaut that he wished to be independent, it put a chill on their relations. Gastaut could, however, be equally contrite, and many are the tales of him taking people to the opera or to dinner by way of apology.
[151] Details in this section are largely taken from my work elsewhere (Shorvon, 'Definition (terminology) and classification'; Weiss and Shorvon, 'International League Against Epilepsy'.
[152] The first attempt to do this was probably that of Herbert Jasper and John Kershman ('Electroencephalographic classification'), recognising that generalised and focal epilepsies could be distinguished electrographically. This distinction was the basis of all future electroclinical classification schemes.
[153] Symonds, 'Classification of the epilepsies'; McNaughton, 'Classification of the epilepsies'; Masland, 'Classification of the epilepsies'; Penfield and Jasper, *Human Brain*.

TABLE 3.5 *The classification scheme of Sir Charles Symonds in 1955: A pre-ILAE scheme*

	Clinical	Anatomical	Physiological	Pathological	Therapeutic
Central epilepsy	Major –generalised Minimal (a) lapses (b) jerks	Central	Bilateral synchronous, symmetrical EEG discharge	Idiopathic (genetic)	– Dione- responsive
Partial epilepsy	Variable, focal onset depending on location	Variable focal	Focal EEG abnormality	Anatomical lesion present	Phenobarbitone, diphenyhydantoin

An example of advanced neurological opinion prior to the ILAE classification schemes. (From Symonds, 'Classification of the epilepsies').

days, by the end of which exhaustion had thoroughly set in and Gastaut had his way. A crucial aspect of the meeting, and part of Gastaut's genius, was the use of actual EEG recordings linked to films of seizures. Gastaut must have been the first (or at least one of the first) to use filming techniques for seizure categorisation, and the classification was based on genuine source material in a way not previously attempted. After a further two days, a new draft materialised,[154] very similar to Gastaut's original, which was then submitted to a newly formed Commission on Terminology consisting of representatives of the American and European branches of the ILAE, the WFN and the IFSECN. This commission met in May 1964 in Heemstede, and Gastaut also published the draft in *Epilepsia*.[155] A personal copy was sent to all neurologists who were members of a national neurological society, and it seems that Gastaut received 170 comments. The draft was then debated at the quadrennial ILAE Congress in Vienna in 1965 and sent back to the commission with various comments before being debated at the ILAE executive meeting in 1967. A shortened summary form of the classification was also published at the end of the 1964 version, but Gastaut disliked this formulation and he suppressed it from later versions (it was, however, simple to use and was rapidly adopted outside specialist epilepsy practice). The final classification scheme was published in 1969 in a supplement to *Epilepsia* as part of the programme of the 1969 New York conference, and then republished in an identical form in *Epilepsia* in 1970.[156] Despite his protestations of wide consultation, Gastaut accepted few amendments to his

---

[154] It is doubtful, from a comparison of the two documents, that Gastaut took much notice of the discussion or points made by the other participants; one suspects that their presence at the meeting was engineered largely to validate his scheme. The Spanish neurologists Luis Oller-Daurella and Luis Oller Ferrer-Vidal commented that there was resistance to the classification scheme which came from 'the Anglo-Saxon countries (especially the USA) and, above all, in Germany' (Olle-Daurella and Oller Ferrer-Vidal, 'Considerations').

[155] Gastaut et al., 'Classification of epileptic seizures' (1964).

[156] Gastaut, 'Classification of epileptic seizures' (1969, 1970).

1964 draft and the 1969 version proved very similar in form and content.[157] Intransigence was one of his hallmarks, and he had bulldozed the classification through in his inimitable fashion, against considerable opposition. At the quadrennial ILAE Congress in New York in 1969, the classification was discussed but does not seem to have been formally approved. Despite the lack of formal recognition, the tagging of the classification with the ILAE name was a publicity coup for the organisation. Indeed, by this single act the ILAE became synonymous with professional authority in epilepsy. This action, more than any other, moved the organisation into the top position in the world of epilepsy, and for this Gastaut must take the lion's share of the credit. Gastaut also produced a dictionary of epilepsy based on this work, which was published by the WHO in 1973, and which again remained the standard dictionary for the rest of the century.[158]

In the 1969/1970 classification scheme (Table 3.6), seizures were defined according to six axes (Gastaut called these 'criteria'): clinical signs, ictal EEG, inter-ictal EEG, anatomy, aetiology and age. In this regard, the ILAE classification was similar to Charles Symonds's classification structure with his five axes: clinical, pathological, anatomical, physiological and therapeutic. The seizures were subdivided into two fundamental groups in both schemes: partial and generalised seizures in Gastaut's, and partial and central in Symonds's. Partial seizures were defined by Gastaut as

> [s]eizures in which the first clinical changes indicate activation of an anatomical and/or functional system of neurones limited to a part of a single hemisphere; in which the inconsistently present electrographic seizure patterns are restricted, at least at their onset, to one region of the scalp (the area corresponding to the cortical representation of the system involved); and in which the initial neuronal discharge usually originates in a narrowly limited or even quite diffuse cortical (the most accessible and vulnerable) part of such a system.[159]

The partial seizure category also included secondarily generalised seizures, which could evolve from either elementary (simple) or complex symptomatology. The generalised seizures could be symmetrical or asymmetrical, tonic or clonic, but were most often tonic–clonic in type. Generalised seizures were defined in Gastaut's scheme as

---

[157] The main differences between the 1964 and the final 1969/1970 versions were changes to the terminology of absence seizures, the inclusion in 1969/1970 of infantile spasms as a generalised seizure type, the absence/presence of alteration of consciousness mentioned with simple/complex partial seizures and the exclusion of the 1964 categories of erratic neonatal seizures.

[158] Gastaut, *Dictionary of Epilepsy*. This work contained more than 700 terms. Part 2 was to be a multilingual index giving the equivalent terms in the different languages, but never seems to have been completed.

[159] Gastaut, 'Classification of epileptic seizures' (1970), pp. 108–9.

TABLE 3.6 *Summary form of ILAE 1964 classification of epileptic seizures*

---

1. Partial seizures or seizures beginning locally
  A. With elementary symptomatology (motor, sensory or autonomic symptoms);
  B. With complex symptomatology (automatism, ideational, psychosensory, psychomotor, etc., symptoms);
  C. Generalised seizures with local onset. (N.B. All partial seizures can develop into generalised seizures, sometimes so rapidly that the local features may not be observable.)
2. Generalised seizures or seizures without local onset
  A. Absences of differing form and duration, including 'absence status'. Absences may occur alone, or in combination with myoclonic jerks, or with increase or loss of postural tone, or with automatisms.
  B. Generalised convulsive seizures, in the form of tonic, clonic, tonic-clonic and/or myoclonic attacks.
3. Unilateral or predominantly unilateral seizures (tonic and/or clonic) in children
4. Erratic seizures in newborn
5. Unclassified seizures

> [s]eizures in which the clinical features do not include any sign or symptom referable to an anatomical and/or functional system localized in one hemisphere, and usually consist of initial impairment of consciousness, motor changes which are generalized or at least bilateral and more or less symmetrical and may be accompanied by an 'en masse' autonomic discharge; in which the electroencephalographic patterns from the start are bilateral, grossly synchronous and symmetrical over the two hemispheres; and in which the responsible neuronal discharge takes place, if not throughout the entire grey matter, then at least in the greater part of it and simultaneously on both sides.

This binary subdivision had originated in the nineteenth century, and the same pattern was followed in the earlier schemes of Symonds, McNaughton[160] and Masland. The classification published by Penfield and Jasper was, not surprisingly, much more surgical, and was based on three parameters: first, and most importantly, a detailed consideration of the clinico-anatomical and electrographic features of seizures; second, aetiology; and third, chronology. The anatomical aspects of seizure discharges were downplayed in Gastaut's scheme, but formed the basis of later classifications, notably those of Hans Lüders. Anatomical schemes are based on the premise that in partial seizures, there is a highly localised focus, but it was Gastaut's insight to point out that in fact there was often a quite diffuse system (a network) involving wide interconnected areas of cortex and deep grey matter underpinning many partial seizures. Because of this, he deliberately rejected the term 'focal', referring to 'partial' as a

---

[160] Francis McNaughton studied medicine at McGill, then Queen Square, then moved to Harvard, and in 1957 was appointed Chair of Neurology at Montreal Neurological Institute.

sign that the concept of a highly localised focus was for many seizures illusory – a distinction now regrettably lost again, as we shall see, in the later ILAE revisions.

Soon after drafting his seizure type classification, Gastaut turned his attention to an altogether more original work: a 'classification of the epilepsies'. In July 1968, no doubt at Gastaut's instigation, the WHO formally asked its experts working on the dictionary of epilepsy to also produce a classification of epilepsy to accompany the classification of seizures. Gastaut asked the ILAE Commission on Terminology to take on this task, as he had done for the classification of seizures, in time for the New York congress in September 1969. This was a nominal request only, for Gastaut had in fact produced a first draft which he circulated in August and November 1968 to the ILAE Commission members and a WHO/IFSECN expert panel. The timescale was ridiculously short, and he again tried to steamroll his classification through. But on this occasion he ran into significant opposition which he failed to overcome. One-third of the members he consulted approved the classification (albeit with reservations), one-third objected to the draft and one-third did not respond. Time was running out, and Gastaut decided to submit his own draft to the New York meeting.[161] It is fairly clear that there was much contention behind the scenes. A week before the meeting, Jerome Merlis, then president of the ILAE, convened and chaired his own International Commission for Classification of the Epilepsies, with members from the WFN, the World Federation of Neurological Societies (WFNS) and the ILAE (including Masland and Gastaut, who were both present). A draft report[162] was produced and presented alongside Gastaut's draft to the New York General Assembly. Bizarrely, a third classification scheme[163] was also produced, by Masland, despite his being a member of the WHO panel and also on Merlis's commission. Gastaut absented himself from the New York congress despite the fact that he was secretary-general at the time, due, as reported by Merlis, to his urgent duties as rector of the University of Marseille. What actually transpired between Merlis, Masland and Gastaut is not recorded, but the ILAE General Assembly was described as 'lively'.[164] In fact, perhaps not surprisingly, no further progress seems to have been made. One suspects there must have been a sense of bitterness and fatigue, for no new efforts were made to produce a classification of the epilepsies for the next ten years.

Both Merlis and Gastaut's schemes were similar, varying mainly in the criteria (axes) used in classification, and both were very similar in structure and conception to that of the classification of epileptic seizures. Terminology was also shared, but with different meanings. Thus, the word 'primary' was

[161] Gastaut, 'Classification of the epilepsies'. [162] Merlis, 'Proposal'.
[163] Masland, 'Comments'. [164] Gastaut, 'Classification of the epilepsies'.

used to refer both to aetiology and to the absence of a focal onset in generalised seizures; the term 'secondarily generalised' applied to seizures, and 'secondary generalised' to epilepsies (this caused confusion then, and still does). Masland's formulation was somewhat different and, from today's perspective, is superior in my view to the other two systems. He collected together all the terms used for 'epilepsy' that were mentioned in the WHO glossary, and attempted to categorise these under four main headings: aetiology, physiology (his term for seizure type/EEG), anatomy and age/precipitant/modifying conditions. Aetiology was subdivided into combined generalised epilepsy (in effect, primary generalised epilepsy), unknown, metabolic and organic. Seizure type/ EEG was divided into generalised from onset, partial from the start, erratic and unilateral. Anatomy was divided into centrencephalic, multiple or diffuse, and partial. Predisposing conditions were divided into age, circadian, relation to female hormonal cycle and reflex epilepsy. Sadly, this classification seems never to have been seriously further discussed.

This raises another issue. Masland had, in 1960, recommended that the term *epilepsy* be 'stricken from the statutes' on the basis that it was not a useful entity given its varied aetiologies and physiologies. Gastaut strongly disagreed, and was a formidable opponent, but similar conclusions had been reached by others both before and since (including, for instance, Wilson, Penrose, Cobb and Myerson). In my view this is a viewpoint that has much force, and is taken up again at the end of this book.

Temporal Lobe Epilepsy

According to the MRC's annual report for 1952, clinical research had to go 'beyond the stage of observation and description of syndromes' and should engage with 'planned investigations of illness'.[165] Yet the former remained the main preoccupation of academic work in clinical epilepsy, hypnotised as it seemed to be by classification and terminology. Defining categories of epilepsy by correlating the clinical features with electrographic patterns, which was Gastaut's particular strength, remained a major thrust of work in epilepsy in the post-war decades.

A number of forms of epilepsy were differentiated using this paradigm. By far the most important new type to be defined in this period was *temporal lobe epilepsy*, an entity which soon assumed a position at the heart of clinical epileptology. It was a topic unwrapped by EEG. Furthermore, by utilising the electro-clinical approach, it was a type of epilepsy which became, and which has remained, the principal neurosurgical target in epilepsy.

That epilepsy could arise in the temporal lobe had been, like so much else, first recognised by Hughlings Jackson in his case report of 'Dr Z', and Jackson

---

[165] Timmerman, 'Clinical research', p. 232.

surmised that this 'particular variety of epilepsy', with dreaminess, absence and cognitive symptoms, had a temporal lobe origin.[166] This concept seemed then to have been largely forgotten until Stauder's publication in 1935 in which he listed symptoms which he attributed to seizures in the temporal lobe (see p. 208). By 1937 Gibbs and Lennox had proposed the name 'psychomotor epilepsy' to refer to this symptom-complex. In 1941 Jasper and Kershman, attempting a classification of seizures based on EEG patterns, recognised that psychomotor seizures were associated with temporal spiking and proposed that the origin of the spikes and seizures was in the temporal lobe or deeper structures.[167] Finally, in 1948, Frederic and Erna Gibbs and Bartolomé Fuster published a landmark paper in which the 'psychomotor type of EEG discharge' was correlated with clinical findings in 300 patients.[168] The paper provided an excellent description of the clinical manifestations of the psychomotor seizure, and the authors located the electrographic discharge in the anterior temporal lobe region. As this was a 'silent area' of the brain, they recommended that in severe cases the discharging area could be surgically removed.

After this slow start, subsequent development was rapid and spectacular. More papers from North America followed, then in 1952 Gastaut jumped on the bandwagon and devoted the 5th Colloque de Marseille to temporal lobe epilepsy. He used the findings of the Marseille colloquium to justify rendering the entire 1953 ILAE congress in Lisbon to the subject of the 'Temporal epilepsies'. The congress took the form of a one-day workshop based on a manuscript Gastaut had written entitled 'So-called 'psychomotor' and 'temporal' epilepsy', which was pre-circulated to twenty discussants who sent in written commentaries. The manuscript (published in *Epilepsia* after the meeting) was divided into six 'critical studies' of contemporary knowledge augmented by Gastaut's own data: clinical symptoms, EEG symptoms, correlations between the clinical and EEG symptoms, surgical anatomical findings, pathogenesis, and methods of treatment. Gastaut concluded with a review of experimentally induced attacks of psychomotor or temporal epilepsy. His requisition of temporal lobe epilepsy, for himself and for the ILAE, followed the same pattern as his work on classification; and, as with the work on classification, he

---

[166] Jackson, 'On a particular variety'.

[167] Jasper and Kershman, 'Electroencephalographic classification'. Gibbs had earlier demonstrated what he thought were generalised discharges during such psychomotor seizures, and an acrimonious debate between the Gibbs school and the Jasper school ensued about whether the psychomotor seizure was focal or generalised.

[168] Gibbs, Gibbs and Fuster, 'Psychomotor epilepsy'. Fuster was training in Chicago as a Rockefeller fellow from Montevideo. Gibbs had earlier, in 1946, presented his findings at the Chicago Neurological Society meeting.

brought the subject into a worldwide spotlight. Perhaps not surprisingly, Gastaut laid great emphasis on classification and terminology when it came to considering psychomotor seizures (he disputed the term 'temporal lobe epilepsy', believing that the epilepsy usually arose in the hippocampus and could arise in other diencephalic structures).[169] The text opened in the following manner:

> An extremely important development has recently occurred in the field of epileptology, viz. the identification of a new form of epilepsy, which has come to occupy a prominent place in nosology. This result is due mainly to the following five causes:
>
> 1) This variety of epilepsy is claimed to be the most frequent of all clinical forms of the disease (from 30 to 80% according to the epileptics concerned: inpatients or outpatients).
> 2) Its clinical symptoms are regarded as highly complex and atypical, comprising psychosensory as well as motor (autonomic, nervous or somatic) manifestations, which is assumed to render the clinical diagnosis very difficult in some cases.
> 3) On the other hand, its electroencephalographic signs are stated to be sufficiently simple and constant to ensure a correct diagnosis by themselves: a focus of negative spikes occupying the anterior temporal region of the scalp, readily demonstrable under the conditions of a standard examination or, at the worst, during activation by sleep or metrazol.
> 4) The mechanism by which it is produced is believed to be as simple as its electroencephalographic signs, since the focus of temporal spikes corresponds with a subjacent lesion involving the temporal lobe; the numerous functions of this lobe explaining the complexity of the clinical symptoms.
> 5) Finally, it is claimed to disappear as a result of specific medical treatment and, when this fails, by excision of the affected temporal lobe, which will cause the symptoms to disappear by removing the lesion. (p. 59)

Gastaut went on to state that '[i]n view of these facts', the interest in the new form of epilepsy would be

> readily understandable ... Thanks to the current medical press, this interest, which initially was confined to specialists alone, is now shared by all medical practitioners. It has, however, spread to them at a time when specialists are commencing to have reservations with regard to the validity of the above-mentioned findings and when a certain number has

---

[169] Gastaut also suggested that temporal lobe epilepsy could be divided into three categories – superficial temporal lobe, hippocampal and diencephalic – although he conceded that there was much overlap and that this was a 'a rough and doubtful classification' ('"Psychomotor" and "temporal" epilepsy').

> even come to doubt the individual character of a 'temporal' epilepsy in
> the literal sense of the word. (p. 59)

This was, he concluded, the rationale both for making the temporal epilepsies the focus of the ILAE's scientific meeting and for opening the topic to discussion.

The three critical studies of clinical and EEG symptoms and their correlations are masterly descriptions of temporal lobe epilepsy, and have, over the subsequent half-century, hardly been added to in any fundamental way. The ictal as well as inter-ictal EEG findings were made possible by the use of intravenous metrazol, which allowed the luxury of direct observation of seizures, at a time just before the widespread use of telemetric technologies. But the validity of this technique was the subject of much critical comment during the discussion.

The critical study of the pathogenesis stressed the importance of 'incisural sclerosis' (p. 61). Gastaut clearly understood that the sclerotic lesion was the cause of and not a consequence of the epilepsy, contrary to the classical opinion of Walther Spielmeyer and others still widely held at that time. How incisural sclerosis arose, though, was contentious. Gastaut felt that head trauma was the commonest cause of temporal lobe epilepsy (50% of cases), resulting in contusional damage to the brain as it was compressed against the sphenoid bone or the free edge of the tentorium. Encephalitis was the second most frequent cause (20–25% of cases). The third cause (5% of cases) was obstetrical injury, and Gastaut completely concurred with Penfield's hypothesis that this resulted in herniation of the temporal lobe over the tentorial edge, causing vascular compression of the anterior choroidal (and other) arteries and ischaemia to the temporal lobe.

In a section on critical study of the methods of treatment, Gastaut reported that anterior temporal lobectomy rendered 50% of patients free of seizures. He realised that even a generous temporal lobectomy did not remove all the epileptogenic structures, and in fact in some cases removed only structures playing a secondary role, although it could remove enough to halt clinical seizures. In this way, Gastaut emphasised that the incisural sclerosis was not, itself, the entire epileptic 'focus', but only part of the epileptogenic network (p. 68). The final study on experimentally induced attacks of psychomotor or temporal epilepsy is a superb summary of contemporary experimental work, deriving mainly from stimulation experiments in unanaesthetised cats and from aluminium oxide lesioning experiments.

Gastaut was at pains to point out that the psychomotor seizure could be produced by discharges in, or stimulation of, a wide variety of structures outside the temporal lobe, and similarly that EEG abnormalities were highly variable. He produced a list of symptoms (derived from the 1952 symposium: as he called it, 'the Assembly for the Exchange of Electroencephalographic Data'; p. 62), which were complex and varied, in great contrast to the clinical simplicity of attacks in the frontal, central, parietal and occipital lobes. Gastaut took this to be a sign of multiple mechanisms and a widely distributed epileptic network which probably extended beyond the temporal lobe. In terms of pathogenesis, it is interesting to note that the possibility of damage during a febrile seizure (prolonged or not) was not mentioned, and indeed febrile seizures were not touched on anywhere in Gastaut's manuscript.

Accompanying the manuscript are the commentaries of seventeen senior figures that are equally noteworthy.[170] Gibbs provided a critique of Gastaut's studies and was clearly very irritated by them. He emphasised the primacy of the anterior temporal lobe (lateral and mesial) in the production of these seizures. Jasper agreed but reiterated Gastaut's emphasis on the anatomically widely distributed nature of the epileptogenic area, stating that 'the periamygdaloid and rhinencephalic portions of the temporal lobe, including the extent of the hippocampal gyrus, and often the pes hippocampi as well . . . are nearly always severely affected in patients with temporal lobe seizures' (p. 83). Margaret Lennox concurred with Gastaut's view. Fulton and MacLean emphasised the importance of limbic structures in relation to epileptic behaviour and the amnesia of the psychomotor seizure. William Lennox also supported Gastaut's view that temporal seizures might be quite widely distributed: 'The brain is too complicated and too well integrated to contain even a phase of epilepsy within a certain brain compartment' (p. 85). Otto Magnus claimed to have been studying temporal lobe epilepsy since 1949 and concurred with Gastaut's views on classification and the anatomical basis of the seizures. Magnus's centre in Holland was reported to have operated on eighteen cases. Giuseppe Pampiglione described his work with sphenoidal electrodes, and he and Gibbs also emphasised the importance of inducing sleep to bring out EEG abnormalities.

William Lennox was the only discussant to mention febrile seizures as the cause of the brain lesion responsible for psychomotor seizures. He wrote:

> Convulsions beginning in childhood may have caused brain lesions which later in life were responsible for psychomotor episodes. In this connection, the febrile convulsions of early childhood are especially suspect . . . Febrile convulsions are especially significant because of the possibility that the infection causes a thrombosis of cerebral vessels in the temporal lobe of the brain. (p. 84)

Murray Falconer described his first sixteen cases of en bloc temporal resection and strongly emphasised his view that hippocampal sclerosis was a cause, not a consequence, of the epilepsy. He also confirmed the developing view of Penfield, in contrast to that of Pearce Bailey, that surgical resection of the uncus

[170] 'Discussion'.

and hippocampus were needed to obtain good results. The most detailed surgical commentary was that of K. W. E. Paine from London, who had reviewed the results of the sixty-eight temporal lobectomies carried out in Montreal by Penfield between 1945 and 1950. He reported that 47% of patients who had been followed for between one and seven years (over 60% for three or more years) had a successful outcome (defined as less than three post-operative seizures, excluding auras, which were recognised to be a common sequela), and that successful outcomes were more likely in patients with unilateral inter-ictal temporal spiking. The operative complications included death in one case, upper quadratic hemianopia in about one-quarter of cases, persistent aphasia in one patient, memory deficit in 30% of patients, severe disabling amnesia in one and mental deterioration, to the extent of confinement in a mental institution, in five patients. Paine disagreed with Gastaut about aetiology, finding trauma and encephalitis to be rare, but considered Gastaut's division of psychomotor epilepsy into three groups –true temporal psychomotor seizures (rare and operable), hippocampal psychomotor epilepsy (common and operable) and diencephalic psychomotor epilepsy (inoperable) – to be very useful. He listed the procedures undertaken in Montreal in assessing a patient and concluded with an insightful comment:

> Even supposing one has the ideal patient with temporal lobe seizures, localized to one temporal lobe by EEG, in whom at operation, it is possible to reproduce his initial phenomenon by stimulation, to delineate accurately his electrographic focus by electrocorticography and to remove the abnormal brain tissue, to show that the electrograms are then normal, then that patient would appear to have about a 60% chance of being completely free of seizures after operation, and a further 30% chance of considerable improvement over his preoperative state. How pleasant it would be to see many of such model patients ... No, the treatment of temporal lobe seizures is hampered by our considerable ignorance of the mechanisms of epilepsy, temporal and otherwise. Excision of abnormal brain can be only a temporary phase in treatment. Surely the neurochemist will come forward in the not too distant future with a less mutilating method. (pp. 90–1)

Penfield was not present in Lisbon, but he sent in written comments reiterating his pathogenic theory of incisural sclerosis. Schwab made the interesting proposal that the seizure phenomenology was a reiteration of '*learned*' patterns of behaviour and proposed the term '*acquired patterned motor* and *sensory epilepsy* or its Latin or Greek equivalent' in place of 'temporal lobe epilepsy' (p. 95 [italics added for emphasis]). The last contribution was by António Subirana from Barcelona, who described two cases in which the ictal phenomenon was a feeling of paradisiacal happiness, similar to that described by Dostoevsky in *The Idiot*: "'The feeling is so wonderful and agreeable that one would gladly give some years of our own life for it, or even life itself!'" ... Our two patients, the one with a malignant glioma and the other with a probable cortical scar, compare this feeling of happiness with a stay in Paradise where all notion of time disappears' (p. 96).

This must have been an extraordinary conference, with the presence of the intellectual leaders in the field, and with conclusions which remain largely uncontested today and cautions which still should be heeded. Subsequently, in 1954, Gastaut organised the fourth colloquium on the topic of pathological anatomy of temporal seizures. A further symposium (confusingly called the Second International Colloquium on Temporal Lobe Epilepsy) was held in Washington in March 1957.[171] The results of an impressive series of experimental studies comprised the first session of this meeting, followed by a series of papers on the pathological and neurochemical aspects. Here, John Cavanagh, Falconer and Alfred Meyer expanded on the relationship between febrile seizures and temporal lobe epilepsy. The next session was on surgical series. Bailey's series of 71 patients, Falconer's of 50 cases and the Montreal series of 244 patients were described from various points of view (clinical, EEG, technical). The last session was concerned with the psychological effects of temporal lobe surgery and two original and interesting papers were included. The first was an exhaustive review by Hrayr Terzian[172] of the effects of bilateral temporal lobe resections; the second, by Marianne Simmel and Sarah Counts, was a detailed account of the psychological sequalae of unilateral surgery (from Bailey's series), with salutary cautions about the long-term results of surgery.

The intensity of the studies of temporal lobe epilepsy in the 1950s was remarkable, and the meetings between 1952 and 1957 must have been exciting affairs, with high-quality scientific and clinical content and the recognition that an important new chapter in epilepsy had been opened. Over this period, the features and treatment of temporal lobe epilepsy were defined in such a way that, it can surely be argued, little of significance has been added since – except perhaps the question of the role of febrile convulsions.

Hippocampal Sclerosis and Febrile Convulsions

Intimately linked to the clinical topic of temporal lobe epilepsy has been the pathological entity known variously as hippocampal sclerosis, mesial temporal sclerosis, Ammon's horn sclerosis or incisural sclerosis. This intriguing pathological finding had been recognised long before the concept of temporal lobe epilepsy emerged. As we have seen, not surprisingly, given its distinguished tradition of descriptive neuropathology, the entity was first identified in

---

[171] The papers in the 1957 colloquium were published in book form: Baldwin and Bailey, *Temporal Lobe Epilepsy*.

[172] Terzian worked with Gastaut and was one of the first to describe Klüver–Bucy syndrome in humans. He was an intellectual figure who was deeply involved in the reformation of Italian psychiatry and its societal connections.

Germany in the late nineteenth century, with notable contributions by Sommer in 1880 and Bratz in 1899, and later by Cécile and Oskar Vogt, Spielmeyer, Willibald Scholz and Stauder. At the time, the lesion was considered to occur in what was then called genuine (or idiopathic) epilepsy and was noted to be frequent in chronic cases. It was assumed by most authorities to be the consequence of epilepsy, and not its cause.

As described earlier, it was in the 1950s that evidence began to accrue that the lesion (whatever its origin) was the cause of temporal lobe epilepsy and not the consequence of chronic epilepsy – a conceptual shift based largely on the fact that surgical resection of hippocampal sclerosis resulted in the cessation of seizures. Penfield had termed this 'incisural sclerosis',[173] and at the Marseille conference he reported that it was present in 100 of his 157 operated patients with temporal lobe epilepsy. However, it was only after the careful pathological analyses of Falconer's series of en bloc temporal lobectomies that it became fully accepted that the lesion was the commonest cause of temporal lobe epilepsy.

Febrile convulsions – convulsions in young children, associated with high temperatures – have been recognised since the time of Hippocrates. In the seventeenth century, Thomas Willis, for instance, provided an excellent description.[174] Until the 1940s, however, febrile convulsions were considered common, largely benign and of not much significance. Alfred Meyer was the first to suggest that Ammon's horn sclerosis was in fact caused by febrile seizures and was consequently the cause of subsequent temporal lobe epilepsy – in effect reconciling Spielmeyer's view that the lesion was the result of seizure-induced anoxia with the idea that it was also the cause of psychomotor epilepsy. Meyer was the pathologist at the Maudsley Hospital, and throughout the 1950s the London and Oxford groups adduced increasing evidence in support of this hypothesis. His proposition was reiterated by Lennox at the Marseilles congress; nonetheless, the theory continued to divide opinion.

J. Gordon Millichap, a contemporary of Lennox and a professor of paediatrics in Chicago, wrote the first monograph on the topic of febrile seizures in 1968.[175] This work provides an estimate of frequency – 3% of the population under five years of age – and an exhaustive literature review of definition and frequency, clinical evaluation, mechanisms, aetiology and treatment. By then, the focus was on recurrence rates and longer-term prognosis. Millichap refuted the theory that febrile seizures predisposed the child to later epilepsy. He reviewed 35 papers in the literature reporting on 5,576 children. He found that 29% of the children developed spontaneous non-febrile seizures and 20% frequent recurrent seizures, but in his view the high rates reflected selection bias and the retrospective nature of the studies. In his own series of 110 children, 4%

[173] Earle, Baldwin and Penfield, 'Incisural sclerosis'.   [174] Willis, *Pathologiae*.
[175] Millichap, *Febrile Convulsions*. This is a comprehensive, if rather pedestrian work which stands in marked stylistic as well as intellectual contrast to Lennox's work.

developed frequent recurrent non-febrile seizures but only 1 child developed psychomotor seizures. Millichap noted, as did everyone else at the time, that those with prolonged febrile seizures, EEG abnormalities and/or frequent febrile seizures were more likely to develop subsequent epilepsy, but he concluded: 'Febrile seizures generally do not predispose to spontaneous seizures . . . Permanent brain damage and hemiparesis as a direct result of the febrile convulsion is a rare complication, occurring in less than two of 1,000 patients' (p. 110). As we shall see, this view was subsequently strongly contested, not least by Jean Aicardi.

Other New Forms of Epilepsy

Another form of epilepsy greatly clarified in this period was *post-traumatic epilepsy*. Its clinical features, and particularly the risk of seizures occurring and recurring after head injury, were studied in detail. Much credit for this must go to Bryan Jennett from Glasgow who, over a period of some decades, carried out definitive research. His focus was on civilian head injury ('non-missile' injury, as he called it), but of course it was the war and the maiming effects of technologically improved munitions which put the issue high on the research agenda. As noted earlier, Penfield's interest in epilepsy was fuelled by his work with Foerster on post-traumatic seizures from the First World War, just as the interest of Earl Walker had been stimulated by the funding for his work with veterans in the Second World War at the Cushing Hospital. Walker wrote a definitive monograph based on his experience at the Cushing Hospital that described the use of pneumoencephalography, scalp EEG, corticography and activated EEG using metrozol. Not surprisingly, as a neurosurgeon he devoted much space to the techniques of surgical treatment, although of 238 patients admitted to the hospital, seizures were controlled medically in 130 and only 40 required surgery. And, in these cases, the epilepsy was fully controlled in about a third.[176]

Bryan Jennett's studies, published in two monographs and a series of papers,[177] were prospective, with long follow-up. Amongst their drawbacks was the fact that the research was carried out before the advent of magnetic resonance imaging (MRI) scanning and mostly before CT scanning, and also that the statistical numeration was simple and devoid of regression or multivariant analyses.

[176] Walker, *Posttraumatic Epilepsy*, pp. 72–4. Control was defined as a six-month period of freedom from seizures. Walker fully acknowledged that the true figure would be possible to ascertain only after a 5- or 10-year follow-up period.

[177] Jennett, *Blunt Head Injuries*; Jennett, *Non-missile Head Injuries*; Jennett, Miller and Braakman, 'Nonmissile depressed skull fracture'; Jennett, 'Acute traumatic intracranial haematoma'. These remain landmark works in the field of post-traumatic epilepsy. Bryan Jennett held the first chair in neurosurgery in Scotland (at the University of Glasgow), and in addition to his work on epilepsy, developed the Glasgow Coma Scale with Graham Teasdale (Teasdale and Jennett, 'Practical scale') and coined the term vegetative state with Fred Plum.

Nevertheless, the findings have stood the test of time and constituted the framework for all future work. Jennett was one of the first to stress the distinction between immediate, early and late seizures. He considered immediate seizures to have a different pathophysiology from that of late seizures, and that their occurrence reflected the acute disturbances of brain homeostasis common in significant head injury. Early seizures also had a different pathogenic basis and a different prognosis, and in Jennett's view the first seven days were 'a natural watershed'.[178] In his first series, 5% of those with significant head injury suffered early seizures. In half, seizures occurred within an hour of the injury, and in 60% within the first day. Status epilepticus developed in 10%. Late seizures occurred in 10% of all cases, 4% in those without early epilepsy and 17% in those with early epilepsy. The risk factors for epilepsy were post-traumatic amnesia of more than 24 hours, depressed skull fracture or intracranial haemorrhage. When late seizures (i.e. 'post-traumatic epilepsy') did develop, they remitted in about a quarter of cases and became severe and intractable in one-third. Interestingly, he correctly identified that the risk of developing late seizures remained elevated for some years after the injury.

In this period, other new forms of epilepsy were described (mainly by Gastaut), including startle-induced epilepsy, hemiconvulsion-hemiplegia-epilepsy syndrome, benign partial epilepsy of childhood with occipital spikes and light-induced epilepsy (photosensitive epilepsy). Two syndromes were the subject of particular study: West Syndrome and Lennox–Gastaut Syndrome.

West Syndrome is a form of epilepsy so named by Gastaut at the 19th Colloque de Marseille, after the description by Dr William West of his son's infantile spasms (a severe form of epilepsy) in *The Lancet* in 1841.[179] When EEG was introduced, Gastaut and Antoine Rémond described the correlation of infantile spasms with what subsequently became known as hypsarrhythmia on the EEG.[180] In 1958, Lucian Sorel and A. Dusaucy-Bauloye from Louvain in Belgium described how adrenocorticotropic hormone (ACTH) could abolish the spasms and the EEG disturbance, and the importance of starting this therapy as soon as possible.[181] ACTH remains a treatment of choice. By 1960 atypical forms of West Syndrome were recognised, as were many of the aetiologies.

Lennox–Gastaut Syndrome has a chequered history. Soon after EEG entered clinical practice, an early success in the task of correlating clinical and EEG features was the identification in 1935, by Gibbs, Lennox and colleagues,[182] of bursts of 3 Hz spike–wave discharges in cases of petit mal. It was then noted that slow spike–wave activity (discharges at less than 3 Hz) was associated with very

---

[178] Jennett, *Non-missile Head Injuries*, p. 27.   [179] West, 'Infantile convulsions'.
[180] Gastaut and Rémond, 'Études électroencéphalographiques'.
[181] Sorel and Dusaucy-Bauloye, 'Traitement spectaculaire par l'ACTH'.
[182] Gibbs, Davis and Lennox, 'Electroencephalogram in epilepsy'. Although, as mentioned earlier, Berger published the EEG during a petit mal seizure in 1933 showing 3 Hz waves without spikes.

different clinical characteristics. Lennox called these spike–wave variants, and he (with Hallowell Davis) noted earlier age of onset, high incidence of mental retardation, signs of brain damage, polymorphic seizures and atypical absences. The concept of an epilepsy syndrome was not fully established at this point. But when Gastaut gathered a large number of cases and devoted a Colloque de Marseille (in 1966) to the problem, he proposed calling it Lennox syndrome, although apparently the participants at the meeting insisted on adding Gastaut's name. Gastaut defined the syndrome as 'a very severe variety of childhood epilepsy which is refractory to treatment and characterized by: (1) frequent tonic seizures and a variant of petit mal absences; (2) pronounced, homogenous mental retardation; (3) inter-ictal EEG records showing pseudo-rhythmical (1.5–2.5 c/s) diffuse slow spike and wave.'[183] It was realised that other seizure types also occurred. The definition depended on what was thought initially to be a unique EEG feature (slow spike and wave). But similar patterns have been subsequently identified in other clinical circumstances, and since then debate has raged about whether this so-called syndrome is really a useful clinical categorisation. What was ignored, of course, was aetiology, and illuminating this would have to wait.

Status Epilepticus

This topic had lain largely dormant since the work of Clark and Prout in 1904, but was revived by Gastaut, who devoted the 10th Colloque de Marseille in 1962 to status epilepticus.[184] It was a time ripe for change and the Colloque contributed in three particular areas. First (inevitably) was in relation to classification. Gastaut suggested a classification which mirrored the classification of epileptic seizures: as he put it, 'there are as many types of status epilepticus as there are epileptic seizures'.[185] This was a major change, for up until the 1940s status epilepticus was a term largely (but not entirely) restricted to convulsive status epilepticus (grand mal status epilepticus). As with much else at the time, it was the EEG which changed the paradigm, for continuous EEG activity was found in various non-convulsive situations. In the years before the Colloque, nosologists had had a field-day describing numerous rare forms and rationalisation was certainly required – an opportunity Gastaut quickly set upon.

The second development was the recognition that status epilepticus could cause cerebral damage, and the Colloque included this too in its programme,

---

[183] Gastaut et al., 'Childhood epileptic encephalopathy'.
[184] The proceedings were published in 1967, the first significant book dedicated to the subject (Gastaut, Roger and Lob, *Les états de mal épileptique*).
[185] Gastaut, 'Classification of status epilepticus'.

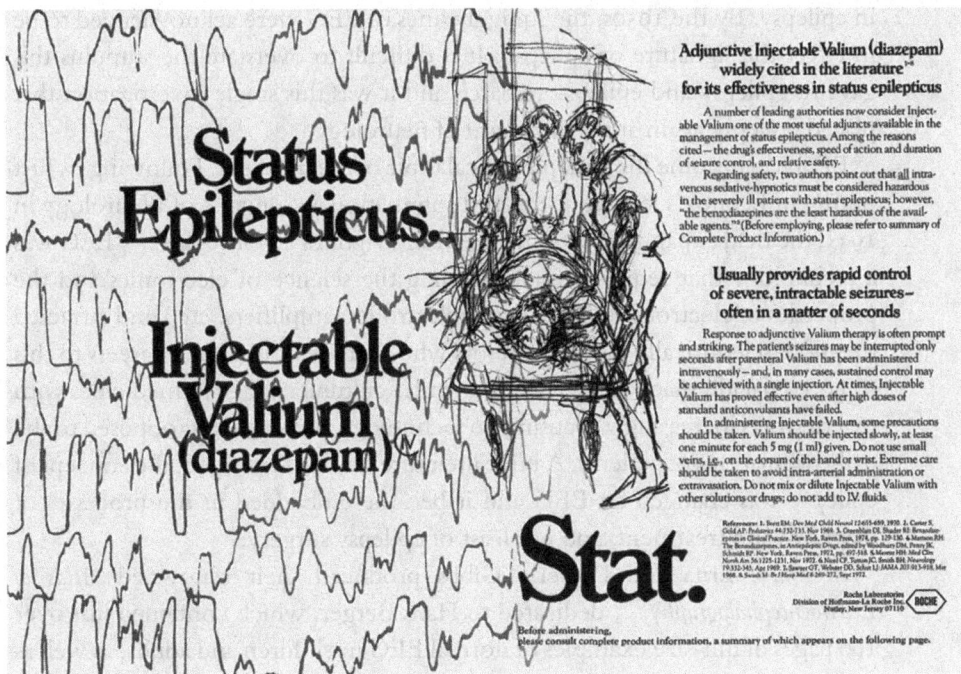

27. The first advert for the use of diazepam in status epilepticus.

although the main steps in understanding the mechanisms of this damage were to be made a few years later.

Finally, the introduction of intravenous benzodiazepines into the treatment of status epilepticus had the potential to revise treatment approaches radically and this too was a topic addressed at the meeting. Henri Gastaut was already a strong advocate of the use of benzodiazepines in status epilepticus. In 1965 he had weighed in with a laudatory report of the use of diazepam[186], and six years later he was even more enthusiastic about the new agent clonazepam, then known as Ro 05–4023 ('[W]e do not hesitate to affirm that RO 05–4023 is by far the most effective agent which we have at present for the treatment of status epilepticus of whatever form and etiology').[187] Other treatment improvements in this period included the use of steroids and intravenous chlormethiazole.

ELECTROENCEPHALOGRAPHY

Despite a general disillusionment creeping in about the value of EEG in neurology and psychiatry in general, there was no concern about its utility

[186] Gastaut et al., 'Treatment of status epilepticus' (1965).
[187] Gastaut et al., 'Treatment of status epilepticus' (1971).

in epilepsy. By the 1950s, the squiggly lines of EEG were acknowledged to be in effect the signature of epilepsy. It is difficult to overstate the stimulus this gave to epilepsy and epilepsy research and it was this single investigation that placed epilepsy again at the vanguard of neurology.

EEG had become the epileptological topic of the moment. Following its first outing in Lennox's lecture at the 2nd International Congress of Neurology in 1935, the field expanded 'with the speed and vigor of a prairie fire'.[188] EEG was a technology that required understanding the science of electronics and the properties of electronic technologies (electrodes, amplifiers, etc.) and attracted the more scientifically minded doctors who then dedicated their careers to this topic – a paradigmatic example of the wider cultural change in medicine, with practitioners increasingly focusing on technology and science as opposed to the daily tribulations of patients. A huge literature on EEG emerged, the concept of epilepsy was changed by EEG and it became embedded in the processes of diagnosis and treatment, and not least of epilepsy surgery.

In 1941, Erna and Frederic Gibbs produced their renowned *Atlas of Electroencephalography*,[189] dedicated to Hans Berger, which contained just over 100 pages of full-size examples of normal EEG in children and adults, as well as EEG in epilepsy, brain tumours, brain injuries, and various other neurological and psychiatric disturbances. In 1950, Denis Hill and Geoffrey Parr edited the first edition of a book which became known as the bible of EEG.[190] The book demonstrated just how technical and scientific EEG was in those days, and how this science was integrated into clinical problems. It was an unparalleled synthesis of the then technical and clinical knowledge (with a reference list of more than 700 articles and books). The non-clinician W. Grey Walter contributed the epilepsy chapter (45 pages) and therein provided a scientific perspective on the ictal and inter-ictal patterns of the main forms of epilepsy. There was no discussion, however, of depth recording, nor of epilepsy surgery or temporal lobe epilepsy. These topics, which were to become the burning clinical themes of the time, would have to wait until the second edition in 1963, with the chapter on epilepsy written by Denis Hill himself. At that time, Britain and the United States led the way in this field, reflecting their already strong traditions in physiology. As a sign of the perceived clinical potential of neurophysiology, a new specialty entitled 'Clinical neurophysiology' was formally established in Britain in the 1950s, removing the study and reporting of EEG from clinical neurology. This was not a pattern of practice followed in Europe, and to many such extreme subspecialisation was seen as detrimental to neurological practice. The non-clinical EEG technician also became vital to the

---

[188] Knott, 'Educational efforts'.   [189] Gibbs and Gibbs, *Atlas of Electroencephalography*.

[190] Hill and Parr, *Electroencephalography*. Sir John Denis Nelson Hill, was a house physician in 1936 when he saw Grey Walter's homemade EEG machine, the first in Britain, and soon realized its potential and during the war, he set up one of the first clinical EEG laboratories.

running of all EEG units and was a profession that developed strongly, especially in the United States.[191] Commercial machines began to be manufactured by instrument companies in the United States, Europe and Japan, and by the mid-1950s, EEG units had been set up in most large teaching hospitals and specialised units.

Technical developments in this period were directed mainly at efforts to record actual seizures and not just the inter-ictal EEG and to link the ictal EEG to the filmed clinical manifestations of a seizure. Early examples of filmed seizures in a clinical setting were provided by Westphal and especially Löwenstein.[192] In 1938, Schwab presented a method of recording both the patient and the EEG onto separate 16mm films and them combining the two onto a single film by using synchronisation markers.[193] In 1953, at the 3rd International EEG, seven techniques for combining visual and EEG data were described; all were expensive, complicated and difficult to achieve. In 1954, Schwab introduced an eighth technique using a prism lens splitter, which simplified the process considerably.[194] However, it was only with the introduction of video technologies in the late 1950s, and then digital video technology in the early 1970s, that procedures for the simultaneous viewing of the film/video and EEG of a patient's seizure became widespread. The first radio-telemetered EEG was introduced by Charles Breakell in 1947 at the Whittingham Hospital, a psychiatric asylum near Nottingham, for use in ambulant patients.[195]

The next technical landmark was the invention of the transistor in 1948. This transformed EEG recording such that within ten years transistors were incorporated into all commercial EEG machines, replacing vacuum-tube amplifiers. Other developments included large-volume data storage on magnetic tape and then, in 1970, the introduction of the PDP-11 mini computer (although enormous by today's standards) which massively increased analysis and storage capabilities.[196] Over the next few years, further technical advances were made in relation to co-registering the EEG and video data, and later to reformatting and displaying both images on a split screen.[197]

---

[191] The history of the role of the EEG technician is well recorded in Knott, 'Educational efforts'. In 1959, the American Society of Electroencephalographic Technicians was organized and published its own journal from 1961.
[192] Westphal, 'kinematographischer Bilder'; Löwenstein, 'klinisch-kinematographische Epilepsiebeobachtung'. Otto Löwenstein emigrated to the USA in 1939 and was presumably an important influence on the subsequent developments by Schwab.
[193] Hunter and Jasper, 'Cinematographic technique'.
[194] Schwab, 'Synchronized moving pictures of patient and EEG'.
[195] Parker and Breakell, 'The radio-electrophysiologogram'.
[196] The author remembers the excitement these machines engendered, first installed at Queen Square in the 1970s.
[197] An early example of such technologies can be seen in a black-and-white 16 mm film: Penry et al., *Absence Seizure*.

In addition to its use in epilepsy (and in localising brain tumours), the value of EEG was also actively explored in the field of human behaviour and psychiatry. In the words of historian Cornelius Borck, 'with the scientific recognition of the EEG as a valid parameter for brain function[,] the entirety of human life from procreation to death could count as [an] object for electro-encephalographic investigation, and indeed almost no human activity was left without a representation in [the] form of an EEG-curve'.[198] EEG had caught the public imagination, and popular media was full of images of electrographic squiggles and brain waves (a term indeed derived from EEG). EEG was used to study such facets as intelligence, personality, psychopathy, psychosis, moral deviancy (e.g. homosexuality) and even psychosomatic illness (e.g. peptic ulcer). The technology achieved particular traction in forensic medicine, especially in America and Britain, and EEG abnormalities were claimed to be found in more than half of psychopathic criminals.[199] This work all eventually came to nought, and indeed much was rubbish, As Adrian put it wryly:

> The development of electrical technique has given a new way of looking about, and so much is going on in the nervous system that it is hard to resist the temptation to record anything that turns up. This method has had the merit of showing many unexpected resemblances in the activity of different parts of the nervous apparatus, but it gives us facts rather than theories, and the facts may not always mean very much.[200]

Very little of the work outside epilepsy (and disturbances of consciousness) endured, but in epilepsy EEG remained a crucial investigation, and so it remains to this day.

By 1960 much of the juice of routine scalp EEG in epilepsy had been squeezed out, but new developments were taking place in another field which were to produce a rich source of electrographic data: the recording of EEG from electrodes placed on the surface of the brain (electrocorticography) or inserted into brain tissue (intracerebral or depth EEG). Penfield used these techniques in his epilepsy surgery programme in Montreal. From there, they spread worldwide. Initially corticography was confined to acute recordings of inter-ictal spikes prior to resection (i.e. in a single operation), but in the late 1940s Penfield and Jasper started to use chronically implanted epidural strip electrodes to record actual seizures. These were inserted in one operation, the wound was then closed and the recordings of EEG continued until enough data had been collected. At that point Penfield would perform a second operation to remove the electrodes and carry out the resection. This became standard practice and, in selected patients, remains so today.

---

[198] Cited in Schirmann, 'Wondrous eyes'.   [199] Silverman, 'Criminal psychopaths'.
[200] Adrian, *Mechanism of Nervous Action*, p. 93.

From the mid-1930s, depth EEG had been used in studies in experimental animals. Recordings in humans began in the mid-1940s, initially during operations for movement disorders,[201] and the first chronic human depth recordings were performed in psychiatric states, in the hope that these would explain the mechanisms of the psychiatric disorders,[202] or in psychiatric patients undergoing leucotomy.[203] It was around then that Reginald Bickford[204] employed depth recordings in epilepsy, first during surgery for post-traumatic seizures, and later in other forms of epilepsy in adults and children.

The use of stereotactic methods for EEG electrode insertion in clinical epilepsy was probably first practised by Ernest Spiegel and Henry Wycis in 1947.[205] By 1950 they had recorded seizure discharges from depth electrodes inserted stereotactically in patients with epilepsy, including petit mal seizures, which they postulated arose in deep structures before spreading to the cortex.[206] Bickford introduced his 'cranial localiser', and others used stereotactic systems which were modified versions of the Horsley–Clarke frame.[207] The next major development occurred in Paris, with the work of psychiatrist-turned-functional neurosurgeon Jean Talairach and neurologist turned electroencephalographer Jean Bancaud.[208] The impetus to study epilepsy came when the neurologist and neuropsychologist Henri Hécaen, having spent a year (1952) in Penfield's unit in Montreal, returned to Paris and convinced the neurosurgeon Gabriel Mazars to start an epilepsy surgical programme. Talairach, who was already working on stereotaxis in movement disorders and pain, was joined by Bancaud, whose prior work was on the neuropsychology of epilepsy. In 1955 they began their joint work on epilepsy. They devised a new method of placing depth electrodes based

[201] For an early report, see Meyers and Hayne, 'Parkinsonism and hemiballismus'.

[202] Delgado, Hamlin and Chapman, 'Psychotic patients'; Heath, 'Correlation of electrical recordings'.

[203] Lüders, 'History of invasive EEG'.

[204] Reginald Bickford graduated from Cambridge University and learned his EEG from Grey Walter and Adrian. During the war, as neuropsychiatric consultant to the Royal Air Force, he developed techniques for acute intracranial recordings. After the war, he was appointed to the Mayo Clinic and then in 1968 to UCSD. It was at the Mayo Clinic that he first performed his human depth studies in epilepsy.

[205] By then, stereotaxis in other indications was quite widespread. Talairach and Wycis both claimed to be the first to devise a stereotactic frame for electrode placement. However, Wycis and his group were the first to publish the method: Spiegel et al., 'Stereotactic apparatus'.

[206] Spiegel and Wycis, 'Thalamic recordings in man'; Wycis, Lee and Spiegel, 'Simultaneous records'; Spiegel, Reyes and Wycis, 'Diencephalic mechanisms'.

[207] Hayne, Belinson and Gibbs, 'Subcortical areas in epilepsy'.

[208] Talairach, trained in Montellier and Paris, although not a neurosurgeon was appointed head of neurosurgery at Hôpital Sainte-Anne; Jean Bancaud trained in Paris, and both created and led what became known as l' Ecole de Sainte-Anne.

on a coordinate system which used the axis joining the anterior and posterior commissures, identified by X-ray ventriculography (as opposed to bony landmarks used in all other methods and originally by Horsley and Clarke).[209] Talairach then developed a system of long-distance stereoradiology, using a double grid for alignment, and simple mathematical methods of correcting for parallax, which allowed safe placement of electrodes away from the position of blood vessels and other structures. He and his close colleagues Pierre Tournoux and Gabor Szikla devised stereotactic atlases showing the position of blood vessels and anatomical structures mapped onto Talairach's grid system.[210] By referring anatomical markers to this axis, he was able, to a large extent, to reduce the variation in the human brain in three-dimensional space (at least in terms of size and orientation, if not shape). Talairach coined the term 'stereoelectroencephalography' (SEEG) for his method, which for the first time allowed reasonably accurate placement of depth electrodes into predefined structures in the brain.[211] In some patients large numbers of electrodes were implanted, and Talairach and his colleagues were able to study the origin and spread of seizures through different brain structures as the seizure evolved electrographically. They used the terms 'epileptogenic zone' and 'irritative zone' to describe the spatial extent of inter-ictal spiking and ictal discharges. A key step in the evolution of this method was the establishment in 1962 of the first 'stereotactic surgical room', designed deliberately to be large enough for teleradiography[212] to be performed at a sufficient distance from the patient to minimise distortion due to parallax error. Intracranial EEG was recorded by multiple electrodes, introduced orthogonally into the brain of patients using the 'Talairach frame'. Initially, they made acute recordings of inter-ictal spikes, but between 1970 and 1973 chronic recordings lasting many days were performed. Unlike corticography, a striking benefit of this investigation was that it was conducted prior to the epilepsy surgical operation, allowing time for detailed analysis of the results and detailed planning of the subsequent operation.

There are however major limitations to the utility depth EEG. First, an intracerebral electrode can sample only a small area around the recording electrode and will miss any nearby epileptic event. Pathways of propagation will be missed for the same reason. This was a crucial limitation, as Ernst

---

[209] A historical assessment of Talairach's work can be found at https://histoire.inserm.fr/. See also Harary and Cosgrove, 'Talairach: A cerebral cartographer'; Chauvel, 'Jean Talairach and Jean Bancaud'.

[210] Talairach et al., *Atlas d'anatomie stéréotaxique*; Talairach and Szikla, *Anatomy of the Telencephalon*. In 1988, a third atlas was produced by Talairach and Pierre Tournoux.

[211] Also publishing the first standard work on this technique: Bancaud et al., *La stéréo-électro-encéphalographie dans l'épilepsie*.

[212] A key feature of the Talairach frame (as opposed to the one used by Wycis) was that two grids were attached at opposite sides of the frame. When the X-ray machine was far enough away to ensure that the path of the X-ray was sufficiently perpendicular to the frame and oriented at right angles to the A-P line, the two grids became superimposed on the X-ray plate.

Niedermeyer pointed out: 'In most cases of severe focal (partial) epileptic seizure disorder, there may be a wide zone of paroxysmal dysfunction with various "subfoci" sometimes apt to appear and disappear in a "will-o'-the-wisp"-like manner.'[213]

Talairach's technological grasp of his subject was superb and his unit rapidly gathered a reputation and a following amongst the students who spent time there. However, his own high expectations of developing functional surgery for epilepsy by making focal lesions stereotactically (as for pain and movement disorders), based on his recordings of the spread of seizure discharges, were not realised. And although his 'anatomo-functional' approach[214] did guide resective surgery, he never provided detailed data on how effective these methods actually proved to be in achieving seizure control.

Throughout this time, those involved with EEG were often entirely focused on the theoretical issues relating to the physics of brain currents and the technological problems of recording electrodes, sensitivity of detection, display, bandwidth and such like, and Talairach's department was an example of this tendency. During the procedures, the patient's hair was entirely shaved, the head fixed in a tight frame, burr holes made according to stereotactic principles and complicated radiological machinery used – all aimed at obtaining the highest-quality recordings. It became a common complaint that, in this extreme example of medicine as technology, the patient as a suffering individual was often neglected and made to feel relegated to the status of an experimental model – a sentiment poignantly illustrated in David B's graphic novel *Epileptic*, which includes scenes from the Talairach unit.[215]

Genetics

As we have seen, the study of genetics in epilepsy was largely extinguished in the aftermath of the Second World War, as the abuses of genetics were seen as reprehensible and a matter of shame. But the topic did not completely disappear. Rather, its focus moved away from degeneration, the neuropathic trait and the more rabid extremes of eugenics – theories which were now discarded

---

[213] Niedermeyer, 'Depth electroencephalography', p. 745. If Hill's book was considered the bible of electroencephalography in the 1950s, then Niedermeyer's textbook, which had gone into seven editions as of 2018 (with evolving authorship), was very much the King James version. Niedermeyer was one of the most influential figures in electroencephalography in the 1960s–1980s. Whilst serving with the German army, he was captured in 1944 and interned as a POW in America. After the end of the war, he returned to Austria to become Chief of Neurology in Innsbruck; in 1952 an EEG machine was delivered there under the Marshal plan, and this sparked his interest in EEG. In 1960 he returned to the USA, this time as an electroencephalographer, eventually to be appointed Encephalographer in Chief at Johns Hopkins, which is where he began the editorship of his famous textbook.

[214] Talairach, 'Mes travaux'.   [215] David B., *Epileptic*.

(a)

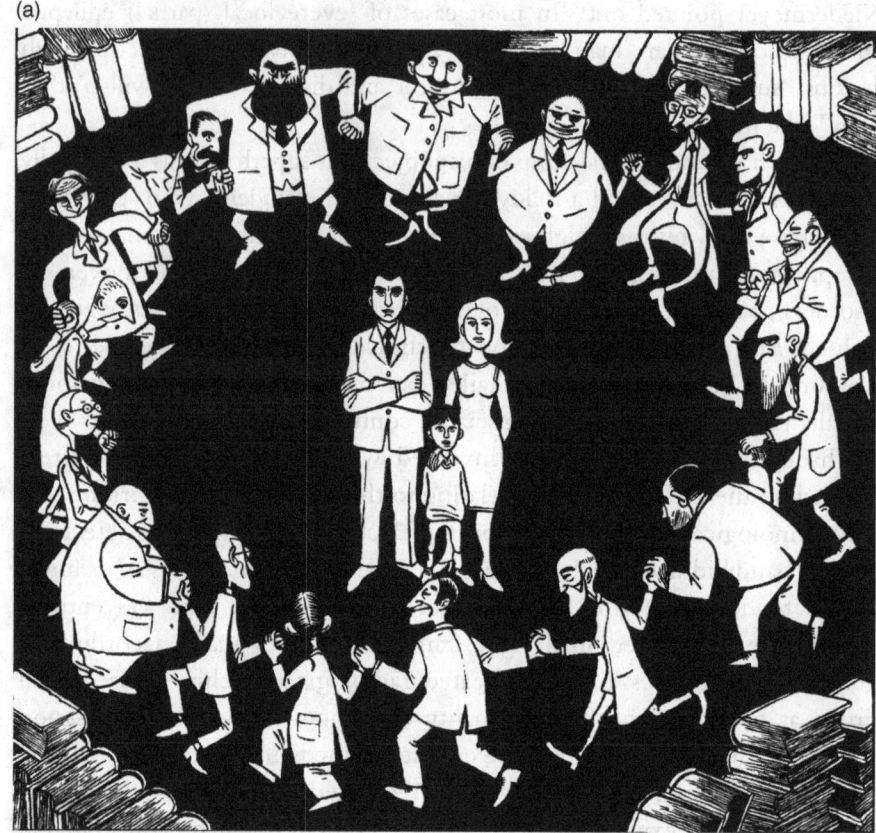

(b)

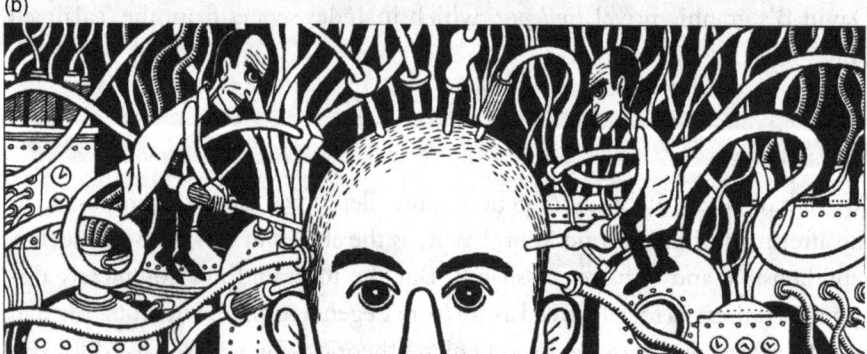

28a,b. What it's like to be a patient. Illustrations from the graphic novel by David B. a. This depicts 'the endless round of doctors'. b. This shows Talairach inserting depth electrodes (From David B, *Epileptic*).

by the same public which only two decades earlier willingly held them to be true. In their place, research revolved around the EEG.

In 1935 Hallowell and Pauline Davis had shown that in healthy identical twins the EEGs were very similar. In 1938, in an influential series of studies, Lennox and the Gibbses showed that EEG dysrhythmias were seen in about 60% of the near relatives of patients with epilepsy, although only 2–3% of these relatives exhibited overt epilepsy.[216] They concluded (erroneously) that electrographic dysrhythmias were a sign of a dominantly inherited gene predisposing to epilepsy, but this predisposition might or might not become manifest. Twenty-five persons carried the predisposition for every one person who developed seizures, and those predisposed were as likely to have epileptic offspring who were what Lennox called 'out and out epileptics'.[217] They further overextrapolated their findings, in 1940 proposing that 12% of the population had a predisposition to epilepsy and that the presence of a dysrhythmia in both parents raised the chance of epilepsy in a family by 35 times. Thus, '[i]f a person with epilepsy marries, his chances of having epileptic offspring will be minimized if he chooses a person whose cortical electrical activity is normal'. The eugenic implications were obvious: 'If, as we believe, our data indicate that dysrhythmia is a dominant trait, then it ... will persist, unless society should assume the herculean task of universal electroencephalographic examinations and the elimination of offspring of the millions who have dysrhythmia'. Lennox implied this was possible despite the 'expense and training required' – but gave no indication that he thought this carried any ethical implications. In Lennox's view, considering the likely dominant nature of the inherited dysrhythmia, breeding-out was an appropriate eugenic solution. Twin studies[218] yielded other interesting findings suggesting Mendelian inheritance, for instance that monozygous twins had very similar records, both in regard to abnormalities and background EEG patterns.[219] However, by the end of his career, Lennox had to conclude with obvious disappointment, that no firm mechanism for the inheritance of epilepsy could be established.[220] Similar conclusions were reached in two large studies from Europe, in 1950 and 1954,[221] which failed to

---

[216] Lennox, Gibbs and Gibbs, 'Cerebral dysrhythmia and epilepsy'.

[217] Lennox, 'Marriage and children for epileptics'.

[218] Lennox was not the first to embark on twin studies in epilepsy. Francis Galton wrote about them and realised their significance and importance (Galton, 'History of twins'). In Munich, Klaus Conrad published a detailed and extensive study on twins with idiopathic and symptomatic epilepsy (1935–8). He showed that 19 out of 22 of the monozygotic twin pairs were concordant with regard to epilepsy, and in 127 dizygotic pairs there was concordance in only approximately 4%. He concluded that heredity did have a determining role in idiopathic epilepsy but only a minor role in symptomatic epilepsy. He was a meticulous researcher. Although the population from which the twins was drawn was institution based, a drawback Conrad recognised, his work stands today as a model of genetic investigation. See Conrad, 'Erbanlage und Epilepsie'.

[219] Lennox, Gibbs and Gibbs, 'Brain-wave pattern'. Where only one twin had epilepsy, they found 74% concordance in basal rhythm, 66% concordance in 3 Hz spike and wave, and much lower concordance in other abnormalities.

[220] Lennox, *Epilepsy and Related Disorders*.

[221] Alström, 'Study of epilepsy'; Harvald, *Heredity in Epilepsy*.

substantiate single-gene explanations of epilepsy. It had thus taken forty years, and a world war, to finally vanquish the confident prediction of Charles Davenport and David Weeks[222] that epilepsy was a Mendelian disorder. In 1960, seemingly naïvely and without irony, Lennox wrote that the 'subject of heredity is perhaps the most controversial of all queries about epilepsy',[223] and concluded, in what was a singular change of mind, that inheritance was less important in epilepsy than in many other common diseases in which the wisdom of marriage was never questioned.

The papers of Montreal-based researchers Julius and Katherine Metrakos, published in 1960 and 1961, presented the most nuanced view at that time of epilepsy genetics.[224] The couple studied approximately 12,000 families with epilepsy, 40 control families and 3,000 EEG recordings on patients, parents and siblings, and came to a number of conclusions which have endured. They found three categories of genes to be involved in epilepsy. The first category comprised genes related to specific diseases in which epilepsy is a part (for instance, tuberose sclerosis). Most of these were inborn errors of metabolism or other forms of symptomatic congenital epilepsy, and in the 1960s rapid progress was being made in identifying them. The second category comprised genes involved in setting the 'convulsion threshold' – in other words, genes which explained the 'predisposition' to epilepsy in a population without other underlying conditions. The third category comprised specific epilepsy genes, and in particular those underlying centrencephalic epilepsy and its EEG appearances. The Metrakoses concluded that centrencephalic epilepsy was caused by an autosomal dominant gene. In this they were mistaken, but otherwise their framework for exploring the genetics of epilepsy remains valid today. They also were the first to point out the age specificity of the genetic expression, with elegant studies of the frequency of spike–wave discharges in different age groups. Although symptomatic epilepsy was far less likely to be familial, the prevalence of epilepsy was found to be slightly higher in close relatives of those with symptomatic epilepsies, and they concluded that there was a weak inherited predisposition even in acquired epilepsy. The Metrakoses also examined the genetic aspects of febrile convulsions and of EEG abnormalities in families of those with febrile convulsions, demonstrating the existence of a genetic predisposition for both convulsions and EEG abnormalities. Finally, they estimated the risk of seizures amongst siblings of individuals with epilepsy. These studies represented a landmark in epilepsy genetics, refining and amending the findings of Lennox. They also marked the beginning of a long tradition

---

[222] Davenport and Weeks, 'Inheritance of epilepsy'.

[223] Lennox, *Epilepsy and Related Disorders*, vol. 1, p. 574.

[224] Metrakos and Metrakos, 'Genetics of convulsive disorders' (1960, 1961). Katherine Metrakos was paediatric neurologist, and her husband Julius a geneticist, at the Montreal Children's Hospital and McGill University.

of genetic investigations in Montreal, continued notably by Fred[225] and Eva Andermann.

In these years, eugenic solutions to epilepsy – by sterilisation or 'euthanasia' – were hardly mentioned. With the exception of Lennox, almost all previous enthusiasts had ceased their public advocacy. By 1960, even Lennox took a more considered approach, calling the 'blanket refusal of the marriage license to epileptics' a childish idea, and he did indeed 'encourage epileptics to marry and have children. However, we stress the individuality of the problem.'[226] He nevertheless retained the view that the severely handicapped – 'poor lumps of mortal clay in human form' – might be allowed to die, but added that 'obviously none would kill'.[227] His last statement on this topic was that '[a] possible reduction of the epileptic population in some future generation through eugenics has long been advocated. However, reduction of radiations in industry, in X-ray therapy, or in war stands first'.[228]

TREATING EPILEPSY

The treatment of epilepsy underwent great changes in this period, not only because of new drugs, but also in terms of improved evaluation and monitoring techniques. It was then that, in many senses, epilepsy therapy adopted the clothes that it continues to wear.

The Randomised Controlled Trial

One technical advance in medical therapeutics raised the quality of clinical research more than any other – the introduction of the randomised clinical trial (RCT) – and this deserves brief special mention.

Recognising that studies were needed with larger numbers, control groups and better statistical methods than were commonly employed, the MRC formed a therapeutics trial committee to address the question of the rigorous testing of new drugs. This move resulted in 1946 in what is considered to be the first RCT: the MRC trial of streptomycin in tuberculosis.[229] It was, in the

---

[225] Frederick Andermann trained in neurology at Montreal and spent his whole professional life at the Montreal Neurological Institute (MNI), where he was instrumental in maintaining the reputation of the institute in the post-Penfield era. His numerous trainees were spread throughout the world, several becoming distinguished epileptologists in their own right, and he made important contributions to many aspects of epilepsy. His work was often carried out with his remarkable physician wife, Eva, also a neurologist at the MNI.

[226] Lennox, *Epilepsy and Related Disorders*, vol. 2, pp. 1001–2.

[227] Lennox, *Epilepsy and Related Disorders*, vol. 2, pp. 1047–8.

[228] Lennox, *Epilepsy and Related Disorders*, vol. 1, p. 574.

[229] Cochrane, 'Randomised controlled trial'.

words of *The Lancet*, 'as near to a laboratory experiment as is practicable'.[230] Austin Bradford Hill, who was credited with inventing the method, had previously written a series of articles in *The Lancet* on basic medical statistics, which was later published as a book.[231] The trial, and the book, were landmarks in medical therapeutics, and practice changed. As *The Lancet* put it: 'Our experience of the last few years proves that writers on clinical subjects are more figure conscious than their elder brothers. It is less common to find startling conclusions from (say) six cases.'[232] The introduction of the RCT was emblematic of increasingly centralised and professionalised research planning and policy which, along with the development of large-scale institutional funding, disciplined clinical research and improved its scientific validity. This proved of profound importance to epilepsy, in which a large number of drugs (in seventy-one proprietary formulations and combinations) were by then being used, none of which had been adequately assessed (see Table 3.7). And as the medical community belatedly appreciated the need for proof and stringency, many were simply to disappear.

At first, epilepsy lagged sorely behind other medical areas, and throughout this period many studies of '(say) six cases' were reported. The first placebo-controlled trial in epilepsy took place in 1952,[233] but the first randomised, blinded and placebo-controlled study had to wait until 1975. This was a small cross-over study of sodium valproate, carried out at the Chalfont Centre for Epilepsy.[234] Ten years later, a definitive multicentre study was carried out in the United States involving 662 adults in 10 Veterans Administration clinics, accompanied by a series of discussion papers by Richard Mattson and colleagues laying out the principles of clinical trial design, which continue to apply today.[235]

---

[230] 'Streptomycin in pulmonary tuberculosis'.

[231] Hill, *Principles of Medical Statistics*. Sir Austin Bradford Hill was Chair of Medical Statistics at the London School of Hygiene and Tropical Medicine.

[232] 'Amateur medical statisticians'. The quotation continued 'and complete reliance on percentages divorced from absolute figures is now the hall-mark not of registered medical practitioners but of broadcasters on war production'. Epilepsy trials were equally poor. In an analysis of all published trials – 155 in all – of phenytoin and carbamazepine (the two most commonly used antiepileptics in 1973), the reports did not state the: dose of drug used in 79%, seizure frequency in 66%, length of time of trial in 28%, seizure type in 23%, age of onset of epilepsy in 95%, duration of epilepsy in 65%, age of patients in 35%, gender in 55%, presence or absence of additional handicaps in 71% or setting in 44%. The number of patients was less than 30 in 30%. Only 1% of the studies were of previously untreated cases (Shorvon, *The Drug Treatment of Epilepsy*).

[233] Handley and Stewart, 'Mysoline'. The control group was dropped only one month after the start of the trial.

[234] Richens and Ahmad, 'Controlled trial'. This trial was randomised (although it is not clear how), and blinded and placebo controlled, in twenty patients. Valproate was shown to be superior to the placebo.

[235] Mattson et al., 'Comparison'. The discussion papers included Delgado Escueta et al., 'Trials for antiepileptic drugs', and Mattson et al., 'Antiepileptic drugs in adults'.

TABLE 3.7 *The drugs used in the treatment of epilepsy in 1955*

Chemical composition	Common or trade (proprietary) names
Barbiturates	
Phenylethyl barbituric acid	Gardenal
Phenylethyl malonylurea	Luminal, Phenobarbital, Phenobarbitone
Methylphenyl barbituric acid	Mephebarbital, Rutonal
Methylphenylethyl barbituric acid	Isonal, Meberal, Prominal
Methyldiethyl barbituric acid	Gemonil
Combinations with barbiturate	
Phenylethyl barbituric acid, belladonna and caffeine	Alepsal
Phenylethyl barbituric acid and amphetamine	Ortenal
Oxazolidine diones	
Trimethyl oxazolidine dione	Absentol, epidone, mino-alleviatin, petilep, trimethadione, Tridione
Dimethylethyl oxazolidine dione	Paramethadione, Paradione
Diphenyl oxazolidine dione	Epidon
Allylmethyl oxazolidine dione	Malidone
Hydantoins	
Diphenyl hydantoin (or diphenyl hydantoin sodium)	Alleviatin, Alepsin, Antipil. Antisacer, Comitiona, Convulsin, Dihydan, Dilantin, Diphentoin, Ditoinate, Epamin, Epanutin, Eptoin, Phenytoine, solantyl
Methyldiphenyl hydantoin	Melantoine
Methylphenylethyl hydantoin	Mesantoin, Phenantoin, Sedantoinal,methoin
Methyldibromophenylethyl hydantoin	Anirrit
Dimethyldithio hydantoin	Thiomedan
Sodium phenylthienyl hydantoin	Thiantoin, Phethenylate
Methylphenyl hydantoin	Nuvarone
Combinations with hydantoins	
Diphenyl hydantoin and phenobarbital	Hydantoinal, comitoina compound
Diphenyl hydantoin, phenobarbital and caffeine	Antisacer compound, apilep
Diphenyl hydantoin, phenobarbital and desoxyephedrine	Isosolantyl, phelantin
Methylphenylethylhydantoin and phenobarbital	Hydantal
Diphenyl hydantoin and methylphenylethyl barbituric acid	Comital, mebaroin
Diphenyl hydantoin, methylphenylethyl barbituric acid and phenobarbital	Comital L
Other types	
Phenylacetylurea	Epiclase, fenilep, phenacemide, Phenurone
Phenylethylhexahydropyrimidine dione	Mysoline, primidone
Benzchlorpropamide	Hibicon, posedrine
Methylalphaphenyl succinimide	Lifene, milontin
Acetazoleamide	Diamox
Glutamic acid (or glutamic acid-HCl)	Acidulin, Glutan-HCl, Glutamicol
Bromides	Large numbers of preparations (in three categories: alkaline bromides and alkaline earths: polybromide; organic bromides; bromide in combination with other agents)

(Derived from: 'International list of antiepilepsy drugs')

The NIH Epilepsy Branch and Antiepileptic Drugs

J. Kiffin Penry made his entrance earlier in this book. Of all his multiple undertakings, it was perhaps his work on antiepileptic drugs which had the greatest impact. This was carried out in his capacity as head of the Epilepsy Branch at NIH, having been appointed in 1966 by his previous tutor, Richard Masland, who must have been very satisfied with the subsequent progress of his protégé. From then until his retirement in 1979 (a period of only thirteen years), Penry and his collaborators radically changed the treatment landscape – and did so in a strategic, planned and comprehensive manner.

As described earlier, in the mid-1960s the pharmaceutical industry had veered away from developing antiepileptic drugs. A survey of pharmaceutical firms conducted by the Epilepsy Branch in 1967[236] found that there were no new antiepileptic drugs under development and that several other drugs had failed to gain approval because of inadequate proof of efficacy. Some companies reported that they had discontinued the screening of new compounds, and others were known to possess anticonvulsant compounds that were not being pursued. One reason was cost, which had increased because of the requirements of the 1962 Kefauver–Harris amendments, but there were others including: insufficient access to pharmacological screening; a feeling amongst the industry that existing drugs, used properly, would suffice in the treatment of epilepsy; the absence of an accepted classification of seizures and well-documented patient populations; and the absence of a rigorous trial methodology compatible with the new regulatory standards. In the twelve-year period from 1961 to 1973, not a single new anticonvulsant drug was marketed in the United States. For Penry and his team at the NIH, this was a matter of great concern.[237]

One of Penry's first acts as head of the Epilepsy Branch was to commission a report from James Coatsworth about the state of clinical trials. The Coatsworth report[238] of 1971 was a notable development in the field of antiepileptic drug therapy. It constituted the first serious look at clinical trials, which made it, one of the first systematic reviews, if not the first, in epilepsy – or, indeed, in medicine. Based on a search of 64 journals, Coatsworth evaluated 800 published reports of 250 separate drug studies (including case reports), of the 13 available antiepileptic drugs, published between 1920 and 1970 which purported to demonstrate the efficacy of an antiepileptic. Coatsworth's analysis demonstrated appallingly bad clinical documentation, design and

---

[236] Public Health Service Advisory Committee on the Epilepsies, *Minutes of Meeting*. This report opened with Sieveking's famous statement that 'there is not a substance in the materia medica, there is scarcely a substance in the world, capable of passing through the gullet of man, that has not at one time or another enjoyed a reputation of being an anti-epileptic'.

[237] For instance, as discussed later, carbamazepine and valproate were by then well established in Europe but were not available in America.

[238] Coatsworth, *Marketed Antiepileptic Drugs*.

methodology. Many of the studies were small, and only three were controlled – each with a cross-over design with randomisation, two being double-blind and one single-blind. Only three studies involved a placebo arm. The lamentable quality of the studies was a shock. And although their authors seemed to consider their anecdotal opinions about the effectiveness of a drug to be valid, Coatsworth sternly dissented. He concluded baldly that almost none of the available antiepileptic drugs had been robustly demonstrated to be effective. Penry agreed with Coatsworth.

The Epilepsy Branch then set to work on an extraordinary range of activities aimed at both raising the standards of evaluation of antiepileptic drugs and improving diagnosis and treatment in routine clinical practice. These included cooperating with the work leading to the ILAE classification of seizures, a vital step in systemising and standardising antiepileptic drug trial parameters; establishing high-quality methodologies for drug trialling and documentation; working to improve the reliability of blood-level measurements of existing antiepileptic drugs; encouraging video-EEG monitoring as a clinical tool and a way of assessing antiepileptic drugs, especially for absence seizures; and funding epidemiological studies of the prevalence of various seizure disorders, as a basis for demonstrating the need for new treatments. He also organised symposia and conferences – and these resulted in a series of important publications.[239] The branch itself then conducted the studies necessary for new drug applications for carbamazepine and clonazepam, which were already licensed in Europe by virtue of clinical trials that did not meet the new US standards.[240] Finally, Penry and his colleagues lobbied publicly for licensing valproate, which was also widely available in Europe but not in the United States. These activities were all to prove extraordinarily successful.

The workshops and symposia were outstanding and memorable events, illustrating Penry's typical modus operandi: meticulous preparation and great attention to detail, but with a wide scope and focus on practical outcomes. The resulting books became standard reference works and were the first significant multi-authored texts in epilepsy. With chapters contributed by the foremost American (and a few European) researchers, detailed data reflecting the state of advanced knowledge at the time was presented, and these were a leading influence on the direction of research over the next decades. Two of the

---

[239] The most significant were: 'Symposium on laboratory evaluation'; Glaser, Penry and Woodbury, *Basic Mechanisms* Woodbury, Penry and Schmidt, *Antiepileptic Drugs*; Purpura et al., *Experimental Models of Epilepsy*; Pippenger, Penry and Kutt, *Quantitative Analysis and Interpretation*; and Glaser, Penry and Woodbury, *Antiepileptic Drugs*. The process leading up to the latter book was an example of Penry's organisational method. A closed workshop was then held in Warrenton, Virginia, in June 1970 to develop plans, contributors were selected from amongst the participants, and a further meeting was then held in Scottsdale, Arizona, in September 1971. The preliminary manuscripts were then submitted for the approval of the editorial board. The editors added new data where pertinent during the editing phase, and the book was published in 1972.

[240] Dreifuss et al., 'Serum clonazepam concentrations'.

books, *Antiepileptic Drugs* and *Antiepileptic Drugs: Mechanisms of Action*, went into further editions.[241] The clinical trials of carbamazepine and clonazepam resulted in licensing of these drugs in 1974 and 1975. Trials were also carried out on sulthiame and albutoin, which showed no effect and these drugs were abandoned. The trial leading to the approval of carbamazepine received the first ILAE Award for Best Controlled Clinical Trial of an Antiepileptic Drug.[242]

The Epilepsy Branch under Penry also established a programme for testing new antiepileptics in synchrony with the FDA's three-phase approach. [243] The goal of Phase 1 was to establish human safety and basic pharmacokinetic parameters in healthy volunteers without epilepsy; Phase 2 would determine whether a given drug seemed to be an anticonvulsant in humans, and to establish a therapeutic range and dose; and Phase 3 would evaluate the efficacy and safety of the drug in short-term and long-term use in a large number of individuals, with adequate variation of characteristics to warrant generalisation of the results to the population in which the drug would be licensed. In Phase 3, blinded, randomised and placebo-controlled trials soon became an absolute requirement. This approach was utterly new in antiepileptic drug testing, and it is a testament to the work of the Epilepsy Branch that the approach remained unchanged in principle over the next five decades.

Penry was equally active in the basic science of epilepsy. He enthusiastically adopted the NIH policies of both stimulating science and supporting industry, believing that these policies would be the best way of improving clinical practice. In 1975, with Ewart Swinyard[244] and Harvey Kupferberg, Penry launched the Antiepileptic Drug Development Program at the University of Utah. This programme provided facilities for academia and industry for screening antiepileptic drugs, with the objective of stimulating pharmaceutical development. The screening consisted of seven different phases.[245] By the end of 1977, more than 43

---

[241] *Antiepileptic Drugs* was published in five editions between 1972 and 2002.

[242] Cereghino, 'Major advances in epilepsy'.

[243] Porter and Kupferberg ('Anticonvulsant Screening Program') point out that Penry's extraordinary energy and enthusiasm fortuitously coincided with a lack of burdensome bureaucracy at NIH at that time.

[244] Ewart Swinyard was a professor and Dean of the College of Pharmacy at the University of Utah.

[245] Drugs progressed from one phase to the next phase only if they showed promise. Phase 1 was a screen for potential efficacy, using the MES (maximal electroshock) and PTZ (pentylene-tetrazol) tests. The first was thought to screen for drugs effective in partial and secondarily generalised seizures, and the second for those effective in primary generalised seizures. In Phase 2, anticonvulsant action and neurotoxicity were quantified, and the median effective dose, time to peak effect and median toxic dose were determined. Phase 3 tested the median hypnotic dose, median lethal dose and toxicity profile in mice. Phase 4 quantified the anticonvulsant activity after oral administration to mice. In Phase 5, test drugs were further characterised using different chemicals to induce seizures in animals. Anticonvulsant properties and toxicity was evaluated in other species in Phase 6, and the lethal doses and effects of prolonged administration in Phase 7. In 2015, the name of the programme was changed to the *Epilepsy Therapy Screening Program* (ETSP), the phases were revised and a wider battery of rodent and in-vitro tests were introduced.

academic medicinal chemists had submitted nearly 800 compounds. By 2000, more than 20,000 compounds had been screened, and the programme continues to this day.[246]

Drug Therapy 1945–1960

In this early post-war period, drugs were usually tested for antiepileptic properties by the random screening of chemicals in unfortunate cats using the model pioneered by Merritt and Putnam. Most of the compounds resulted from the synthesis of biologically active chemical families (i.e. in chemically similar compounds).[247] Examples included the barbiturate, oxazolidinedione, hydantoin and succinimide families of compounds (Table 3.8). Such an approach had the disadvantage, obviously, of focusing too much on what became known as me-too compounds (drugs with similar effects) and, as it turned out, on compounds with a similar mechanism of action, although at the time the actual mechanisms of action were almost entirely unknown. Later, in the 1960s, the steric molecular conformation of drugs was found to be important,[248] but structure–activity relationships were based usually on what was essentially intuitive and empirical guesswork.

In his magnum opus of 1960,[249] Lennox provided a glimpse of the then gold-standard treatment approaches in epilepsy, grouping them into three: hygiene, drugs and surgery. Hygiene (lifestyle issues and diet) still occupied first place and was not merely the footnote it was to become in later decades. His recommendations were much the same as those of many earlier authors in the previous 100 years, put in a way that no doubt would have amused the ancients: 'The close relationship of measures that make for good health is exemplified by the fact that Hygeia, the goddess of health, was no other than the daughter of Aesculapius, the god of medicine' (p. 820). Lennox was scornful of most diets: 'good health does not depend on meaningless taboos' (p. 823) and 'the patient should eat what other members of the family eat' (p. 821). He did however endorse the value of the ketogenic diet, which of course he had worked on years earlier:

> In spite of the proven value of the ketogenic diet, it is little used today, except in certain long-established centers, such as the Mayo and Johns Hopkins

---

[246] See Porter and Kupferberg, 'Anticonvulsant Screening Program'. The programme made a major contribution to the development of felbamate, topiramate, rufinamide, lacosamide and retigabine, and some contribution to vigabatrin, lamotrigine, oxcarbazepine and gabapentin.

[247] Some drugs being developed for another indication were then found, following screening, to be useful in epilepsy. Trimethadione and carbamazepine, for instance, were originally under investigation for use in pain and depression, and valproate as a solvent.

[248] In epilepsy, diazepam and phenytoin are examples of drugs with dissimilar chemistry, but similar molecular and steric conformation (Camerman and Camerman, 'Diphenylhydantoin and diazepam').

[249] Lennox and Lennox, *Epilepsy and Related Disorders*, vol. 2, p. 820.

TABLE 3.8 *New anticonvulsant drugs marketed in the USA and Europe between 1945 and 1951*

Year of first	Trade introduction name	Scientific name	Manufacturing company
1946	Tridione	Trimethadione	Abbott
1947	Mesantoin	Mephenytoin	Sandoz
1949	Paradione	Paramethadione	Abbott
1950	Thiantoin	Phenthenylate	Lilly
1951	Phenurone	Phenacemide	Abbott
1952	Gemonil	Metharbital	Abbott
1952	Hibicon	Benzchlorpropanamide, Beclamide	Lederle
1953	Milontin	Phensuximide	Parke, Davis
1954	Mysoline	Primidone	ICI
1957	Peganone	Ethotoin	Abbott
1951	Celontin	Methsuximide	Parke, Davis

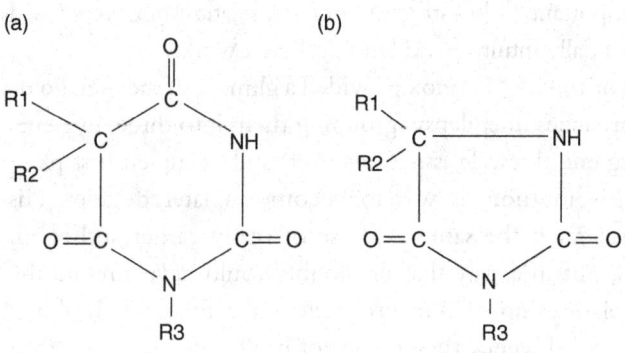

(a) (b)

Barbiturate	R1	R2	R3	Hydantoin
Veronal	Ethyl	Ethyl	H	(Too toxic)
Phenobarbitone	Ethyl	Ethyl	H	Nirvanol
Mebaral, Prominal	Phenyl	Ethyl	Methyl	Mesantoin
(Not synthesised)	Phenyl	Phenyl	H	Phenytoin

29. The similarity in chemical structure between barbiturates (a) and hydantoins (b), and their derivatives.

Clinics and the colonies of Denmark and Holland. The reasons are obvious: effective medicines are now available. The diet is limited and distasteful to the patient, and time-consuming and expensive for the parent. (p. 829)[250]

---

[250] In the Heemstede epilepsy colony, about 30–50% of patients received the diet between 1945–52 and then its use began to fade, disappearing altogether around 1960 (SEIN in-house newsletter – personal communication from Walter van Emde Boas).

He also noted, based on his earlier work, that dehydration was ineffective and starvation helped temporarily, but it was not a permanent solution. Activity was encouraged, and he thought electroconvulsive therapy might have some place: 'To hold a drowning man under the water seems no more illogical than to give an epileptic a convulsant drug. Yet fire can be fought with fire, and cowpox prevents smallpox' (p. 833).

The focus of this chapter, however, was on drug therapy, and it occupied 100 pages of his book. Lennox made 'fifteen suggestions . . . as possible guide lines leading towards successful drug therapy' (p. 835). These included: 'Treat the patient', not just his symptoms; 'fit the treatment to the fit'; 'individualize dosage'; 'prescribe adequate dosage'; and '[watch] the waves' (i.e. the EEG) (pp. 835–40). These principles are the origin of much which has been written since and remain largely true today. In a subsection titled 'A century of hope' (p. 851), Lennox listed 16 drugs that he called his 'therapeutic arsenal' (Table 3.9). Bromides were by then 'little used' (p. 855). Barbiturates were still mentioned with enthusiasm. He noted that 2,500 barbiturate compounds had

TABLE 3.9 *Lennox's 'therapeutic arsenal'*

Non-commercial official name	Patented trade name
For grand mal and psychomotor seizures	
Bromides	Bromides
Phenobarbital[a]	Luminal
Methobarbital	Mebaral
Diphenylhydantoin[a]	Dilantin
Mesantoin	Mesantoin
Ethotoin	Peganone
Primidone[a]	Mysoline
Phenacemide	Phenurone
Methsuximide[a]	Celontin
Acetazoleamide[b]	Diamox
For petit mal seizures	
Trimethadione[b]	Tridione
Paramethadione[a]	Paradione
Phensuximide[a]	Milontin
Ethylmethylsuccinimide	Zarontin
Quinacrine hydrochloride	Atabrine
Metharbital	Gemonil

[a] Drugs of initial choice
[b] Drugs of second choice
Phenurone and diamox were noted to be often effective against petit mal as well, and phensuximide to be often effective against grand mal.
(Lennox and Lennox, *Epilepsy*, Vol. 2, pp. 845–89)

been synthesised, of which 50 were marketed, and that phenobarbital was the most frequently used in epilepsy. Mephobarbital (Mebaral, produced by Winthrop-Stearns) was 'the only barbiturate besides phenobarbital effective against epilepsy' (p. 860; although in this, Lennox was incorrect), and one which seemed to have more effect on petit mal. However, and perhaps not surprisingly, he was most enthusiastic about phenytoin (Dilantin), which he considered a more potent anticonvulsant than phenobarbital, its discovery in 1938 being 'for epileptics a year of jubilee' (p. 861). He noted that in Europe phenobarbital was still preferred (citing Gastaut), but for him Dilantin was 'the drug of choice for the control of psychomotor seizures and convulsions'. It also had the 'advantage of a minimal hypnotic effect' (p. 862). 'A therapeutic "bull's-eye" may be scored with Dilantin even for a person with long-standing convulsions previously unrelieved by phenobarbital' (p. 865), but care was needed with dosing and the range of side effects.

By 1960, Lennox had also come to value Mesantoin (manufactured by Sandoz, and a close structural sister of phenytoin), which was preferred by one-half of patients over phenytoin for more effective control or fewer side effects, although 'the number of reported cases of aplastic anemia dulls enthusiasm for this medicine' (p. 869). To Lennox, 'Mesantoin and Dilantin are Damon and Pythias in respect to their suitability for joint action. Similarity of action gives a doubled therapeutic effect; the dissimilarity of their side reactions keeps these within bounds.' He sometimes recommended their joint use. Ethotoin (Peganone) according to Lennox was one of 1,500 compounds screened by Abbott Laboratories in the previous eight years, but it did not seem to induce much enthusiasm.

Primidone (Mysoline) was 'especially welcomed as a contribution from abroad, by the Imperial Chemical Industries of England' (p. 872), but it did have a tendency to cause side effects on initiation: '"I feel just awful, all over," wails a person who is plunged into the treatment' (p. 872). Lennox seemed to have favoured large doses, and he mentioned one young woman with out-of-control attacks who finally gained complete control with 600 mg of phenytoin and 2,000 mg of primidone – enormous dosages by today's standard.

Next came phenacemide (Phenurone), which was 'what in athletics might be called a triple threat because, more than any other drug, it acts against each of the three main types of seizures, and especially against the most feared psycho-motor seizures. However, it is also a triple threat to the patient himself because of possible effect on the marrow, the liver, or the psyche' (p. 874). Given 1 chance in 250 of not surviving this treatment, Lennox asked, 'Is the risk too great?' In fact, he prefaced his list of drugs with a section on the question of drug-induced fatalities, opining that '[a]granulocytosis may be an "act of God," coming or going without any explanation that man can offer' (p. 847). Although, to the physician today, Lennox seemed rather shockingly unconcerned about these fatal reactions, his was the first major epilepsy book to give aplastic anaemia, severe skin and blood reactions a detailed consideration.

He found methsuximide (Celontin) to be useful in petit mal, likening it 'to a "pusher" locomotive that helps a train up a long grade' (p. 875). Acetazoleamide (Diamox, produced by Lederle) had possibly less 'staying power' than the diones or succinimide drugs, but it reminded Lennox of the 'excitement that began in the 1920's over the relationship of seizures to fasting, ketosis, dehydration, and later to the relationship of the tension of carbon dioxide to cerebral circulation, to petits, and especially to the alternate spike–wave discharges of the EEG' (p. 876), which of course were all areas which Lennox had researched.

The oxazolidinediones were an early group of compounds to emerge in the euphoria that followed phenytoin. Trimethadione (Tridione) was one of the first and subsequently, within Parke-Davis, Charles Miller and co-workers systematically explored other succinimides. Three derivatives were identified, licensed and marketed: phensuximide (Milontin, 1953), methsuximide (Celontin, 1957) and the ethyl derivative, ethosuximide (1958). Lennox was excited by trimethadione (Tridione), which 'heads the list of drugs that are peculiarly beneficial to persons subject to petits, and less distinctly for the other members of the petit mal triad ... World-wide acceptance of Tridione was attained more quickly than acceptance of Dilantin [but] Tridione had no competitor' (p. 879). However, 'while harmonizing the brain waves, Tridione may play havoc with the blood-forming organs', and Lennox recommended monthly blood counts but warned of the 'fickleness of the peripheral blood' (p. 881). When patients with petit mal failed to respond to Tridione, '[t]he circuit of other drugs in the group against petits must be called on, single or in combination: Paradione, Milontin, Diamox, Atabrine, even caffeine and Phenurone' (p. 882). Paramethadione (Paradione) was somewhat better than trimethadione for the treatment of petit mal though worse for grand mal, but it was safer. Ethlymethlysuccinimide (Zarontin) was still an experimental drug when Lennox's book was published, but he mentioned its first trial,[251] which employed a high dose of 1,750 mg/day, and the fact that 24% of patients experienced 80–99% control of seizures – an unprecedented effect. The drug's side-effect profile took longer to be recognised, with the first cases of fatal allergy noted only in the 1960s. But it remains a mainline treatment, even today, which is true of very few other drugs in Lennox's survey.

Corticosteroids, and particularly ACTH, were also introduced into clinical epilepsy practice in 1950, when reports of ACTH's efficacy in childhood epilepsy began to be made. The dramatic effect in infantile spasms was reported in 1958, and ACTH has since remained first-line therapy for this indication.

---

[251] Zimmerman and Burgemeister, 'Petit mal epilepsy'.

For a time, steroids were widely used in other types of epilepsy and in status epilepticus. Paraldehyde became another drug widely used in status epilepticus and in alcohol withdrawal seizures at mid-century, not least for its safety and remarkable efficacy. Introduced into clinical practice in 1882, its anticonvulsant action was first reported in 1940. Its intravenous use in status epilepticus required a complex series of glass tubing (it degrades plastic), with a striking resemblance to a school chemistry lesson; its lingering odour permeating all corners of a ward is still seared in my memory as a madeleine of the then contemporary practice. Chlormethiazole was also popular in status epilepticus after the first report of its use in 1963,[252] and by 1970 it had become a standard second-line therapy. But its tendency to accumulate dangerously meant that by the 1990s it was only occasionally used, and now not at all, as other safer alternatives entered clinical practice.

As for the mechanisms of action of these drugs, Lennox admitted that little was known. He was also cautious about their overall effectiveness, and realised that selection bias, duration of follow-up and severity of side effects might all potentially distort his views. His own experience of 680 'office patients' surveyed retrospectively by questionnaire was that 24% had seizures arrested for 18 months or more, 49% showed a 50–99% improvement, 17% were somewhat improved (<50%), 6% were about the same and 4% were worse (p. 891).

So what can one make of this? Lennox had enormous experience, was foremost among key opinion leaders and was courted by the two pharmaceutical companies most active in the field of epilepsy: Abbott and Parke-Davis. His opinion on the relative merits and disadvantages of the drugs carried enormous weight but was based on his (vast) personal experience rather than any gold-standard evidence. That is a pity, as the RCT methodology was well known by then but not mentioned once in his book. Nevertheless, a guide to the practice of the period, *Epilepsy and Related Disorders* was (and is) surely without parallel.

By the time Lennox's book was published in 1960, the field was moving on, and Lennox himself failed to make any reference to what was probably the most important advance in applied clinical therapeutics of the time – the ability to measure the serum levels of drugs and application of the technique to epilepsy therapy. Like so much of epilepsy science, the methodology was technology driven. Before the early 1940s, few (if any) analytical methods of assaying drugs in biological fluids were available. The first were colorimetric methods (used for sulphonamides). Later, attempts were made to use chemical and ion-exchange chromatography and spectrometry for phenytoin, but initially these were too insensitive. The major breakthrough was in 1956, when suitable spectrophotometric and colorimetric procedures were introduced. In 1965, a

[252] Poiré et al., 'Traitement des états de mal épileptiques'.

phenytoin assay using thin-layer chromatography linked to colorimetry was described. That same year a benzophenone-extraction procedure was introduced, followed in 1968 by a gas-liquid chromatographic method. These developments led to the systematic measurement of antiepileptic drug serum levels in the clinic, and a series of studies showed a relationship between effectiveness and blood levels of phenytoin and phenobarbital, as well as a relationship to toxicity. The measurements of blood level also allowed assessment of absorption, distribution, metabolism and excretion and these were parameters that were routinely accounted for in clinical practice by the late 1960s. Again, most work was carried out on phenytoin, a fortunate choice, as phenytoin has an interesting metabolic and pharmacokinetic profile and exhibits saturation kinetics which render its serum-level measurements more useful clinically than those of any other antiepileptic drug. A classic paper by Henn Kutt and colleagues in 1964[253] was particularly influential in showing a tight relationship between phenytoin blood level and effectiveness and toxicity. But the same close relationship between blood levels and effect does not apply to many other drugs, and had phenytoin not been chosen as a study-drug it is possible that the whole field of therapeutic drug monitoring in epilepsy might have died on the vine. Nevertheless, by the end of the 1960s, a fairly comprehensive definition of the pharmacokinetic parameters of all the available antiepileptic drugs had been achieved and became a requirement of the regulatory authorities. The full flowering of this field occurred though in later decades (see pp. 445–8).

Four New Drugs

The decade 1958–68 was to prove a golden age of new drug licensing in epilepsy in Europe, unrivalled before or since – a result of the pharmaceutical optimism, rising wealth and the new energy in the field of epilepsy (Table 3.10).

Although Lennox had caught the early stirrings of ethosuximide, which was to have an enduring effect in epilepsy, there were three other new drugs (and drug groups) – carbamazepine, valproate and the benzodiazepines – discovered in the 1960s, a few years after the publication of Lennox's book, which would transform epilepsy and render his therapeutic opinions largely redundant.[254]

Carbamazepine was developed in the laboratories of the Swiss pharmaceutical firm Geigy in 1953. Trade-named Tegretol, it was the first of the antiepileptic drugs to produce huge profits for its manufacturer. Carbamazepine was discovered in the search for a psychoactive drug following the success of chlorpromazine. Changes to the chlorpromazine molecule led to the discovery

[253] Kutt et al., 'Diphenylhydantoin metabolism'.
[254] Details from Shorvon, 'Drug treatment of epilepsy'.

TABLE 3.10 *New drugs for epilepsy licensed in 1958–68: a golden decade*

Date	Trade name	Scientific name	Manufacturer
1958	Zarontin	Ethosuximide	Parke, Davis
1960	Librium	Chlordiazepoxide	Roche
1962	Ospolot	Sulthiame	Bayer
1963	Valium	Diazepam	Roche
1965	Tegretol	Carbamazepine	Geigy
1967	Epilim, Depakene Depakote*	Valproate	Sanofi-Labaz
1968	Rivotril	Clonazepam	Roche

* Epilim is the brand name for sodium valproate; Depakine is the brand name for valproic acid; and Depakote is the brand name for valproate semisodium, a stable coordination compound containing a 1:1 mixture of sodium valproate and valproic acid.

first of the tricyclic drugs, such as imipramine, which were found to have value in depression. Then, substitution of the basic side chain at the N5 position of the tricyclic ring by a carboxamide moiety led to the discovery of carbamazepine. This was found to have more potent effects in the maximal electroshock model than any other of the similar compounds being produced (although only a small effect in the pentylenetetrazol model). It was first investigated as a drug for depression and psychosis, then pain, and when its effects on neuralgic pain were discovered it was licensed and marketed for trigeminal neuralgia in 1962. Its antiepileptic effects had been investigated clinically in 1959 and were first reported in 1963, and the drug soon gained a reputation in Europe as a promising new antiepileptic. One of the first controlled and single-blinded (but not randomised) trials in epilepsy was undertaken at a hospital for the mentally subnormal in England in 1966.[255] Tegretol was substituted for existing therapy with phenobarbitone in 50% of the subjects and compared to the continuation of phenobarbital in the other 50%. Identical white tablets were produced that contained phenobarbital, phenytoin, primidone and carbamazepine, and staff and patients were blinded to which drug was being taken. The study was conducted over 18 months in 45 patients. Carbamazepine was found to have an equivalent antiepileptic action to phenobarbital, phenytoin and primidone, given either separately or in combination. Although it was hoped that there would also be a psychotropic effect, no difference between the groups was noted. Four patients on carbamazepine died during the study, but this was felt by the investigators (one of whom worked for Geigy) to be no more than would be expected by chance. In 1965 the drug was approved for use as an anticonvulsant in the United Kingdom, and then Europe, although approval in the United States was delayed until 1974.

[255] Bird et al., 'Tegretol (carbamazepine)'.

By 1975 carbamazepine had become one of the most-prescribed drugs world-wide, and its effectiveness against partial seizures and generalised tonic–clonic seizures has never been bettered. Even now, fifty years after its introduction, it remains the gold standard and the drug to beat for any new compound. It was soon found to cause a mild rash in at least 5% of persons and, rarely, more severe dermatological disturbances, with occasional fatalities.[256] Aplastic anaemia was also found to occur in about 1 per 100,000 and serious hepatic failure in 15 per 100,000 exposed persons. Minor side effects were quickly spotted, and occurred particularly on starting the drug. But once a person was established on therapy, studies showed significantly better side-effect profiles than in the case of pheny-toin or phenobarbital. Carbamazepine is involved in many pharmacokinetic interactions, the importance of which were fully recognised by the late 1970s, and it remains, after phenytoin, the compound for which therapeutic drug monitoring (TDM) is most valuable. In 1972 carbamazepine epoxide was deter-mined to be its major metabolite. Its toxicity and efficacy were fully appreciated by 1980 and measurement of the plasma levels of epoxide as well as the parent drug were recognised to be needed clinically. Like phenytoin, carbamazepine prescribing required (and still requires) skilful handling. Consequently, the introduction of these drugs and the need for pharmacokinetic monitoring proved a useful justification for the promotion of specialisation and epilepsy clinics.

Dipropylacetic acid (valproate) was synthesised in 1881 and had been used for about eighty years as an organic solvent. In 1962, Laboratoire Berthier, a small pharmaceutical company in Grenoble led by two brothers, les frères Meunier, decided to test a series of compounds in the rat, in collaboration with George Carraz of the University of Grenoble. Dipropylacetic acid was chosen as the solvent. When all the compounds were apparently found to be antiepileptic in this model, the Meunier brothers decided to test the solvent alone and it became immediately obvious that it was this that conferred the antiepileptic action. The laboratory proceeded to develop valproate in-house. In 1963, a first experimental study of the compound was conducted in sixteen rabbits given the convulsant cardiazol. In those days, there were few restrictions in Europe on the human testing of novel agents, and the first clinical study was reported in 1964. It was soon apparent that more resources than were possible in the Meuniers' small laboratory were needed. As a result, the drug was sold on and licensed in the mid-1960s by the French pharmaceutical company Sanofi-Labaz. It was then extensively promoted, and in 1967 valproate was approved in France, and soon after in other European countries.[257] By 1970 valproate was being widely used in Europe but its licence in the United States was delayed. This

[256] The propensity to cause a severe dermatological reaction was found in 2006 to have a genetic basis.

[257] Spain, 1970; Belgium and Holland, 1971; Britain, Switzerland and Italy, 1972; in various formulations, under the trade names of Epilim, Depakine and Depakote.

became a cause célèbre, with Kiffin Penry leading a campaign to the US Senate, and the FDA took the unprecedented step of requiring the Abbott pharmaceutical company to supply data in order that the drug could be considered for licensing. The drug was eventually approved in 1976, albeit only for the treatment of absence seizures. The battle for approval was turned into a 1987 ABC television film, *Fight for Life*, which emphasised the arbitrariness of regulatory approval and the political nature of regulatory decisions (Penry was portrayed as 'Dr Keith', played by Robert Benson).

In 1975 Daniel Simon and Penry published a major review of the drug,[258] and this formed the basis of the subsequent FDA approval. They located reports of 13 clinical trials, including 2 double-blind cross-over trials, and performed what was an early meta-analysis of 10 trials in 1,020 patients. The results showed a reduction in tonic–clonic, myoclonic and absence seizures in more than 50% of patients, and in about one-third of patients with partial seizures. The effect of valproate on abolishing photosensitivity and spike–wave paroxysms on EEG, and its effects in atypical absence, were also recognised. By 1980 valproate was being routinely recommended as first-line therapy. From the earliest days, anxiety was expressed about the safety of the drug. Sedation was soon reported, as was encephalopathy (two patients in the initial trials were rendered comatose). Other serious side effects were not identified until the 1980s and 1990s, and the drug's teratogenicity, described in the next chapter, became the subject of large-scale litigation.

By the 1970s, epilepsy led the therapeutics drive in neurology and, partly because of phenytoin, carbamazepine and valproate, epilepsy had risen to the top of the neurological agenda again. These three drugs remain the most-cited and most-studied compounds in the history of epilepsy.

In psychiatry, the potential for drug therapy was proving even more exciting. The development of antipsychotics and tricyclic antidepressants transformed the specialty, as described earlier, but in the 1960s another psychopharmaceutical discovery burst onto the scene and one that was also to have a profound influence on epilepsy. The 1,4-benzodiazepine drugs (chlordiazepoxide, diazepam, clonazepam) had, even more than barbiturates, an extraordinary impact on many aspects of Western culture and way of life. Valium entered the folklore of the age (for instance, as the 'little yellow pills' in the famous Rolling Stones' song 'Mother's Little Helper'), and these drugs helped fuel both a revolution in biological psychiatry and the societal reaction, the anti-psychiatry movement of the 1960s. The story of their discovery offers an intriguing insight into the process of mid-century drug development.

The first reports of the clinical effects of chlorpromazine were published in 1952 and its obvious commercial importance and rapid success sparked a race

---

[258] Simon and Penry, 'Sodium di-N-propylacetate'.

amongst pharmaceutical companies to discover other psychoactive drugs which might have improved properties. The Swiss pharmaceutical giant Roche was a leader in the field and had developed a range of animal-testing models for assessing sedative properties. In the mid-1950s Leo Sternbach, a medicinal chemist in charge of a company laboratory in New Jersey, decided to investigate the pharmaceutical actions of a group of compounds he had created, which came to be known as benzodiazepines. They were attractive candidates as they were readily produced, capable of generating whole families of compounds through chemical manipulation and largely unstudied in pharmacology. They had the 'look', as Sternbach later put it, of being biologically active. He started with benzheptoxdiazines and synthesised a range of derivatives with different side-chain products. Initially, no biological action was found and Sternbach's laboratory was asked by Roche management to focus on other research areas. In cleaning up, his technician found a few hundred milligrams of crystallised compounds, prepared in 1955, which were thought to be quinazoline 3-oxides. Sternbach decided to submit these for animal screening, and the drugs were found to have powerful sedative effects. Sternbach pressed on. He found that the compounds were not in fact quinazoline oxides; they had a seven-membered diazepine ring. In May 1958, a broad patent was filed for the 2-amino-1,4-benzodiazepine 4-oxides and various substituents in the benzo and phenyl rings, and granted in July 1959. An intensive pharmacological programme of work ensued, and the first compound, given the generic name chlordiazepoxide, proved superior to its derivatives and was submitted for licensing to the FDA. In 1960, in short order, the compound was approved and licensed under the name Librium. Sternbach carried on with his chemical exploration and discovered that the N-oxide (at the 4-position) was not necessary for the pharmacological action, contrary to the then-current hypothesis regarding mechanisms of action; rather, the biological activity depended on the presence of a chlorine in the 7-position. With additional manipulation, another compound, given the name diazepam, was discovered and found to have a broader spectrum of activity than Librium, with stronger antiepileptic and muscle-relaxant properties and very low toxicity. Following clinical studies, the drug was licensed in 1963 under the name Valium. In the next fifteen years, more than 4,000 related compounds were synthesised and screened and by 1978, twenty-three compounds had been licensed worldwide (including eight in the United States). Such a programme was only possible in the research factories of the largest multinational pharmaceutical companies,[259] and it was this model of drug development that led to the global dominance of the mega pharma companies.

[259] Details taken from Sternbach's own retrospective accounts – published repetitiously in amongst others: 'Benzodiazepine story' (1978); 'Benzodiazepine story' (1979); 'Story of the benzodiazepines' (1980).

The benzodiazepines were found on random screening to be effective in epilepsy. The anticonvulsant effect of Librium was first reported in humans in 1960 and that of diazepam in 1962. Gastaut was enthusiastic about this class of drugs (and his views on their value in status epilepticus are described earlier). In 1982, in a characteristically definitive statement, Gastaut reviewed the overall experience with benzodiazepines and proclaimed that he had tested twenty-one of the agents since 1965 and considered them 'to be clearly distinguished from all other types of anticonvulsant drugs'.[260] Three in particular had exceptional anticonvulsant properties: clonazepam, flunitrazepam and clobazam. He by then recognised their disadvantages as well, noting that although the drugs were effective in all types of seizures, they were less so than other agents displaying more specific actions (i.e. valproate and ethosuximide in primary generalised epilepsy, and phenytoin and carbamazepine in partial epilepsy). The advantages of the benzodiazepines were rapid action intravenously and their lack of parenchymal toxicity, but their shortcomings were tolerance and side effects such as sedation. Gastaut concluded that although they were the treatment of first choice in acute epilepsy (such as status epilepticus), they were less efficacious in chronic epilepsy and indicated from onset only in Lennox syndrome. In other epilepsies they should be given only after failure of other more appropriate anticonvulsants. His assessment still stands today.

Surgical Treatment For Epilepsy

As we saw earlier, by the mid-1930s, although neurosurgery was a growing specialty practised in quite a few European and North American centres, epilepsy surgery was still hardly performed. This was to change, though, with the introduction of EEG. This provided, for the surgeon, ancillary evidence of the site of the focus and confirmation of the clinical diagnosis and was a huge stimulus. For the first time an objective method seemed to afford 'visualisation' of epilepsy in the brain. And it was the temporal lobe which was to be the target of most interest.

Precedence in science is important, and controversy exists about who was first to resect mesial temporal structures in a temporal lobectomy.[261] As mentioned earlier, at the meeting of the Chicago Neurological Society in 1946, Gibbs presented his data showing that the psychomotor seizure was accompanied by a specific spike focus in the region of the anterior temporal lobe, and

---

[260] Gastaut, 'Effect of benzodiazepines'.

[261] This is a key point, as it is clear that removal of the mesial structures is in many cases responsible for the success of the operation. See the interesting contributions of Nicholas Moran ('History of temporal lobectomy') and Jerome Engel ('Temporal lobe surgery'). The key papers by Arthur Morris were 'Treatment of psychomotor epilepsy' and 'Temporal lobectomy'. Interestingly, Penfield's books and papers of the period make not a single reference to Morris's publications, although no doubt he must have been aware of them.

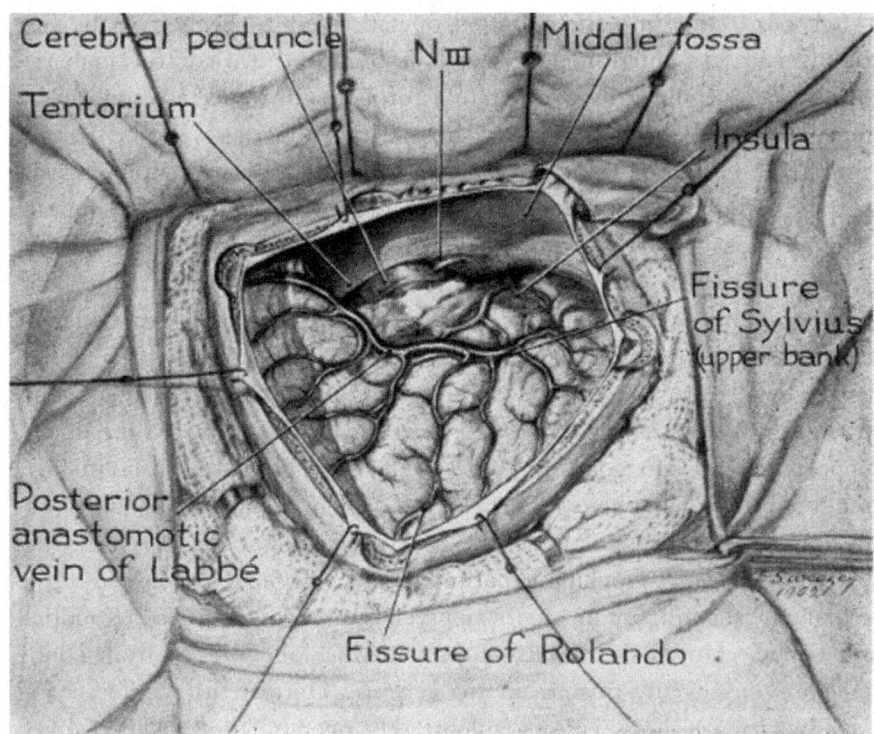

30. A surgeon's view of the 'Montreal' method of temporal lobectomy (after excision of mesial temporal structures). (From: Feindel et al., 'Epilepsy surgery').

in1948 he published his definitive paper linking the anterior temporal EEG discharge to psychomotor seizures.[262] He thereafter persuaded his surgical colleague, Percival Bailey, to resect the anterior temporal lobe in such patients on the basis that this was a silent area, that it was removed without difficulty in cases of tumour and that without further intervention patients with severe psychomotor epilepsy would be 'goners' – ostracised, unemployable and likely to develop other psychiatric disorders. This was not the first time that surgery was contemplated to remove an 'electrical focus' with no evidence of a pathological lesion (precedence goes to Lennox[263]), but it was obviously a momentous step - essentially a leap in the dark. Bailey agreed, and on 12

---

[262] Gibbs and Lennox had coined the phrase 'psychomotor seizure' by 1937, but initially described generalised discharges associated with it.

[263] Dr Jason Mixter, neurosurgeon, performed a two-stage, bilateral frontal lobe resection on a patient with petit mal and frontal foci in a paper in 1938. This was claimed by Lennox to be the first case in which resection was based entirely on EEG evidence (Gibbs, Gibbs, and Lennox, 'Cerebral dysrhythmias of epilepsy'). The patient was said to have improved, but a subsequent note by Lennox in 1960 reported an ultimately poor outcome requiring placement in an institution, where he died (see Lennox, *Epilepsy and Related Disorders*, vol. 2, p. 901). Percival Bailey was the neurosurgeon at the University of Chicago (see his interesting biography by Bucy, 'Bailey').

March 1947 (after an earlier limited operation on 26 February), the first patient had his anterior temporal lobe removed to control epilepsy. Resection was guided by peroperative corticography, and resection of the mesial temporal lobes was deliberately avoided because of the risk of amnesia.[264] One of Bailey's residents assisting in surgery was John Green, who soon after moved to Phoenix where he began his own series of temporal lobe resections in July 1948. In 1951, Bailey and Gibbs wrote up their first twenty-eight patients, partly because Arthur Morris, at Georgetown University, gave the Davidson Lecture in 1949 on his own experience of various temporal resections guided by corticography. He had written up five cases in detail in 1950, and, in a second paper in 1956, Morris claimed that his first case was operated on August 12 1946 and that he removed the uncus, hippocampus and amygdala. In 1951 Green also published the 'preliminary' results of resection in twenty-three patients, which 'in some cases include[ed] the hippocampal gyrus and uncus (the anterior portion)'.[265] In 1957, in what was surely a deeply shocking experiment, and a deplorable example of the lack of ethical constraint in American psychosurgery of the period, Kendrick and Gibbs reported the results of 72 temporal lobe and 33 frontal lobe resections in seventy-five psychotic persons. Thirteen had epilepsy and sixty-two had psychosis without epilepsy. The operations were all performed with depth EEG recordings and 'discharging areas' were removed. Twenty-four patients had bilateral resection temporal lobe resections and twenty-four unilateral resections, and in most of these mesial structures were apparently resected. In almost all the patients with psychosis without epilepsy, spiking in the deep structures of the temporal lobes and orbital frontal lobes was observed (as had been the case in Robert Heath's report in 1954) and was the rationale for operation. Of the thirteen cases with epilepsy, four only were relieved of seizures and there is no comment on the effects on psychosis. Shockingly, in some recalcitrant cases bilateral frontal and bilateral anterior and mesial temporal excisions seem to have been carried out.[266]

Meanwhile, across the great lakes in Montreal, in 1938, Herbert Jasper established an EEG service dedicated to selecting patients for Penfield to operate upon and providing preoperative corticography.[267] In 1950, with Herman Flanigin, Penfield reviewed seventy-five temporal lobe operations on sixty-eight patients that he had performed between 1939 and 1949. In this group, hippocampal resection was carried out in only two patients and uncal

[264] Their early work is meticulously described in Hermann and Stone's excellent 'Historical review'.

[265] Green, Duisberg and McGrath, 'Focal epilepsy'. Bruce Hermann has commented, however, based on personal knowledge, that Green did not resect the hippocampus itself until 1956.

[266] Kendrick and Gibbs, 'Origin, spread and neurosurgical treatment'.

[267] Jasper published an early, extensive and influential review which defined the application of EEG to epilepsy surgery: Jasper, 'Electroencephalography'.

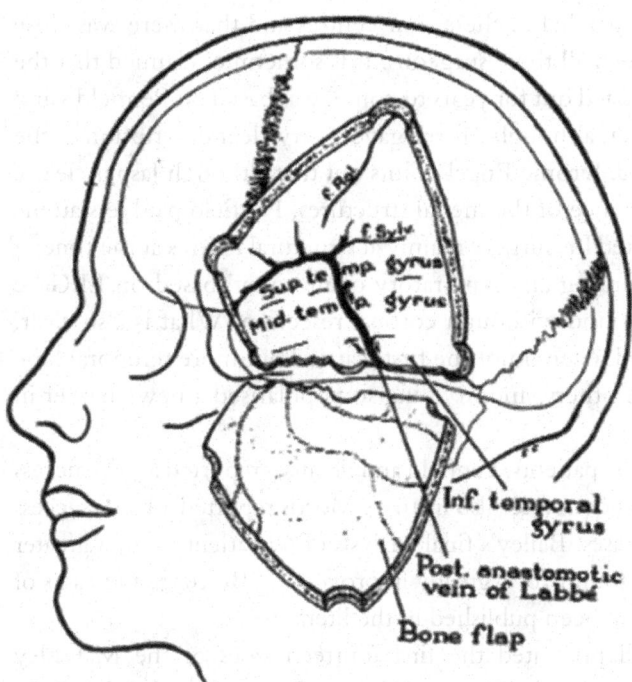

31. Penfield's subtotal anterior-mesial temporal lobectomy, (From: Feindel et al., 'Epilepsy surgery').

resection in ten.[268] His practice obviously changed around this time, for in his next report of the eighty-one cases operated on between 1949 and 1952, Penfield reported that most had had a routine removal of the uncus, amygdala and hippocampus as well as the anterolateral temporal cortex. Penfield and Maitland Baldwin[269] published their standard technique for 'subtotal temporal lobectomy', which included resection of mesial structures, in October 1952. They concluded that 'the abnormal, sclerotic area of the cortex, which must be removed in most cases, lies in the deepest, the most inferior and mesial portion of the [temporal] lobe' (p. 625). In his later series, Penfield also reported that he had reoperated on 'a number' of his earlier temporal lobe patients in order to excise the hippocampus, sometimes with conversion of failure to success, including one of the 1939–49 series.

Thus, it is not clear whether the crown for performing the first hippocampal surgery in epilepsy can be claimed by Green, Penfield, Morris or even Bailey. Morris's claim that his first mesial resection was in August 1946, if true, would give him this honour. But it must also be recognised that changes were made to

---

[268] Penfield and Flanigin, 'Surgical therapy'. Herman Flanigin spent several years as a trainee with Penfield and Jasper in Montreal, then returned to Oklahoma, Arkansas, and in 1980 established an Epilepsy Surgery Program at the Medical College of Georgia.

[269] Penfield and Baldwin, 'Temporal lobe seizures'.

surgical techniques in parallel in these four centres and that there was close communication between all these surgeons. It is sometimes claimed that the standard operation, carried out for years to come, was based on Penfield's and Baldwin's paper of 1952, although Morris gave a very clear description of the same operation in 1950. Jerome Engel points out that although Jasper clearly understood the importance of the mesial structures, Penfield paid less attention to EEG and directed his surgery mainly at structural lesions at the time; if no lesion was found during an 'exploratory craniotomy' based on EEG he would close up the wound without a cortical resection. What is also clear, though, is that Penfield, even if not the first, carried out more temporal lobe operations than all the others, and in doing so popularised a new chapter in epilepsy therapy.[270]

In the 1950 series of 68 patients, Penfield and Flanigin reported a 53% success rate and 27% seizure freedom rate; also in 1950, Morris reported a 100% success rate in his 5 operated cases. Bailey's final analysis of 60 patients with a greater than 5-year follow-up found 30% 'greatly improved'.[271] By 1953, 132 cases of temporal lobectomy had been published in the literature.

In 1953, Denis Hill presented the first fourteen cases of the Maudsley Hospital group operated on by Murray Falconer from 1951 (the first from Europe).[272] One patient (the first patient) died a few days after the operation, but of the others ten were free of seizures (although auras persisted in three). These initial cases were drawn from a psychiatric service, and great attention was paid to the psychological consequences of surgery, noting striking changes in behaviour that occurred after operating – usually beneficial changes, but not always (see pp. 304–6). Hill ended this paper with a thought which has repeatedly been made ever since, although it has been difficult to action: 'In the long run it may prove wiser to operate early and prevent the personality change, rather than to wait until the symptoms become flagrant.'[273]

After the third patient, Falconer perfected the en bloc resection of the mesial and neocortical structures, in which the anterior 5.5–6.5 cm of the temporal lobe, including the hippocampal and mesial temporal structures, was removed in one piece.[274] This allowed detailed neuropathology to be carried out, in a way, for instance, that was not possible in Montreal. For the first time, surgical outcome could be correlated with the pathological finding of hippocampal sclerosis – the pathology colourfully called the 'fatal flaw' by David Taylor. Using this technique, Falconer showed unequivocally that hippocampal sclerosis was the commonest cause of temporal lobe epilepsy, not its consequence,

---

[270] However, to counter the tendency for hagiography vis-à-vis Penfield, see Moran, 'History of temporal lobectomy', and Engel, 'Temporal lobe surgery'.
[271] Bailey, 'Surgical treatment'.   [272] Hill, 'Discussion'.   [273] Hill, 'Discussion'.
[274] See Meyer and Falconer, 'Pathological findings'.

and that its removal was at the heart of successful temporal lobe surgery.[275] He was proved correct. In 1951 Lennox also proposed replacing the term 'psycho-motor epilepsy' with 'temporal lobe epilepsy', given the specificity of the clinical symptoms.[276] Thenceforward, both terms were used synonymously.

By 1970 quite a few units in the United States were carrying out temporal lobectomy, usually with corticography on the Montreal model, and were providing outcome figures. The definitive statement, however, came from Theodore Rasmussen in Montreal. He had first trained in neurosurgery with Penfield and at the Mayo Clinic, and then spent seven years as Professor of Neurological Surgery at the University of Chicago. In 1954 he returned to Montreal as chair of neurology and neurosurgery at McGill, and when Penfield retired in 1960, Rasmussen assumed the directorship of the MNI. In 1963 the Montreal Neurological Hospital was founded, and Rasmussen was appointed its first director-general. Between 1955 and the end of his surgical career in 1980, Rasmussen had performed more epilepsy surgery than any of his con-temporaries. In 1969 he reported on 1,690 resective operations in 1,450 patients, who were operated on primarily for epilepsy, rather than tumours or other lesions requiring treatment in their own right.[277] The site of operation was based on EEG and clinical grounds, and the surgery was, as a rule, carried out under local anaesthetic. Using preoperative corticography, post-excision spiking cortex was usually then also resected (a policy which became known as 'chasing the spikes'). The mortality rate was <2%. Twenty per cent of the patients had a tumour, usually identified pre-operatively. In about a third of patients the epilepsy was considered due to birth trauma or anoxia, and in about a quarter of cases the cause was not established. In 508 patients with non-tumoral temporal lobe epilepsy, with follow-up of two or more years, 69% were greatly improved and 46% were seizure-free. After frontal lobe resection, 59% and 32% of 184 cases were improved or seizure-free; 61% and 37% of 56 patients after central resection; and 65% and 45% of 77 cases after parietal resection.

In 1983, Rasmussen published a further analysis of 1,210 patients with tem-poral lobe epilepsy operated on at the MNI between 1928 and 1980,[278] many with long-term follow-up. Of these, 1,034 patients were non-tumoral, 169 had tumours and 7 had major vascular malformations. Of those followed for more than two years post-operatively, 37% of the 894 non-tumoral evaluable patients had become and remained seizure-free (or had only auras), and a further 26% of

[275] The en bloc resection also allowed identification of other hippocampal lesions in the remaining patients, including hamartoma, dysplasias and post-infective changes (Meyer, Falconer and Beck, 'Pathological findings').

[276] Lennox, 'Psychomotor triad'.

[277] Rasmussen, 'Focal epilepsy'. This was Rasmussen's definitive statement on surgery, based on all the cases operated on by Penfield and himself (and others) up to 1967.

[278] Rasmussen, 'Results, lessons, and problems'.

patients had a marked reduction in seizure tendency. Of the evaluable tumoral patients, 46% were seizure-free and 30% exhibited a reduction in seizure tendency. Most of these patients had only inter-ictal EEG recordings as facilities for EEG telemetry had been introduced only relatively lately. Rasmussen made the interesting clinical observation that at surgery, electrographic seizure discharges confined to the hippocampus seldom resulted in clinically overt seizures, and clinical signs developed only when the discharges spread to involve the amygdala or temporal neocortex. He pointed out, too, that even amongst those who had spiking on the post-excision cortical electrogram, most became seizure-free. The psychological or behavioural effects of surgery were not discussed.

In Rasmussen's view, 'more was better'. It was the size of the resection and the completeness of removal of the epileptogenic zone, defined by preoperative corticography, that influenced outcome more than the pathological basis or anatomical location. Not everyone agreed, and similar outcomes were obtained by Falconer's temporal lobe series of 200 cases without extensive corticography to guide his en bloc resections. For Falconer, the underlying pathology had the greatest bearing on outcome.

Rasmussen also worked on hemispherectomy, including for the syndrome which carries his name,[279] and frontal lobe resections for epilepsy as well as on more general neurosurgery. Always in the shadow of Penfield's achievements, Rasmussen's contribution has perhaps been underestimated, not least the role of his work in transforming epilepsy surgery into an almost routine procedure.

Stereotactic surgery[280] was another approach to epilepsy surgery explored in the 1940s and 1950s, with growing interest by a number of surgeons in the United States and in Europe.[281] Ernest Spiegel and Henry Wycis were probably the first to use ventricular system landmarks (outlined by ventriculography) to guide stereotaxis, and they published a stereotactic atlas, including charts of the variability of certain structures, predating Talairach's more celebrated work. Spiegel coined the term 'stereoencephalotomy' for the lesioning that was performed largely in psychiatric and emotional disorders, as an alternative to frontal leucotomy and in movement disorders, as well as for petit mal and grand mal epilepsy. As with Kendrick's operations, those of Spiegel and Wycis' were experiments seemingly conducted without any form of ethical oversight or constraint, and a variety of stereotactic procedures were undertaken. These included operations on patients with petit mal epilepsy, in whom bilateral lesions were placed in the region of the

---

[279] Rasmussen Syndrome is an unusual progressive focal encephalitis, confined to one hemisphere, that causes severe focal epilepsy and often epilepsia partialis continua. An international symposium on the topic was published in 1991: Andermann, *Rasmussen's Syndrome*.

[280] Surgery carried out through a burr hole in which a small key target area is destroyed by thermal coagulation or some other method, and which does not require a large craniotomy or the resection of large amounts of brain tissue. The target was initially precisely defined in three-dimensional space by the use of a stereotactic frame attached to the head.

[281] See Mark and Sweet discussion: www.youtube.com/watch?v=obWq7d95Mig

mass intermedia of the medial thalamus, on the basis that Jasper had postulated this region to be the origin of petit mal seizures, or the hypothalamus.[282] The assessment of outcome was risible, with no mention of complications and only brief, uncontrolled descriptions of the effects on seizure frequency. Some of the patients (it is not clear how many) were psychotic and institutionalised, and one wonders how secure the seizure classification was. There were no descriptions of any demographic features or details of prior epilepsy. The effect on behaviour was equally poorly documented. One patient was said to have 'favorable changes in his personality pattern' (p. 475).

In various centres in Europe and North America, a range of targets were chosen for stereotactic ablation, often seemingly without any specific justification. These targets included the fornices, pallidum, putamen, internal medullary lamina, hypothalamus, cingulum, fields of Forel, amygdala, fornix, lenticular nucleus, the mass intermedia and anterior, ventrolateral and centromedian nuclei of the thalamus. Outcomes were reported frequently for single or small numbers of patients, and a large and totally uncontrolled literature accumulated.[283] In recollections published in 1975, Sixto Obrador noted that functional neurosurgery became widespread in this period,[284] with most stereotaxy performed to control pain or disorders of movement. Riechert in Freiberg, for instance, reported in 1975 that he had performed well over 3,000 operations for diverse disorders.[285] Regarding lesioning for epilepsy, Riechert wrote:

> Of the epileptic group of diseases it appeared to us, considering the success of resection of the temporal lobe, that a stereotactic operation for temporal lobe epilepsy would be successful and more easily tolerated than the open operation. Here we went on the assumption that the most important efference of the epileptogenetic cornu ammonis is the fornix. Epileptic potentials are conducted over this structure to the diencephalon. Another pathway passes through the anterior commissure. In suitable cases of temporal-lobe epilepsy after previous stimulation and recording, we interrupt the fornix at its intersection with the anterior commissure below the foramen of Monroi. In some patients the amygdaloid nucleus or the hippocampus was also eliminated. Several reports have been made on the results of this operation which we called 'fornicotomy'. (p. 401–2)

[282] Spiegel, Wycis and Reyes, 'Diencephalic mechanisms'.

[283] See, for instance, Umbach, 'Fornicotomy for temporal epilepsy'.

[284] Obrador was an enthusiastic supporter of stereotactic psychosurgery. Trained by Spiegel and Wycis, and based in Madrid, he carried out many novel operations, often on a nebulous theoretical basis. He mentioned having visited stereotactic centres, for instance, in Boston, Los Angeles, San Francisco, London, Newcastle, Birmingham, Edinburgh, Madrid, Barcelona, Valencia, Seville, Santander, Málaga, Moscow, Leningrad, Berlin, Freiberg, Helsinki, Copenhagen, Zurich, Bratislava, Granada, Santiago de Chile, Mexico and Tokyo. Many others also existed (Obrador, 'Personal recollections').

[285] Riechert, 'Development of human stereotactic surgery'.

He did not report any outcomes, and it seems likely that despite its widespread use in other conditions, stereotactic epilepsy surgery did not catch on and was performed on relatively few persons with epilepsy. One can presume that this was largely because such surgery was quickly found to fail. Certainly no large-scale detailed outcome statistics were ever published. It is not hard to disagree with Falconer's prediction of 1973 that, as the techniques had no pathological justification, 'they will fall into oblivion, as have many of the psychosurgical procedures practiced during and immediately after the Second World War'.[286]

Falconer's comments raise what was seen as a very significant issue for epilepsy surgery in that period: the need to avoid the moniker of 'psychosurgery' (although his early temporal lobectomies at the Maudsley could certainly have been described thus). Pearce Bailey had stressed this point in relation to resective epilepsy surgery, but it was an even more pressing issue in stereotactic surgery, which was the dominant psychosurgical technique. Slowly the public were waking up to the potential abuses of psychosurgery, and some surgeons ran into trouble. The experiments of Heath in Tulane for instance were the subject of a US Senate subcommittee as well as massive public outrage. In Britain, the Birmingham neurosurgeon Eric Turner, who had devised several types of temporal lobotomies for the control of epilepsy and its behavioural disorders, also became entangled with accusations over psychosurgery. As a result, his ideas were not pursued.[287]

Stereotactic surgery, in the sense of therapeutic lesioning to cure epilepsy, may have fallen quickly out of favour. But stereotaxis for the placement of electrodes to record EEG as a prelude to resective surgery did not. The technique became, and remains, a major application of stereotaxis in epilepsy. Jean Talairach and Jean Bancaud were leaders in this field, at the Sainte-Anne Hospital in Paris as we have seen earlier and although their highly technological 'anatomo-electro-clinical correlations' were admired for their precision, it is notable how few papers were ever published reporting in any detail the outcomes of their surgery.[288]

---

[286] Falconer, 'Reversibility by temporal-lobe resection'.

[287] See Turner, 'New approach'; Gould, 'Surgery of last result'.

[288] Notwithstanding the lack of outcome data, the influence of the St Anne group spread by the training in Paris of a whole generation of surgeons in the SEEG approach, which remains widely used especially in the French and Italian epilepsy surgery centres. In this sense, the Paris centre rivalled that of Montreal. Amongst the new generation were Patrick Chauvel and Philippe Kahane, in France; Claudio Munari, in Italy, who spent several years with Bancaud and Talairach before returning to Milan to form the first epilepsy surgery programme; Gazi Yaşargil, who combined SEEG evaluation with surgery carried out using the operating microscope and devised the selective amygdalo-hippocampectomy, and Heinz Gregor Wieser, both in Zurich. In North America, André Olivier in Montreal, John Van Buren at NIH and Paul Crandall in Los Angeles imported the technique. Mark Rayport, one of Penfield's last residents, spent time at Sainte-Anne in the late 1960s as a visiting professor

Other operations also began to be applied to the problems of epilepsy. Hemispherectomy[289] was first carried out by Walter Dandy in 1923 for the resection of a glioma, and was first employed to treat epilepsy in 1938 by Kenneth McKenzie. In South Africa, Rowland Krynauw reported its value in twelve children with infantile hemiplegia and epilepsy in 1951. Since then, hemispherectomy has retained a place especially in the treatment of children with infantile hemiplegia and severe unilateral epilepsy due to large brain pathologies, and for Rasmussen's syndrome of unilateral encephalitis. The early operations consisted of resecting most of the grey matter of one hemisphere and were known as 'anatomical hemispherectomies'. By 1961, 267 cases had been reported in the world literature, the mortality of surgery was quite high (7%), but the epilepsy was markedly improved in more than 80% of survivors.

The surgical division of the corpus callosum for epilepsy was first suggested in 1886 by Victor Horsley, who is said to have carried out the operation in primates. The first clinical callosotomies for epilepsy were carried out in 1939 by William van Wagenen at the University of Rochester Medical Center in New York. He reported on ten cases, with 'satisfactory' outcome in seven.[290] In the same year, Theodore Erickson from Montreal reported that he had observed experimentally in primates that callosal section, and also transcortical section in the central region at right angles to the central sulcus, isolated an epileptic focus and interrupted the spread of epileptic discharges into the other hemisphere.[291] One can assume that van Wagenen was aware of this work, but both the experimental and clinical findings were published almost simultaneously. These clinical cases were notable, too, for the careful post-operative psychological studies by van Wagenen's psychiatric colleague Andrew Akelaitis.[292] He, and subsequent psychologists, were fascinated by the operative creation of a 'split brain' in which one hemisphere received no information from the other. This stimulated a profusion of esoteric psychological findings. Following these early reports, no further operations of this type appear to have been carried out until 1962,[293] when Joseph Bogen and colleagues devised

and translated the 1988 atlas into English. He was one of the first to adopt SEEG in North America. Working in Ohio with his wife Shirley Ferguson, a psychiatrist, he combined the Montreal and Sainte-Anne methods, but also emphasised the psychodynamic aspects and behavioural consequences of epilepsy surgery.

[289] The resection of large areas of brain tissue from one hemisphere.

[290] Van Wagenen and Herren, 'Epileptic attack'.

[291] Erickson, 'Spread of epileptic discharges'.

[292] A. J. Akelaitis, 'Corpus callosum. II'; 'Corpus callosum. VII'; 'Anterior commissure'.

[293] Why this is so is not clear. Bogen has suggested that the reason might have been the interruption of the Second World War, unfavourable outcomes or the growing conviction of the times that the reticular formation was of particular importance in seizure spread (Bogen, 'Callosotomy for epilepsy'). However, van Wegenen's colleague Frank Smith stated that 'Van Wagenen always was sorry about what he did to those patients ... For over a

more extensive versions of the operation, with the severance of the anterior fibres initially and then a completed callosotomy if the initial operation was ineffective.

THE EXPERIENCE OF HAVING EPILEPSY

In the post-war period attitudes to, and prejudices about, epilepsy greatly changed. Although obviously not shared by all people in all situations, as attitudes depend on individual and national experience, it is quite clear that, generally speaking, the public perceptions of epilepsy became more sympathetic and less injurious. The reasons for this defy simple explanation, but no doubt include the greater scientific understanding of the organic basis of epilepsy, not least due to EEG, leading to the perception that it was not an inherited mental disease, nor inevitably associated with abnormal intellect or personality, nor linked to cognitive or behavioural decline. But perhaps most fundamental was the political and social impact of the ideals of liberal democracy and respect for human rights.[294]

America was spared most of the desolation of World War Two, and it was there and not in Europe that academic interest in the social impact of disease matured, that the use of new survey techniques was pioneered and also where the first serious attempts at political lobbying were made, particularly by the lay American Epilepsy League and its sister professional association, the American League Against Epilepsy.

Lennox had become a key person in the fight against stigma, realising the handicap of epilepsy to be more social than physical, based on unreasoned fear of convulsions and popular prejudice and misinformation regarding the intelligence and personality especially of non-institutionalised patients. Education was, in his view, a key focus for affirmative action. In 1947, Lennox, Merle McBride and Gertrude Potter[295] published an investigation of educational opportunities, and offered advice to schools and colleges and recommendations for action. Their survey of 1,676 schools of higher education revealed that only 0.05% of students had epilepsy, which Lennox considered to be one-tenth of the population prevalence and one-third of the number who might have received higher education were it not for popular prejudice. Twenty per

decade there were persons in Boston who referred to us as "the West Coast butchers"' (Mathews, Linskey and Binder, 'William P. van Wagenen').

[294] The Nuremberg trials were fundamental to this change. As a direct consequence of the judgements made there, the UN General Assembly affirmed that 'crimes against humanity' and 'genocide' became entities in international law. Following this, in December 1948 the United Nations adopted the Universal Declaration of Human Rights, and in 1953 the European Convention on Human Rights was signed into law. The latter was also in part a reaction against Stalinism in the Soviet Union.

[295] Lennox, McBri[d]e and Potter, 'Higher education of epileptics' [nb: Merle McBride's surname was misspelt McBribe on the title page of this article].

cent of schools denied admission to epileptics outright, and 27% would admit them only conditionally. Only 21% of children with epilepsy were in regular classes.[296] 'Hindrances to climbing the educational ladder increase with its height'. Lennox and his colleagues wrote:

> [P]hysicians who treat many epileptics are acutely aware that in many colleges mere mention of the word 'epilepsy' automatically closes the entrance door (or opens the exit door) for patients who are both intelligent and eager ... With regard to the intelligence of epileptics, common opinion that seizures and mental retardation go hand in hand in grossly untrue ... There is no distinctive 'epileptic personality'.[297]

As part of a concerted effort by the American chapter and lay organisations, efforts were made to counter public attitudes. On 24 May 1945, Lennox testified before the Committee of Labor of the House of Representatives, where he pointed out that seven of the attitudes of 'Dame Rumor' were false, namely: the cause is a complete mystery; epilepsy gets progressively worse; mental impairment is inevitable; the outlook of essential epilepsy is worse than acquired epilepsy; no epileptic should marry; inactivity is the best treatment; and no effective treatment is known.[298]

Lennox's work illustrates another important post-war development in epilepsy: the use of survey data as a research instrument, which he also helped pioneer. Surveys had been carried out since the nineteenth century, but it was only in the 1920s that formal methodologies were devised, and, when social surveys of public opinion evolved in the 1940s, epilepsy was in the vanguard. Notable were a series of five-yearly surveys of attitudes and knowledge about epilepsy carried out amongst the American public, which were amongst the first national surveys designed by George Gallop.[299] They demonstrated that there was a shift in opinion during the post-war years as attitudes towards epilepsy became progressively more liberal. Throughout this thirty-year period, those familiar with epilepsy (90–95% of the population) were asked three questions designed by Lennox, Merritt and William Caveness.[300] To the

---

[296] As a sign of changing attitudes, by 1958 this figure had risen to 76%.

[297] Lennox, McBri[d]e and Potter, 'Higher education of epileptics'.

[298] Collier, 'Social implications and management', p. 67.

[299] These surveys were conducted by William Caveness and colleagues in 1949, 1954, 1959, 1964, 1969, 1974 and 1979 with the assistance of George Gallup of the American Institute of Public Opinion. Gallup went on to become the doyen of survey technique. The importance of the 'survey' (broadly interpreted) in medicine is emphasised in Armstrong, *Political Anatomy*.

[300] The responses to these questions changed progressively in the years 1948, 1954, 1959, 1964, 1969, 1974, 1979: To the question 'Would you object to having any of your children in school or at play associate with someone who sometimes has seizures (fits)?', the answer was 'no' in 57%, 68%, 67%, 77%, 81%, 84% and 89% respectively; to the question 'Do you think epilepsy is a form of insanity or not?', the answer was 'no' in 59%, 68%, 74%, 79%, 81%, 86%, 92%; and to the question 'Do you think epileptics should be employed in jobs like other people?', the answer was 'yes' in 45%, 60%, 75%, 82%, 76%, 81%, 79%.

question 'Would you object to having any of your children in school or at play associate with someone who sometimes has seizures (fits)?', 57% answered 'no' in 1949, a figure which rose to 89% in 1979. To the question 'Do you think epilepsy is a form of insanity or not?', the number answering 'no' changed from 59% to 92%. And to the question 'Do you think epileptics should or should not be employed in jobs like other people?', the number answering 'yes' rose from 45% to 79%. The most favourable opinions were found amongst the better educated, those with better jobs, and the younger and urban members of the population. However, even in 1969, when asked what they thought was the cause of epilepsy, a small number of people surprisingly still clung to the view that epilepsy was the result of demonic possession, radioactive fallout or children drinking alcoholic beverages, or that it was infectious. Even in 1979, 18% would not permit their children to marry someone with epilepsy, and 6% would prohibit their children from playing with someone with epilepsy.[301] The authors considered that the evolution of more enlightened opinion could be due to educational efforts by professional and lay societies, improved treatment, better employment opportunities and changes in legislation. Surprisingly, they seem to have ignored the rise of more liberal social and cultural attitudes generally. Whatever the reasons, it is clear that, overall, post-war attitudes were more enlightened than those in the pre-war years and became more so over the thirty-year period. The same questions were posed in Germany, Spain and Britain in 1967–8, and similar prejudices were found.[302] Stimulated by this work, there followed a veritable flood of surveys and reports of stigma in epilepsy worldwide, especially after the 1980s.

Legal hurdles against employment, education, driving, immigration, child-bearing and marriage had grown up in many countries during the interwar years, and slowly these, too, were modified or repealed. The legal framework around epilepsy was the topic of a book published in 1956 by Roscoe Barrow, Dean of the University of Cincinnati College of Law, and Howard Fabing, a neurologist who chaired the Legislation Committee of the American League Against Epilepsy (which sponsored the book).[303] This was a landmark in the post-war history of epilepsy. It was the first full-scale study of laws in relation to epilepsy. Barrow and Fabing's key point was that these laws resulted in the perpetuation of stigma, which was *the major hurdle* preventing social integration for persons with epilepsy. They recognised that the laws were misconceived and highly discriminatory, based as they were on previously held misconceptions that epilepsy was inherited, incurable, associated with mental defect and mental illness, degenerates to dementia or mental illness, and that the offspring

---

[301] Caveness, 'Public attitudes toward epilepsy'; Caveness et al., 'Attitudes toward epilepsy in 1964'; Caveness, Merritt and Gallup, 'Twenty years'; Caveness and Gallup Jr, 'Thirty years'.
[302] Bagley, 'Social prejudice'.   [303] Barrow and Fabing, *Epilepsy and the Law.*

of those with epilepsy will inherit the condition. As Pearce Bailey (then director of NINDS) put it in his foreword to the book:

> Epilepsy is an anomaly in medicine. Although seizures may now be controlled by drugs in a large majority of cases, the improved medical condition of the patient may have little bearing on improving his social and economic opportunities … they stand isolated from the main stream of normal living – socially, economically and psychologically … The problem of isolation of the epileptic is not a new one nor are the prejudices that have created the problem. Yet little progress has been made toward the restoration to the epileptic of those human rights which should be his natural heritage. The epileptic himself is unwilling to organize for this effort, for to do so is publicly to announce his disability, when his every desire is to hide it … One way to reduce prejudice seems to be to focus on its legally unjust manifestations. (p. vii)

Barrow and Fabing realised that many of the discriminatory laws had their origins in the eugenics movement. In US immigration laws, 'epileptics' were grouped with 'the feeble-minded, insane, alcoholics, lepers, prostitutes and paupers' (p. 88) and excluded from migration to the United States. They noted that, at the time of writing, seventeen US states still had prohibitions on marriage and still linked epilepsy, insanity and mental deficiency together. Six states declared it a crime for someone with epilepsy to marry, and in some states violation of the statute rendered the marriage unlawful or void. The authors pointed out the obvious fact that the laws were unsound from the genetic and scientific points of view, as well as being morally and socially wrong, and yet 'epileptics continue to live under anachronistic legal restraints imposed sixty years ago and in a social climate which associates epilepsy with idiocy and insanity' (p. 2). Moreover, '[i]t was well known that, as a rule, employers do not knowingly employ epileptics' and 'social attitude towards epileptics and the anachronistic epilepsy laws drive unknown thousands "underground"' (p. 3). Barrow and Fabing argued that stigma was largely due to the association with mental illness:

> Our laws set epileptics apart as a special group in society and contributed greatly to the stigma against epilepsy. Eugenic marriage and sterilization laws apply equally to 'idiots', 'epileptics' and the 'insane' … It must be recognized that it is especially difficult to overcome the social attitude towards any mental condition requiring institutional care. Now that institutional care is rarely necessary in the case of epilepsy, this condition should be dissociated from mental illness and mental defects in order that the stigma against epilepsy may be uprooted. In forcing epileptics into the same legal mould with the mentally defective and mentally ill who require institutional care, separating them only by a comma, the laws condition society to associate and to equate these mental conditions with epilepsy

... If the stigma against epileptics is to be removed, recent medical
discoveries in treating epilepsy must be translated into legal reform. (p. 8)

Regarding sterilisation, they noted that twenty states had laws applicable to
epilepsy, and in five of these the laws applied to all epileptics, not just those in
institutions – remarkably without consideration of aetiology or seizure control,
with decisions made in the absence of medical input. Similar stigma and unfairness was found in relation to the laws governing driver's licensing and worker's
compensation. In their liberal and humane book, Barrow and Fabing presented a
range of sensible and forward-looking recommendations and concluded:

Medical progress in the control of epileptic seizures has rendered our
epilepsy laws anachronistic ... [R]eform will enable us to carry forward
the education of our people in the true nature of epilepsy, and thus to
remove the illogical stigma against the disorder. The social and vocational
rehabilitation of our 1,500,000 epileptics can then be achieved. Thus, a
large group of our people who are presently denied a normal, productive
life will be enabled to make a full contribution to society ... [Their
proposals] are a challenge to remold our epilepsy laws to implement the
medical gains of the past quarter century in the treatment of one of man's
age-old, stigmatized diseases. This is a blueprint for social action which
will permit us to atone for more than 2,000 years of error in the management of the epileptic patient. (p. 109)

Stigma had by then become a focus for sociological study. Important books
were Erving Goffman's *Asylums* (1961) and *Stigma* (1963),[304] which achieved
wide readership and turned the spotlight on asylums and the prejudice shown
to the mentally ill.

One cause of stigma, often overlooked, was the nature of medical practice,
and the medical profession became a target of just criticism in these and other
works of the period. It was indeed the case that a new form of medical
authoritarianism had grown up, in parallel with the greater power of medical
treatment. The style of practice, particularly in neurology, remained austere
and hierarchical, a pattern shared more or less throughout Europe and the
United States. What it was like to be a trainee neurologist in the French system
in the 1950s was well described in memoirs by Jean Aicardi.[305] To Aicardi, the
system was a highly elitist system in which the pinnacle of success was gaining a
place at one of the Parisian *grandes écoles* and a titular professorship at the public
teaching hospitals in Paris – the Hopitaux de l'Assistance Publique de la Ville de
Paris. Competition was fierce; who you knew and what connections you had
were vital. The professor, often known as 'Dieu', was 'a formidable and largely
unapproachable authority figure with whom opportunity for dialogue was
typically non-existent'. He (it was always a 'he') gave magisterial lectures,

---

[304] Goffman, *Asylums*; *Stigma*.   [305] Aicardi, 'My circuitous path'.

using a blackboard – no slides or videos – and sometimes demonstrating a patient with his or her face masked.[306] The senior professors made a considerable fortune in their private practices and were not often seen on the wards.[307] Their public patients were treated as if they were being done a favour. An even more hierarchical system applied in the German-speaking countries of Europe, where the treatment of trainees was often quite hostile. In Britain, at the time, although the hierarchy was much flatter, the Professor of Neurology at the National Hospital in the early post-war decades had a grip on the careers of the trainees throughout the country, not least because they spent part of their training at the hospital and because of the small number of neurologists country-wide. In all Western countries, the paternalistic attitude towards patients had lessened somewhat in the post-war period compared with the interwar years, but it still marred many consultations in epilepsy. The dramatic social cataclysms of the late 1960s did have an effect, however, and the style of epilepsy medicine was to change completely in the subsequent decades.

The Writings of Margiad Evans

Remarkably, in the first half of the twentieth century, no work of literary merit, to my knowledge, was written in which the author admitted to having epilepsy and in which he or she described what it was like to have the condition. This makes all the more striking the extraordinary frankness and vividness with which Margiad Evans embarked on this task. Already a celebrated poet and novelist, Evans suffered her first epileptic seizure in May 1950, and eight years later succumbed to the inoperable brain tumour that caused it. The years between 1950 and 1954 were a period of intense emotional upheaval for her as she struggled to come to terms with increasingly severe epilepsy. During this time she wrote two autobiographical books centred on her epilepsy – *A Ray of Darkness* (1952) and *The Nightingale Silenced* (1954) – both extraordinary testaments. Few, if any, before or after, have described their experience of epilepsy with such clarity and sensitivity. She was, she wrote in *The Nightingale Silenced*, 'like a steel rope' (p. 85), and certainly she showed astonishing strength in the face of frequent, devastating seizures. But, at the same time, her descriptions were sensitive and perceptive, with a beautiful sense of language. It is this combination which makes her two books of unparalleled value as authentic authorial

---

[306] Earlier, patients were displayed, filmed and photographed, often naked. When this practice died out is not clear, although it seems still to have been common even into the 1940s in Germany.

[307] Niall Quinn has described his time as a trainee in Paris in 1978. Professors were rarely seen on the wards, but exceptions were made for patients from top châteaux families or a viticulteur from Burgundy (Quinn, 'Year at the Salpêtrière', p. 28).

description, imaginative interpretation and evaluation. Both books were based on her diary entries, much of which were written as poetry. The purpose of the books, she felt, was to absorb the deeper experience of her epilepsy in order to learn. 'Certainly', she wrote in *A Ray of Darkness*, 'I could not pretend there was any moral or philosophical value in this book. I have nothing to teach from my epilepsy' (p. 10; although she also wrote that the book contained 'clues' for neurologists to the epilepsy experience). But this was to underestimate the value of her writing. She saw the illness as a voyage and the sufferer,

> like Melville's Ishmael in the crow's nest, looks out on the wondrous Pacific calms, the deeps and the waves he must sail without head knowledge. For in disease there *are* wondrous calms and profound lulls: there are thoughts and contemplations of which no other deeps can give us hints and the voyage, to the sufferer, may even be beautiful though he never again see land and home. (pp. 11–12)

A Ray of Darkness is a story of the early years of Evans's epilepsy and its precursors, which she felt assisted understanding. She described events which, in retrospect, she recognised as minor seizures:

> It caused no pain, it lasted a few seconds, I saw and heard and moved while it happened. I have often crossed a room, and, while not losing sight or bearings, not known *how* I crossed it. The sequence of consciousness was so little broken by it, that after it had happened it seemed not an atom of time or myself had been missing, and I only knew it had happened again by the numb sensation in the centre of the brain which followed it . . . I do, however, remember laughing to my husband about my 'little wheel, going off again'. It seemed like a tiny wheel – the wheel, say, of a watch, whirring at blurring speed, quite soundlessly, in my head while I went on with whatever I was doing, guided by the *consciousness left over* rather than the consciousness of the moment . . . The wheel would then cease, and there was a loud silence such as follows a blow on a drum . . . I have, if I may so illustrate it, left myself on one side and come to myself on the other, while feeling an atom of time divided the two selves. (pp. 39–40)

She was interested in the 'double bodiedness' (p. 40; a not uncommon conception of people with epilepsy). Her detailed description of her first convulsive fit demonstrates her perceptive and poetical genius. It was an event in which she felt she 'had fallen through Time, Continuity and Being' (p. 78). She wrote of the period after the seizure as 'an extraordinary blank. The next mental process is terrible, the brain held and let go, held and let go, a confused mess of atmosphere and memory. It worked, but like an engine, an engine misfiring and unsteered' (p. 80). She had images floating into her mind – for instance of a 'jug, a blue-banded, quart milk-jug – bobbing up and down in me, and again it was amazingly solid, was seen and then snatched away and then seen again as though held up in the air before me, as, I have since imagined, religious maniacs behold their sins' (p. 80).

After her second convulsion six months later, in October 1950, she documented its undermining effect on her confidence, life and work:

> I have been incredulous of all things firm and material. The light has held patches of invisible blackness. Time has become as rotten as worm-eaten wood, the earth under me is full of trapdoors and the sense of being, which is life and all that surrounds and creates, a thing taken and given irresponsibly and without warning as children snatch at a toy. Sight, hearing, touch, consciousness torn from one like a nest of a bird. (p. 122)

She wondered: 'Is epilepsy a religious or a moral disease? Is it possible that it is my *fault*?' (p. 97). She railed at the dire effects of the antiepileptic drugs which 'make me apathetic, have faded and dulled and dimmed the powers of imagination and concentration' (p. 189). She described the moment before a seizure:

> The utmost source of terror to me was never the summons but this awful yet *silly* moment, when the being tries to laugh it off, to leave it behind, to walk irresponsibly away ... The next instant I fall into nothing. This horrible light-heartedness and ghastly gaiety are not sensual – they are emotional. That is why they leave an impression which is ineffaceable, unforgettable and utterly fearful. (pp. 155–6)

She used her writing as a method to communicate the meaning and feeling of the experience of epilepsy, but was anxious that she could not: 'Language is demanded by epilepsy, as by poetry, that simply does not exist; and no amount of agility can create it ... Language can, however, ... suggest that greater, wordless language within from which mental and spiritual discovery issues. It can suggest truths which are the more certain for being inarticulate' (p. 167).

Not everyone understood, and a ludicrous vituperative review of *A Ray of Darkness* in the newsletter of the British Epilepsy Association accused her of egotism, claiming that her experience was too personal and not enough like that of others with epilepsy to provide any insight. It is difficult to think of a more ignorant review, but it greatly upset her. In an exchange with the Association, she found out that the piece had been written by a 'brilliant young scientist' and was told by George Burden that 'epileptics would be afraid of the book' given the way the condition was described. Others felt differently. To some acclaim, she broadcast a talk on epilepsy, titled 'A Silver Lining', on BBC radio on 19 March 1953, urging a more positive response to the disease. Lennox wrote of her book: 'No other epileptic writer, poet, mystic or activist has shared his experience so explicitly and so generously, or has used words so deftly in tracing a way through the deep passages where brain, mind and spirit join.'[308] He was absolutely correct. Pearl S. Buck, the 1938 Nobel laureate for literature, also reviewed the book, this time perceptively:

> Margiad Evans is a poet with a mind of unusual clarity and sensitivity. For such a mind to be attacked by the tragic blows of epilepsy would be unendurable, except that Miss Evans is more than a poet and a fine mind. She is a person of character, rich and profound, and she accepts her affliction not only with fortitude, but also with grace and understanding ... she shares with the reader the experience of her suffering, and this without a trace of self-pity.[309]

Evans made at least two bonds in the world of epilepsy. Lennox became a close friend, correspondent and admirer, and made fulsome reference to her writing in his own book on epilepsy. Frederick Golla (Dr 'T' in her books) was her physician at the Burden Institute, and Evans developed a close and intimate relationship both with Golla and with his daughter Yolande.

Evans's second book, *The Nightingale Silenced*, was written in 1954, after her epilepsy had dramatically worsened, but was published only in 2020 (as it was essentially still only in manuscript form at her death).[310] She wrote it whilst an inpatient at the Burden Institute under Golla, and it was at this time that the full horror of her epilepsy was unfolding. The book was her 'outside inside story as requested by Lennox' (p. xxxi) and, with the hurtful criticism of the British Epilepsy Association of her previous book in mind, it opens with a poem entitled 'The Egotist'. The book richly and evocatively describes her experience of epilepsy as it entered its severest stage. In the moment before a seizure developed, for instance:

> [in] the eerie presages of a bad seizure [it is] as though everything stops inside you: it was then already too late to do anything ... The sight was unaltered, only there was no sound ... [then] my left arm was fighting the air which suddenly seemed all squares and angles. The spots on the walls had got into my eyes, and something in the middle of my head was getting smaller and smaller. I didn't feel myself fall, but I knew when they thrust the spatula into my mouth. Then I went out and stopped trying so desperately to get into that bed which had stretched its white oblong in front of me like a new tomb ... it seemed that blow after blow was rained on my head: and though it didn't hurt in the sense that physical pain is understood, all I can say is that there are other forms of pain ....my

---

[308] Letter to Margiad Evans from William Lennox, 21 March 1953, Cited by J. Pratt, 'Introduction,' *The Nightingale Silenced*, p. xxix.

[309] Cover note to *A Ray of Darkness* in the 1953 American edition. Cited by Pratt, Introduction, *The Nightingale Silenced and Other Late Unpublished Writings*, pp. xxix–xxx

[310] It was edited and put into publishable form, collected together with letters and a journal, by her nephew Jim Pratt, who also contributed a most interesting introduction, from which many details in this text are taken. Pratt's collection is published in the Welsh Women's Classics series (although strictly speaking Evans was not Welsh).

> surroundings fought me and seemed to come horribly close. Then at last
> there was no space left even inside my head ... My perceptions were not
> acute and ordinary. They were psychic or poetic ... Fear. Dread. Horror.
> I was shaking with these and extreme misery ... I remember praying to
> the epileptic Saint Theresa for a little oblivion ... Death I did not fear; but
> feared that I would live. (p.163)

She had the day before told Golla that the seizures were 'strong'. He answered,
'So am I' (p. 165), and she felt protected.

Her epilepsy descended into a state of near status epilepticus and she was

> nursed in the Central Hall of the Institute on the floor on a mattress with
> other mattresses round me, and at intervals I would return from sleep or
> unconsciousness for another convulsion. The contortions formed me to
> turn away from those who were helping me when I wanted most of all to
> turn to them, to be held and comforted like a child. (p.167)

As the epilepsy receded, Golla told her that 'attacks like this can always
be stopped' (p.167). Her seizures then worsened again: 'The convulsions
now seemed to centre in my mouth, my hands and my heels, and to
affect my hearing, for the world went curiously silent as if in snow ...
My chest was like a wheel going over stones' (p.168). The psychic
effects interested her more than the physical effects. She noted that
because the internal life is changed by epilepsy, the visual value of
external things is also changed:

> When the disruption of the brain in the acute state of epilepsy approaches,
> ... the appearance of one's home and the scenery about one's home
> undergoes this great invisible change from the particular or descriptive to
> the evocative or dreadful ... An appalling terror which nobody who has
> not experienced it could believe, a terror amounting to panic seemed to
> emanate from every piece of furniture, every book, every saucepan. Like
> 'Jungle Fear' it was everywhere. Touch only deepened it. The more real
> the object surrounded by the unreal horror became, the worse it was. Had
> there been some hallucination, *something* unusual, it might have been
> easier. But the objects I knew did not want my body; it was my mind
> they wanted to destroy. (pp.142–3)

In his foreword to the 2020 edition of *The Nightingale Silenced*, Peter Wolf notes
that Evans uses oxymoron as a literary device to contrast the mental images
conjured up by her epilepsy with that of her conscious life – for instance, of
'black sunlight', 'voiceless call' and 'red snow' (pp. xi–xiii). Evans also envis-
aged her seizures as a terrific alien power and suggested that the ancient view of
epilepsy as demonic possession arose not from the onlookers of sufferers in fits
but from the sufferers themselves, 'Epilepsy was once called Possession ...
Possession it may be. But it is the Possession by the sufferer of epilepsy, not his by

the seizure'[311] – as Wolf points out, a unique and thought-provoking notion (p. xi). He also highlights Evans's insistence that patients with epilepsy have knowledge which doctors do not possess, and that the patients' view is often under-recognised and under-valued. Evans's trust in and respect for her doctors (especially Golla and her local Dr Y) was a sign of the times. Another notable feature of the times was her view that that those with epilepsy had 'a certain peculiar temperament', which included a tendency 'to brood on real or fancied wrongs . . . [experience] periods of heated expansion or inspiration, and those of cold contraction and uninspired misery . . . [being] too "garrulous" . . . the mind seems to expand in all directions at once . . . [be] an egotist, a supreme egotist, but not by nature selfish'.[312] She brooded profoundly on death, nature and the natural world, and the mystical nature of God. To Evans, the experience of epilepsy had positive features, allowing her to see the world and nature more clearly and precisely: 'Happiness is divine. / But too much health is like too much light: it blinds' (p. 30).

In Wolf's view, Evans's two books together are 'probably the most comprehensive literary self-report of epilepsy available'.[313] I think this is so. Furthermore, her books provide an intensely poetic and sensitive vision, at once authentic and accurate to an extent unequalled in any other literary writing. Evans herself, however, refers to two other writers – Dostoyevski and the Swedish writer Ludvig Nordstrom – who had, in her view, an understanding of what epilepsy felt like. She (and Lennox) seem to had corresponded with Gunnar Qvarnstrom, whose biography of Ludvig Nordstrom[314] focuses on the central role of that authors' probable epilepsy and the impact of epilepsy on his 'visional experiences'.

Epilepsy in Other Literature, Television and Film

In this early post-war period, epilepsy did feature in other creative works, with various themes explored. The long link between epilepsy and religion, evident in almost all the nineteenth-century novels involving epilepsy, for instance, was still very much present in mid-twentieth-century fiction. This is well demonstrated by Muriel Spark, who converted to Roman Catholicism and, like Dostoevsky, dealt with the subtle and complex questions of Christianity and faith in the apparently sublunary lives of her characters.[315] Ronald Bridges, the central character in Spark's novel The Bachelors (1960),

---

[311]   A Ray of Darkness, p. 11.   [312]   A Ray of Darkness, pp. 13, 14, 19, 26.

[313]   The Nightingale Silenced, p. xiii.

[314]   Qvarnström, Från Öbacka till Urbs. Nordstrom never publicly admitted to having epilepsy, but this was 'more-than-possible' in her view (The Nightingale Silenced, p. 135).

[315]   See Gilliatt, 'The dashing novellas of Muriel Spark'. Gilliatt was herself the wife of a professor of neurology. Spark may have become interested in the symbolic aspect of epilepsy when she witnessed a seizure in the street.

has epilepsy and is involved in spiritualism and metaphysics. Her written descriptions of his epileptic seizures are extremely realistic. Although she did not herself have epilepsy, it is clear that the condition interested her and that she must have had some personal acquaintance with it. Spark uses epilepsy as a metaphor for conversion and transcendence. Ronald Bridges was a convert to Catholicism who wanted to become a priest but was not able to do so because of his epilepsy. His counsellor suggested that instead of embracing the priesthood, he should become 'a first-rate epileptic' (p. 7). He, too, was an outsider, a bachelor, but his seizures provided him with insight into faith and compassion. His epilepsy also prevented his marriage, which was portrayed as a central purpose of human existence. Ronald's epilepsy combines the natural and supernatural and gave him a wisdom not shared with others, such as his ability to detect forgery, upon which the plot turns. Epilepsy in Spark's book was also a form of demonic possession (in moments of Ronald's self-reflection, 'obsessive images of his early epileptic years bore down upon him and he felt himself ... as one possessed by a demon', p. 8). Following Spark's conversion to Roman Catholicism, her interest in spiritualism intensified and a misfortune such as epilepsy was increasingly linked to damnation, with Ronald and his epilepsy being a metaphor for the flawed relationship between God and man. In the course of the book, Ronald underwent a transfiguration through his relationship with his protagonist Patrick Seton (Satan?) and became possessed by his evil. The book also highlighted the isolation, the sense of being 'other' and the loneliness of epilepsy. At the climax of the novel, whilst testifying in court against Seton that 'I have never, so far as I know made a mistake in a case of forgery' (p. 177), Ronald collapsed in an epileptic seizure:

> [He] swayed ... and fell two steps before he got to the bottom. There he foamed at the mouth. His eyes turned upward, and the drum-like kicking of his heels began on the polished wooden floor ... 'Is this man a medium?', said the judge. 'Put something between his teeth,' said Martin Bowles, in the tones of a zoophobic veterinary practitioner. 'He's an epileptic.' (pp. 185–6)

At the end of the book, Ronald goes

> home to bed. He slept heavily and woke at midnight, and went to walk off his demons ... [Thinking of his single bachelor friends, they were] fruitless souls, crumbling tinder, like his own self which did not bear thinking of. But it is all demonology, he thought, ... and to do with creatures of the air, and there are others besides ourselves, ... who lie in their beds like happy countries that have no history. (pp. 201–2)

A second theme, an antidote to modern scientific medicine, was a strain of romanticism, often expressed in the context of left-wing anti-capitalistic sentiment, which became a significant force in the creative arts of the 1960s and 1970s. Illness was viewed as a form of personal expression rather than as a defect of nature, depending as much on person and personality as on any physiological mechanism. John Berger's book *A Fortunate Man* (1967) expresses this well. The hero, John Sassal, a GP in southern England, had a childhood dream to live as a Conrad hero, the master of a schooner, and saw diseases as a mysterious and dangerous sea. He found with his scientific knowledge that he could beat sickness, but that often his patients remained ill and unhappy. He could cure disease, but he could not cure his patients. To Berger, cultural deprivation was the cause of much disease, and (as a Marxist critic) at its core lay capitalism. To Sassal, contemporary medicine depersonalised both doctor and patient with its technology, its fragmentary treatment and its specialisation, and as an institution was overwhelmingly venal. To Berger, self-awareness and moral choice were needed to avoid the diseases of ignorance and dependence – and epilepsy surely was high on the list of conditions to which this applied.

The portrayal of epilepsy and of epilepsy doctors was simplified, sometimes to the point of caricature, in film and especially in television dramas, which in that period often had a strong documentary element. More sophisticated filmic approaches had to wait until the late twentieth century. Probably the first TV depiction of epilepsy occurred in the pseudo-documentary series 'Medic', which, in rather clumsy illustrative story lines, highlighted the laudatory work of doctors. In one episode, aired in 1955 (*Boy in the Storm*), a 17-year-old orphan named Robert has epilepsy which was described as a 'condition designed to blight and destroy his entire existence'. His guardian, an aunt, had kept him in virtual isolation since childhood due to fear, shame and ignorance. After she had died, a visionary doctor assessed him with EEG and a Rorschach test and placed him on antiepileptics. Robert's seizures stopped, and he was thought 'safe' to be given over to a foster family (a psychologist mother who has lost her son in the Korean War). The film tries to dispel the stigma of epilepsy by showing that it is 'nothing to do with being crazy', but rather is an electrochemical event in the brain. Modern science and treatment can cure epilepsy, and the sufferer can be returned to 'normality'. The analogy of the dam (from Lennox) is used to explain this. Robert was assured that he could marry, and he (calling himself the 'Mad Hatter') fell in love with the EEG technician (calling her the 'Queen of Hearts'). Whether this love is ever requited was not revealed, perhaps being a step too far.

Such TV documentaries invariable portrayed doctors as white males, besuited and Brylcreamed, pontificating on the triumphs of scientific medicine to their adoring and grateful patients (for instance, the neurologist in *Boy in the Storm* and Dr Kildare in the 1940 film *Dr Kildare's Crisis*). In documentaries, the same impression is gained, for instance, by the neurosurgeon in episode 2 of the BBC's 'Physical Mental Health Treatments' (1957), who discussed frontal lobotomy as if it were a minor operation, quite uncritically and with the effortless sense of superiority and professional smugness which seems to have characterised medicine in those days. Similar examples in period dramas included the portrayal of Professor Theodore Meynert's 1888 ward rounds in *Freud: The Secret Passion* (1962), and that of Dr Lewis Yealland, the Second World War neurologist at the National Hospital, Queen Square in the film *Regeneration* (of 1997, and in the book of 1991 by Pat Barker on which the film is based). The neurologist's arrogance, typical of the wartime and early post-war period, as well as the inadequacy of his style of physical treatment (more akin to torture than medicine) were brutally exposed. Comedy scriptwriters poked fun at this style, a classic example being the ward round scene in *Doctor in Love* (1960). One struggles to find real depictions of doctors who exhibit any self-doubt, humility or any sense of apology about the limitations of their medicine. Lawrence and Toba Kerson, in their review of film,[316] make another interesting point – that seizures were sometimes used to highlight qualities such as care and tenderness in others, but that the 'others' are seldom doctors and furthermore are usually female (for instance, the EEG technician in *Boy in a Storm*).

THE INTERNATIONAL EPILEPSY MOVEMENT

The post-war years were of great importance to the ILAE. In the 1945 volume of *Epilepsia*, Lennox bid farewell to the 'blackness of war' without much ado and looked forward to renewed interactions with the League's transatlantic friends.[317] Two thousand copies of *Epilepsia* were printed that year, and advertising (for Dilantin) appeared for the first time. The British branch was reconstituted and held its first meeting in December 1945. In 1946 Holland and Argentina formed branches of the League, making, with the Scandinavian branch, a total of five.

Of these, the American branch was now the largest by far. It held its first post-war meeting on 13–14 December 1946 in New York, jointly with the Association for Research in Nervous and Mental Disease, of which Lennox was president. Although badged as a meeting of the ILAE, there were no international delegates and only five non-Americans amongst the faculty of eighty. It was, however, a remarkable meeting, with a programme demonstrating the range and scope of American epileptology and the newly released power of American academic epileptology, led by the Boston group. It also reflected the optimism and hegemony of the United States in the new world

---

[316] Kerson and Kerson, 'Truly enthralling'.   [317] 'The League and *Epilepsia*'.

order.[318] There were forty-four lectures from members of the American branch, and one given by a foreign invited speaker (an intriguing talk by Grey Walter entitled 'Analytical Means of Discovering the Origin and Nature of Epileptic Disturbances'). The papers from the American branch included contributions by Penfield, Jasper, Margaret as well as William Lennox, Merritt, the Gibbses, Earl Walker, Bailey, Ziskind, Livingston, Schwab, Potter and Fay. As Lennox wrote: 'This two day session covered the various aspects of research in epilepsy with a completeness never attempted before',[319] a statement with which it is hard to disagree. The programme included investigations into history and aetiology and experimental studies dealing with transmission of nerve impulses and electrophysiological aspects. Major emphases of the conference were on EEG and newer therapies such as diphenylene hydantoin, mesantoin, tridione and paradione. Post-traumatic epilepsy as a by-product of war was considered in five papers, including new techniques for operative surgery. Four papers dealt with psychosocial studies.

The American *Layman's League Against Epilepsy* had also made great progress during the war years. Founded in 1939/40, it was incorporated in 1942 and then changed its name to 'the American Epilepsy League, Inc.' in 1944/5. By 1946, it had 1,989 members, 7,000 or more sets of printed material had been distributed (articles, pamphlets and books), 10 articles had been published in the professional literature and 3 nationwide surveys had been completed. Chapters were being set up locally (at the city, state and regional levels), and sample bylaws were produced for these chapters centrally. In 1945, the Layman's League Against Epilepsy and the American League Against Epilepsy together made presentations to a congressional labour subcommittee which was investigating aid to the physically handicapped (the Kelly Committee). This was probably the first time that a dual approach by both a professional and a lay organisation was made. The potential power of such a lobby – recognised early by Lennox – was clearly demonstrated (see p.205).

At the 1946 ILAE meeting, Lennox also successfully moved that the lay organisation should be named an affiliate of the ILAE and share editorial as well as financial responsibility for the publication of *Epilepsia*. As if to kick off this collaboration, Lennox published the aforementioned article 'The Higher Education of Epileptics' with McBride and Potter of the American Epilepsy League, as the only article in that issue of the Journal.[320]

---

[318] The proceedings were published as a 654-page book: Lennox, Merritt and Bamford, *Epilepsy*.

[319] W. Lennox, 'The international league'.

[320] Lennox, McBri[d]e and Potter, 'Higher education of epileptics'.

The first truly international meeting of the post-war ILAE was held in Paris in 1949. This meeting was held in conjunction with the congress of the larger and more prestigious organisations: the International Neurological Congress and the International Society of Electroencephalography. The ILAE had no separate programme, but there were 3 sessions on epilepsy and 27 papers. In attendance were 1,038 participants from 44 nations, and the speakers included the post-war leaders of epilepsy: Lennox, Gastaut, Penfield, Jasper, Putnam and Walker. The meeting was a watershed for epilepsy for many reasons: it was the first with a large international audience, and the first in which the ILAE featured strongly in the congresses of the larger neurological societies. It was the last time the ILAE had as its president a non-specialist in epilepsy (Macdonald Critchley, a general neurologist[321]). It also marked the beginning of the end of the full engagement of the American branch, for it seems that with Lennox's retirement, the American Epilepsy League began to lose interest in international affairs.[322] It withdrew its funding from *Epilepsia*, effectively terminating the second series, which ceased publication in 1950. It is not known what Lennox's views about this were, but he must have been disappointed as it ended the arrangement he had negotiated and which was crucial to the survival of the journal during and after the war. Publication restarted (as the third series) in 1952, with the journal comprising one volume a year and concentrating on critical reviews rather than original research, but not co-funded by the lay organisation. It again ceased publication, after only three years, in 1955.

In 1953, the next (eighth) quadrennial meeting of the ILAE was held in Lisbon and, as discussed earlier, was devoted entirely to the topic of temporal lobe epilepsy. Gastaut was by then ILAE secretary-general and, by force of character, was largely directing the organisation's affairs. The ninth quadrennial meeting, in 1957, was in Brussels, and it was there that the world of clinical neuroscience began to reorganise itself with the foundation of the WFN. Gastaut was involved in organising the meeting, and the ILAE's profile was rising because of his presence. By now it had an increasingly European outlook and, at a time when the Cold War was at its height, America seemed to be drawing in its horns. In 1957 the American chapter changed its name to the American Epilepsy Society (AES), a name Lennox described as 'colorless and unco-operative',[323] and ever since has remained semi-detached from the ILAE.

Epilepsia was again resuscitated in 1959/60 with the publication of the first volume of the 'fourth series'. Sir Francis Walshe was appointed editor-in-chief

---

[321] Critchley, a physician at the National Hospital, Queen Square, was president of the ILAE from 1949 to 1953 and later president of the WFN between 1966 and 1973.

[322] It was a time of internal reorganisation and name change, and these seem to have trumped any interest in foreign activity.

[323] Lennox, *Epilepsy and Related Disorders*, vol. 2, p. 1036.

and the editorial policy again changed, this time with the express aim of being a scientific journal and publishing original research. It got off to a good start, putting out interesting and high-quality papers from its very first issue.

After Brussels, the next quadrennial meetings took place in Rome in 1961, Vienna in 1965, New York in 1969 and Barcelona in 1973, all held in conjunction with other congresses of neurology and or neurophysiology. The Barcelona congress was described by Masland as 'one of the largest assemblies of neurologists from around the world',[324] and conferences were now firmly embedded in the calendars of neurologists, psychiatrists and other medical specialists. Part of the reason was the fact that transcontinental and transatlantic travel was becoming easy and affordable.[325] Medicine was becoming, even more than before, a global village.

Founding the International Bureau for Epilepsy

The idea of an international laymen's epilepsy organisation, in partnership with the professional body, originated in 1939 when Lennox, as president of the ILAE, wrote to Hans Jacob Schou, the ILAE secretary-general, suggesting that 'a special branch of the League, an association of laymen interested in epilepsy be formed' as 'it is a well-known fact that in all civilized countries there is among laymen a growing interest in disease'.[326] Lennox continued that in 'all countries with a high standard of education there are so many intelligent epileptics that they will join our League Against Epilepsy. What is more natural than the idea that those who suffer from the disease themselves should be the most active in assisting the physicians in combating it?'[327] War intervened, and no such international branch was set up.

As we have seen, however, Lennox did succeed in setting up an active and successful American organisation (the Layman's League Against Epilepsy), and a second national lay organisation was then established in Britain in July 1950. This organisation, the British Epilepsy Association (BEA), rapidly became a significant force in the cause of epilepsy. National organisations then followed in many countries, but no further moves to form an international movement were made until 1961. Then, at the 10th quadrennial meeting of the ILAE in Rome, a special gathering was arranged by the BEA titled 'The Role of the Lay

---

[324] In 38th issue of the IBE Newsletter, 1973 (ILAE Archive, Wellcome Trust).

[325] The trip across the Atlantic for professional exchanges had previously been made by ship, but the introduction of Boeing 707 passenger services in the 1960s and the rapid rise of national airlines made travel easy and routine.

[326] Schou, 'Subjects for discussion'. It is interesting that Lennox, who after all had worked as a missionary in China, should think that in 'non-civilised' countries there might be no interest amongst the laity in epilepsy.

[327] Lennox, cited in Schou, 'Subjects for discussion'.

Organisations in the Treatment of Epilepsy'.[328] A key figure in persuading the ILAE to hold the assembly was George Burden,[329] who was then general secretary of the BEA. At the meeting, descriptions of the activities of their organisations were given by Ellen Grass, president of the American Epilepsy Federation; Irene Gairdner, honorary secretary of the BEA; and Mrs Kilgour, the honorary secretary of the Scottish Epilepsy Association. Dr Mosovich, of Argentina, resuscitating Lennox's pre-war aspirations, proposed a motion to establish an 'international bureau' to '[c]analize all possible information about associations to help people with epilepsy and distribute this by means of a newsletter at a certain fixed period and make information available on how to organize a laymen's league and how this should be financed'. He also suggested that an international film library about epilepsy be created and that the emblem of this association should be the 'candle already adopted by the British Epilepsy Association and by associations in Australia, Canada, Sweden and New Zealand'.[330] The ILAE board then met with Burden, and a small pump-priming grant was awarded.

The Bureau immediately became active, with an office based in London and a rapidly developing programme, including the production of a widely praised film and patient literature. In 1966, at a meeting in Wiesbaden, the International Bureau Against Epilepsy was formally established, not as 'the social arm' of the ILAE, as had been the original conception, but as an independent organisation. Its very success caused political tensions with the League. Following the Wiesbaden meeting, Lorentz de Haas,[331] president of the ILAE, wrote to the ILAE executive: 'The Bureau has since carried out a variety of tasks and developed laudable activities ... It is perhaps understandable that the Bureau has done so in a position of considerable independence. The question, however, is whether this independence has not assumed proportions reaching farther than has ever been the intention of the Committee of

[328] Details from the ILAE Archive held by the Wellcome Trust in London (see Weiss and Shorvon, 'International League Against Epilepsy').

[329] George Burden graduated from the London School of Economics and worked as a psychiatric social worker in London at the Kings and the Maudsley Hospitals, where he developed his interest in epilepsy. In 1958 he joined the British Epilepsy Association as its first full-time secretary, and in 1961 he was appointed secretary general of the newly formed IBE. He worked tirelessly in this role, travelling the world to promote local organisations and setting up travelling epilepsy workshops. He initiated the International Epilepsy Symposiums. He was also politically active as the Labour Mayor of a London borough and an unsuccessful parliamentary candidate. He was a quiet, kind and committed man, with an exceptional ability to relate to people with disability (see obituary in *The Times* newspaper in September 1999).

[330] See Weiss and Shorvon, 'International League Against Epilepsy'.

[331] Albert Marie Lorentz de Haas trained with Lennox, was appointed Medical Director of the Alexander van der Leeuw Kliniek in Amsterdam and then succeeded B. Ch. Ledeboer as medical director of Meer and Bosch in Heemstede.

the International League.' Gastaut and Burden had already crossed swords on various topics, and De Haas continued in a threatening fashion:

> While we may gratefully acknowledge all that the International Bureau in London has so far done, we must bear in mind (as must the Bureau) that it is closely linked to the League and owes its appellation 'International' to the League. Should the Bureau fail to understand this, then the League could in fact establish another bureau at any time, anywhere in the world.[332]

At the ILAE General Assembly in Vienna, Gastaut launched a tirade in an equally undiplomatic fashion: 'You know that for a long time I have considered that the Bureau's insufferable independence diminished the effectiveness of the League, and that this competition between two organisations that have the same goals is ridiculous and intolerable.'[333]

Difficult relations between lay and professional organisations are not uncommon, and usually reflect personality clashes (this was certainly the case in respect to the relationship of Burden and Gastaut), differences in priorities and struggles over which side should set agendas and policies. All contributed to the poor relations between the ILAE and IBE. Finances also played a key part. The ILAE was always financially more secure than the IBE, not only because medical professionals were more prosperous than the average patient but also because of access to sponsorship from the pharmaceutical industry. Eventually, relationships settled down, and a series of annual joint meetings – the 'European Symposia' – were initiated to focus on the social aspects of epilepsy, with the first meeting in Paris in 1967.

This squabbling between the League and its newborn infant was unbecoming. It was also a sign that as the ILAE became larger and more organised, it had become more bureaucratic. Personality and politics seriously intruded on its work, and the strong but abrasive personality of Gastaut magnified the problems It must have annoyed him to find that he could not browbeat laypeople in the way he could his doctor colleagues. This was not an auspicious start to what should have been a joyous birth, and, as we shall see, 'Entente' was never 'cordiale' and further problems were soon to develop.

Nor was the relationship with the Bureau the only source of dissention at the time. In 1962 Walshe resigned the editorship of *Epilepsia*, alluding to difficulties with Gastaut and with the AES. Walshe had a difficult personality, as had Gastaut, and they clashed over many topics; after resigning, Walshe had little further to do with the epilepsy movement. A similarly vicious personal row took place between the ILAE executive and its treasurer, the Dutch neurologist

---

[332] A. M. Lorentz de Haas to the ILAE Executive Committee, 7 July 1966, ILAE Archive, Wellcome Trust.

[333] Henri Gastaut, 13 July 1966, ILAE Archive, Wellcome Trust.

Otto Magnus. The row had been simmering for some years but came to a head when, in 1972, Magnus was forced to resign after being accused (probably unfairly) of improper use of funds. These bitter internal fights were not only the result of personality differences, but were tinged also with the politics of nationalism. In particular, tensions arose between America and Europe, perhaps coloured by the international tensions of the Cold War and the civil disturbances in the United States over the Vietnam War. International relations everywhere seemed mired in conflict.

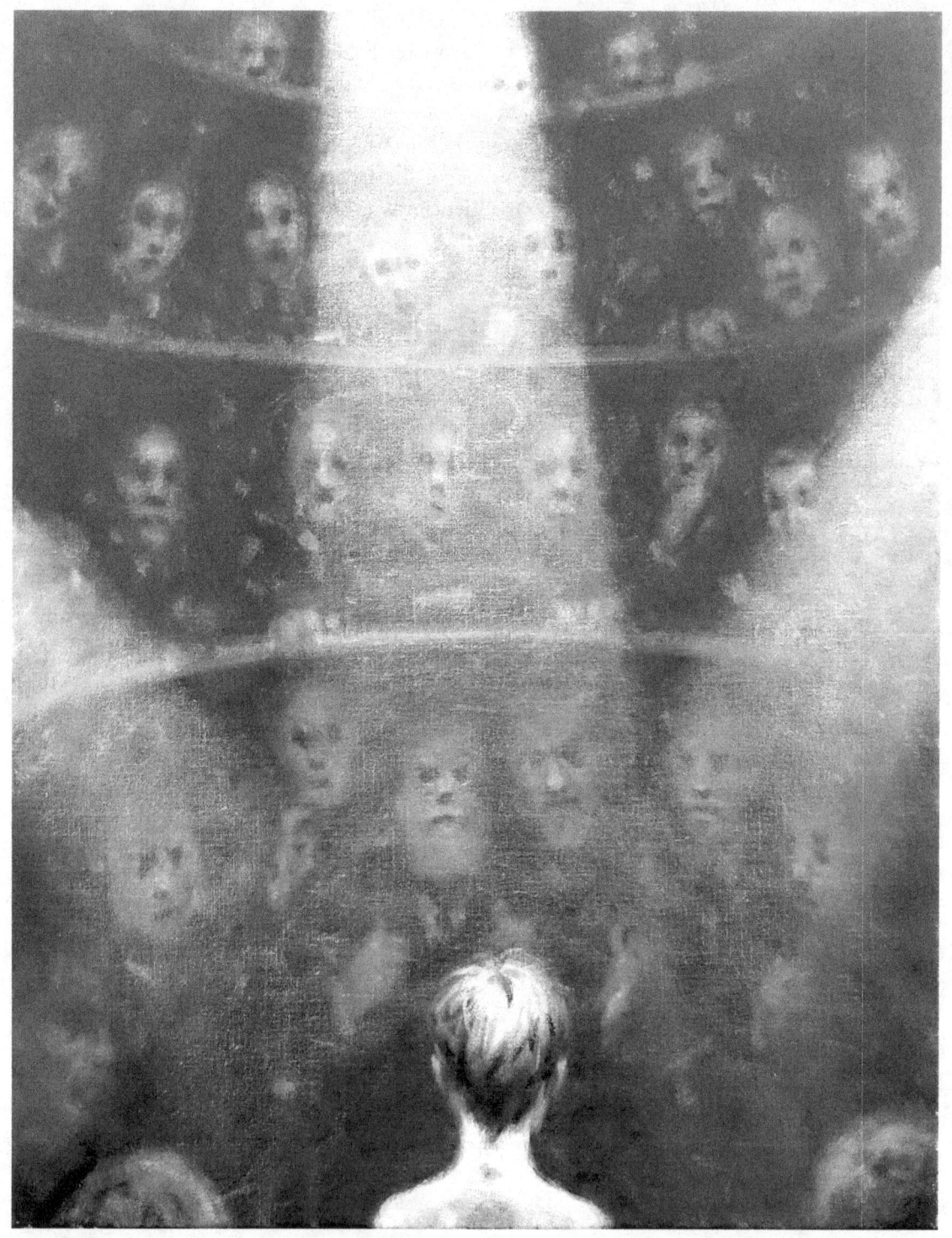

32. 'What is it like to be me?' The consultation style of the early post-war years (A painting by David Cobley, 2021).

FOUR

1970–1995: EPILEPSY IN A GLOBALISED WORLD

CHANGING OF THE GUARD

In these years, the social changes (that 'profound revolution in human affairs')[1] emerging in the earlier post-war period, were now in full flower. In the Western world, by 1970, the middle classes had expanded and were better off and better educated than in any previous era, the working class had declined and consumerism in medicine was changing the relationship of doctor and patient. A cultural revolution upended many social norms. The contraceptive pill had changed sexual behaviour, students led anti-war and civil rights movements and traditional governments in Europe (notably in France) were under challenge. A feminist movement was reborn, and a 'new left' emerged that campaigned for personal freedom and social emancipation. Within this setting, more liberal and more respectful attitudes developed towards the disabled, including those with epilepsy. Perhaps for the first time in history, people with disabilities were publicly and loudly acknowledged to have the same rights as their able-bodied peers. Along with other medical conditions, epilepsy was the topic of much medical and social debate. In the developing world, too, epilepsy was moving up the agenda of health concerns, due partly to rapid urbanisation and the often intensive activity of lay organisations dedicated to improving the care of those with epilepsy, a rise accelerated by a focus on research in epidemiology and healthcare delivery.

[1] Hobsbawm, *Age of Extremes*, p. 286.

The field of epilepsy was, in general, becoming more professionalised and more organised. This was partly due to the work of the International League Against Epilepsy and International Bureau for Epilepsy, as well as government and non-governmental agencies. Much of the development was the result of the new technology of computing, which not only transformed industry and science but was becoming integral to the day-to-day practice of medicine and its administrative bureaucracies. The first hospital computer systems were introduced around 1970 and soon underpinned every aspect of the medical process. Personal computers and the evolution of the Internet had a dramatic effect on medical communication.[2] They changed the professional lives of doctors by ramping up information exchange at every level and were to have an equalising effect across the world, rendering geography less relevant.

All, though, was not progress. The world economy underwent dramatic fluctuations which had a significant knock-on effect on healthcare spending. The progressive expansion of wealth between 1945 and 1972 (the golden age of capitalism) was brought to an abrupt end by the quadrupling of oil prices in 1973 and the subsequent recession in many Western countries. Over the next two decades, growth faltered, with the threat of high inflation, and then returned – only to be followed by further recessions in the early 1980s and again in 1991 interposed with the booms of the yuppie years. In Europe, government-funded healthcare systems came under financial strain, a problem exacerbated by an ageing population and the escalating cost of high-technology medicine. A more critical public view of medicine had begun to emerge, denting the optimism of the immediate post-war years. Fewer new landmark discoveries and a willingness to question medical authority helped to bring about this shift. In parallel, the ideologies of social democracy which had formed the basis of the political and economic systems guiding most of Western Europe (and others in the Western world) were eroded, not least by the policies of Margaret Thatcher and Ronald Reagan, and began to be replaced, from the 1980s, by the creep of neoliberalism with significant ramifications for healthcare, regulation and the free flow of the medical market. The hegemony of capitalism was strengthened by the weakening and then collapse of the Soviet Union in 1991 and the economic integration of developing countries. Globalisation of business and the rise of multinational companies, drove economic and technological growth in the medical technologies and pharmaceutical sectors. Between 1970 and 2000, the percentage of gross world

---

[2] From small beginnings in the late 1960s, as a private network, it is astonishing how rapidly information exchange on the Internet developed: a standard Internet protocol, of TCP/IP (1982); the domain name system (1983); 2,000 computers linked to the Internet (1985); 20,000 hosts (1987); a standard mark-up language, HTML (1990); introduction of the World Wide Web by CERN (1991); 600 websites and 2 million interconnected computers (1993); Windows (1994) by Microsoft; Google search engine (1998).

product that comprised exports doubled, and pharmaceutical and medical technology firms were in the vanguard of this expansion. High-technology medicine continued to develop because it was a lucrative business in healthcare systems where fees were paid for investigation, but less glamorous medical topics were starved of funds. Medical priorities and the clinical protocols became heavily dependent on economic factors, and business engaged with healthcare to a greater extent than at any time in history and for the primary purpose of profit. These developments were to prove a curate's egg in the field of epilepsy.

By now, and for the first time, epilepsy had become a specific focus of biomedical science. This process was stimulated by the increasing priority given to laboratory research in universities and industry. Basic research, not only in the life sciences but also in physics and mathematics, increasingly turned towards medicine, no doubt in recognition of the rich pickings of the expanding healthcare economy. New pharmaceutical and new medical neuroimaging technologies flourished.

The achievements of modern medicine confirmed the supremacy of specialist and science-driven medicine. Neurology had become fully established as a specialty in all Western countries, and epilepsy as a sub-specialty in many. Patients with epilepsy benefitted from more attention from the growing number of specialists, new modes of investigation and new therapies; these profoundly influenced their prospects.

Epilepsy became less 'invisible', public attitudes changed and stigma was reduced. The international epilepsy movement extended its reach around the world and became more influential and attention began to focus on the problems of epilepsy in the developing world. However, modern technological medicine had its downsides; consultations certainly became less holistic and less personalised as scientific medicine developed, and narrow clinical protocols and guidelines introduced a sameness and uniformity against which some railed.

AETIOLOGY AND SYNDROMES

Two parallel developments occurred during this period which were to change fundamentally the *concept of epilepsy*. First was a new emphasis on aetiology, and especially the structural causes of epilepsy brought about by the introduction of CT and MRI; second was the idea of the epileptic syndrome, and with it a new classification of the epilepsies.

The emphasis on aetiology, presaged by Kinnier Wilson, became the dominant focus of clinical research by the 1980s. In previous decades, under the spell of EEG, epilepsy had been conceptualised as a cerebral dysrhythmia and an essentially functional disorder, but the new imaging technologies of CT and MRI turned the spotlight on structure as well as function. Opinion moved back to the view that there was often (some even suggested always) a structural change in the brain that underlay epilepsy. The the type of structural aetiologies and the imaging technologies are described later in this chapter, but first we must consider the question of the 'epilepsy syndrome'.

The Epilepsy Syndromes and the 1989 Classification of the Epilepsies

A largely Gallic initiative, reflecting impatience with the narrowness of the seizure-type approach to diagnosis, the second major conceptual change of this period was the notion of epilepsy syndrome. This was to become the predominant preoccupation of epilepsy nosologists in the last two decades of the twentieth century.

As we have seen, an early attempt to classify 'the epilepsies' and to distinguish this from a classification of epileptic seizures was made in 1969 when Henri Gastaut attempted to steamroller through his proposed new classification of the epilepsies to complement his classification of seizures. However, the idea garnered little support. No further action was taken until 1981, when ILAE president Mogens Dam established a new Commission on Classification and Terminology, chaired by Peter Wolf. In parallel, a workshop along the lines of the Marseilles Colloquia was organised by Joseph Roger, previously a student of Gastaut. At the workshop, held in Marseilles on 7–10 July 1983, a series of *epilepsy syndromes* were defined (Table 4.1).[3] The workshop proceedings, outlining the proposed syndromes, became known as the *Guide Bleu* of epileptology,[4] and following its publication the ILAE commission in 1985 published new proposals for a Classification of the Epilepsies and Epileptic Syndromes. After some revision, this was presented to the General Assembly of the ILAE in New Delhi in 1989, where it was approved.[5] A syndrome was defined as

> [a]n epileptic disorder characterized by a cluster of signs and symptoms customarily occurring together; these include such items as type of seizure, etiology, anatomy, precipitating factors, age of onset, severity, chronicity, diurnal and circadian cycling, and sometimes prognosis. However, in contradistinction to a disease, a syndrome does not necessarily have a common etiology and prognosis.

Another difference from 'a disease' (discussed further later) was that a syndrome does not have the same societal connotations, and 'having a syndrome' was (and is) generally perceived to be better than 'having a disease'.

---

[3] Interestingly, a co-organiser was André Perret from the pharmaceutical company Sanofi. It was in pharma's interest to create 'new diseases' (see Moynihan and Henry, 'Fight against disease mongering'). Were similar motives considered by Sanofi's strategists?

[4] Roger et al., *Epileptic Syndromes in Infancy*.

[5] Commission, 'Proposal for revised classification'.

TABLE 4.1 *The twenty recognised epilepsy syndromes from the 1989 classification of epilepsies and syndromes*

Benign childhood epilepsy with centro–temporal spikes
Childhood epilepsy with occipital paroxysms
Primary reading epilepsy
Chronic progressive epilepsia partialis continua of childhood
Benign neonatal familial convulsions
Benign neonatal convulsions
Benign myoclonic epilepsy in infancy
Childhood absence epilepsy
Juvenile absence epilepsy
Juvenile myoclonic epilepsy
Epilepsy with grand mal (generalised tonic–clonic) seizures on awakening
West Syndrome
Lennox–Gastaut Syndrome
Epilepsy with myoclonic–astatic seizures
Epilepsy with myoclonic absence
Early myoclonic encephalopathy
Early infantile encephalopathy with suppression bursts
Severe myoclonic epilepsy in infancy
Epilepsy with continuous spike–waves during slow–wave sleep
Acquired epileptic aphasia; and febrile convulsions

Source: Commission on Classification and Terminology of the International League Against Epilepsy, 'Proposal for revised classification of epilepsies and epileptic syndromes'.

The 1989 classification divided the 'epilepsies' into four categories, with twenty syndromes fitted into this new classificatory framework (Table 4.2). The syndromic approach appealed especially to those involved in paediatric practice, and most syndromes became widely accepted and taken up into routine clinical practice.[6] The classification however was not as successful. Its four categories were very similar to the seizure-type categories, and, as could perhaps have been predicted, this caused enormous confusion; non-specialists particularly failed to appreciate the difference, and the scheme never entered routine neurological parlance.

---

[6] *Idiopathic Generalised Epilepsy* (IGE) is a paradigmatic example of the advantages and problems of a syndrome approach in three ways. First, it has relatively distinctive and clear-cut clinical features: three generalised seizure types (myoclonic, absence and tonic–clonic seizures), a diurnal pattern (on awakening or at night), frequent precipitation (by flashing lights, stress, tiredness or fatigue), typical EEG patterns and specific drug treatment. Second, its cause was, and is still, obscure, and although the syndrome is presumed to be genetic, intensive large-scale studies have failed to identify any clear-cut causal factor – and in this sense it cannot be considered 'a disease'. Third, like all syndromes it was susceptible to a lumper–splitter (and, frankly, rather pointless) controversy about whether it is a single entity or has 'subtypes' – for instance childhood absence epilepsy, juvenile myoclonic epilepsy, juvenile absence epilepsy and epilepsy with grand mal seizures on awakening.

TABLE 4.2   *The major subdivisions of the 1989 classification of epilepsies and epileptic syndromes*

1. **Localisation-related epilepsies and syndromes**	1.1 Idiopathic
	1.2 Symptomatic
	1.3 Cryptogenic
2. **Generalised epilepsies and syndromes**	2.1. Idiopathic
	2.2 Cryptogenic or symptomatic
	2.3 Symptomatic
3. **Epilepsies and syndromes undetermined whether focal or generalised**	3.1 With both generalised and focal seizures
	3.2 Without unequivocal generalised or focal features
4. **Special syndromes**	

Source: Commission on Classification and Terminology of the International League Against Epilepsy, 'Proposal for revised classification of epilepsies and epileptic syndromes'.

The development of syndromes raised two critical nosological problems, which have continued to dog the field. First is the fact – and the stated ILAE position – that the main difference between a 'syndrome' and 'disease' is that the latter requires a defined aetiology. However, this distinction is blurred and unsatisfactory – not least by the existence of many 'idiopathic' diseases and the increasing number of 'syndromes' for which a single aetiology has been uncovered; this is a topic taken up again in the Epilogue.

Second is the infuriatingly imprecise criteria that had been used for defining an entity as a syndrome. The boundaries of many of the syndromes were indefinite, and endless debate ensued between 'splitters', who liked to create new syndromes out of subtle phenotypic variations, and 'lumpers', who liked to consider all the variations as simply epilepsy (these debates continue). The least contentious conditions that were labelled syndromes ended up being those later found to have a single genetic cause, and thus more appropriately considered as diseases and not syndromes at all (e.g. benign neonatal convulsions, severe myoclonic epilepsy of infancy and Rett syndrome).

THE BASIC SCIENCE OF EPILEPSY

The circus of nosology could rotate endlessly, but of much more fundamental importance to epilepsy were the explosive advances in molecular biology. Basic scientific research in epilepsy entered a phase of rapid growth. Most important were the discoveries made in the molecular chemistry and physiology of epileptic discharges and in relation to ion channels, neurotransmitters and receptors. These discoveries stimulated the search for new drugs and a better understanding of the mechanisms of antiepileptic drug action. Molecular genetics, another field of intense laboratory activity after the 1950s, had relatively little direct effect on epilepsy in this period; for its main impact, which was to prove profound, was to come later.

The number of people employed in scientific endeavours, and the number of laboratories, rapidly increased. In 1910 the total number of British and German physicists and chemists amounted to only 8,000 persons (with not many elsewhere). But by 1980, 5 million persons worldwide were estimated to be engaged in scientific research and development, mainly in the United States and Europe. By 1970 a typical Western country had more than 1,000 scientists per million of population (compared to around 30 per million in African countries).

The leading laboratories were based in the North American, Japanese and European universities, and in the global pharmaceutical companies. In the United States and in Britain, the direction of research was partly the result of the decisions made in earlier decades by the National Institutes of Health (NIH) and the Medical Research Council (MRC), which prioritised laboratory clinical research and which focused on neurochemistry and neurophysiology. A similar stimulus occurred in France and Germany through their national bodies. Funding was made available to university departments through central and project grants, and the resulting work reflected the new and much more organised approach to basic science.[7]

By 1975 there was general agreement in the scientific community that epilepsy was due to a disordered balance of excitation and inhibition.[8] This simple idea guided thought throughout this period. The previous interest in acetylcholine and its metabolism in epilepsy (what might be called the acetylcholine wave) had abated, and the pharmaceutical industry and universities turned their gaze first to inhibitory mechanisms, and particularly to gamma aminobutyric acid (GABA) neurotransmission, and thereafter to excitation, especially involving the neurotransmitter glutamate. A third strand of research in the field of the molecular mechanisms of ionic conduction also gathered force in the 1980s. In the 1970s and 1980s, huge resources were committed to

---

[7] The difference in the approach to funding in Britain and America is described in detail in chapter 6 ('Styles of medical research') and chapter 7 ('Theoretical perspective') in Hollingsworth, *Political Economy of Medicine*. Hollingsworth noted that US government support was more generous, that it was spread over more institutions and that there were more organisations to apply to for research grants. On the other hand, British research was more focused and of an overall higher quality, primarily 'because fewer persons of marginal abilities were able to engage in medical research' (p. 235). By 1978, 43% of all biomedical articles were from the United States, the greatest contributor, with Britain second.

[8] Although it was recognised, too, that this was not always simply excessive excitation and in some situations, such as absence seizures, the seizures might be due to inadequate inhibition.

the study of these processes in healthy individuals, and in epilepsy and other diseases.

It was in the late 1960s and early 1970s that the role of GABA as the most important inhibitory neurotransmitter in the mammalian central nervous system was appreciated. This small achiral molecule (with a molecular weight of 103) was first synthesised in 1883, and by 1910 had been found in other biological tissues. However, its presence in the brain was not described until 1950. Initial studies in crustaceans suggested it might have inhibitory actions, and early investigations of GABA in the human brain produced contrary results. Indeed, by 1960 considerable evidence had been gathered purporting to show that GABA was not a human neurotransmitter. It was only in 1967 that Krešimir Krnjević and Susan Schwartz[9] provided unequivocal evidence of its role as an inhibitory transmitter. This was further supported by data obtained on the natural alkaloid bicuculline, which blocks the action of GABA.[10] It became apparent that a variety of drugs could bind to the receptor, including general anaesthetics and neurosteroids, and most notably the barbiturates and benzodiazepines.[11] Exponential growth in research on GABA (the 'GABA wave') followed, not least in the laboratories of the pharmaceutical industry, in the hope of finding GABAergic drugs which were sedatives and anxiolytics (these being bigger markets than epilepsy) as well as antiepileptics. The GABA-A receptor was cloned in 1987,[12] and was shown to lead to an influx of chloride ions and to hyperpolarisation of the membrane. The molecular structure of the GABA-A receptor was described at the end of the 1980s by Richard Olsen and Allan Tobin.[13]

It had been known since the 1930s that the brain also had high concentrations of glutamate, and in fact dietary glutamate and glutamine were tried as treatments for epilepsy in the 1940s. In 1954 Takashi Hayashi showed that intracerebral injections of glutamate produced convulsions, and he speculated that it might be a neurotransmitter. It was first thought to be inhibitory, as it was known to have a structure somewhat similar to GABA. Then, in the early 1960s, its excitatory action was demonstrated by David Curtis, John Phillis and Jeffrey Watkins using microelectrophoresis in spinal neurons (a technique pioneered by Bernard Katz in 1950). Still, many considered it to be a non-specific brain metabolite, and only in the late 1970s was it accepted that glutamate was the principal excitatory transmitter within the mammalian nervous system. In 1977 it was unequivocally demonstrated that glutamate exerted its effects via synaptic neurotransmission,

[9] Krnjević and Schwartz, 'Action of g-aminobutyric acid'.
[10] Curtis et al., 'Central inhibition'.   [11] Haefely et al., 'Possible involvement of GABA'.
[12] Schofield et al., 'Receptor super-family'.
[13] Olsen and Tobin, 'GABAA receptors'. The GABA receptor was found to comprise of five subunits. Each subunit consists of four transmembrane domains, and a large N-terminal and short C-terminal in extracellular domains. Many genetic variants have been described.

and not – as was the prevailing view – via a direct and non-specific action on neurons. Key to this work was the discovery of new selective agonists/antagonists, and three different forms of ionotropic post-synaptic glutamate receptors were identified (named after potent agonists: N-methyl-D-aspartate (NMDA), α-amino-3-hydroxy-5-methyl-4-isoxazolepropionic acid (AMPA) and kainate).[14] In the early 1980s, metabotropic glutamate receptors were also identified. NMDA and AMPA receptor antagonists were shown to exhibit excellent anticonvulsant effects in experimental models. In 1986 it was demonstrated that NMDA receptor activation resulted in calcium influx into the cell, raising the possibility that NMDA antagonists might also prevent brain damage caused by prolonged seizures. These efforts were followed by intense study in the 1980s and 1990s (the 'glutamate wave') in the search for glutamate antagonists which might be useful in controlling epilepsy and preventing cerebral damage, as well as therapeutic action in the more lucrative targets of schizophrenia and behavioural disturbances.

Throughout this period, it was known that epileptic discharges were critically dependant on voltage-gated and transmitter-gated ion channels (ionotropic receptors). The main synaptic mechanism of inhibition was the inhibitory post-synaptic potential (IPSP); that of excitation, the excitatory post-synaptic potential (EPSP). By 1980 the IPSP had been shown to be mediated by the GABA receptor, which, when stimulated, opens ion channels allowing an influx of chloride ions with resultant hyperpolarisation. By the 1990s the IPSP had been shown to have two components – one fast, one slow – thought to be mediated by different types of GABA receptors (GABA-A and GABA-B, respectively). Another level of inhibition, which functions over a period of minutes, was what was then known as the ATP (adenosine-triphosphate)-dependent sodium–potassium exchange pump. The EPSP was known to be produced by glutamate at the NMDA receptor, and to a lesser extent at the AMPA and kainate receptors, and these were differently distributed in different brain regions (and studied most in the hippocampus), but a fuller understanding of these mechanisms had to wait until after the 1990s.

The physiological feature most characteristic of epilepsy was the EEG 'spike'. The essential cellular features of the spike produced by strychnine application to the cortex of animals had been established by 1959, and those produced by application of penicillin by 1961. In both cases, the neuron responded to the convulsant with a brief and rapid burst of repetitive action potentials. The newly developed technology of sufficiently thin glass microelectrodes allowing recordings to be made from the interior of the cell showed that the bursts of action potentials were due to a large shift in

---

[14] Watkins and Jane, 'The glutamate story'.

the resting membrane potential – the paroxysmal depolarisation shift (PDS).[15] Some cells exhibited 'bursting' behaviour (i.e. a run or burst of multiple action potentials in response to a single depolarisation), and this was thought to be mediated by a variety of ionic currents. When a number of cells in the region demonstrate a PDS, an inter-ictal spike is formed. The physiological and neurochemical mechanisms underpinning the PDS were studied in the 1970s in 'brain slices' from the hippocampus. These were thin slices (about 4,000 microns thick) which could be adequately oxygenated in vitro and yet preserved their essential structure.[16] Using the slices, it became clear that blocking the action of GABA resulted in a PDS and epileptiform spikes. In hippocampal slices, the PDS was found to occur particularly in CA3 pyramidal cells in the hippocampus (and some cells in layers IV and V of the cortex), which also featured 'intrinsic burst generators'. It was believed likely that abnormalities which affected the kinetics of the intrinsic bursting mechanism were somehow important in generating epileptic discharges, and by 1987 the role of ion conductance in 'setting' the level of depolarisation was fully established. Key to this discovery was the invention of patch clamping to measure the flow of current through single ion channels.[17] It was discovered that ion channels could be modified by noradrenaline, acetylcholine and dopamine, and these chemicals, too, were the subject of experimentation; mutant channels in the fruit fly *drosophila* were common experimental models as it had been estimated that three-quarters of the genes causing human disease existed in the fly as well.

It was also realised that the individual cells producing fast repetitive discharges could not cause seizures on their own, but if many such cells were synchronised, seizures might result. Synchronisation therefore was also intensively studied, at the synaptic and non-synaptic levels, and it became clear that networks of interconnected neurons (neural networks) were needed to explain epilepsy. In chronic epilepsy, 'sprouting' of new synapses in the CA3 region occurred after seizures and was thought to be one possible mechanism for propagation and persistence of seizures. At the systems level, using mathematical modelling it was also shown that because of the network characteristics in the hippocampus, a wave of epileptic activity could be generated even if relatively few CA2 or CA3 cells were hyperexcitable – provided the cells

---

[15] The term was possibly first used and defined in 1964 (Matsimoto and Ajmone-Marsan, 'Interictal manifestations').

[16] The brain slice played a pivotal role in developing and exploring the action of antiepileptic drugs, as well as the basic mechanisms of the epilepsies.

[17] This technique was described in 1978 by Erwin Neher and Bert Sakmann, who shared the 1991 Nobel Prize for Physiology or Medicine for describing the function of single ion channels. Neher, Sakmann and Steinbach, 'Extracellular patch clamp'.

were connected to several others and excitation was powerful enough to stimulate the connected cells.

In the 1980s, attention turned to the complex physiology of glutamatergic neurons.[18] Activation of the AMPA and kainate receptors was found to contribute to the fast component of the PDS, and the NMDA receptor to the slow component. The chemical basis of excitation was thought likely to be largely due to glutamate action at the NMDA receptor, but ephaptic (i.e. non-synaptic) transmission was also recognised and noted to be important. In addition, changes were noted in the AMPA and kainate receptor densities in resected hippocampal tissue from chronic epilepsy, but their significance was not established. In 1982, MK801 was found to be a pure non-competitive NMDA receptor antagonist and was trialled as a clinical anticonvulsant, but its side-effects including psychosis and cognitive disruption prevented its clinical development; and a similar fate was suffered by other seemingly promising NMDA receptor antagonists. They were, however, extensively used to characterise glutamate receptor function in animal models.

By 1995 it was obvious that there were likely to be multiple underlying mechanisms of epileptic phenomena, and that the process of unravelling these had begun but was far from completion. For focal epilepsy, the predominant belief was that at the epileptic focus, epileptic seizures were due to neuronal hyperexcitability (either impaired synaptic inhibition or enhanced synaptic excitation) associated with some form of synaptic reorganisation. Moreover, some areas, notably the hippocampus and limbic structures, were especially vulnerable. Primary generalised seizures, on the other hand, were known to have a completely different pathophysiology related to circuits involving the premotor cortex and thalamus. At this time, whilst it was clear that either enhanced glutamatergic action or impaired GABAergic action could produce seizures, there was no evidence that either was actually the cause of human epilepsy. Almost nothing was known about the genetic basis of the underlying hyperexcitability of epilepsy, despite the fact that a number of inbred models had been developed that exhibited features of epilepsy. Nor were any 'epilepsy genes' known.

The spread of epileptic discharges in secondary generalisation was studied experimentally using multiple depth recordings and lesioning. These experiments showed that the substantia nigra, globus pallidus, thalamic nuclei, mesencephalic reticular formation and other brainstem sites were all involved in discharge spread from the hippocampus and neocortex. Large neural networks, widely distributed throughout the brain, were implicated. Certain neurons were also shown to have a predilection for rhythmical activity and could serve

---

[18] Although the role of glutamate in inducing seizures was first described in 1951 by Okamoto, 'Epileptogenic action of glutamate'.

as pacemakers for cerebral activity. Most neurochemical research focused on calcium currents in the thalamus. These low-threshold currents proved to be the pacemaker in absence epilepsy, and work moved to the study of the calcium channel. By 1995, the voltage-gated calcium channels in the thalamus were divided into different types (L, N, T and P), distinguished by their pattern of voltage-dependent activation and inactivation, their rate of inactivation and their agonist or antagonist pharmacology.

The 1980s also put pay to Penfield and Jasper's idea that loss of consciousness at the onset was due to seizure activity in the deep midline structures of the brain. Rather, it was shown that bilateral application of strychnine, pentylenetetrazol (PTZ) or oestrogens onto the premotor cortex of cats or monkeys produced the same EEG pattern. Moreover, the pattern was preserved even if the cortex was disconnected from the thalamus but interconnected by the corpus callosum. Pierre Gloor[19] proposed that spike–wave discharges were an abnormal response of the cortex to the thalamocortical volleys which would normally produce the EEG phenomenon known as spindles. Also in the 1980s, a variety of inbred strains of mice and rats demonstrated spontaneous spike–wave activity (the 'tottering mice' model in 1979, and the GAERS and WAG rat models in the 1980s) which produced motor arrest. These showed that genetic defects could lead to alteration of neuronal function as well as to altered ionic currents. Other models included the photosensitive baboon *Papio papio*, audiogenic seizures in mice, seizures in Mongolian gerbils and seizures due to lateral geniculate nucleus kindling in the cat. Evidence from these models suggested that primary generalised tonic–clonic, myoclonic and absence seizures could arise from abnormalities in a wide range of cerebral structures, including the brainstem, thalamic nuclei or cortex.

Even by 1980, understanding of the mechanism of action of antiepileptic drugs was still rudimentary. The antiepileptic mechanisms of carbamazepine, ethosuximide, barbiturates and valproate were unknown, and only preliminary data was available on effects of benzodiazepines on GABAergic transmission. By the early 1970s phenytoin was known to 'stabilise' membranes; the landmark finding that the drug inhibited sodium conductance in the giant squid axon was made in 1972.[20] However, despite much work in the next decade, it

---

[19] Gloor's definitive monograph was *The Temporal Lobe and Limbic System* (1997), finished by colleagues at the MRI after Gloor suffered a disabling stroke. Gloor was born in Switzerland, graduated in Basel and then moved to the Montreal Neurological Institute, where he succeeded Jasper as Chief of Neurophysiology and became a leading authority on the human temporal lobe.

[20] Lipicky, Gilbert and Stillman, 'Diphenylhydantoin inhibition'. This paper builds on the classic work of Hodgkin and Huxley on the squid giant axon, which formed the basis of much future work on sodium and potassium conductance using the voltage-clamp method (Hodgkin and Huxley, 'Conduction and excitation in nerve').

was not clear that this was the basis of the antiepileptic effects. Other candidates were effects on calcium conductance, reuptake of neurotransmitters and glial function. Enormous progress was made after 1980, and by 1995 the following mechanisms had been identified as the predominant explanation of antiepileptic action: sodium channel blockade (phenytoin, carbamazepine and, weakly, lamotrigine); GABAergic enhancement by binding to the GABA receptor (benzodiazepine and barbiturates); action at the T-type calcium channel (trimethadione and ethosuximide, although now somewhat contested); and action at the NMDA receptor (felbamate). Whether valproate exerted its primary action at the sodium channel or GABA receptor, or elsewhere, was not known, and still is not. The inhibition of sustained repetitive firing by phenytoin and carbamazepine at the sodium channel was voltage and use dependent. Drug binding to the GABA receptor had been studied in great detail. For instance, it was known that the benzodiazepine and barbiturate binding sites were distinct and that, at high doses, barbiturates increased chloride conduction even in the absence of GABA. It was also known that some drugs, such as tiagabine (then undergoing development), acted by preventing GABA reuptake and that others, such as Vigabatrin, acted by inhibiting GABA metabolism by inactivating the enzyme GABA transaminase.

There was a sense of real excitement in the basic science field as discovery was piled on discovery, but the findings seemed to have only distant relevance to clinical practice and few of the basic findings were translated into clinically useful tools or insights.

The Basic Science of Genetics

Outside the field of epilepsy, laboratory science was advancing on all fronts, and one area in particular was to become of great importance to epilepsy – the science of genetics (a timeline of genetic discovery is shown in Table 4.3). Here it is worth summarising briefly the waves then forming which were to later surge in a dramatic fashion over the whole of the epilepsy landscape.

The greatest scientific discovery in the biology of the second half of the twentieth century, surely, was the elucidation of the molecular 'mechanism of inheritance'. This was an extraordinary scientific achievement, progressing rapidly through a series of landmark discoveries. It began with the identification of the double-helix structure of DNA[21] in 1953 and the realisation that the two strands of helix unravel when the sperm and the egg combine and one strand from each parent recombines to form a new double helix which acts as the

[21] DNA is a polymer consisting of a long chain of 'nucelotides'. Each nucleotide consists of a sugar molecule (ribose in RNA or deoxyribose in DNA) attached to a phosphate group and a nitrogen-containing base. The bases used in DNA are adenine (A), cytosine (C), guanine (G) and thymine (T). In RNA, the base uracil (U) takes the place of thymine.

TABLE 4.3 *Timeline of discovery in basic genetics*

1859	Publication of Charles Darwin's *On the Origin of Species by Means of Natural Selection, or the Preservation of Favored Races in the Struggle for Life*
1865	Gregor Mendel demonstrates that heredity is transmitted in discrete units and established principles of segregation and dominance
1869	DNA isolated from cells by Frederick Miescher
1883	August Weismann proposed the germ plasm theory of inheritance, that hereditary information was carried only in sperm and egg cells, challenging Lamarckism and pangenesis
1902	Walter Sutton proposed the chromosome theory of heredity showing that chromosomes occur in matched pairs, with one strand inherited from the father and one from the mother
1902	Archibald Garrod demonstrated the principle of inborn error of metabolism with the example of alkaptonuria
1905	William Bateson coined the term genetic
1908	Hardy-Weinberg equation undermined much popular eugenic theory
1909	Wilhelm Johannsen coined the word 'gene'
1910	Albrecht Kossel describes the five bases occurring in nucleotides (adenine, cytosine, guanine, thymine, uracil)
1911	Thomas Hunt Morgan showed that chromosomes carry genes, and described genetic linkage
1911	Alfred Sturtevant describes linkage mapping
1918	Publication of the *Correlation Between Relatives on the Supposition of Mendelian Inheritance* by Ronald Fisher
1931	Cross-over of chromosomal material was identified as a cause of recombination
1941	George Beadle and Edward Tatum proposed the one gene one enzyme hypothesis, and showed that mutations in genes cause errors in specific steps in biochemical pathways
1944	Oswad Avery isolates DNA and suggested that it is DNA which carries hereditary material
1951	Rosalind Franklin produced the first clear X-ray diffraction images of DNA
1952	Alfred Hershey and Martha Chase, working on viruses, confirmed that genes were made of DNA (and not protein)
1953	Francis H. Crick and James D. Watson described the double-helix structure of DNA
1955	Joe Hin Tjio defined 46 as the exact number of chromosomes in human cells
1957	Crick proposed that the DNA sequence is a code for the 20 amino acids forming mammalian proteins
1959	Jerome Lejeune discovered the first chromosomal abnormality in disease: trisomy in Down syndrome
1961	Francis Crick and Sydney Brenner showed how the trios of DNA bases coded for the 20 amino acids that constitute human proteins
1961	Robert Guthrie developed a method to test newborns for the metabolic defect phenylketonuria (PKU)
1961	Sydney Brenner, François Jacob and Matthew Meselson discovered that mRNA takes information from DNA in the nucleus to the protein-making machinery in the cytoplasm (the ribosomes)
1966	Marshall Nirenberg demonstrated the nucleic acid sequences that determined the 20 kinds of amino acids in proteins
1966	Publication of first edition of *Mendelian Inheritance in Man* by Victor McKusick

(continued)

TABLE 4.3 *(continued)*

1972	Walter Fiers published the first gene sequence (a bacteriophage)
1975	Fred Sanger invented a method for rapid gene sequencing, which revolutionised the field and became the most common sequencing method
1975	Southern blotting developed
1977	Introns discovered (non-coding regions)
1981	For the first time, genes were inserted into laboratory animals – 'transgenic' animals – providing a way of studying the function of individual genes
1981	Human mitochondrial DNA was sequenced
1983	Huntington disease was the first human disease to be mapped to a specific chromosomal location,
1983	Polymerase chain reaction (PCR) was invented
1986	Positional cloning of the first disease gene (chronic granulomatous disease)
1986	Automatic DNA sequencing developed
1989	Use of microsatellites as genetic markers
1994	The first gene with mutations to be associated with increased susceptibility to a human disease (breast cancer) was identified
1990	The Human Genome Project was launched
1992	Microsatellite map of human genome completed
1993	MicroRNA was first described
1996	Dolly the sheep was the first mammal to be cloned from an adult cell
1999	The full genetic sequence of a human chromosome (chromosome 22) was published for the first time, containing 33.5 million base pairs
2003	Human Genome Project was completed: 2.85 billion nucleotides, with a surprisingly small number of protein-encoding genes (between 20,000 and 25,000). Also found that similar genes with the same functions present in different species
2005	First draft of the human haplotype map is published
2006	Copy number variation of human genome is described
2007	First large GWAS study of common diseases is published
2010	First draft of the Neanderthal genome
2012	CRISPR-Cas9 gene editing
2016	First commercially available $1,000 whole genome sequencing service
2017	First gene therapy approval by FDA

(This list is of selected discoveries which were to have an impact on epilepsy).

genetic 'code' of an offspring. In 1955, the number of human chromosomes (46) was correctly identified for the first time, and it was realised that a variation of even one base in the DNA string could lead to a specific alteration in the structure of a protein that could be the cause of genetic disease (first in the haemoglobin molecule as a cause of sickle cell disease). In 1957, Francis Crick[22] proposed that the sequence of the 4 bases in DNA was a code for the sequence of the 20 amino acids that form mammalian proteins. Other discoveries followed in quick succession. In 1961, Crick and Sydney Brenner proposed that it is the string of three nucleotides (triplets) that code for one amino acid, and by 1966

---

[22] Crick shared the 1962 Nobel Prize in Physiology or Medicine with James Watson and Maurice Wilkins for their discoveries relating to the molecular structure of nucleic acids.

the unique triplet code for each of the twenty amino acids in human proteins had been identified. It was then shown that messenger RNA takes information from DNA to the protein-making machinery (the 'ribosomes') in each cell. It was also recognised that there were operator and repressor genes which could switch on and off under environmental and genetic influences to regulate gene expression, providing some explanation of how different cells with the same DNA produce different proteins. By 1970 the basic mechanisms of genetics and how genetic variants could translate into disease had been revealed. A universal terminology had been established, and the field boomeranged.[23]

Advancing technology then underpinned further discovery. Sanger sequencing was developed in 1975, rendering the identification of the DNA codes (the 'sequence' of nucleotide bases in DNA) feasible in human research. In 1977 introns and exomes were identified, and in 1982 a genetic database of DNA sequence data was opened by NIH. In 1983 the first human disease gene defect (in Huntington's disease) was mapped to a chromosome, and in 1993 the defective gene was identified (with a coding defect that proved not to be a mutation but an expanded sequence of repeating triplet nucleotide bases, an unforeseen disease mechanism which became to be known as a repeat disorder). The first human genetic map was produced in 1987, and in 1990 the Human Genome Project was launched as a collaborative effort of governments and charities, with the objective of sequencing the entire human genome (the entire sequence of nucleotide bases) as well as those of other model organisms (yeast, roundworm and fruit fly). This culminated in 2003, on the fiftieth anniversary of the discovery of the DNA double helix, in a draft of the human genome – a reference sequence of more than 3 billion nucleotide bases. The enabling technology was automated high-speed sequencing – a next-generation version of the Sanger sequencing of the 1970s.

The commercial potential of genetics was quickly recognised. The first biotechnology company, Cetus, was formed in 1971 in California and in 1985 discovered a way of commercially amplifying DNA by a polymerase chain reaction (PCR) so as to render the amount of DNA suitable for genetic testing and genetic experiments. Other companies were soon formed. In 1990 the first gene therapy was approved in America to treat combined immunodeficiency disease, the first cloned mammal was created in 1996 (Dolly the sheep) in Edinburgh and in 1998, Celera Genomics was launched to compete with the Human Genome Project and to license the genome commercially. In 2017 the first gene therapy was approved by the FDA, and later by other regulatory agencies. The genie was truly out of the bottle.

The completion of the Human Genome Project lead to the advent of *Genome Wide Association studies* (GWAS) in 2007. Technology rapidly advanced

---

[23] See, for instance, Crick, *What Mad Pursuit*.

with the development of powerful sequencing methods, and by 2016, commercially available genome sequencing at less than $1,000 per genome was offered to the public. Thus, with breath-taking speed, the 'new genetics' emerged – a novel science which was to have a profound effect on epilepsy after 1995.

'New genetics' symbolised the power of science, and also the power of industry in the capitalistic environment that translated science into markets and profit. There were inevitable implications of these discoveries at all levels of society, and slowly the media and the public began to appreciate the enormity of their impact and their huge potential for understanding and mitigating human disease. All, though, was not positive. In the mid-1970s, public concern began to be expressed at the technologies of recombinant DNA, the patenting of recombinant products and genetic engineering, but essentially business interests effectively neutered any serious government control.[24] Many people were also horrified at the patenting of naturally occurring genes, and this remains a fraught concern. As cloning and gene therapy developed, embryo research and gene therapy sparked additional anxiety. As sequencing become more powerful, the pace of research into the genetics of human disease picked up, and by the 1990s 'gene-hunts' had become competitive races by researchers, with little heed to the social or ethical consequences of their endeavours.[25] So complex were the technologies, that both the social and medical responses to these developments were plagued with miscomprehension.

The impact of these discoveries on epilepsy is described in the next chapter. It is perhaps surprising to see how long it took for clinical epilepsy researchers to grasp their potential. Contributing to this was the fact that, as with most clinical science, the application of genetics to human epilepsy depended more on the introduction of available technologies than on the development of new scientific hypotheses – emphasising once again the applied nature of most of the contemporary human epilepsy research.

PSYCHIATRY OF EPILEPSY

By the 1970s the psychiatry of epilepsy had also moved on. Psychiatry had ceded its position as the dominant specialty for epilepsy, perhaps both a cause and a consequence of the growing medical and public opinion that epilepsy was no longer to be considered a 'mental disorder'. Although psychiatrists still took primary responsibility for those whose epilepsy was complicated by learning disability or behavioural disorder, the majority of

---

[24] See Howard and Rifkin, *Who Shall Play God?*; Glasner, *Splicing Life.*
[25] Cook-Deegan, *Gene Wars*, p. 6.

specialist consultations were by then based in neurology clinics. As a result of the impact of drug therapy, clinical psychiatric practice was now also a largely outpatient exercise, and the alienist tradition in epilepsy, predominant throughout the whole of the earlier history, had well and truly ended. Psychoanalysis, too, was now mostly relegated to the outer reaches of the medical universe. As epilepsy had evolved to be seen as a primarily neurological topic, the role of psychiatric research had contracted to the study and treatment of its psychiatric complications rather than of the condition itself.

Amongst the most important trends of that period was the rise in interest in quantitation and measurement. This had risen strongly up the psychiatric agenda in an attempt to give the specialty seemingly scientific credentials, and as a reaction against what was by then generally perceived to be Freudian pseudo-science. Indeed, 'scales' became the bread and butter of psychiatric medicine, not only focused on IQ (a rather discredited concept) as in the past, but now on specific cognitive attributes, behaviour and mood. One such application was to that relic of previous ages – the concept of the epileptic personality, though not focused on idiopathic epilepsy as in the past but on temporal lobe epilepsy. The work of Norman Geschwind, and David Bear and Paul Fedio,[26] stands out. Geschwind used scales to identify a new behavioural syndrome (the 'Geschwind Syndrome') which he found to be associated with temporal lobe epilepsy, although it has to be said that its features closely resembled those found of the early-twentieth-century descriptions of the epileptic personality:

> increased concern with philosophical, moral or religious issues, often in striking contrast to the patient's educational background, an increased rate of religious conversions (or strongly justified, rather than casual, lack of religious feeling), hypergraphia (a tendency to highly detailed writing often of a religious or philosophical nature), hyposexuality (diminished sex drive sometimes associated with changes in sexual taste), and irritability of varying degree.[27]

Geschwind later postulated, on shaky evidence, that it was the presence of the spike focus that caused the behavioural syndrome. He took the view that since electrical stimulation of limbic structures clearly altered behaviour, spike discharges could do so as well, and, influenced by contemporary experimental

---

[26] Geshwind trained in Harvard and spent time at the National Hospital, Queen Square. He was appointed Professor of Neurology at Harvard Medical School, Neurologist in Chief at Beth Israel Hospital and a Professor at the Massachusetts Institute of Technology. Waxman and Geschwind, 'Interictal behavior syndrome'; Bear and Fedio, 'Quantitative analysis'; MacLean, 'Papez theory of emotion'.

[27] Geschwind, 'Behavioural change'.

work on kindling, he attributed the behavioural changes to 'kindling by the electrographic spikes'.[28] However, the extent to which any of these personality features are in fact due to organic processes (such as kindling) or to psychological or social factors was then (and still remains) entirely unclear.

Bear and Fedio's inventory[29] was a scale designed to identify traits associated with temporal lobe epilepsy in which eighteen personality features were identified which were considered more common in patients with temporal lobe epilepsy than in other forms of epilepsy or in normal controls. Not all authorities agreed with their formulation and this remains a controversial area, but the inventory is still widely used clinically. Bear attributed these features to 'sensory-limbic hyperconnection' – in effect the converse of Klüver–Bucy syndrome in primates, which resulted from bilateral temporal lobe ablation.[30] Whether this explanation holds water is doubtful, and, as is the case with epilepsy psychosis, the mechanisms remain essentially unknown.

The heavy dependence on quantitative scales was also to become a predominant feature of the approach of clinical psychology to epilepsy (and to other disease areas). In the early twentieth century IQ testing had been introduced into epilepsy studies to categorise levels of mental handicap, but it was only in the post-war years that more sophisticated quantitative neuro-psychological batteries aimed at specific cognitive functions were established. The Halstead battery, originally designed for assessing head-injured patients,[31] was extended with the addition of the Wechsler Adult Intelligence Scale, as a general measure of intellectual functioning, and the Minnesota Multiphasic Personality, as a measure of emotional functioning, into the Halstead–Reitan Neuropsychological Test Battery. This became commonly used in the clinical practice of epilepsy. Then in 1978 Carl Dodrill[32] modified the battery to be used specifically for epilepsy, introducing, in 1980, the Washington Psychosocial Seizure Inventory. The inventory sought to quantify psychosocial

---

[28] Geschwind, 'behavioural change'.   [29] Bear and Fedio, 'Quantitative analysis'

[30] Bear, 'Temporal lobe epilepsy'. The eighteen characteristics attributed by Bear and Fedio to temporal lobe epilepsy were: emotionality, grandiosity, sadness, anger, aggression, altered sexual interest, guilt, hypermoralism, obsessionalism, circumstantiality, viscosity, sense of personal destiny, hypergraphia, religiosity, philosophic interest, passivity, humorlessness and paranoia. This list is also remarkably similar to the traits ascribed to the 'epileptic personality' in the late nineteenth and early twentieth centuries.

[31] Ward Halstead was appointed Professor of Psychology at the University of Chicago. He and his student Ralph Reitan developed the Halstead–Reitan battery: a series of neuropsychological tests for studying cognitive and behavioural functions that was widely used in epilepsy. Halstead set up a neuropsychological laboratory and devised his battery primarily for evaluating head-injured and lobotomised patients. Halstead's landmark work was *Brain and Intelligence: A Quantitative Study of the Frontal Lobes* (1947).

[32] Dodrill modified the Halstead–Reitan test battery to include the Stroop Test, Wechsler Memory Scale and Seashore Tonal Memory Test. The resulting battery included sixteen discriminative measures: Dodrill, 'Neuropsychological battery for epilepsy'.

adjustment, in a post-Meyerian model, into seven domains: family background, emotional adjustment, interpersonal adjustment, vocational adjustment, financial status, adjustment to seizures and medical management. Other questionnaires, designed for more general usage, became also widely used in epilepsy, included those measuring behaviour (such as the Bear–Fedio Inventory), affective states (for instance, the Beck Depression Inventory) and the numerous cognitive scales used in neuropsychometric assessment.

The scientific mind likes nothing more than figures, and these quantitative measures were highly seductive. Nonetheless, quantitation is not infrequently spurious, both conceptually (for instance, by the abstraction of intelligence or emotion into a single number and the use of these numbers to segregate and to rank) and methodologically, with many studies failing to recognise the strong influence of selection bias. Although the more sophisticated scales had some validity, the use of simplistic scales to quantify complex behaviour was a pseudo-science, a form of reductionism that in the past had led to the excesses of biological determinism, to the detriment of many individuals. And many of the findings from psychological work in this period, based on these scales, neither endured nor contributed much to the treatment nor to any fundamental understanding of epilepsy.

This specific link between temporal lobe epilepsy and personality change was not universally accepted, with some considering that no specific personality features exist in epilepsy and others that the so-called temporal lobe features occur in epilepsy of all types.[33] A particular personality structure was also proposed in patients with idiopathic generalised epilepsy (primary generalised epilepsy), characterised by impulsivity, risk taking, irresponsibility, self-interest and distractibility,[34] but again with little consensus.

The psychiatric features of seizures themselves were also explored. A wide range of affective changes, delusions and hallucinations were reported. The widespread use of depth EEG for preoperative assessment threw up some interesting findings, which built on the earlier work of the biological determinists described in the preceding chapter. Well-documented case reports were published of epileptic patients experiencing episodic rage and associated

---

[33] For reviews of work on the psychiatry of epilepsy, see Ettinger and Kanner, *Psychiatric Issues in Epilepsy*, and Devinsky and D'Esposito, *Cognitive and Behavioral Disorders*.

[34] First proposed by Janz, *Die Epilepsien*. Janz was widely considered the father of post-war German epileptology, and celebrated for his meticulous clinical observation and judgement. After his military service he trained in neurology; in 1983 he was appointed Chief of Neurology at the Free University in Berlin, and in 1988 Professor Emeritus. His book became the standard German work on epilepsy, but surprisingly has not been translated into English. Juvenile Myoclonic Epilepsy is sometimes called 'Janz syndrome' in view of his detailed descriptions, although it had been well described by others (not least Herpin, Gowers and Muskens). He served as Vice-President of the ILAE (1973–81). He was an erudite man and amongst his interests outside epilepsy was the anthropology of Victor von Weizsäcker, whose Collected Works he edited.

psychotic features during prolonged hippocampal seizures (amounting to non-convulsive status epilepticus) occurring at a time when the scalp EEG was unremarkable. These findings supported the suggestions made in previous decades that some episodic behavioural responses in epilepsy might be due to seizure activity itself in deep-seated areas of the brain.[35]

The link between epilepsy and aggression also continued to interest researchers, especially in relation to temporal lobe epilepsy. However, different studies found wide variation in the rates of aggression – due mainly to the selection bias of the study population, the definition of 'aggression' and, to some extent, the preconceptions of the authors. Henri Gastaut, for instance, estimated that 50% of his temporal lobe epilepsy patients showed 'paroxysmal rages',[36] whereas in an outpatient survey of 666 patients, Simon Currie and co-workers reported a rate of aggression of only 7%.[37] A further distinction was made between the aggression that occurs during or in the aftermath of a seizure (ictal aggression) and the inter-ictal aggression that occurs independent of seizures. It was conceded, however, that this distinction was not straightfor-ward. For instance, when EEG abnormalities are taken into account,[38] the distinction between ictal and post-ictal states is to some extent blurred, echoing the nineteenth-century view that aggressive outbursts (furor epilepticus) could be epileptic equivalents or larval epilepsy.[39]

In accord with the political and cultural trends of the 1970s, however, many rejected the uber-deterministic biological approaches to aberrant behaviours which had flourished in the 1950s and 1960s. Sociology provided a different perspective, viewing abnormal behaviour in epilepsy as a sign of conscious or unconscious deviance from social norms with societal, not biological, causes. Christopher Bagley[40] sought to integrate the sociological, psychological and neurological elements into a unified explanatory model, seeing abnormal

---

[35] The literature on these points is discussed in two papers: Elliott, Joyce and Shorvon, 'Delusions, illusions and hallucinations' parts 1 and 2. Of particular interest was the later work of Heinz Wieser, who used telemetered depth recordings to demonstrate that episodes of seizure activity in limbic structures, without changes on the scalp EEG, were associated with behaviour change. A wide range of hallucinatory symptoms occurred during electrographic seizure activity in limbic structures at times when there was no overt seizure. It is interesting to note that the more complex hallucinatory states are not very anatomically specific. Repeated seizures or stimulation of a single area, even within the same patient, can produce different psychic responses, whilst stimulation of widely distinct areas in the limbic system within the same individual can produce remarkably similar phenomena.

[36] Gastaut et al., 'Étude du comportement'.   [37] Currie et al., 'Clinical course and prognosis'.

[38] See, for instance, Wieser, 'Limbic seizures and psychopathology'. Wieser reported aggressive behaviour occurring without any evidence of a clinical seizure or any scalp EEG changes, although depth EEG showed spikes and subclinical 'seizure activity' in the temporal lobe. Heinz Gregor Wieser exported the St Anne tradition of multiple intracranial electrode recordings to Zurich, where he worked with the neurosurgeon Gazi Yaşargil.

[39] See Esquirol, Des maladies mentales.   [40] Bagley, Child with Epilepsy.

(deviant) behavioural traits to be the result of a complex mixture of an genetic and physical causes, upbringing and education, and early experiences and responses to rejection and stigma (an approach similar to that of Adolf Meyer decades earlier): 'In the final analysis we have to consider the uniqueness of each individual in our matrix. Our social matrix is a matrix of individuals interacting with one other, and in so doing forming agreement on the kinds of roles which are to make up a social system, and how these roles are to be performed' (p. 276). This is a more nuanced approach than biological explanations of behaviour, or simplistic psychometric questionnaires, but equally difficult to prove – and the position taken by individual psychiatrists on this matter was much based on philosophical, social and political persuasion.[41]

In relation to criminality, attitudes had also moved on. The viewpoint of Lombroso, for instance, that criminality was an inherited trait associated with epilepsy was thoroughly discarded. The 1970s studies of John Gunn were influential in showing that criminality was not an 'epileptic trait', and also in pointing out that crimes were most unlikely to be committed during epileptic seizures.[42] Studies of prison populations did show a higher prevalence of patients with epilepsy than expected, but it was widely accepted that the high prevalence was due to sociological factors rather than the intrinsic biology of epilepsy. Furthermore, when methodological biases were removed, the suggestion of a specific link with temporal lobe epilepsy disappeared.[43]

In the law courts, criminal acts during a seizure, although rare, did pose a legal problem. In British and Commonwealth law (and similar considerations applied in the United States and Germany, for instance), the M'Naghten Rule of 1843, named after the accused murderer Daniel M'Naghten, established that a person committing a crime during, or in the aftermath, of a seizure was, at the time of the crime, temporarily *insane* – rather than being of *no mind*. The difference was important, for if the crime occurred when there was 'no mind', the person should be acquitted, whereas if it occurred during 'insanity', the person required admission to a secure hospital. A series of cases challenged this interpretation, and in 1961 Lord Justice Tom Denning of the Court of Appeal argued: 'It seems to me that any mental disorder which has manifested itself in violence and is prone to recur is a disease of the mind. At any rate, it is the sort of disease for which a person should be detained in hospital rather being given an unqualified acquittal.'[44] Not all agreed, and many continued to call for a change in the law – but none was forthcoming. This is an area, and not

---

[41] Similarly, theoretical frameworks in the area of stigma produced more meaningful findings than simple attitudinal questionnaires.

[42] Gunn and Fenton, 'Epilepsy, automatism, and crime'; Gunn and Bonn, 'Criminality and violence'.

[43] Stevens and Hermann, 'State of the evidence'; Kligman and Goldberg, 'Epilepsy and aggression'.

[44] *Bratty* v. *Attorney General.*

uniquely so, where the law and medical opinion remain wholly out of step. In parallel, criteria were developed in the 1970s to determine whether or not a violent act was committed during an epileptic seizure,[45] in an attempt to prevent epilepsy being used inappropriately as a defence. The EEG, too, assumed a greater importance than was justified in the law courts, with psychiatrists overemphasising minor changes taken as evidence of either of psychopathic tendencies or of epilepsy itself.[46] All these aspects raise difficult issues about the nature and limits of criminal responsibility in epilepsy (and other brain disorders) that continue to resonate to this day.

NEUROLOGY OF EPILEPSY

By 1970 epilepsy had been fully incorporated into the neurological fold. The result was a much more medical approach to its study than ever before. With the rise of funding for academic medicine, and the new emphasis on research as a criteria for medical advancement, clinical investigation was given an enormous boost and the epilepsy literature burgeoned, with the number of published studies increasing threefold between 1970 and 1995; a selection is described here of the research areas which advanced most and in which research has endured.

Epidemiology and Prognosis of Epilepsy: The Advent of Cohort Studies

The epidemiology of epilepsy was put, during this period, on a much more secure footing, thanks largely to better methodologies and statistical analysis, and in particular to the advent of prospective longitudinal cohort studies.[47]

The first classic epidemiological study of epilepsy was reported in 1959, by Kurland, based on work done in Rochester, Minnesota (Table 4.4). Prior to this, there were no large-scale studies of epilepsy in which all cases (or, at least, all diagnosed cases) were included within a well-defined population frame. The Mayo Clinic Diagnostic Index was searched for cases of convulsive disorders among residents of the community in the period 1945–54, inclusive.[48] Kurland concluded that as the only neurologists and EEG facilities in the county were at the clinic, there was an 'almost complete identification of the epileptics in the local population', although in retrospect this seems over-optimistic (as the study did not

---

[45] These include such factors as a prior diagnosis of epilepsy; short-lived episode; habitually aggressive automatisms; the presence of amnesia for the event; a lack of planning, concealment or premeditation; and the simple nature of the crime (i.e. not involving complex thought).

[46] For an interesting discussion of the use of EEG in the American courtroom, see Hughes, *EEG in Clinical Practice*, pp. 197–212.

[47] These are reviewed in Shorvon and Goodridge, 'Longitudinal cohort studies'.

[48] Kurland, 'Incidence and prevalence'; Hauser and Kurland, 'Epidemiology of epilepsy.

TABLE 4.4   *Findings from the landmark epidemiological study from Rochester Minnesota*

Incidence of epilepsy (age adjusted)	31/100,000/yr
Incidence in first five years	152/100,000/yr
Incidence in adult life	20/100,000/yr
Prevalence (age adjusted)	3.8/1000
Identifiable underlying cause	36%
New cases classified as tonic–clonic seizures	55%

(Based on 194 cases. Derived from Kurland, 'The incidence and prevalence of convulsive disorders' published in 1959)

include those attending psychiatrists, general physicians, primary care physicians and those undiagnosed or untreated) and the figures provided are surely minimum estimates. The 194 cases were classified as grand mal, petit mal or focal seizures, and the grand mal cases were divided into primary (without identified cause) and secondary (with apparent cause) categories. In 1975 a second study was undertaken in Rochester, using the record linkage system, this time encompassing the period between 1935 and 1967; 1448 cases were found. The mean annual incidence rate of epilepsy was 48.7/100,000, a rate highest in childhood, falling in mid-life and rising again in the elderly. The fact that the rate was higher than in the first study was attributed to better case ascertainment. This and other investigations reported prevalence rates of around 1–3/1,000. Another figure of interest was the *lifetime prevalence rate* of around 6%.[49]

The Rochester study is open to many lines of criticism, and it certainly fails to meet the gold standard of epidemiology today. But at the time, it provided the best available figures, and it became (and remains) a standard reference. It also stimulated more activity. By 1982 more methodologically sound studies had been published from Denmark, Great Britain, Iceland, Israel, Japan, Norway, Poland and the United States, with incidence rates varying between 1–30/100,000 (children, 80/100,000) and prevalence rates between 1–9/1,000 (children, 30/1,000). Lifetime prevalence rates from Great Britain, Iceland and the United States showed rates of around 5%.[50] In the developing world, epidemiological studies were also published from many cities and countries, usually finding higher incidence and prevalence rates than in the West, although less stringent methodology rendered some of these findings unreliable.

Nevertheless, a consensus arose that epilepsy is a common condition throughout the world, with incidence rates in most locations varying between

[49] This is more accurately known as the 'cumulative incidence rate'. This statistical measure was introduced by D. L. Crombie and colleagues (in Crombie et al, 'Survey of the epilepsies'), who calculated that 4% of a population will have at least one seizure and 3% a diagnosis of epilepsy at some point in their lives.

[50] Zieliński, 'Epidemiology'.

40–70/100,000 and prevalence rates of 4–10/1,000. Genuine variations in figures depend on the age structure of a population, as epilepsy is more common in children than in adults; on socioeconomic factors affecting health and healthcare; and, to some extent, on differences in underlying aetiologies. Although figures from the developing world were found to be generally higher than in the developed world, the biological aspects of epilepsy were not found to vary much from country to country, and the similarities of such features as seizure type, age of onset and frequency of seizures were more notable than their differences. However, many studies lacked sophistication, and it seems quite possible that unique features of epilepsy in some locations were overlooked and remain still to be detected.

The prognosis of epilepsy was another topic that attracted considerable attention. A starting point for work on this topic was Ernst Rodin's *Prognosis of Patients with Epilepsy* (1968), which provided an extensive review of studies of prognosis over the previous fifty years and added findings from the author's institutionalised patients.[51] Rodin came to the pessimistic view that only around a third of patients could hope to achieve long-term remission of seizures. He also concluded that the longer the follow-up, the worse the prognosis, and that ultimately 80% of patients with epilepsy were likely to have a chronic disorder, even given short-term remissions. These views reflected the orthodox opinion of the time, but were unduly gloomy. In fact, the long-term prognosis is substantially better than this, and the main reason for Rodin's pessimism was selection bias which, as evinced earlier, had been the curse of many earlier epilepsy statistics.

It was the cohort studies of unselected patients that gave the truer estimate of prognosis. The first notable such study, published in 1979, was again from the Mayo Clinic.[52] Using a retrospective record linkage system, 475 patients were identified whose history stretched over at least 5 years (including 141 with a history of more than 20 years). At 5 years after diagnosis, 42% of cases were in a greater than 5-year remission, rising to 65% at 10 years and 70% at 20 years (and only 6% of patients who had been in 5-year remission later relapsed). Eventually, more than three-quarters of patients were in terminal remission and about half had discontinued antiepileptic drugs. Although the methodology of this study can be criticised, it was nevertheless the first published study to suggest that the overall prognosis of epilepsy was much more favourable than previous orthodox opinion would have it.

The Mayo Clinic study was followed in 1981 by the first study of prognosis in a truly population-based cohort. This used the record system of a general

---

[51] Is it far-fetched to note that the use of the word 'patients' not 'people' in the title of the book is indicative of Rodin's conservative and old-fashioned views? It ran contrary to the then strong campaign to use the term 'people with epilepsy' in place of 'epileptics'.

[52] Annegers, Hauser and Elveback, 'Remission of seizures and relapse'.

practice covering 6,000 persons in a population around the town of Tonbridge in the south of England: 122 patients with a history of epilepsy or epileptic seizures were identified, representing a lifetime prevalence of epilepsy of 20.3/ 1,000. By 10 years after the onset of epilepsy, about two-thirds of patients, and by 20 years 80% of patients, were in remission. The pattern of epilepsy over time was reported for the first time: 18% of patients had experienced only a single seizure; 49% of patients had active seizures for a period, then entered terminal remission (the 'burst pattern'); 21% had no remission at all after the onset of their seizures (the 'continuous pattern'); and in 12% remission periods were followed by relapses (the 'intermittent pattern').[53]

Both of these studies took a backward look at existing prospectively collected data. In 1983 a true prospective study, the National General Practice Study of Epilepsy (NGPSE), was launched. After follow-up for nine years, around two-thirds of patients had entered long-term remission, and after twenty-two years 84% were in terminal remission. All three studies showed that the prognosis of newly diagnosed epilepsy is better than often thought, and that it was early in the course of epilepsy that remission, if it was going to happen, usually occurred; conversely, the longer the seizures remained active, the worse the ultimate prognosis (notwithstanding this, significant numbers of patients did enter remission even after many years of seizures).[54] Other population-based studies followed throughout the decade, and roughly similar results were reported by all. Cohort studies were also carried out on febrile seizures, the outcome of monotherapy and the risk of withdrawal of antiepileptic drug therapy in those in remission.

These initial cohort studies were performed by individual research groups. At the same time, however, government-based population statistics were being used to provide information about epilepsy. An early example was the National Child Development study in Britain, a prospective cohort study of all persons born in one week in March 1958 (17,415 children) who were then studied at the ages of 7, 11 and 16. Amongst 15,496 of these children, a clear-cut diagnosis of epilepsy had been established in 64 (a prevalence rate of 4.1/1,000) by the age of 11.[55] After the 1990s, computerised databases made their entry into the field of epidemiology, transforming the topic again by allowing studies to be made of huge numbers, often of whole national populations, thus removing any vestige of selection bias; these rapidly replaced the manual case finding and follow-up of the earlier studies.

---

[53] Goodridge and Shorvon, 'Epileptic seizures'.
[54] In many ways, these findings confirmed the intuition of Aldren Turner (Turner, *Epilepsy*, pp. 216–19).
[55] Ross, Peckham and Butler, 'Epilepsy in childhood'.

Heredity and Epilepsy

Despite the remarkable advances being made in the basic science of genetics, the question of heredity in epilepsy had become becalmed, and to today's eyes the approach looks oddly old-fashioned. In 1980, as a swansong of his time directing the Epilepsy Branch of the NINDS, Penry published a book with Michael Newmark summarising the state of contemporary knowledge.[56] They listed the twenty-nine inherited inborn errors of metabolism and the thirty-four other inherited neurological diseases then recognised to be Mendelian disorders, and the five chromosomal disorders, which included epilepsy amongst their manifestations. At that time, apart from four types of progressive myoclonic epilepsy, no pure forms of Mendelian epilepsy had been found.[57] Of epilepsy in general, the authors reviewed thirty-six preceding genetic studies and noted that many found no evidence of inheritance. Nevertheless, they concluded that up to 40% of cases of epilepsy had a family history, and up to 10% of offspring or siblings had a history of seizures. Furthermore, in studies of generalised tonic–clonic seizures (two studies), absence seizures (five studies) and febrile seizures (fifteen studies), rates were twice as high. Photosensitivity and EEG patterns were also found to have an inherited element. Finally, they reviewed data on twins, finding that thirteen clinical and ten electroencephalographic twin studies showed concordance rates of up to 90% in monozygotic twins and 10–15% in dizygotic twins. The difference between monozygotic and dizygotic rates was taken as the best evidence of the existence of inheritance, although it was accepted by then that this must be in a polygenic manner. Penry and Newmark discuss mechanisms and biomarkers, such as the HLA (Human Leucocyte antigen) types, but come to no firm conclusions. All in all, this review was a sterling effort but found little which moved the field forward. As the authors noted in the preface, 'In spite of the importance of the genetics of epilepsy, a consistent and coherent approach to the subject has not been formulated. Many of the current data are contradictory, and several significant clinical problems remain to be solved' (p. v). Few could disagree. Epilepsy genetics was in the doldrums and surprisingly not exploiting the dramatic advances being made in the basic genetic sciences. This was to change fundamentally after the mid-1990s.

---

[56] Newmark and Penry, *Genetics of Epilepsy*.

[57] In those days, the progressive myoclonic epilepsies were divided into four groups, very different from the classification today. The four groups were Unverricht type with Lafora body, Lundborg type, Hartung type, and an unclassifiable variable group. 'Pure genetic epilepsy' is a term used to define those conditions in which epileptic seizures are the only, or at least the predominant, symptom of a genetic defect.

Febrile Seizures and the Rise of Paediatric Epilepsy

Febrile convulsions appeared in the 1989 classification as a 'special syndrome'. They had remained a subject of intense interest in the decades after 1970, not least because of the question of whether these childhood convulsions predisposed to the development of later temporal lobe epilepsy (Alfred Meyer's hypothesis). To investigate this question further, and to mitigate the problem of selection bias, a series of very large-scale, prospective cohort studies were carried out in the 1970s and 1980s, in which bias was minimised.[58] In all these studies, the risk of subsequent epilepsy after febrile seizures was found to be very low. In the British Birth Study, for instance, of 16,004 neonatal survivors (8.5% of all infants born in one week in April 1970) and followed prospectively, 13,135 were assessed at the age of 5 and 10 years. Of 14,676 children, 398 (2.7%) had febrile convulsions of whom 16 were known to be neurologically abnormal before the seizure. Of the remaining 382, only 13 had one or more subsequent non-febrile seizure, and only 9 developed epilepsy. Similarly, the National Collaborative Perinatal Project, a study of 1,706 children with febrile seizures followed prospectively for seven years, found that one-third had a recurrence of febrile seizures, but only 1% developed epilepsy. These studies confirmed previous findings that it was only the prolonged or unilateral febrile convulsions that were particularly associated with temporal lobe epilepsy. In 1988, Sheila Wallace published a book reviewing the entire topic.[59] She confirmed the association, but took the view that in most cases the febrile seizure did not cause the epilepsy. Rather, both were manifestations of a pre-existing predisposition.

Meanwhile, experimental animal studies were showing conclusively that prolonged seizures could indeed damage the brain. In 1973, for example, Brian Meldrum demonstrated that it was not the hypoglycaemia nor hypoxia associated with seizures, but the seizures themselves which were the main cause of damage. He used the term 'excitotoxic' damage.[60] He showed that burst firing sustained for more than thirty minutes (but not shorter seizures) led to selective neuronal necrosis in the hippocampus, amygdala and cortex. In the 1980s he suggested that the mechanism of cell death was mitochondrial poisoning from calcium influx due to excessive glutamatergic activity, which triggered cellular necrosis and apoptosis. An enormous body of work by others followed that

---

[58] The most important such community-based studies were the National Collaborative Perinatal Project from the United States and the National Child Development Study from the United Kingdom.

[59] Wallace, *Child with Febrile Seizures*.

[60] Meldrum's classic experiments with baboons were landmarks in the field. See Meldrum and Horton, 'Status epilepticus in primates'; Meldrum and Brierley, 'Epileptic seizures in primates'; Meldrum, Vigouroux and Brierley, 'Systemic factors and epileptic brain damage'; Meldrum, 'Cell damage in epilepsy'.

confirmed Meldrum's findings. In a kainic acid model of epilepsy, Yehezkel Ben-Ari showed that the induced damage was similar to the pattern of cellular loss in hippocampal sclerosis and that the animals experiencing this damage went on to have spontaneous limbic seizures.[61] It was also found that, in response to epileptic seizures, 'axon sprouting' and the creation of new synapses occurred, as well as other structural changes, such as loss of dendritic spines, distorted dendrites, neuronal death and gliosis. In the hippocampus, the dentate hilar cells were thought to be particularly vulnerable due to low levels of the calcium-binding proteins calbindin and parvalbumin. Chronic epilepsy was therefore conceived to be associated with reorganisation of neuronal and synaptic pathways and not simply a non-specific loss of neurons. Although experimental models indicated that experimentally induced seizures could cause mesial temporal lobe damage and that this damage could then go on to cause spontaneous seizures (i.e. epilepsy), clinicians were still divided on this point. Only when serial human MRI scanning showed that prolonged seizures did indeed induce hippocampal sclerosis was the hypothesis that prolonged febrile seizures could result in temporal lobe epilepsy universally accepted (some fifty years after it was first postulated).

Paediatric neurology also formed as a specialty and developed strongly in the 1950s and 1960s, both in the United States and in Europe.[62] In Paris, Stéphane Thieffry formed the first paediatric neurology unit (in fact, if not in name) in 1951 at the Hôpital des Enfants Malades, and it was in Paris that the figure of Jean Aicardi, who became the doyen of paediatric epilepsy of his generation, deserves particular mention.[63] Aicardi helped define three new epilepsy syndromes (Rett syndrome, Aicardi syndrome, Aicardi–Goutières syndrome; and also the syndrome of alternating hemiplegia of childhood), and wrote standard textbooks of childhood neurology and epileptology.[64] In 1970 and 1983, he showed that febrile seizures

---

[61] Ben-Ari, 'Limbic seizure and brain damage'.

[62] Although some general paediatricians had developed an interest in neurology; one example of importance in epilepsy was Cornelia de Lange in Amsterdam (who (remarkably still steeped in classics) described 'typus degenerativus Amstelodamensis' in 1933, later known as 'Cornelia de Lange syndrome').

[63] Jean Aicardi worked as neurologist at l'Hôpital des Enfants Malades, initially under Thieffry, and it was there that he gained his experience as a child neurologist, as well as at L' Hôpital Saint-Vincent de Paul. He also served in Thieffry's research unit, at INSERM, and was appointed Director of Research there from 1986–91. On his retirement in 1992, took up the position of Honorary Professor of Child Neurology at Institute of Child Health in London. He published more than 250 papers in international journals and helped train a cohort of child neurologists, including Charlotte Dravet, Alexis Arzimanoglou and Renzo Guerrini, who themselves became leading figures in paediatric epileptology. He was the epitome of the civilised academic – modest, generous and immensely knowledgeable – and was universally admired.

[64] Aicardi's monographs include *Diseases of the Nervous System in Childhood* (1992, 1998, 2009); *Epilepsy in Children* (1986, 1994); *Aicardi's Epilepsy in Children* (with Arzimanoglou and Guerrini; 2004); and *Movement Disorders in Children* (with Fernandez Alvarez; 2001).

prolonged beyond thirty minutes were associated with poor outcomes, including subsequent epilepsy and the HHE syndrome.[65] These findings led Aicardi to press for more urgent treatment of febrile seizures than was commonly the practice, leading to acrimonious exchanges with American colleagues who disagreed. Aicardi was subsequently proved right, and his trenchant advocacy resulted in a significant change to clinical practice which must have prevented the development of chronic epilepsy in many children worldwide.

Mortality and Sudden Death in Epilepsy

People with epilepsy have been known to be at risk of premature death ever since the time of Hippocrates. In the sixteenth and seventeenth centuries, the London bills of mortality, which were early if not the first attempts at a statistical treatment of death rates,[66] listed the falling sickness or convulsions as a relatively common cause of death. In 1904, L. Pierce Clark had written that the 'epileptic was foredoomed to die in status'.[67] In 1907, Turner reported a study by William Spratling showing that 40% of deaths among 150 Craig Colony inmates with idiopathic epilepsy were the direct result of epilepsy, the mean age of death being 29 years.[68] As the twentieth century drew on, however, in part due to the liberalising and destigmatising mood of the post–Second World War period, epilepsy came to be seen as a chronic but not fatal condition. Indeed, once progressive aetiologies were discounted, life expectancy was considered to be much the same as in the general population. In the 1970s, the finding that the prevalence of epilepsy was less than the cumulative incidence raised the possibility that death rates in epilepsy were in fact greater than suspected. In 1974 Janusz Zieliński published a review of mortality in epilepsy and the results from one of the first epidemiological surveys reporting death rates in the modern era (it was from Warsaw). He found the death rate in those with epilepsy to be 1.8 times that in the general population, and 3.5 times that in persons under 50 years of age. The mean lifespan was 12.5 years after onset of seizures – 20 years shorter than in the general population.[69] Similar findings from a range of other populations followed, and death rates were found to be greatest in those with neurological handicap or symptomatic epilepsy. Zieliński stressed the importance of the underlying aetiology, and demonstrated that although most deaths were due primarily to this, epilepsy itself was the cause in 14%. Having established figures on incidence, prevalence

---

[65] Aicardi and Chevrie, 'Convulsive status epilepticus'; Aicardi and Chevrie, 'Consequences of status'.

[66] Weekly mortality statistics from London, published first in 1592 (and from 1613 by the Worshipful Company of Parish Clerks).

[67] Clark, 'Status epilepticus'.   [68] Turner, *Epilepsy*, p. 116.

[69] Zieliński, 'Epilepsy and mortality rate'.

and prognosis, the focus of the existing cohort studies of epilepsy moved to mortality rates. The record linkage study from the Mayo Clinic found an overall standardised mortality ratio (SMR) of 2.3 and the NGPSE reported an overall SMR of 2.6 after a prospective follow-up of 22.8 years; this was also the only study to provide life-expectancy figures in epilepsy.[70]

Death due to epilepsy itself had been considered initially to be largely the result of accidents or status epilepticus. But in the 1960s interest switched to the phenomenon of sudden unexplained death in epilepsy (SUDEP). In fact, it had long been recognised that patients with epilepsy might die suddenly. Spratling, for instance, described epilepsy as a 'disease which destroys life, suddenly and without warning through a single, brief attack, unaided by an accident . . . such as suffocation, or fracture of the skull . . . and does so in from 3 to 4 per cent of all who suffer from it';[71] Turner also remarked on sudden death, which he attributed usually to asphyxiation. The phenomenon, however, had been largely ignored until 1971, when a study from Cleveland of the circumstances surrounding death in nineteen cases demonstrated that 'natural death' in epilepsy was not often due to suffocation, drew a parallel with crib death (cot death) and was the first to suggest that death might be due to primary respiratory arrest or an autonomic mechanism.[72] This landmark study triggered considerable further research. In 1984 Leestma and colleagues, pathologists from Chicago, published an analysis of 66 cases of sudden unexpected death in people with epilepsy,[73] and in 1989 reported a further study and used the term 'SUDEP' for the first time. They estimated that SUDEP accounted for the death of 1/370–1/110 persons with epilepsy.[74] It was then a series of studies by Lina Nashef and colleagues in the 1980s that moved this phenomenon to the centre stage of epilepsy. Nashef researched the circumstances and frequencies of sudden death in various populations and, later, the mechanisms in a series of elegant studies of seizures recorded using EEG telemetry. These studies demonstrated that SUDEP almost always occurred after tonic–clonic seizures, was usually unwitnessed and often at night, and it as postulated that death in most cases was due to respiratory arrest following a seizure. Nashef suggested that SUDEP was most commonly the result of the profound cerebral inhibitory drive that occurred in the aftermath of seizures. This inhibitory drive was essential to terminate a seizure, but on occasions also switched off respiration. Other less common mechanisms proposed included cardiac arrhythmia and autonomic dysfunction. These conclusions have largely stood the test of time.

[70] Gaitatzis et al., 'Life expectancy'. This paper provided the gold standard data not only in clinical practice but also for medico-legal purposes, as in the final decades of the twentieth century, physicians and hospitals became increasingly entangled in litigation.

[71] Spratling, *Epilepsy and Its Treatment*, p. 304.

[72] Hirsch and Martin, 'Unexpected death in young epileptics'.

[73] Leestma et al., 'Sudden unexpected death'.

[74] Leestma et al., 'Sudden unexpected death'; Leestma et al., 'Unexpected death in epilepsy'.

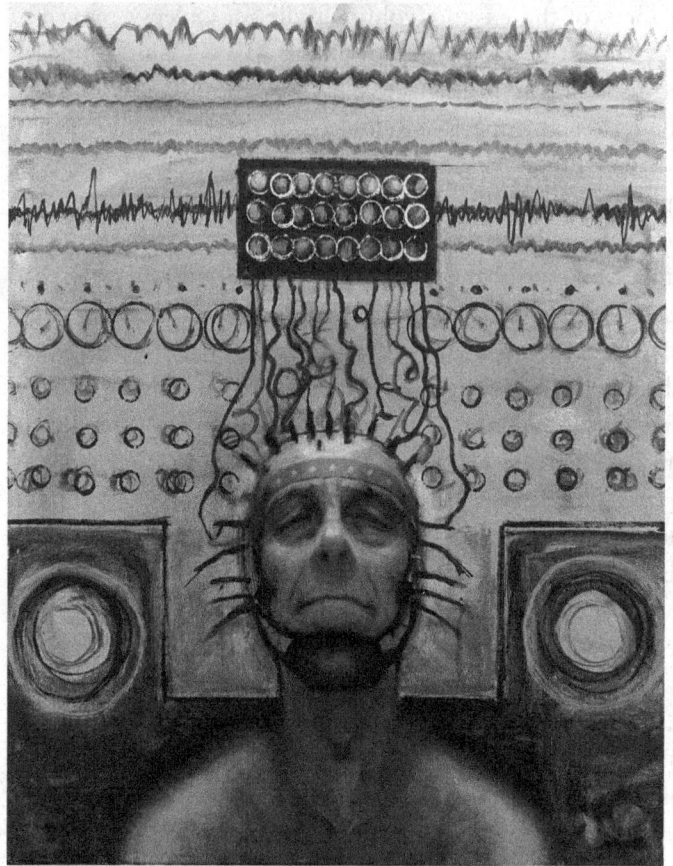

33. 'Wired up'. (A painting by David Cobley, 2021).

Video-EEG Telemetry and Invasive EEG

By 1970 it was clear that almost nothing further of fundamental significance to epilepsy clinical practice was going to be learned from scalp inter-ictal EEG.[75] Consequently, technically minded neurophysiologists turned their attention to two other avenues of research: the digital storage of colossal amounts of data and the computerised analysis of this data. As we saw in the preceding chapter, new methods for recording, analysing and storing EEG data followed – all heavily dependent on rapidly advancing new technologies in the field of computing, video/film and electronics. As a result of these technological advances, long-term patient monitoring became, for the first time, feasible in normal clinical practice.

From the very first use of EEG in epilepsy, it was known that the EEG signs of epilepsy were episodic, and that a single 'routine' EEG, recorded for only

---

[75] A selective timeline of the history of EEG and associated fields was published in 1998 (Swartz and Goldensohn, 'Timeline').

30–40 minutes, frequently missed abnormalities. More than 50% of routine EEGs in newly diagnosed epileptic patients were normal, and 15% remained normal even after ten recordings. It was also realised that recording the ictal EEG (i.e. that during a seizure) was far more informative than recording inter-ictal abnormalities and so attention moved to methods for long-term recording. Many of the developments were in the USA, where in the 1950s and 1960s, the most advanced EEG technologies were developed. In 1954 in Houston, for instance, Peter Kellaway,[76] one of the pioneering electroencephalographers of his time, was recording depth EEGs for periods of more than 8–10 hours for the purposes of epilepsy surgical assessment.[77] However, 10 hours of EEG, even at a slow paper speed (1.5 cm/sec), generated more than half a kilometre of paper, and this fact alone limited the practical value of prolonged recordings. The field opened out as recording onto computer tape rather than paper became possible, as new transmission and recording methods (including radio telemetry) and methods for integrating EEG recording with time-locked video were developed.[78]

By 1973 monitoring units had been established at NIH in Bethesda, at the University of California in Los Angeles and at the National Hospital in London, amongst others. By the end of the 1970s a typical system had three low-light monochrome cameras (whole-body, face close-up and EEG), with reformatting to make a composite picture of these multiple views. This technology enabled detailed off-line analysis of seizure phenomenology, and minutely documented descriptions of absence seizures, complex partial seizures and infantile spasms were published along with data on the frequency and duration of absence seizures. Diagnosis and differentiation from pseudo-seizures became more accurate, and the selection of cases for surgical treatment became based on ictal recordings, which provided more accurate information on the localisation of seizures than was possible with inter-ictal data alone.

Miniaturisation of recorders also allowed ambulatory recordings, trialled initially in the mid-1970s and within a few years a cost-effective commercial system from Oxford Medical Systems had become available, in which four EEG channels were recorded onto a cassette recorder carried around by the patient. This was found useful for diagnosis and assessment, and then later for the automatic quantification of spike–wave discharges in absence epilepsy. Cable telemetry was also in wide use by 1973, and by the 1980s it had replaced radio systems in most hospitals. This consisted of a head-mounted EEG

---

[76] See Mizrahi, Pedley and Apple, 'In memoriam Peter Kellaway'.

[77] Kellaway also recorded the EEG of astronaut Fred Bauman for 55 hours during the Gemini VII orbital space mission in 1965, and went on to determine the quality of sleep in weightlessness by recording 400 hours of EEGs during Spacelab missions.

[78] Video was seen by all to have significant advantages over cine film. These advantages included monitoring by closed-circuit television, immediate review, playback and reusable tape.

preamplifier and multiplexer unit connected by a long cable (up to 8 metres) to a reading station. The multiplexer reduced the 16 signal lines to 1 to facilitate transmission through a single twisted wire, and a demultiplexer then reconstructed the original EEG signals for write-out. A 'seizure button' could be incorporated into the system so that patients were able to mark the record whenever they felt that a seizure was occurring or about to occur.

The early prolonged recording systems were all built in-house, but by the early 1980s commercial systems were available and affordable (a reasonable system could then be bought for around $35,000) and video–EEG telemetry moved from the confines of research institutes to become available in many hospitals. The major centres still clung to their home-made equipment, but this was slowly replaced as commercial machines became increasingly refined. 8- and 16-channel ambulatory cassette recorders became commercially available and computerised data reduction systems and automated seizure-detection methods were developed. In 1985 the journal *Electroencephalography and Clinical Neurophysiology* published a supplement of more than 400 pages devoted to long-term monitoring in epilepsy.[79]

The second avenue of development in those years was in the field of invasive EEG for surgical purposes. From the late 1970s, in part encouraged by the experience of the Sainte-Anne school, neurophysiologists became much more adventurous in their use of intracranial recordings as part of the surgical evaluation. In the 1970s and 1980s, the rapid developments in solid-state electronics broadened the field by the miniaturisation of equipment. New techniques and materials for fabricating microelectrodes were formulated. By 1990, rigid or flexible nichrome depth electrodes were being produced which were compatible with MRI imaging and which could accommodate up to eighteen contacts along their length, along with subdural strips, subdural grids, epidural strips and grids, and epidural pegs. These electrodes could be used for stimulation as well as recording. Increasingly complex EEG assessments of patients were made, with sometimes up to sixty-four channels of EEG being recorded for days or weeks on end, requiring enormous data-storage capacity and many person-hours of EEG interpretation. These were used primarily to assess patients for epilepsy surgery, although in some centres (for instance, in Amsterdam), invasive neurophysiology was developed initially for lesioning white matter tracts in psychosurgery, and only later extended to epilepsy.[80]

---

[79] Gotman, Ives and Gloor, *Long-Term Monitoring in Epilepsy*. This work provided detailed technical specifications as well as summaries of its applications of the new technologies.

[80] There was a distinguished Dutch tradition of neurophysiology, which was always strikingly internationalist in outlook. Colin Binnie, the English neurophysiologist, spent ten years in Heemstede as Director of Meer and Bosch, and both there and in London became a leading international figure, contributing notable technical and clinical advances, including studies on photosensitivity and on inter-ictal EEG changes demonstrating that inter-ictal spiking subtly

Other technical advances took place in preamplifiers, computerised data storage, video–EEG synchronisation with a digital clock, slow-motion replay, infra-red cameras for night recording and automated EEG analysis. How much of this was driven by clinical utility, or just technophilic enthusiasm, is perhaps arguable, but in these years the revolution in electronics and computing stimulated a new dynamism in the hitherto stolid field of neurophysiology.

Imaging Epilepsy

More far-reaching than any new neurophysiological technology, though, were advances in neuroimaging. We have seen how plain radiology, followed by ventriculography and angiography, had earlier contributed to moving the concept of epilepsy from that of an idiopathic disease to that of a symptomatic condition. However, it was to be two further developments in the field of radiology which were to have the most radical effect: computerised axial tomography (CT) and magnetic resonance imaging (MRI). Both technologies were the fruit of the post-war rise of computing, electronics and related technologies and the application of the striking theoretical developments that had taken place in the field of particle physics. Both CT and MRI had an impact on epilepsy, but it was MRI in particular that profoundly changed epilepsy practice, much as EEG had done in the 1940s.

CT scanning was developed, almost single-handedly, by Godfrey Hounsfield,[81] a British electronics engineer. Hounsfield had worked in the field of radar research during the war and later in the development of computers. He then turned his attention to medical imaging and immediately saw that conventional X-ray had three basic limitations:

> Firstly, it is impossible to display within the framework of a two-dimensional X-ray picture all the information contained in the three-dimensional scene under view. Objects situated in depth, i.e. in the third dimension, superimpose, causing confusion to the viewer. Secondly, conventional X-rays cannot distinguish between soft tissues. In general, a radiogram differentiates only between bone and air, as in the lungs. Variations in soft tissues such as the liver and pancreas are not discernible at all and certain other organs may be rendered visible only through the use of radio-opaque dyes. Thirdly, when conventional X-ray methods are used, it is not possible to measure in a quantitative way the separate densities of the individual substances through which the X-ray has passed.

impaired motor performance. Binnie was also instrumental in the early clinical development of lamotrigine.

[81] Largely self-taught, and without a university degree, Hounsfield won the 1979 Nobel Prize for Physiology or Medicine for the invention and development of CT, and later was also a pioneer of MRI.

> The radiogram records the mean absorption by all the various tissues which the X-ray has penetrated. This is of little use for quantitative measurement.[82]

Hounsfield proceeded to devise a computer program to reconstruct sets of X-ray measurements taken at a multitude of different angles, using iterative algebraic techniques. The reconstruction was displayed as 'slices' through the head (like slices in a loaf of bread). Because of the huge number of measurements, the sensitivity of the X-ray was greatly enhanced, and brain tissue could easily be differentiated from bone and from the CSF surrounding the brain and in the ventricles. Hounsfield was working not in a university, but for the British company EMI, which had no previous interest in medical imaging. He obtained partial funding from the MRC, which saw the potential of the project. He initially used gamma rays, but these proved insensitive and he began to experiment with X-rays. He scanned human cadaveric brains and after several years of experimentation was ready to apply the technology clinically. The MRC put Hounsfield in touch with James Bull, a neuroradiologist working in London, who referred him onto his colleague James Ambrose at the Atkinson Morley Hospital in London, where the first patient was scanned on 1 October 1971. The scan was conducted at each of 180 degrees around her head. A total of 28,000 readings were taken, recorded on magnetic tape and then taxied across London for analysis by an EMI computer. The scan revealed a frontal brain tumour, which was then promptly resected. The extraordinary potential of this technique, and its huge advantages over the other technologies of the time, was obvious to all. EMI built five more EMI scanners, as they were then known, and shipped them to other hospitals in London, Manchester and Glasgow, and to the Mayo Clinic and Massachusetts General Hospital. Bull presented the findings of his CT scanning at the international radiological meeting in Chicago in November 1972, where the effect was said to have been electrifying. The technique improved rapidly, and EMI scanners started to be produced in large numbers. By 1974 there were 40 scanners in US hospitals; by 1976, 475; and by 1980, 1,471. In 1980, 46% of large US hospitals (>300 beds) had a scanner installed; 19% were located out of hospital in private clinics, but there was a singular dearth in the large public hospitals (8% had a scanner), in Veterans Administration hospitals (10% had a scanner) and in rural areas. This was a market now driven by economics.[83] The US government decided that a US manufacturer should be involved. General Electric geared up, and the US government employed protectionist measures. This had the effect of removing EMI from the market in what turned into a ruthless and cutthroat international race.

---

[82] Hounsfield, 'Computer medical imaging'.
[83] 'Policy implications of the computed tomography (CT) scanner'.

The impact of CT in epilepsy may have been less than in other areas of neurology, but it was still very significant. At the 21st International Congress on Electroencephalography and Epilepsy, organised by Gastaut and held in Marseille in September 1975, the results from 1,702 patients from 7 research groups were described. CT abnormalities were found in about two-thirds of cases. Gastaut published his own findings in detail in *Epilepsia* in 1976, based on 500 consecutive patients seen in his clinic in whom CT had been performed over the previous six months. All of these patients also had EEG and seizures classified according to the ILAE system.[84] Organic lesions were found in 55% of cases. In a study of 1,000 cases a year later,[85] Gastaut, with his son as co-author, found normal CT scans in 89% of those with primary generalised epilepsy (and in the remainder only atrophic lesions), and in only 23% of those with secondary generalised epilepsies and 37% of those with partial epilepsy. Gastaut père and fils also reported the results for various epilepsy syndromes and different aetiologies, pointing out that CT scanning picked up 20% of lesions missed by all other methods. They predicted, correctly, that CT would be ordered as often as an EEG in clinical practice – a notable tribute to the imaging technology from a staunch neurophysiologist.

MRI followed hot on the heels of CT. It can be described without exaggeration as a technological tidal wave breaking over neurology. The effect of MRI has proved to be greater than any other technological advance in epilepsy up to this time, with the arguable exception of EEG.[86] MRI was first known as nuclear magnetic resonance (NMR) imaging, but the term 'nuclear' in that cold-war era was thought to worry patients, and the manufacturers realised had negative marketing connotations, and so the name was changed. Its origins were in NMR spectroscopy which had been developed first in the field of chemistry,[87] and then extended to biology in the mid-1950s for both excised tissue and later live animals. Raymond Damadian, a research physician in New York, became the first to use NMR in medicine – making claims, later shown to be unsubstantiated, that he could accurately screen for cancer. In 1971 he did show that tumours and normal tissue had different NMR characteristics, and his company, the FONAR Corporation, introduced the first commercial NMR scanner in 1980. But this device had no spatial resolution,

---

[84] Gastaut, 'Conclusions'.

[85] Gastaut and Gastaut, 'Computerized axial tomography'. Gastaut also showed oedema followed by atrophy over a two-month period in a case of hemiclonic status epilepticus in a one-year-old – the first case in which the atrophy and cell loss following status epilepticus was visualised.

[86] A popular history of MRI is told in Kevles, *Naked to the Bone*, and Rinck, *Magnetic Resonance in Medicine*.

[87] Thanks to work by such figures as Wolfgang Pauli, Otto Stern, Isidor Rabi, Felix Bloch and Edward Purcell. For their efforts they were awarded the Nobel Prize in Physics in 1945, 1943, 1944, 1952 and 1952, respectively.

was not tomography and was not of much use clinically. The next key step was the encoding of the NMR image spatially. Two scientists – Paul Lauterbur of New York and Peter Mansfield of Nottingham – independently developed methods of localising the signal in 3D space. Much of the early ground-breaking work at this stage was carried out in Britain, with the leading research groups based at the Universities of Nottingham, Aberdeen, Oxford and Imperial College London. In 1977 an NMR machine was built for humans, and Mansfield and Henry Maudsley produced the first in vivo image of human anatomy – a finger; then, a second Nottingham-based group imaged a wrist. In 1978 Mansfield produced a scan of the human abdomen. The first image of a human brain was published by Ian Young, working at EMI in London in 1978.[88] Meanwhile, in Aberdeen, John Mallard and colleagues built a whole-body MRI machine for experimental research. In vivo MRI spectroscopy was also pioneered by George Radda and colleagues in Oxford from 1974. At that stage, although much of the developmental work in MRI was carried out in Britain, the parlous state of the British industrial economy and the lack of opportunity led many of the researchers to emigrate to America.[89]

This was the prelude to clinical scanning. The first MRI scanner for clinical use, manufactured by EMI, was put in place in 1978 at Hammersmith Hospital in London by the research group of Robert Steiner, Graeme Bydder and Ian Young, and the first brains scan were performed that year. The first series of neurology patients studied by MRI was reported from Hammersmith Hospital using the 0.5 Tesla EMI NMR system in 1982.[90]

The potential for NMR was obvious and, as with CT, an intense commer-cial scramble developed. Although the first manufacturing companies were British, the US market was the prize. The first US scanner was placed in a private office in Cleveland in 1980, and by the end of 1984 American hospitals had acquired an estimated 108–150 scanners. By 1990, 91% of all MRI scanners were sold in the United States (and 77% of all CT scanners). The Food and Drug Administration held up its approval of MRI as a clinical tool until US manufacturers had geared up,[91] and, as with CT, the British manufacturer EMI was squeezed out of the market. Rapid technological advances ensued, with improved hardware and a host of new imaging protocols, including the first functional MRI (fMRI) images in 1991 by John Belliveau. By then the quality of structural MRI images had rapidly improved, and the superiority of MRI over CT for most applications was beyond doubt. As a result, in the 1990s, sales

---

[88] Clow and Young, 'First NMR scan'.
[89] Christie and Tansey, 'Making the human body transparent'.
[90] Bydder et al., 'NMR imaging of the brain'.
[91] A ferocious battle between manufacturers ensued. EMI patents were sold to Picker, which was then bought by Philips. M&D Aberdeen failed to flourish. General Electric acquired Technicare in 1985, the French company CGR in 1988 and the Israeli company Elscint in 1998, and became the largest manufacturer. Oxford Magnets produced all the early magnets.

began to skyrocket, and by 2004, 75 million scans had been produced by 10,000 MRI scanners worldwide. The first gadolinium contrast agents were patented in 1981 in Berlin, and the first images of humans using this were made at Hammersmith Hospital in 1984. The first Nobel Prize in Physiology or Medicine in the field of MRI was awarded jointly to Lauterbur and Mansfield in 2003.[92]

Lauterbur commented that physicists and chemists were awarded the prize, not physicians, and this was no accident. Moreover, although medicine was the beneficiary, the revolutionary advances (in Kuhn's words) were those being made in engineering and basic physics. The place of physicians was in the relatively mundane process of applying these technologies to clinical problems – an altogether less intellectually challenging process. This may sound a little unfair, but there is no doubt that in the field of human MRI all the major developments occurred in the basic sciences of physics and chemistry. In contrast was the situation in EEG, where physicians played a foremost part, a change reflecting the post-war industrialisation and commercialisation of bio-medical technology.

In the early years of brain MRI, the technology was thought by some to be no better than CT for epilepsy.[93] By 1990, this was clearly not the case. MRI had been shown to reliably detect and quantify hippocampal sclerosis,[94] and to be greatly superior to CT in the detection of small lesions such as cavernomas, small tumours, congenital malformations and dysplasias. In 1992, the first meeting devoted to MRI and epilepsy – a NATO Advanced Research Workshop – was held in London. The purpose of the workshop was to review progress and suggest directions for further research; participants came from eleven countries. It had only been just over ten years since the first report of MRI in neurology, and enormous strides had been made. These were detailed in the proceedings of the workshop, published in 1994.[95] In the first chapter, the central clinical questions which were being addressed, or which might be addressed in the future, were laid out in five areas (diagnosis, pathophysiology, treatment, prognosis and prevention). The current state of research in these areas, for both MRI and MR spectroscopy, was described in the book's remaining fifty-three chapters. Progress had been remarkable, and there was by then no doubt that the technology represented a paradigm shift in epilepsy. The workshop participants spent one day at the Chalfont Centre for Epilepsy,

---

[92] The prizes were richly deserved, although they brought an extraordinary reaction from Damadian, who was bitterly disappointed by his exclusion and posted advertisements in the newspapers complaining of the injustice.
[93] Sperling et al., 'Magnetic resonance imaging'.
[94] Cook et al., 'Hippocampal studies'; Jack Jr et al., 'Temporal lobe seizures'.
[95] Shorvon et al., *Magnetic Resonance Scanning and Epilepsy*.

where the first MRI scanner dedicated entirely to epilepsy research was installed in 1992.

The leading centres of MRI research in epilepsy were then in London, Montreal, Erlangen and several American centres. But soon research was also underway in many other academic units in Europe and North America, and MRI scanning was soon being employed clinically and academically in neuroscience centres around the world.

In terms of establishing the aetiological diagnosis of epilepsy, MRI was without peer. For the first time, a non-invasive investigation was available that could reliably detect mesial temporal sclerosis, small lesions and a whole range of congenital anomalies. The MRI characteristics of these lesions were quickly defined, and within a few years research was well advanced in correlating the imaging findings with clinical and EEG features. MRI also proved crucial in identifying epilepsy-induced cerebral damage, such as that resulting from prolonged febrile seizures, with initial work in 1992 and extended over the subsequent decade. The entire practice of medicine in relation to epilepsy, as well as the approach to pathological investigation, changed as a result. The proceedings of the NATO workshop showed that almost all the major principles accepted today had already been defined by 1992 – a sign of the extraordinary progress made the previous decade. The field had been effectively harvested and subsequent work in clinical MRI in epilepsy was incremental. Research then began to focus on subtle structural variations in gyration and sulcation, and changes in idiopathic generalised epilepsy and in the pathways of seizure spread, but all these lines of inquiry proved to be relatively unproductive.

MRI had also become the fundamental investigation in epilepsy surgery, influencing surgical technique, rendering surgery more accurate and precise, and for the first time enabling post-operative confirmation of the extent of resection. The latter was important as it became rapidly evident that the previous estimates of many surgeons of exactly what they had resected at the time of surgery were often wildly inaccurate. An important step was the introduction of 'frameless stereotaxy', using MRI with fiducial markers placed on the scalp. The heavy and cumbersome stereotactic frame soon became a museum relic. Reports of MRI findings in hippocampal sclerosis related the size and extent of hippocampal damage to surgical outcome, the extent of surgical resection and the bilaterality of hippocampal damage.[96] Similarly, MRI had proved invaluable in planning and carrying out resective surgery of foreign tissue lesions. So-called multimodel imaging studies correlating clinical symptoms, EEG, CT, positron emission tomography (PET), magnetoencephalography, single-photon emission computed tomography (SPECT) and angiography

---

[96] See, for instance, 'Cook et al., 'Hippocample volumetry'; Jack Jr et al., 'Temporal lobe seizures'; Jackson et al., 'Detection of hippocampal pathology'.

also commenced around this time and were to occupy clinical researchers in subsequent decades, not least as computerised methods for co-registering data from these different investigations became available.

Other technical developments were also underway. The value of new MRI sequences, such as fluid-attenuated inversion recovery and diffusion-weighted scanning, were already established by 1992. Others were to follow, although none of these were to make a particular impact in the field of epilepsy. By 1994, 1.5 Tesla MRI scanners had been shown to be superior to those with lower field strengths in almost all aspects, and higher field scanners (for instance 3 T or 7 T) had yet to be introduced; but even now, some thirty years later, 1.5 T scanners remain the workhorses of neurology.

Not all MRI techniques proved beneficial. Post-processing techniques and three-dimensional analyses were in the works, including fractal analysis, shape and texture analysis, flattening of image projection and three-dimensional rendering, but most proved to have limited clinical utility (being more like rather sophisticated computer games). MR spectroscopy and chemical shift imaging was intensively investigated, but again – in the field of epilepsy, at least – ultimately proved of very little benefit. Functional MRI using BOLD (blood-oxygenation-level-dependent) imaging had been described by Seiji Ogawa in 1990. Its first experimental use in humans followed in 1992 and it seemed to have great promise in advancing the understanding epileptic seizures, which, after all, were transient 'functional' events, but this technique too has failed to make much impact.

MRI is an exemplar case study of technical innovation in medicine. The original discoveries were in the field of basic science – in this case, physics, computing, electronics, engineering and chemistry – with no connection to medicine. Development of the science took place over decades. A tentative introduction into the medical arena was made jointly by university-based academics in the basic sciences and medicine – and the basic science was turned into an applied science. Commercial industry rapidly converted early promise into very large profits with massive marketing and sales. Within a few years, the main parameters of the clinical utility had been established by a few landmark publications. A bandwagon effect ensued, and within ten years or so teams around the world were carrying out research, usually incremental in nature. Vast numbers of papers found their way into publication (PubMed lists around 500 articles on the topic of MRI and epilepsy in the ten years after the first clinical article was published in 1982; and then 4,000 articles in the next 10 years), many of questionable value. Where expensive technology is concerned, commercial interests overwhelmed the field and hijacked academic development. This pattern was characteristic of all fields of radiology, EEG and post-war genetic research. Within the maelstrom of medical, technological and commercial interests, it is notable that patients were the one group entirely excluded from decision-making.

HEALTHCARE FOR EPILEPSY

By the 1970s, the European welfare state had become fully ensconced. By thus extending the role of government, healthcare itself had entered the bear pit of economics and political debate. Health economics had risen up the agenda as medicine became more commercialised and as public expectations of health-care rose, fuelled not only by politicians but also by medical over-promotion. There were diverse patterns of provision and funding.[97] By 1981, in Britain only 3% of healthcare was paid out of income or savings; 96% was paid out of central taxation. In Belgium, Denmark, Germany, France and Holland most healthcare was paid for via insurance schemes, in Spain by insurance supple-mented with taxation, and in Italy and Ireland by taxation supplemented with insurance. Insurance schemes were usually compulsory, but some excluded categories of chronic illness. Most of these welfare systems required direct payments by patients. The amounts varied, but were usually small. The organ-isation of healthcare was local or regional in some countries and national in others, and details such as waiting times, access to services, equity and quality varied from country to country. In some countries, such as Britain, almost all specialised practice took place in hospitals. In others, the division between specialist and general practitioners was less clear-cut; in Germany, for instance, more than half of specialists practised outside hospitals. Hospitals were owned by the state in Britain,[98] but other countries offered different mixes of national, regional and private ownership. Each system had advantages and disadvantages, but much turned on finance. Levels of funding varied considerably, but budgetary pressure was a feature of each, with cost containment most strongly exercised in taxation-based systems. Systems relying on central taxation minimised regional differences and provided superior equity of access, but there was more diversity and responsiveness in the decentralised insurance-based systems.

For most patients with chronic diseases such as epilepsy, the introduction of universal healthcare was a boon, and the overall provision of care for epilepsy greatly improved under all of these schemes. Outpatient clinics in neurological units became the norm. For the first time in the history of the condition, patients had relatively easy access to specialists and to effective treatment. By 1970, new patients were generally admitted to hospital for initial investigations, and routine cases were subsequently followed up in outpatient clinics,

[97] Vaizey, *National Health*.
[98] Six of the eight colonies continued to be run by voluntary organisations, but with central funding.

sometimes for years on end.[99] Access to investigation, treatment and the full range of facilities opened up even to the poor and the destitute. It is easy to forget how remarkable this change was.

Medical practice evolved with the introduction of new treatments and new investigatory modalities, reducing the need for hospital admissions. By the end of the 1980s, admission into neurological beds for epilepsy in most countries was confined largely to emergencies for status epilepticus, diagnostic evaluation of complex epilepsy (often based around a telemetry unit) and surgery. New cases of epilepsy and routine follow-up of those with chronic epilepsy were by then dealt with entirely in an outpatient setting.[100] CT and MRI replaced the older and more invasive tests such as angiography or air encephalography, which had been routinely performed in the early post-war period.[101] As the reach of medicine increased, in Western countries at least, the number and size of hospitals grew rapidly. The United States, for instance, had only 149 general hospitals in 1873 and more than 7,000 by 1970. Hospitals, though, were expensive items and the number of hospital beds became a political issue as centrally funded health services struggled with the inflationary cost. By then most patients in many Western countries were used to being treated without significant cost both by their general practitioners and as outpatients in the medical or neurology departments of general hospitals. And, as access increased, the stigma of epilepsy lessened.

Asylums, Colonies and Special Centres for Epilepsy

In Britain, in 1948, at the start of the NHS, 40% of all hospital beds were occupied by the 'mentally defective'. But, with the closure of asylums, numbers fell precipitously,[102] from 135,000 in 1961 to around 30,000 in 2000.[103]

[99] In Britain, for instance, outpatient visits rose from 40 million in 1955 to more than 50 million in 1980 (Vaizey, *National Health*).

[100] The first outpatient clinic for epilepsy was set up in the 1860s at the National Hospital, Queen Square in London, and the basic structure of outpatient care has hardly changed in form since then. However, access to such outpatient facilities did greatly increase. By the 1970s it was normal for patients who developed epilepsy to be referred to specialist clinics – a privilege which in practice was available only to a few in the pre-war years.

[101] The air encephalography suite at the National Hospital, Queen Square, for instance, closed in the mid-1980s.

[102] In Britain, the Mental Deficiency Act of 1913 was replaced in 1959 by a new Mental Health Act, which in the era of psychotropic medication had led to the dissolution of the asylums, the assimilation of psychiatric care into the wider hospital system and had given the medical profession more discretionary powers. As public anxiety over mental illness rose, another Mental Health Act was passed in 1983 which then limited medical powers, introduced more legal duties and emphasised the rights of patients. The evolution of post-war legislation is in part evidence of the success of the lay movements in changing policy.

[103] In the 1960s, it was predicted that all hospitals would close quickly and that patients would be supported in community care. But community resources were never properly provided, and the closure of large hospitals proved slow and difficult.

Community care was promised to deal with those who would previously have been committed to an institution. Therapeutic communities were set up, and the mentally ill were given far more autonomy. However, in practice, community services were insufficient and the closing of asylums failed to improve the predicament of many vulnerable patients.

Similarly, in the United States, in 1956 more than 560,000 Americans were confined in state psychiatric institutions. The Kennedy and Johnson administrations enacted a series of laws that provided generous funding for totally new community mental health centres providing 'street psychiatry'. Asylum after asylum was closed, and by 1977 the number of asylum residents had fallen to 176,000.[104] The ambitious programmes for community care were initially successful, but the Nixon and Ford administrations cut funding radically and many mentally ill and handicapped patients were left destitute with no services at all. In Britain care was usually crammed into existing facilities, but in the United States new facilities were scheduled. Yet when economic conditions worsened and right-wing monetarist governments were elected, the plans faltered and many patients suffered badly. The same pressures applied in most other Western countries, the most extreme example being in Italy where Italian Law 180, passed in 1978, aimed to abolish mental hospitals entirely. Initially the public responded with enthusiasm, and an 'atmosphere of carnival and general rejoicing' reigned.[105] But as community facilities failed to materialise, there were catastrophic consequences in many regions.[106]

In the 1980s the pendulum again began to swing. The public repeatedly voiced concern over crime and nuisance from long-term patients released into the community and who could not cope. But the clock could not be turned back. Pressure to take troublesome patients out of communities resulted in a rise in the numbers of mentally ill in prisons, where care was even worse. It was hoped that moving persons from mental hospitals into community facilities would also be cheaper, and it was for this reason that deinstitutionalisation was promoted by a bizarre coalition of civil libertarians on the left and fiscal conservatives on the right. But, depending on what was put in its place, cost savings proved elusive. There is now a general consensus that the closure of the hospitals

---

[104] In 2010 there were only 37,000 state psychiatric beds in the United States. Most were short-term or acute inpatient units in general medical hospitals. In 1977 the US Commission for the Control of Epilepsy and Its Consequences (*Plan for Nationwide Action*, vol. 1, p. 734), had reported that there were 176,000 beds in US institutions for the mentally retarded which included beds for those with epilepsy.

[105] Heptinstall, 'Psichiatria democratica'.

[106] Jones, *Asylums and After*, pp. 216–22. She points out that 'it is much easier to destroy the existing services than to create better ones' (p. 221).

went too far, and no appropriate large-scale formula for community care of those with learning disabilities has been found anywhere in the Western world.[107]

In Europe, the epilepsy colonies – albeit almost all ridding their names of the word 'colony' – largely survived (in contrast to the United States, where all were closed down), mainly because their expertise in epilepsy care was not shared with hospitals or community facilities. By the 1960s and 1970s, partly due to pressure from the anti-asylum movement, and partly because of concern about costs, the therapeutic and rehabilitative roles of the colonies were emphasised over their custodial functions. As a result, although the numbers of residential beds continued to decrease, the colonies did not disappear. In Britain, for instance, by 1969 there were still 2,129 residents in epilepsy colonies. In 1972, in response to the specially commissioned Reid Report, residential space was converted into short-term accommodation housing what were now termed Special Centres for Epilepsy, which were in effect neuro-logical units for diagnosis and treatment, with facilities for short-term (three to six months) rehabilitation, in a residential setting, and for 'assessments under everyday living and working conditions'. For children, the residential units also incorporated special schooling.[108] The thrust of the Reid Report was that, to survive, epilepsy colonies should evolve into such special centres,[109] and similar transformations, with the establishment of hospital facilities side by side with residential care, occurred in colonies throughout Europe.[110] The prototype colony at Bethel even developed invasive monitoring and a surgical assessment unit. In the view of John and Mary Laidlaw,[111] the Special Centre should provide mainly for people with epilepsy who are 'very nearly, but not quite' independent due to the problems peculiar to epilepsy (p. 543). These were persons who were independent in most aspects of daily living and who were employable in sheltered situations. It was the hope that most of the persons

[107] For a discussion of the 'disaster' of what purported to be community care, see Murphy, *After the Asylums*.

[108] Cited in *Reid Report*, col. 474. The Special Centres were encouraged to be jointly managed lay charities and NHS hospitals. An example was (and still is) the Chalfont Centre for Epilepsy, which was established jointly by the National Hospital, Queen Square and the National Society for Epilepsy. By 1995 the assessment unit admitted more than 1,000 patients a year and provided EEG telemetry and a dedicated MRI scanning unit. For the development of the centre over 100 years, see Barclay, *A Caring Community*. The Reid report recommendations were influenced by similar developments in Holland, where eight special centres of varying size and sophistication had already been established.

[109] In keeping with the changing social ethos, the recommendations included special mention of children, unmarried mothers (e.g. that they should not be barred from using the services) and the elderly. Non-medical aspects, such as local authority accommodation, employment and staffing, were also emphasised. Although six Special Centres were recommended, only three materialized: at Chalfont, Bootham Park Hospital in York and the Park Hospital in Oxford (for children).

[110] See Steinhoff, Chatrou and Hjalfrim, 'European Association of Epilepsy Centres'.

[111] See Laidlaw and Laidlaw, 'People with epilepsy', first and second editions. Laidlaw was director of the Chalfont Centre for Epilepsy; his wife, Mary, was the senior nursing officer.

admitted to a special centre would be able, after rehabilitation, to leave and to live independently, although how often true rehabilitation was achieved remained arguable. For the more disabled, however, epilepsy colonies still provided a vital function, but with a new ethos of care not containment. As the Laidlaws put it, the longer-term residents should

> feel that the centre offers them not a prison to which they are sent, but a community in which they want to stay because it provides a better quality of life than they could find elsewhere . . . We suggest that there are those who would prefer to live as first-class citizens in a therapeutic community rather than to exist as third-class citizens in the open community.

The United States took a different path. Early in the century the colonies had become generally larger and more institutionalised than their European equivalents, and took on a more custodial and less homely guise. In the post-war years, as fewer and fewer 'sane' epileptics, or those with recent-onset epilepsy, were taken into colony care, the inmates were increasingly drawn from those with severe mental deficiency and behavioural problems (exactly as the Laidlaws cautioned against). The colonies in effect became indistinguishable from the large mental hospitals and suffered from the same problems of institutionalisation and the same abuses. As a result, when deinstitutionalisation became accepted societal dogma, all (or almost all) the epilepsy colonies were closed down. Some became non-residential 'developmental centers' (a form of day-care centre), taking in persons with mental handicap and a wider range of problems, many without epilepsy. It was partly to fill the gap caused by this wholesale restructuring that a new solution was proposed for people with epilepsy: the Comprehensive Epilepsy Program. For a trial period the National Institute of Neurological and Communicative Disorders and Stroke established five such programmes to 'incorporate principles of the level of care and provide tertiary care in a multidisciplinary regional manner, tying together existing services, operating outreach programmes, educational programmes at all levels and conducting all this in a research setting'.[112] A paradigmatic example was the Comprehensive Epilepsy Program at the University of Virginia.[113] It was focused around a new diagnostic, treatment and rehabilitation unit at the Blue Ridge Hospital (an old tuberculosis sanatorium) in a poor rural area of Virginia with

---

[112] Dreifuss, 'Comprehensive epilepsy program'.

[113] This facility was administratively linked to the tertiary care neurology unit at the University of Virginia in Charlottesville (US Commission, *Plan for Nationwide Action*, vol. 2, pp. 1104–10; and described in some detail in Dreifuss, 'Comprehensive epilepsy program'. The author remembers travelling with Dreifuss in his old jalopy into the backwaters of rural Virginia, where de bono satellite clinics were held. These services provided succour to largely indigent people in a country where primary care was non-existent and secondary care was financially out of reach.

fifteen inpatient beds, EEG telemetry and drug monitoring, as well as rehabilitation facilities for education, recreation and activities of daily living. The average length of stay was sixty days. Education was provided by seminars and literature, and close contact was maintained with a residential rehabilitation training centre for the handicapped some miles away. The staff also provided twelve satellite or field clinics as a form of outreach in rural and isolated communities. The concept of 'levels of care' was employed, meaning that the intensity of care was tailored to the individual patient. The whole enterprise was funded largely by NINDS and state agencies. Run by its visionary director, Fritz Dreifuss, the Virginia programme proved very successful. But after the cuts legislated by the Reagan administration, the service disintegrated and the Blue Ridge centre eventually closed in 1996. The focus towards the medicalised care of the least handicapped was reasserted.[114] When J. Kiffin Penry retired as chief of the Epilepsy Branch at NIH, he was replaced by Roger Porter, who expanded the hospital-based elements of the comprehensive programmes. This resulted in forty epilepsy centres, based in large university hospitals,[115] providing tertiary medical care and, in some, EEG telemetry[116] and neurosurgical facilities, but without the more comprehensive residential and rehabilitation aspects of the Virginia programme. There, and in many other locations, facilities for those with epilepsy and learning disability were significantly curtailed.

Governmental Reports on Epilepsy Care

As governments reluctantly took on the responsibility of healthcare for epilepsy, government reports on the care of epilepsy proliferated. This reflected the increasing politicisation of care and the growing medical interest in the topic of epilepsy, as well as the fact that care provision was now often seen as wholly inadequate by a population with growing expectations. In the United States, as a result of lobbying by the Epilepsy Foundation of America, a Commission for the Control of Epilepsy and Its Consequences was established in 1975, with Richard Masland as Executive Director and David Daly as Chair. The commission published a 6-volume report (of over 2,500 pages, with more than 200 recommendations) in 1977 and 1978 – the massive and rambling Plan for Nationwide Action on Epilepsy.[117] As the title implied, the report

---

[114] One suspects that this was partly due to the lack of interest in mental handicap shown by most neurologists; as epilepsy care moved from psychiatry to neurology, those with epilepsy and mental handicap often fell through the cracks.

[115] Rowland, *NINDS at 50*, p. 77.

[116] By 1981, for instance, there were twenty-nine video-EEG telemetry units in operation throughout the country.

[117] US Commission, *Plan for Nationwide Action*. After publication, two conferences (Living Well with Epilepsy, I and II) were held in 1977 and 2003 to assess progress and to identify gaps for continuing public health action.

presented a more or less coordinated plan for the whole spectrum of epilepsy services, although in the United States, where healthcare is the least centralised of any Western nation, such a plan was difficult to implement. In the event, many of the recommendations were not acted upon, but the report did substantially raise the profile of epilepsy services, and improvements resulted. The commission's recommendations focused on specialisation of epilepsy services and served to fuel rapid growth in specialised medical services.

In Britain, where healthcare was centralised more than in most other countries, five government reports were devoted to epilepsy between 1953 and 2000.[118] The 1953 Cohen report was short (thirty-one pages in all) and made twenty-three recommendations encapsulating the new mood of liberalism and welfare. These recommendations emphasised the welfare of adults and children with epilepsy, in addition to medical services, involved multiple levels of NHS and social services, and included the establishment of a range of special facilities: regional hospital epilepsy clinics; special investigatory clinics for epileptics with behaviour problems; long-stay treatment and rehabilitation centres; resettlement clinics; long-stay hospital units for epileptic children with 'exceptionally bad behaviour disorders'; and hostels for 'epileptics who are ready to try out their ability in employment, but who still require some care' (p. 12). In a rather visionary way, and before widespread public criticism of asylums, it was recommended that the epilepsy colonies should be 'as much therapeutic as custodial', be more concerned with medical care and rehabilitation with the ultimate goal of returning individuals to a normal life in the community, and either incorporated into the NHS or at least be associated with NHS hospital services.[119] Little action resulted, as the Reid Report, published in 1969 as a follow-up to the Cohen Report, made clear. The Reid Report came to seventy-four pages and made fifty-six recommendations. In addition to the special centres – the report's most innovative recommendation – it proposed a 'basic framework of care' which included epilepsy clinics in district hospitals, multidisciplinary teams and attention to public attitudes. In accord with the prevailing philosophy regarding institutional care, it recommended that the epilepsy colonies should plan for a continuing reduction and in effect phase

[118] Ministry of Health, *National Assistance Act*; Central Health Services Council, *Medical Care of Epileptics*; Reid Report, *People with Epilepsy*; *Report of the Working Group*; Clinical Standards Advisory Group, *Services*. See also Shorvon, 'Specialized services'.

[119] Amongst the other recommendations made were that: children should as far as possible be educated at ordinary schools; the greatest care should be taken that' children not be unnecessarily 'labelled' as epileptics' (p. 12); when institutional care was needed, the type of institution chosen should be that most suited to the major disability, which may or may not be epilepsy.

themselves out, with existing residents moved into community care where possible. The report also recommended that progress should be reviewed regularly, resulting in the Winterton Report (1986) and then the Clinical Standards Advisory Group (CSAG) Report (2000) which was a comprehensive attempt to design a 'joined up' service linking the community and hospital services.

The changes in epilepsy care that did occur very much reflected the changing social attitudes to all forms of illness and handicap. The initial emphasis of health service planning was bureaucratic and administrative, but the tone slowly evolved in the post-1980 consumerist world to give greater weight to the user's perspective. All the reports reiterated the advantages of specialisation and also of combining medical and social services, as epilepsy was acknowledged to have unique claims on both.

TREATING EPILEPSY

Between 1970 and 1995 epilepsy treatment evolved beyond all recognition, not so much because of new drugs —and it was only in the latter years of this period that a clutch of new compounds did enter clinical practice – but because of advances in clinical therapeutics.

Pharmacokinetics and Drug Level Monitoring

Three technologies had transformed the practice of epilepsy during the post-war period. Two of them – EEG and neuroimaging – have already been described. The third – the ability to measure and monitor antiepileptic drug levels in blood – was less glamorous, yet it proved of greater direct importance to medical (drug) therapy in epilepsy than either of the other two. It also transformed experimental study and drug development. Advances in this field permitted small concentrations of drugs and metabolites in body fluids to be measured accurately. This resulted in intensive studies of the pharmacokinetics of antiepileptic drugs. Investigations were performed and published of such processes as: drug absorption into the blood stream and into the brain; the metabolism of the drug; its distribution in the body; its excretion and elimination from the body; the metabolites created from the drug; and the interference (interaction) of these processes by other drugs.

The blood level of a drug in a person can act as a guide to its activity, as a surrogate measure for the cerebral concentration of the drug. A range of new laboratory technologies, including mass spectrometry, high-performance liquid chromatography, radioimmunoassay and enzyme immunoassay, introduced blood level testing into clinical practice. Whole laboratories were set up in hospitals in the United States and

34. An early advertisement for the EMIT assay method for estimating anticonvulsant drug serum levels. The 'window' refers to the 'therapeutic range'.

Europe to service clinical needs. These developments were detailed in *Antiepileptic Drugs: Quantitative Analysis and Interpretation*, published under the auspices of the NIH in 1978, which demonstrated how prominent the study of pharmacokinetics had become.[120] Of the fifty-nine chapters in the first edition, thirty-four are wholly devoted to pharmacokinetics, and it featured in at least half of the remaining twenty-five chapters. In the final chapter, Richard Schmidt provides the rationale for this emphasis, noting that blood level monitoring

---

[120] Pippenger, Penry and Kutt, *Antiepileptic Drugs*.

could add precision to the assessment of drug effectiveness and toxicity and had become a practical reality for routine application. He pointed to the importance of the 'therapeutic range', the wide individual variations in dose/level relationship, enzyme induction, drug interactions, narrow therapeutic windows, effects on protein binding of thyroid hormones and effects on vitamin D. These issues remained pertinent, and the parameters hardly changed over the next fifty years.

As pharmacokinetic parameters vary greatly from individual to individual, it became accepted that the blood level of some drugs was a better guide to therapy than dosage. The *therapeutic range* was defined (albeit on relatively shaky evidence) as the range of levels within which a drug was most likely to control seizures without adverse effects. In theory, levels below the range were less likely to exert an antiepileptic effect, and levels above the range were more likely to result in side effects. The classic early studies were confined to measurements of phenytoin.[121]

It soon became clear that a good understanding of the pharmacokinetics of all drugs was vital for effective clinical prescribing in many situations, and, as a result, a large industry developed around blood level measurement.[122] Armed with pharmacokinetic information, clinicians could now take a 'scientific' approach to drug prescription for the first time. Furthermore, as the interpretation of drug level measurement was perceived to be beyond the competence of the general neurologist, the development further spurred the subspecialisation of epilepsy within neurology and paediatrics, as well as the formation of a new specialty of clinical pharmacology within medicine.[123]

By the late 1970s, therapeutic drug monitoring (TDM; the measurement of blood levels), as it became known, was in widespread clinical usage. A full range of pharmacokinetic parameters and measures was established.[124] Studies had also been made of 'special populations', such as children, the elderly, those with renal and hepatic disease, and pregnant women. By the early 1980s the characterisation of the hepatic enzyme system had largely been completed, and

---

[121] Kutt and McDowell, 'Management of epilepsy'.

[122] In the 1960s and 1970s, many companies developed TDM products using enzyme immunoassay and enzyme-multiplied immunoassay technique technologies.

[123] James Shannon was appointed scientific director of the NIH in 1949, and established the institute's first Laboratory of Clinical Pharmacology. It was there that the early applications of clinical pharmacology were developed. Departments of clinical pharmacology followed in the 1960s at Hammersmith Hospital (Colin Dollery), University College London (Desmond Laurence), Nashville (John Oates), Kansas City (Dan Azarnoff), San Francisco (Ken Melmon), Atlanta/Chicago (Leon Goldberg) and Stockholm (Folke Sjöqvist) Several of the early leaders of clinical pharmacology specialised in epilepsy (including, for instance, Alan Richens in London). The origins of clinical pharmacology are charted in Dollery, 'Clinical pharmacology'.

[124] See Richens, 'Clinical pharmacology'.

relevant factors affecting blood levels, both environmental and genetic, were intensively studied. A large literature arose related to drug interactions at the level of absorption, protein binding, induction of metabolism, inhibition of metabolism and renal excretion.

In these early years, external quality control of assays became an issue, and an innovative scheme was established by Alan Richens from St Bartholomew's hospital in London.[125] Every three months or so, each participating laboratory was sent a set of samples. The laboratory measured them and sent the results back to Richens, and was then informed whether the measurements were accurate to within 95% confidence limits.[126]

Phenytoin was the first drug studied, and this proved a fortuitous choice. Drug level monitoring in blood proved more valuable in the case of phenytoin than for any other antiepileptic,[127] for various reasons: its clinical useful therapeutic range, saturable kinetics, reliance on hepatic metabolism, propensity for drug interactions and the marked individual variation in dose–level relations. It became the exemplar drug for the new speciality of clinical pharmacology, and reputations and careers were made on the back of pharmacokinetic studies of this drug. Epilepsy also benefitted, rising up the neurological pecking order as a topic requiring precision prescribing.

Drug–drug interaction studies of phenytoin were also the first to be performed. These started in the mid-1960s, and by 1980 phenytoin interactions, for instance, were recorded with more than fifty different drugs. The finding of a massive interaction between sulthiame and phenytoin was largely responsible for the removal of sulthiame from the pharmacopoeia. Interaction studies with other drugs followed, and the list of drug–drug interactions progressively enlarged as new drugs were introduced.

The regulatory agencies also responded to the new pharmacokinetic studies by requiring the pharmaceutical industry to provide more and more interaction and pharmacokinetic data on their new drugs prior to licensing, and made decisions about dosing regimes, warnings and contraindications based on these data. The related topic of pharmacodynamics – the study of the effect of the drug on brain function – is potentially more important than pharmacokinetics, but in this period it was hardly studied and far less understood.

---

[125] By 1977, the St Bartholomew's Hospital Quality Control Scheme for Antiepileptic Drugs involved 190 laboratories in the United Kingdom, most other Western European countries, South Africa, South America, Australia and Malaysia. Alan Richens – was one of the first clinical pharmacologists to specialise in the field of epilepsy and one of his PhD students at the Chalfont Centre for Epilepsy was Emilio Perucca, who later became ILAE president.

[126] Richens, 'Drug level monitoring'.

[127] The concept of the therapeutic range has little or no value for many other drugs, including the benzodiazepines and sodium valproate.

Clinical Therapeutics and the Rise of Monotherapy

In the era before pharmacokinetics, clinical therapeutics was based on clinical impression, and fashion largely dictated the choice of treatment. For instance, for no obvious reason, phenobarbital was more popular in France, phenytoin in the United States and carbamazepine in Scandinavia, and officially recommended indications for certain individual drugs varied from country to country. It was also universal practice to prescribe multiple drugs simultaneously (polytherapy), both in newly diagnosed patients and in those with chronic epilepsy. Some combinations of drugs were available in a single tablet (e.g. Garoin, which contained 50 mg of phenobarbital and 100 mg of phenytoin) and were popular choices for initial therapy. The extent of polytherapy in epilepsy was evident from a survey in four European countries, which found that 11,720 patients, randomly selected from inpatient and outpatient populations, were receiving 3.2 drugs per patient, of which 84% were anticonvulsants.[128]

The introduction of TDM enabled greater precision. In the late 1970s a new trend developed, with practice moving away from polytherapy to the use of single drug treatment (monotherapy) using drug level monitoring to guide dosage. Monotherapy clearly reduced side effects and, crucially, was found to be as efficacious in many patients as polytherapy.[129] As a result, almost all treatment protocols of the period were rewritten to advise that monotherapy should be the rule in new patients and used wherever possible in those with chronic epilepsy. This was a landmark in clinical therapeutics and resulted in an enormous shift in practice. By mid-2000, the PubMed database contained more than 2,300 references to anticonvulsant monotherapy, and monotherapy became a theme in many national and international ILAE conferences and workshops. Although striking in its simplicity, monotherapy had become a byword for advanced therapy. In the 1980s most combination preparations of antiepileptic drugs were removed from the major markets of Western Europe and the United States.

Toward the end of the decade, regulatory authorities joined the monotherapy bandwagon and requested monotherapy trials, without which the licence for a new drug would be granted only for use as adjunctive therapy (i.e. in combination with another drug). This requirement can be viewed rather cynically as a mechanism for restricting spending on novel drugs, for no drug has been shown to be effective in polytherapy but not monotherapy. In the late 1990s, as a counter-balance to monotherapy, the concept of rational polytherapy has been proposed – in other words, combinations of drugs with

---

[128] Guelaen, Van Der Kleijn and Woudstra, 'Statistical analysis'.
[129] See Shorvon and Reynolds, 'Unnecessary polypharmacy'; Shorvon and Reynolds, 'Reduction of polypharmacy'; Reynolds et al., 'Phenytoin monotherapy for epilepsy'.

different modes of action that might have a synergistic as opposed simply to an additive effect. There proved not a shred of robust clinical evidence to support this idea, and 'rational polytherapy' never caught on in routine clinical practice.

Toxicity and Side Effects of Antiepileptic Drugs

Side effects of antiepileptic drugs had been a clinical issue since the time of bromides, but the medical view in the early part of the century was that significant toxicity was expected, acceptable and something patients had to tolerate. In the 1960s, William Lennox could still write that drug-induced fatalities might be an 'act of God' – although, of course, the patient's opinion on such matters was never considered.[130]

With time, however, interest in epilepsy therapeutics increasingly turned to the topic of side effects. Three categories were recognised. The commonest were the acute side effects related to brain function (neurotoxicity) and included drowsiness, imbalance and slowing of mental response. Whilst in the past these effects were considered inevitable – and indeed, as mentioned earlier, sedation was considered a sine qua non of anticonvulsant effect – TDM had shown that, for some drugs, these effects could be minimised whilst maintaining effectiveness by using blood levels to guide dosing. The second category, the chronic long-term side effects, were also common, and found to be much less related to the moment-by-moment dose or blood level and more to the total amount of drug administered over months or years (the drug load). Such effects included drug-induced folate deficiency and vitamin D deficiency; changes in skin and connective tissue; and bone, hepatic, haematological and endocrine changes. These effects were found to be more prevalent with anticonvulsant polytherapy – indeed, avoiding these side effects was a key advantage of monotherapy – but were generally less severe with the newer drugs than with bromide, barbiturate or phenytoin. Acute allergic reactions – 'idiosyncratic side effects' – were a third category of side effect, also largely unrelated to dose, and were occasionally fatal.

In 1975 an influential review was published by Edward Reynolds, later president of the ILAE, summarising the core literature. Citing more than 250 references, Reynolds pointed out that some effects were subtle and easily overlooked, and that it had taken many years (often several decades) of widespread prescription even for common side effects to be recognised. He concluded:

> Although any paper devoted to toxicity without reference to therapeutic effects is in danger of appearing unnecessarily alarmist, and it is not disputed that some of these complications are less disabling than poorly

---

[130] Lennox, *Epilepsy and Related Disorders*, vol. 2, p. 847.

controlled seizures, the fact remains that far too many patients suffer more from the treatment than the disease. Treatment which is life-long, potentially harmful, and influenced by so many factors, known and unknown, needs constant supervision. With increasing awareness and understanding of chronic effects, and the regular use of drug levels and other metabolic markers (e.g., folate, alkaline phosphatase, and calcium levels), it should be possible to improve therapeutic efficiency and to strike a better balance between the burdens of the disease and the complications of therapy.[131]

This was well said, and from then on drug toxicity became a common topic of conferences and papers in medical circles. Numerous papers on these topics were published,[132] confirming the shifting agenda, and acknowledgement of these issues no doubt improved the lives of many patients.

Another category of side effect was teratogenicity (drug-induced congenital defects in the growing foetus caused by the ingestion of the drug by the mother when pregnant). The dire effects of thalidomide, which came to light in 1961, electrified public interest and resulted in the setting up of registers of congenital abnormalities in most countries. At this stage, few drugs other than thalidomide were known to be seriously teratogenic (cytotoxic folate antagonists were an exception), but slowly suspicions grew about the whole class of anticonvulsant drugs. Epilepsy was a common condition in women of childbearing age, and as antiepileptic drugs were commonly taken through pregnancy they were soon in the forefront of the new and rapidly developing field of teratogenicity. In 1968, in a letter to *The Lancet*, Roy Meadow described three infants with cleft palate and lip born to mothers on antiepileptic drugs, associated with congenital heart lesions, minor skeletal abnormalities, and dysmorphic facial and skeletal features.[133] He concluded that 'before creating anxiety about useful drugs, it would be helpful to know if other people have encountered this association'. With this mild and tentative letter, a whole new chapter in epilepsy therapeutics was opened. Further small case reports and series were published, and, over the next fifteen years, twenty large-scale epidemiological studies were carried out which showed significant increases in the rate of congenital malformations in children of mothers with epilepsy. This topic quickly rose up the epilepsy agenda, resulting in more than 500 papers published between 1970 and 1985, conference presentations and at least one book.[134] The risk of congenital abnormalities of the lip or heart was found to be about 10 times that in the unexposed population, and congenital heart defects 4 times. The overall risk of malformations was thought to be in the region of 5% of all exposed pregnancies.

---

[131] Reynolds, 'Chronic antiepileptic toxicity'.
[132] See, for instance, Trimble, 'Anticonvulsant drugs; Trimble, *Psychopharmacology of Epilepsy*.
[133] Meadow, 'Anticonvulsant drugs'. Sir Samuel Roy Meadow is a British paediatrician, an admirer of the child psychoanalyst Anna Freud and best known for his work on Munchausen by proxy and child abuse.
[134] Janz et al., *Epilepsy, Pregnancy and the Child*.

In 1982 a large, well-conducted epidemiological study in the Rhône-Alps region of France found an increased risk of spina bifida, a serious malformation of the spine and nervous system, in infants of mothers taking valproate.[135] The risk in valproate-exposed infants was calculated to be 1.2%, compared to 0.06% in infants of unexposed mothers. Moreover, it turned out that 35% of epileptic mothers in the region were being treated with valproate, and 60% of children with spina bifida had been exposed to the drug in utero. Up until this time, valproate was thought to be extremely safe, and indeed to be a drug of choice in pregnancy but the recognition of the full range of valproate's teratogenic effects would have to wait another thirty years, vindicating Reynolds's warning that it can take many years for side effects to be fully recognised.

By the 1990s most neurologists should have been aware that both epileptic seizures and drug treatment carried risks in pregnancy; that, ideally, pre-conception counselling should be performed (although this was rarely done at the time); that polytherapy should be avoided and that low doses of anti-epileptics were preferable; that folate supplementation should be given; that if one pregnancy was affected, there were higher risks in the second; and that days 18–40 after conception were the most risky. Still, many babies born in these years were damaged by anticonvulsant treatment taken by their mothers, and there was understandable outrage against the medical profession.

New Antiepileptic Drugs Introduced into Clinical Practice Between 1970 and 1994

After the flood of new drug introductions in the 1960s – in many ways the golden age of new anticonvulsant drugs – a severe drought ensued. The only new licensings between 1970 and 1989 were of clobazam, introduced in 1975 in Europe, and progabide (a drug which never became popular) in 1985 in

TABLE 4.5 *Antiepileptic drugs licensed between 1970 and 1995: The 'second generation antiepileptic drugs'*

Year of first licence	Proprietary name	Country where first licenced	Manufacturer
1975	Clobazam	UK/Germany	Hoeschst
1985	Progabide	France	Sanofi
1989	Vigabatrin	UK	Marion Merrill Dow
1989	Zonisamide	Japan	Dianippon
1990	Oxcarbazepine	Denmark	Novartis
1990	Lamotrigine	Ireland	Wellcome
1993	Felbamate	USA	Carter-Wallace
1994	Gabapentin	USA/UK	Parke-Davis

[135] Bjerkedal et al., 'Valproic acid'.

France. The reasons are complex, but include the perceived difficulty in licensing a drug after the tightening of the regulatory environment in the 1960s, the economic depressions of the 1970s and a general feeling that this was a small and crowded market already too full of existing drug therapies to make investment worthwhile. By 1985, however, the advancing basic science of GABergic and glutaminergic synaptic action had revived an interest within the pharmaceutical industry in identifying compounds which acted on the processes of neurotransmission. Drought was followed by plenty, and the five years after 1989 were a period of intense activity in the field of antiepileptic pharmacology (Table 4.5).

By then, pharmaceutical marketing methods had become highly sophisticated, and industry was spending huge sums to strengthen its hold on the medical world. Money was given to sponsor medical conferences,[136] medical publications and educational events; to cover the expenses of travel and

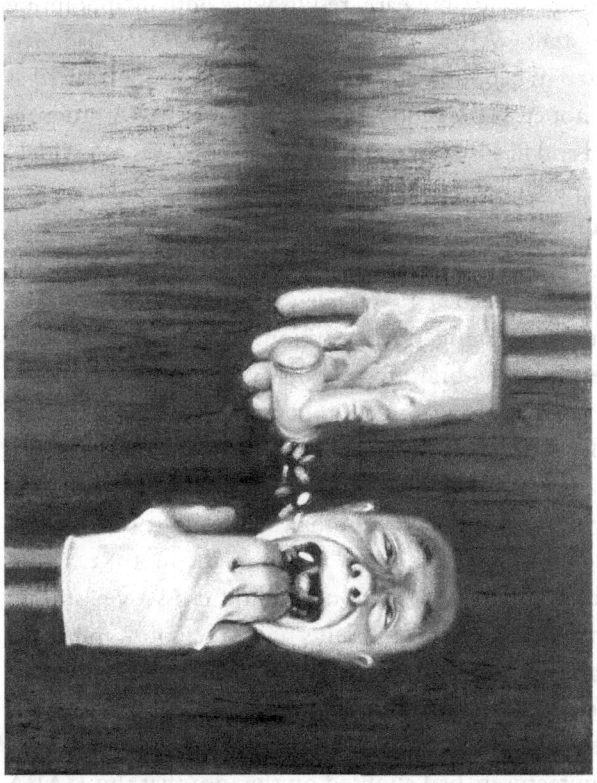

35. Please tell me this is really going to make me better' (A painting by David Cobley, 2021).

---

[136] The 1993 and 1995 International Epilepsy Congresses each included eight satellite symposia, organised by the pharmaceutical industry, which paid the ILAE handsomely for the privilege.

accommodation for doctors attending conferences, and sometimes lavish entertainment; and as grants and fees to so-called key opinion leaders (KOPs). The international epilepsy conference circuit flourished as never before, and the coffers of the ILAE, whose congresses were by then pre-eminent in the field of epilepsy, rapidly expanded. A band of high-profile doctors flew around the world, supported by industry, singing the praises of one drug after another, with presentations largely sculpted by pharmaceutical marketing companies. As one notorious doctor quipped in the 1990s when challenged that his lectures always favoured the company sponsoring the talk, 'It's Monday, so it must be gabapentin'. The basic marketing idea to be implanted was that these second-generation antiepileptics should replace the older workhorses (especially carbamazepine and valproate) and were modern, more effective and safer. As it turned out, newer did not always mean better, although it took decades for this to be recognised.

The 'GABA wave' of the 1970s was widely expected to produce dividends in the shape of novel GABAergic drugs, but early results were both disappointing and also confusing. The potent GABA agonists muscimol and THIP had pro-epileptic effects when tested in baboons, and GABA itself could not be used as an antiepileptic as it does not cross the blood–brain barrier. A GABA prodrug, progabide, was developed and licensed in several countries but was not widely taken up, and then a well publicised breakthrough did occur.

Vigabatrin, a compound devised at the Centre de Recherche Merrell International in Strasbourg, proved to be an irreversible inhibitor of the enzyme GABA transaminase (GABA-T) which catabolises GABA at the GABAergic synapse, thus prolonging GABA action. Vigabatrin was soon shown to raise GABA levels in the brain in rodents and in mice and subse-quently to afford protection in mice against audiogenic seizures. A year later, the agent's positive effects in the photosensitive baboon model were reported.[137] By the early 1980s, three years after the discovery of its neuro-chemical action, vigabatrin was being used in human studies. The first Phase 2 single-blind efficacy studies were carried out in Denmark in 1983.[138] By 1989, four short-term single-blind and six double-blind cross-over studies had been conducted in a total of 274 patients (a sufficient number in a development programme in those days) and the drug was licensed in Europe (but not in America). It was launched in 1989, first in the United Kingdom and then in Denmark, and soon after in sixty countries. Early on in its development, the manufacturers had alighted on the idea that this GABA agonist action was a rational design, and a lavish marketing campaign for vigabatrin was conceived around the slogan of 'rational therapy'. Sponsorship

---

[137] Meldrum and Horton, 'Blockade of epileptic responses'.
[138] Gram, Lyon and Dam, 'Gamma-vinyl-GABA'.

money poured into the clinical epilepsy world, and the marketing of vigabatrin was deemed a huge success. In those heady years, few were the medical meetings not sponsored by the company Marion Merrill Dow, whose hospitality and largesse were overwhelming and whose influence seemed to be everywhere.

The speed at which the drug was licensed was perhaps surprising, for there were toxicological concerns from the outset. Early pathology studies had shown the development of vacuoles within the myelin (a constituent of all neurons) in the brains of mice, rats and dogs treated with high doses of vigabatrin, but not in monkeys. Studies of human brain tissue (removed at epilepsy surgery) did not show similar effects, but anxiety over neurotoxicity hung over the drug in many quarters right through the 1990s. The mechanism of vacuolation, an unusual effect, was and remains obscure. Psychosis and other severe psychiatric symptoms began also to be reported in some early human subjects treated with the drug, and its propensity to cause marked psychiatric reactions and aggression was later to become widely established. Despite this, by the mid-1990s vigabatrin still was widely used and heavily marketed – although not in the United States, where the FDA showed more caution than the European agencies.

In January 1997, Mark Lawden, a neurologist from Leicester, reported severe constriction of the visual field[139] in three patients taking vigabatrin.[140] The report appeared just as the FDA had decided to issue an approvable letter for use of the drug in the United States, a decision rapidly retracted (later, the FDA complimented itself on not having licensed the drug). A rash of further cases was discovered, and by 1999 it had become clear that vigabatrin causes visual field constriction in around 30–50% of users and that the effects are irreversible. In 1999, the Committee for Proprietary Medicinal Products of the European Medicines Agency recommended that marketing authorisations for vigabatrin be maintained only under specific and highly restrictive conditions,[141] and sales of the drug plummeted as the drug fell into disuse. It further transpired that a monitoring study of vigabatrin prescription events conducted between 1991 and 1994 had identified four cases of bilateral, persistent visual field defects for which there was no alternative cause; this observation was neither well publicised nor acted upon. The inevitable lawsuits then took place to determine whether the company knew or should have known about the risk to vision, and were settled for undisclosed sums.

Another theory which has not stood the test of time was that folate deficiency may be antiepileptic. However, based on this idea, researchers at the

---

[139] At its worst causing 'tunnel vision', in which the periphery of vision is entirely lost and only central vision remains.
[140] Eke, Talbot and Lawden, 'Vigabatrin'.
[141] Committee for Proprietary Medicinal Products, *Opinion*.

Wellcome Research Laboratories decided in the 1980s to examine the anti-epileptic effect of anti-folate drugs. It proved a wild goose chase in terms of mechanism, but the goose did lay one golden egg. Among a whole series of compounds studied, one – BW430C (later named lamotrigine) – showed promise in a number of conventional animal models of epilepsy. The toxicological testing was slower than predicted and, hemmed in by regulatory restrictions, the first human studies were of single-dose effects on inter-ictal EEG abnormalities and photosensitivity. Eventually, six Phase 3 trials using a cross-over design were carried out. It was an erratic clinical development programme, but ultimately successful, and the drug was licensed first in Ireland in 1990, in the United Kingdom in 1991 and then in other countries in Europe. A parallel group study was completed in the United States (216 patients), and the drug was licensed there as well in December 1994. The lamotrigine programme marked the last time that cross-over designs were used in definitive epilepsy drug studies, as the FDA thereafter favoured the parallel group design.[142] After marketing, more trials were carried out, and a meta-analysis showed that the drug actually had only a relatively modest effect (an approximately 25% reduction in seizures).

One problem not identified in the short-term studies, but soon to become very apparent, was the propensity of lamotrigine to cause an allergic rash in a surprisingly high proportion of initial patients (more than 10% in the placebo-controlled trials). Occasionally, the reaction extended to complete exfoliation and was sometimes fatal.[143] The rash was also found to be more common in children, which resulted in the regulatory requirement for complex dosing regimens depending on age and co-medication. Ironically, although introduced as an anti-folate antiepileptic, the drug turned out not to have a strong anti-folate action. After further years of experimentation, it was concluded that the effects of lamotrigine were due to its sodium-channel-blocking properties – in other words, a similar mechanism of action to that of the older-generation antiepileptics phenytoin and carbamazepine. Despite what was considered by many to be an initially relatively poor performance, lamotrigine was heavily marketed as a novel and exciting antiepileptic drug. The marketing was more efficacious than the clinical trials, and sales grew rapidly, first in Britain and later in continental Europe and the United States. By 1994 lamotrigine had been used by more than 80,000 people in 40 different countries. Taking up the mantle from Merrill Dow from the early 1990s, Wellcome and its successors Glaxo Wellcome and GlaxoSmithKline sponsored extravagant meetings, journal articles and supplements, and provided many epilepsy activities with financial support.

---

[142] In fact, in the case of lamotrigine, the cross-over designs in small numbers of patients produced much the same results as the parallel group design in much larger numbers of patients. One wonders whether this decision should be reconsidered.

[143] Rzany et al., 'Risk of Stevens-Johnson syndrome'.

Several years after its launch, it became apparent that lamotrigine had value in treating not only the partial epilepsies, its initial licensed indication, but also the generalised epilepsies, both primary and secondary. At the time, treatment of generalised epilepsy was dominated by valproate and soon an aggressive advertising battle was launched by Glaxo Wellcome, with lamotrigine profiled as the drug 'for women with epilepsy' – no weight gain, no ovarian cysts, no teratogenicity (in contrast to valproate) and, for good measure, no interactions with the contraceptive pill (in contrast to carbamazepine). Women with epilepsy became a hot topic, and a remarkable number of publications and conferences, partly subsidised by the industry, were subsequently devoted to the subject.

Early on in its antiepileptic drug development programme, NIH had identified one important compound: 2-phenyl-1,3-propanediol dicarbamate (felbamate). It had been synthesised at the Wallace Laboratories in the 1950s as a relative of meprobamate in the search for new sedative drugs. But when it appeared to have little promise as a sedative, the compound was shelved for many years. Later, when screened by the NIH program, the drug was found to have very low toxicity ('This drug does not kill rats', as Harvey Kupferberg put it), and had a promising profile of antiepileptic drug activity in both rats and mice. Its pharmacokinetics were rapidly defined, and it soon progressed into clinical trials. In 1991, the first Phase 2 studies, funded by NIH, were reported and were soon followed by two monotherapy studies in 1992–3. By the mid-1990s, eight major double-blind placebo-controlled studies had been carried out. The trials had innovative designs, and the development programme was controversial, but the FDA recommended the drug for approval in December 1992. This was the first new antiepileptic drug approved in the United States for fifteen years, and the move was influenced by the general political pressure to get an 'American' drug to market. The launch in July 1993 was followed by a truly massive advertising campaign. The basic message was that here was a new, highly effective American drug with a remarkable lack of toxicity.

Advertisements of an attractive women walking in a flower-strewn meadow with the caption 'Seizure control that is easy to live with' appeared in the national press. The culmination of the press campaign, in August 1993, was a *Time* magazine feature article, headlined 'Taming the brain storms', about Lynn Tiscia, a 38-year-old Connecticut homemaker and mother of two boys, whose uncontrolled seizures and quality of life were dramatically improved by felbamate. 'I'm back!', says Tiscia. 'It's me . . . My sister tells me she finally likes me again. She even lent me her car. My mother yells at me again. It's great.'[144] The article had a photo of the beaming Lynn with her children in Doolittle

[144] 'Taming the brain storms'.

Park playground. The campaign was very effective: as Lynn Tiscia signed off, sales of felbamate took off.

In clinical trials, 1,600 people were exposed to felbamate, over half for nine months or more, and no significant haematological or hepatic changes were noted. Within the first year of launch, by August 1994, more than 110,000 patient exposures had resulted. In January 1994, the first case of aplastic anaemia was noticed and by the end of 1994, 34 cases were reported. In retrospect, 23 cases definitely related to felbamate had occurred, with 14 deaths. Eighteen patients also developed hepatic failure, with five deaths definitely attributable to felbamate. By August 1994, the FDA recommended suspending use of the drug. A planned launch of the drug in Europe, with a major conference planned in Spain by the European licensee Schering-Plough, was cancelled at the last minute. In US courts more than 100 lawsuits were launched, mostly from people not claiming a bad reaction to the drug but rather emotional distress or damages due to the forced withdrawal. Carter-Wallace went out of business. This was an unhappy episode in the history of antiepileptic drug therapy; however, when the dust settled, the overall risk of marrow depression was found to be between 27 and 300 per million patients treated, and of hepatic failure between 1 in 26,000–34,000 persons – a higher risk than that of carbamazepine but not orders of magnitude greater.[145] The drug was a casualty of incautious claims and aggressive advertising, and a prime example of the principle that the value and risks of a new antiepileptic may take years to establish. The excessive marketing and subsequent public and regulatory reaction resulted in a lost opportunity for what might have proved to be a useful drug in some situations.

Another new drug licensed in this period was gabapentin, an analogue of GABA, whose structure was deliberately twisted in the laboratory to increase its penetration into the brain. The initial clinical studies concerned spasticity and rigidity. But later three proof-of-concept (Phase 2a) studies demonstrated antiepileptic activity, and then double-blind randomised clinical studies, with an obtuse and unusual statistical approach, were published. In 1994 gabapentin was licensed in the United States and the United Kingdom. Although the compound was developed as a GABA analogue, in fact its antiepileptic effects are due to an entirely different mechanism: binding to the $\alpha 2\delta$ subunit of the neuronal voltage-dependent calcium channel (this mechanism of action was discovered a decade or more after licensing). Gabapentin was also trialled in eight non-epilepsy indications, including bipolar disease, mood disorders and neuralgic pain, but not licensed at the time. Within a few years it became one of Pfizer's bestselling products. According to one estimate, 90% of prescriptions for gabapentin were for non-epilepsy (i.e. non-licensed) indications and

---

[145] Bialer et al., 'EILAT VIII'.

particularly in the large market for pain; by 2003 it was one of the 50 most-prescribed drugs in the United States (with sales rising from $97.5 million in 1995 to nearly $2.7 billion in 2003). However, in 2004 the company was fined very large sums of money to settle a range of civil and criminal charges related to illicit marketing of the epilepsy drug for off-label uses. It continued to be manufactured by Pfizer, which obtained a licensed indication for neuralgic pain. But, after a few years of routine clinical experience, it gained a reputation as largely ineffective in epilepsy and fell out of common usage. Quite why the trials were more positive than routine use is an unanswered question and deserved more scrutiny.

Oxcarbazepine was first synthesised in 1966. Its structure is very close to that of carbamazepine, and it has the same mechanism of action. The clinical effects of oxcarbazepine were found to be also almost indistinguishable from the older drug, although it had fewer interactions and a lower risk of allergy. Licensed first in Denmark in 1990 and then over the next ten years in other European countries and the United States, oxcarbazepine became a moderately commonly prescribed antiepileptic. Total sales, however, were and are still far below those of carbamazepine.

Drug Treatment by 1995

Between 1960 and 1995, the drug treatment of epilepsy had become highly systematised, not least because of the plethora of medical conferences in that period and the publication of books focused on drug therapy. And drug treatment took the form that was to apply for the next three decades at least, with the following principles. First, certain drugs were specific for certain seizure types. In practice, the specificity applied mainly to generalised seizures, and for partial seizures almost all drugs were considered as good (or bad) as each other. Second, certain drugs were defined as 'first-line' therapy and others restricted to a second-line or 'adjunctive' position. Further old-fashioned therapies were still available, but were rapidly falling out of use.[146] The first-line therapies were (with dates of first licensing) carbamazepine (1962), valproate (1961), phenytoin (1939), phenobarbital (1912), clonazepam (1968; 1975 in the USA), clobazam (1975; 2011 in the USA) and ethosuximide (1958). Third, treatment was differentiated into categories of patient: newly diagnosed patients with drug-naïve epilepsy – all were to receive monotherapy with

---

[146] These included (with their dates of first licensing): other hydantoins – ethotoin (1956), methoin (1956), deltoin (1966) and albutoin (1967); other barbiturates – methylphenobarbital (1932), dimethoxy-methyl phenobarbitone (1975); other succinimides – phensuximide (1951), methsuximide (1951); oxazolidinediones – troxidone (1945), paramethadione (1954); sulphonamides – acetazolamide (1955) and sulthiame (1960); and other drugs – pheneturide (1949) and beclamide (1956).

Potassium bromide 1857	Phenobarbital (Luminal®) 1912	Phenytoin (Dilantin®) 1938
K$^+$ Br$^-$		
Valproic acid (Epilim®) 1967	Carbamazepine (Tegretol®) 1965	Ethosuximide (Zarontin®) 1958
Tiagabine (Gabitril®) 1996	Zonisamide (Zonegran®) 1989	Pregabalin (Lyrica®) 2004
Lamotrigine (Lamictal®) 1991	Topiramate (Topamax®) 1995	Vigabatrin (Sabril®) 1989
Gabapentin (Neurontin®) 1994	Felbamate (Felbatol®) 1990	Oxcarbazepine (Trileptal®) 1990
Retigabine (Trobalt®) 2010	Rufinamide (Inovelonl®) 2007	Levetiracetam (Keppra®) 1999

36. 'Chemical structure of antiepileptic drugs with trade names and date of introduction.

one of the first-line drugs; chronic uncontrolled epilepsy – monotherapy or limited polytherapy was advocated, with trials of different drugs when one failed; epilepsy in remission – drug withdrawal could be considered after two years or more without seizures, but there was always a risk (albeit reducing over time) of recurrence. Fourth, epilepsy specialists were urged to pay great attention to the pharmacokinetic properties of antiepileptic drugs in their prescribing. Similarly, drug licensing required detailed pharmacokinetic data, and several potentially useful drugs failed to achieve a licence because of poor kinetic properties. Finally, as it became clearer that the drugs did not differ markedly in terms of efficacy, it was their side effects that had become central to decisions about drug-choice.

Surgical Treatment of Epilepsy

In 1983, Arthur Ward, editor-in-chief of *Epilepsia*, provided a useful analysis of the then position of resective epilepsy surgery.[147] He pointed out that the basic concept of resective surgery had not changed since Wilder Penfield's time (actually, since the time of Victor Horsley), and that it depended on the resection of 'the focus' identified by clinical, EEG and CT findings. Regarding outcome, he cited Rasmussen's 1983 series (see pp. 371–2), by far the largest at that date, which he rightly viewed as the gold standard for what could be achieved. Ward considered resection to be potentially possible in anyone with drug-resistant focal seizures. Yet, despite Ward's estimate that there were 54,000 candidates for surgery in the United States (and Engel in 1992 put the figure nearer to 100,000)[148] only 100 operations a year took place. In Ward's view, this underutilisation was due to misconceptions regarding effectiveness, the economic cost and the lack of information about the availability of surgery. Ward was a surgeon and had taken a surgical stance which ignored the reluctance of doctors and patients to believe that a significant quantity of brain tissue – 15% of total brain area in the case of temporal lobectomy – could be resected without adverse effects and a general anxiety that the adverse effects were being overlooked or ignored, which in most surgical series was indeed the case.

In specialised units, epilepsy surgery had begun to be widely available and had been given a major boost by the introduction of MRI scanning and the establishment of EEG telemetry units. In the United States, surgical units sprang up in many locations (thirty-seven American units participated in the 1986 Palm Desert meeting, and no doubt there were other active centres who were absent). In Europe too, and elsewhere, epilepsy surgery began to flourish,

---

[147] Ward, 'Surgical therapy of epilepsy'.
[148] Engel and Shewmon, 'Who should be considered as a surgical candidate', p. 26.

led by individual surgeons who were often trained in established units in other countries – thus introducing an international flavour to epilepsy surgery, reflecting its highly specialised nature (eleven centres participated in the Palm Desert meeting, five from Europe, three from Japan, two from Australia and one from Brazil).[149] The numbers of patients operated upon, though, were often quite small at most of these units, with surgery frequently dependant on a single neurosurgeon who might perform only a handful of cases a year.

In some countries epilepsy surgery had started around the turn of the twentieth century, stimulated by the example of Horsley, but had ceased, and then restarted again in the years after World War Two. Switzerland provides a good example of this. Emil Kocher, a close friend of Horsley, had introduced surgery for epilepsy in the 1890s, but it then petered out. It was resuscitated in the 1960s under the leadership of Hugo Krayenbühl,[150] and in 1967 the Turkish-born surgeon Mahmut Gazi Yaşargil was appointed in Zurich, where he introduced the operating microscope into epilepsy surgery, perfected a new trans-sylvian approach to temporal lobectomy and introduced the 'selective temporal lobectomy' which involved the resection of mesial structures whilst retaining lateral temporal cortex. With Wieser, he developed a thriving epilepsy surgery centre in Zurich, and on his retirement a similar style of surgery was carried on by Yasuhiro Yonekawa, one of his erstwhile trainees. A comparable picture emerged in Holland, which had a long tradition of advanced services for epilepsy. The first operations were carried out between 1889–93, following Horsley's example, but presumably because of disappointing results, epilepsy surgery then ceased until 1938 when the young surgeon Arnaud Cornelis de Vet carried out his first epilepsy operation. Between 1949 and his retirement in 1969, he had operated on 213 patients, 78 with psychomotor epilepsy, based on the Montreal approach. In 1976, Colin Binnie introduced video-EEG monitoring, and in 1990 Walter van Embe Boas, who had trained with Fred Andermann in Montreal expanded the epilepsy surgery programme. In total, between 1973 and 2005, 775 epilepsy surgeries were conducted in Holland, in one of the largest programmes in Europe[151]. In Britain, similarly, after Horsley's time, surgery became restricted to occasional operations on post-traumatic epilepsy until the 1950s, when interest again developed – largely on the Montreal example and stimulated particularly by stereotaxis and functional surgery. At the London Hospital, Douglas Northfield conducted fifty temporal lobectomies using subdural and depth electrodes (thirty by 1958), and small surgical programmes were developed in

---

[149] Schijns et al., 'Epilepsy surgery in Europe'; Lüders, *Textbook of Epilepsy Surgery*.

[150] Hugo Krayenbühl was trained by Cairns at the London Hospital. He returned to Zurich in 1936 and was there appointed to the first Chair in Neurosurgery in Switzerland in 1948.

[151] Details taken from Van Emde Boas and Boon, 'Epilepsy Surgery in the Netherlands and Belgium'.

other centres in London and in Birmingham, Cardiff, Edinburgh, Liverpool, Newcastle and Oxford. At the Maudsley Hospital, in 1951, Falconer initiated a programme of temporal lobe surgery which was then continued on his retirement by his trainee, Charles Polkey. In the 1980s, the National Hospital, Queen Square restarted a surgical programme for adults,[152] and at the Hospital for Sick Children, Great Ormond Street, a parallel paediatric programme was initiated, with both hospitals publishing the results of large series in subsequent decades.

In other countries, epilepsy surgery developed in the post-war period and often, after a stuttering start became fully established decades later, frequently on the initiative of a single individual. In Sweden, for example, Herbert Olivecrona[153] carried out epilepsy operations in the 1950s, but thereafter surgery was only occasionally performed until the 1980s, when it was boosted by the appointment in Umea of Herbert Silfvenius, who had earlier trained in Montreal. Similarly, in Denmark operations were carried out in the 1950s, the numbers then dwindled in the 1970s and 1980s (not least because of public opposition to psychosurgery) and then surgery was revitalised by Mogens Dam, later ILAE President, in the late 1980s. In Italy, several operations were performed in 1955, after which epilepsy surgery virtually disappeared. But it restarted in 1994 when Munari, trained by Bancaud and Talairach in Paris, set up a comprehensive epilepsy centre in Milan,[154] the first in the country, and in which he introduced SEEG on the French model. In Ireland, a surgical programme was started by H. M. Carey, who had trained at the Karolinska in stereotactic neurosurgery with Lars Leksell[155] and in Zurich with Yaşargil. In Germany, modern surgery started in the mid-1980s, and a survey in 2004 showed 14 programmes and about 500 surgeries per year. In Norway, epilepsy surgery was started in 1949 by the neurosurgeon Kristian Kristiansen,[156] who trained with Penfield. In Greece, epilepsy surgery started in 2001 and in Finland between 1988–99 in Kuopio and then in Helsinki.

---

[152] The team was led by the neurosurgeon David Thomas, the neurophysiologist David Fish and the neurologist Simon Shorvon and neuropsychiatrist Michael Trimble.

[153] Olivecrona trained with Cushing and practised in Stockholm, becoming the first Professor of Neurosurgery at the Karolinska Institutet.

[154] With the neurophysiologist L. Tassi and neurologist Guiiano Avanzini. Avanzini made distinguished contributions to clinical and experimental epilepsy, and served both as Treasurer and President of the ILAE between 1997–2005.

[155] Lars Leksell developed his novel arc-centred stereotactic frame (in contrast to the Spiegel-Wycis Cartesian corordinate system) and subsequently developed focused radiosurgery using what was termed a 'gamma knife'.

[156] Kristian Kristiansen was trained by Arne Torkidsen, became involved in the resistance against German occupation in the war and had to flee to London to join the Norwegian government in exile. Between 1947 and 1949 he trained further with Penfield in Montreal. He was appointed Professor of Neurosurgery in Oslo in 1961.

Outside Europe, surgery also began to flourish, often established by individuals trained in London, Montreal or one of the American centres. The situation in Australia was a prime example. Peter Bladin[157] was the pioneer, setting up a surgical programme and appointing the next generation of epilepsy specialists who were all to become international figures, such as Sam Berkovic, who trained in epilepsy in Montreal, and Ingrid Scheffer and Graeme Jackson, who both trained in epilepsy in London. In the early 1980s, three other Melbourne hospitals set up epilepsy services, including that of Mark Cook, also trained in epilepsy in London, at the Royal Melbourne Hospital, which became a leading and innovative international centre. Between 1969 and 1991, more than 200 temporal lobe resections were carried out in Melbourne, and between 1990 and 1997, 226 temporal lobe and 40 extratemporal lobe epilepsy surgeries were performed. Epilepsy service also developed in Sydney, in 1989 in Perth, and later in other states.

Non-resective surgical techniques also evolved, especially in relation to hemispherectomy. As we have seen, by 1960 the operation was quite widely employed and considered relatively safe – an assessment which, however, proved overly optimistic. The classical operation left a large subdural cavity, and as time passed slow leakage of blood into the cavity caused haemosiderosis and hydrocephalus – disastrous complications that occurred in up to one-third of cases and resulted in severe, progressive and untreatable disability and inevitable death. The classical operation was therefore abandoned around 1970 and variants which avoided these complications were devised. The first was the 'functional hemispherectomy', first described in 1974 by Rasmussen, in which the cortex was undercut so that its connections with the rest of the brain were severed. As there was little removal of brain tissue, no cavity was formed, and late deterioration was thus avoided. Other functional variants, mainly concerned with reducing the amount of tissue removal, were then subsequently proposed. With all such operations, viable, potentially sentient but disconnected brain tissue is left in situ and this has seemingly obvious ethical implications; however, these have been little debated. Another anatomical variant was devised by Christopher Adams in Oxford in 1983, in which the hemispherectomy cavity was created extradurally, not subdurally, and this also considerably reduced the risk of complications. All these operations are nevertheless mutilating. No other neurosurgical procedures remove (or disconnect) so much brain tissue, and hemispherectomy could be a success only if employed in situations where there was little normal functioning brain tissue in the hemisphere to be resected or disconnected. Although life-saving in severe infantile epilepsies, and effective in controlling epilepsy, patients were left with multiple neurological problems, and control of seizures was achieved only at a price.

[157] See Bladin, 'Reflections on a life in epilepsy'.

By the late 1970s and 1980s, section of the corpus callosum was another non-resective surgery that had become quite widely adopted. In 1982 a conference was held in Dartmouth in which various centres reported their clinical and experimental results,[158] painting an optimistic picture of surgical progress. However, by 1990 the fashion for this operation too was diminishing when, just as in van Wagenen's surgery, long-term results were recognised to be poor and most of these operations were deemed futile.[159] The operation was then almost entirely superseded by vagal nerve stimulation. This involved a simple and safe non-cerebral operation and rapidly became a popular option, although its effects on seizures were modest (with almost no patient gaining seizure control), palliative rather than curative, and even in that regard frequently completely ineffective.

Another new non-resective surgical procedure devised in this period was the so-called multiple subpial transection (sometimes called the Morrell procedure after its originator, Frank Morrell).[160] This involved the creation of parallel rows of cortical incisions 4–5 mm deep, over the area of the epileptic focus, which produced an effect on the brain surface similar to that of a ploughed field. The rationale was that the transections severed only the horizontal connections between brain cells, thereby preventing the recruitment of neighbouring neurons essential for the production of synchronised epileptic discharges, whilst preserving normal functions which are largely dependent on vertically oriented fibres. In practice, however, it became clear that fibres in all orientations are cut, and it is not clear whether improvements in epilepsy were due simply to non-specific damage to the cortex. It had been hoped that the transections would be particularly useful in areas of the brain where resection would result in significant neurological deficit (so-called 'eloquent cortex'), such as the primary motor, sensory or language areas of the brain. However, early enthusiasm for the operation was rapidly tempered, and the idea that significant neurological damage or symptoms could be avoided did not stand the test of time.[161]

The EEG assessment for epilepsy surgery also underwent great changes during this period. In the early 1960s an inter-ictal scalp EEG was usually all that was required. Once prolonged video-EEG recordings became possible, ictal EEG was considered a prerequisite for surgery on the basis that inter-ictal EEG was unreliable as a method of localisation (which it clearly is, despite early claims to the contrary). Invasive EEG began then to be increasingly pursued,

---

[158] Reeves and Roberts, *Epilepsy and the Corpus Callosum*.

[159] At the time of writing, this is now a rarely performed operation, confined to cases of the severe Lennox–Gastaut type of epilepsy or to epilepsies due to large unilateral acquired frontal lesions in which resection is sometimes combined with an anterior callosotomy.

[160] Morrell, Walter and Bleck, 'Multiple subpial transection'.

[161] It is now an operation mainly carried out only around the edge of a resection cavity of a lesion adjacent to eloquent cortex.

TABLE 4.6 *Reported number of surgeries carried out for epilepsy: From responses to the questionnaires from the Palm Desert meetings in 1986 and 1992*

Type of surgery	Before 1986	1986–1990
Anterior Temporal lobectomy	2336 (68%)	4862 (59%)
Amygdalohippocampectomy	ND	568 (7%)
Extratemporal resection	825 (24%)	1073 (13%)
Lesionectomy	ND	440 (5%)
Hemispherectomy and large multilobar resections	88 (3%)	448 (5%)
Corpus callosotomy	197 (6%)	843 (10%)
Total	**3446**	**8234**

(nb: These are the numbers of surgeries reported, but it has to be noted that such figures are often overestimates).
(From: Engel, *The Surgical Treatment of the Epilepsies* and 'Update')

and in the 1980s a number of epilepsy surgical centres arose with invasive EEG telemetry at their centre. By the 1980s EEG data was correlated with data from CT scanning, PET and SPECT scanning, digital angiography and magnetoencephalography. Complex technical protocols were promoted by the leading surgical teams, but still only small numbers of patients were actually operated on.

The take-up of epilepsy surgery was stimulated to the greatest extent by the arrival of MRI on the epilepsy stage. The visualisation of structural pathologies which previously were not possible to detect gave surgeons new confidence. To the surgical mind, if an abnormality could be *seen* and not just inferred, then the temptation to remove (resect) it was much stronger. By the early 1990s, methods had been established for quantitatively assessing, with great accuracy, the extent and position of the structural changes of hippocampal sclerosis, and this in particular boosted the lure of temporal lobe surgery.[162]

Epilepsy surgery, from its inception, had its champions and advocates. In this period, Jerome (Pete) Engel was one of these. He hosted the two Palm Desert conferences and considered that almost all the centres conducting epilepsy surgery in the world were represented there.[163] In 1986, 44 worldwide centres completed his questionnaire, and 113 in 1992 (with results summarised in Table 4.6). The numbers of cases reported by these centres to have been operated upon had roughly tripled – no doubt as a result of the widespread introduction of MRI and also perhaps Engel's strong promotion. In America, 26 epilepsy surgery programmes reported performing approximately 500 therapeutic surgical procedures in 1985, and by 1990 this had risen to 67 programmes performing approximately 1,500 procedures in total. Around two-thirds of patients with temporal lobe resection, neocortical resection and

[162] See Cook et al., 'Hippocampal studies'; Jackson et al., 'Detection of hippocampal pathology'.
[163] For the 1986 conference findings, see Engel, *Surgical Treatment of the Epilepsies*, p. 727; for the 1992 conference findings, see Engel, 'Update'

hemispherectomy were said to be seizure-free (at least in the short term), but only 7% of those undergoing callosotomy. Despite the threefold increase in the number of operated cases, there were large numbers of potential candidates for surgical treatment who were not offered this option; Engel estimated this to amount to 100,000 persons in America alone, with 5,000 new cases being added each year. Although some considered the figure to be an exaggeration, Engel's message was clear and compelling, and he and the ILAE campaigned vigorously for more surgical activity.

It was initially thought that MRI would reduce the need for invasive EEG, but in fact the fascination of correlating findings from MRI and invasive EEG proved too seductive to resist.[164] In addition, angiography was used to plan the position of the implanted electrodes, making depth recordings much safer. Increasingly complex and expensive protocols were adopted for presurgical assessment, but, in marked contrast to pharmaceutical treatment, regulatory oversight was minimal then and remains so. Furthermore, no controlled assessments of the incremental value of these new and complex protocols were then (or since) performed and it remains quite unclear, to this author at least, whether intensive EEG examinations were really necessary on the scale at which they were (and still are) undertaken. Neither the side effects nor the gain in efficacy had been fully explored. In some centres at least, the commercial potential of this approach and the attraction of monetary profit have dominated clinical decision-making.

The establishment of multidisciplinary teams (MDTs) – involving specialists in neurosurgery, neurology, pathology, neurophysiology, neuropsychiatry and neuropsychology – was another feature key to the success of epilepsy surgery. Such teams were established in a number of worldwide units, each with a different emphasis. The paradigmatic early examples were the MNI, where Penfield was joined by neurophysiologist Herbert Jasper and psychologist Brenda Milner, amongst others; the Sainte-Anne Hospital in Paris, where from the beginning neurosurgeons, neurologists, psychologists and neuro-physiologists collaborated and devised the anatomo-electro-clinical method; and the Maudsley Hospital in London, where Murray Falconer was joined by prominent figures in the fields of pathology, psychiatry and neurophysiology, and where many aspects the pathological basis and psychiatric consequences of temporal lobe epilepsy had been defined. In this sense, epilepsy led the surgical world.

---

[164] At the Palm Desert conferences in 1986 and 1992, the circulated questionnaire also enquired about presurgical evaluation. By 1992 ictal video-EEG telemetry was always recorded in around three-quarters of patients, but only 2–3% of centres always performed depth EEG (compared to 11% in 1986), and between a third and a half never did (similar figures applied to the use of strips and grids, functional imaging, and PET and SPECT scanning [Engel, 'Update']). MRI was not enquired about, but presumably was done in all cases.

In this period, the approach to resective epilepsy surgery developed in two different directions, especially after the advent of MRI. In North America and in the United Kingdom, where MRI studies were most intensive, the emphasis of surgical assessment was on the visualisation of structural lesions and the correlation of the lesion to the epileptogenic focus. Conversely, the French and Italian programmes were focused more on neurophysiological processes and the existence of epileptogenic networks. In all centres, though, increasing emphasis was placed on intracranial recordings and on advanced MRI techniques, and as time passed the two approaches have moved closer together.

Ward ended his 1983 review with 'clues to the future', predicting that for patients in whom resection was not feasible, chronic stimulation of subcortical targets to provide inhibitory input into the epileptic focus would be beneficial (he seemed to favour the fields of Forel, as proposed by Sid Watkins some fifty years earlier) or stereotactic lesioning, for instance in the cingulum. This preference was slightly surprising, as stimulation of those deep structures had been in vogue and then abandoned. In fact, Ward's predictions were partly correct and a new wave of brain stimulation did develop some decades later, but as with the earlier attempts, has so far failed to make much impact. Paradigmatic, though of the futility of prophesy, Ward did not mention MRI once in his review, and hardly mentioned invasive EEG, yet it was these technologies that advanced epilepsy surgery to the greatest extent..

EPILEPSY IN THE WIDER WORLD

In the first half of the twentieth century, most scientific and large-scale clinical research in epilepsy was conducted in the United States, Britain, continental Europe and Japan, where the professional leaders in the field were also based. In other developed areas of the world, little epilepsy research was performed. Moreover, the small literature from developing countries was in part contributed by sociologists or anthropologists with a special interest in traditional treatments and beliefs.

By the mid-1970s, however, medicine had moved a long way down the path to becoming the global village it now is.[165] Western concepts and practices percolated across the world, and were embraced especially by the educated and upwardly mobile classes. The growth of international institutions, mainly instruments of global capitalism, the rapid rise in air travel and rising standards of living all raked the ground, enabling the flowering of social and medical change in diverse parts of the world. In the field of epilepsy, another factor was

---

[165] The term 'global village' was coined in 1964 by Marshall McLuhan, writing on the cultural impact of modern communication technologies. See McLuhan and Powers, *Global Village*. It is equally applicable to the highly efficient and globalised information networks of medicine.

the increasing reach of the pharmaceutical industry, which developed new markets and funded professional activities to promote products – to such an extent, in fact, that the industry in many countries controlled almost the entire epilepsy treatment agenda through its marketing and promotional efforts. The World Health Organization (WHO) and World Bank were the most influential international institutions, and both created policies which favoured the implementation of Western medical practice, for instance in the field of pharmaceuticals. In epilepsy, as in other conditions, the WHO focus was largely on primary healthcare, stimulating research into the management of epilepsy by non-medical healthcare workers in rural areas and the production of simple manuals of epilepsy treatment.[166] Then, following the economic recessions of the mid-1980s, the expenditure on health by the World Bank began to dwarf that of the WHO. The momentum shifted to health sector reform, focusing on financing and organisational issues to maximise efficiency and effectiveness. The international professional organisations also moved to the fore, and the ILAE and the IBE in particular played growing roles in guiding epilepsy policy in many developing countries.

As a further consequence of the forces of medical globalisation the medical concepts, care and treatment of epilepsy began to exhibit a sameness throughout the world which was in some ways regrettable. What was lost in this process is not possible to know, but loss there must have been.

The development of epilepsy in Australia, India and Zimbabwe serve as illustrations of the worldwide trends.

Epilepsy in Australia

Prior to the European settlement of the continent, almost nothing was recorded about epilepsy in Australia, although Mervyn Eadie quotes Gustave Hogg's observation that the Tasmanian aboriginals knew about 'madness and convulsions [which were] believed to be due to an evil spirit'.[167] In the colonial era a system of training and the style of medical practice were entirely transplanted from the mother country. Institutions and hospitals similar to those in Britain were set up, and almost all the early neurologists spent a year or more of their training in Britain, and to a lesser extent in North America. Their resulting epileptology remained closely aligned to Western models throughout the century.

---

[166] Amongst these were the studies of ICBERG (International Community Based Epilepsy Research Group), which were the topic of an entire session at the League's International Congress in New Delhi in 1989. See also Shorvon et al., *Management of Epilepsy*.

[167] Eadie, *Flowering of a Waratah*, p. 1. An excellent history of the development of neurology in Australia that provided much source material for the text.

During the late nineteenth century, rapidly expanding Australian towns made no special provision for epilepsy. There were no neurologists, and people with epilepsy were either kept at home or consulted private doctors in the community. Where home care was not possible, many ended up in gaols (in 1877, for instance, in the state of Victoria, 7–18% of all prisoners had epilepsy),[168] at least until provision could be made in the newly founded lunatic asylums. As in the European capitals, public disquiet was expressed repeatedly about the management and abuses of the asylum system. Asylums became the subject of reports and commissions, although no specific action regarding epilepsy was ever taken.

In this period, all medical officers were government appointees. Medical schools were set up all over the country, and a system of medical education and clinical practice was established based on the British model. The *Australian Medical Journal* was founded in 1856 as the forum for Australian medicine,[169] but for the next eight decades it contained almost no reference to epilepsy. One early paper reported a presentation made on 3 March 1886 by the prominent and fashionable Victorian physician William Springthorpe to the Medical Society of Victoria, describing his experience of twenty-one patients with epilepsy. Springthorpe referred to concepts of the cause, pathogenesis and treatment of epilepsy which were very much in line with contemporary European thought and with no specifically Australian features.[170] The first, and for many years the only, epilepsy facility in Australia was the Talbot Colony Farm for Epileptics, founded in 1907 after a campaign by the National Council of Women of Victoria. The colony was built and run along the lines of the colonies at Bielefeld in Germany and Chalfont in England, and its founders were fully apprised of the principles of the colony movement in Europe.[171] Agricultural work was provided for the males, domestic and indoor work for the females (sewing mostly) and a special school for children. Medical and

---

[168] Bladin, 'A century of prejudice'. Conditions in the prisons must have been terrible. Bladin reports that no treatment is mentioned, and the death rate was said to be extremely high (30% of all epileptics in Ballarat goal, for instance, in 1900).

[169] Renamed several times. Since 1914 it has been published under the title *Medical Journal of Australia*.

[170] Springthorpe was a celebrated physician who had spent several years of postgraduate training at the National Hospital, Queen Square and was clearly fully apprised of Jackson's and Gowers's writings. His treatment recommendations included: the removal of peripheral irritants; potassium bromide and, if this failed, zinc oxide, belladonna, cannabis, digitalis; ligature around an affected limb as a counter irritant in focal seizures; caffeine and nitroglycerine in petit mal; and a seton tied in the nape of the neck, a treatment he attributed to Samuel Wilks (cited in Bladin, 'John William Springthorpe').

[171] An important influence was the publication of the 1893 report of the Charity Organisation Society ('*The Epileptic and Crippled Child and Adult*'), which was almost certainly widely read in Australia at the time.

academic input was minimal.[172] In 1961, when the colony closed, it was still the only epilepsy facility in the country. In 1936 a report from Australia provided a glimpse of the distribution of care for epilepsy patients in the state of Victoria:

> There are about 150–160 epileptics at the Talbot Colony. Practically none of them can be regarded as sane. In the institutions of the Mental Hygiene Department there are 230 epileptics with Congenital Mental Deficiency, and there are 210 more who can be regarded as insane. I happen to know 2 or 3 sane epileptics and doubtless there are a fairly large number of epileptics who can be regarded as responsible. My view is that for these, private medical attention is all that is required. They will not go to a clinic – they will not go to a colony. It is only when there is disorder of conduct, irresponsibility, mental deficiency or deterioration resulting from epilepsy that the question of colony or institutional treatment arises.[173]

Up until the Second World War, and during the war, there was little evidence of any specialist clinical work for epilepsy, nor of any basic research, and no specialised civilian or military neurologists. Epilepsy was hardly mentioned in the official Australian records.[174] It is interesting, too, that epilepsy was very rarely referred to in the eugenic publications of the period. Indeed, epilepsy seems to have been thoroughly under the radar.

It was the development of neurology in Australia that led to a flowering of specialised epilepsy work. The first neurologists in Australia emerged in the 1940s, amongst whom was Edward Graeme Robertson, a graduate in medicine from Melbourne who trained in neurology in London. He returned to the Royal Melbourne Hospital and was appointed there and to the Royal Children's Hospital as a neurologist in 1944. At the time there were two neurologists in Melbourne, one in Sydney and none elsewhere. Robertson was the first Australian neurologist to write on epilepsy, publishing several clinical articles on the condition.[175] By 1950, eight neurologists had been appointed in Australia, and over the subsequent decade, as the specialty

---

[172] As a medical facility, it seems to have failed to live up to its promise. By 1928 Springthorpe noted there were 'quite a number of patients [who] would do equally well as chronic dements in a chronic asylum at a saving of expense'. He called for the 'admission of a better class of patient, less deficient mentally and more open to improvement'. See Bladin, *Prejudice and Progress*, p. 134.

[173] 'Institutions for the care and treatment of epilepsy in different countries of the world'.

[174] Walker, *Clinical Problems of War*. Epilepsy was mentioned as being 'incompatible with capacity for service', and isolated seizures were thought to be rare presentations of malaria or electrolyte disturbance (pp. 308–9). Apparent convulsions were also noted to be an occasional symptom of hysteria (p. 689).

[175] Perhaps the best clinical paper from Australia was that of Robertson, 'Epilepsy as a symptom'. Robertson described the different types of seizure patterns arising in different cerebral locations, but this was work carried out when he was in London. On returning to Australia, one senses that the facilities for research were not available and that clinical work was too pressing for any further academic study.

developed an elevated academic status, appointments began to be made in most of the larger Australian medical schools. By 1960, the number of neurologists had increased to twenty-six, almost all of whom had done their postgraduate neurology training in Britain, most for at least part of their time at the National Hospital, Queen Square.

The first physician to develop specialised epilepsy services in Australia was the neurologist Peter Bladin, who was appointed to the Austin Hospital in Melbourne in 1965 to head up the new neurology department.[176] In 1959–60, he obtained his postgraduate qualifications at the National Hospital, Queen Square, but found that it was the psychiatrists (especially Denis Hill) and the neurosurgeons at the Maudsley Hospital, and not the neurologists at the National Hospital, who were most interested in epilepsy. On his return to Melbourne, Bladin worked to recruit a multidisciplinary team. In the mid-1970s he set up an epilepsy programme based on the Maudsley and Montreal models, but with a particular focus on the psychological and social aspects of the disease. Bladin made meticulous studies of outcome that confirmed what Hill and Pond had noted in the 1960s: that successful surgery was not simply a matter of controlling seizures. It also involved an adjustment to life after epilepsy and dealing with what Bladin and colleagues famously named 'the burden of normality'.[177] Citing Ferguson and the Rayports' observation that epilepsy 'may serve both as a weapon and as a shield', Bladin and his co-authors wrote that on being rendered seizure-free, some patients are 'effectively disarmed, no longer receiving the consideration extended to the chronically ill. New intrapersonal and interpersonal demands may be required of the patient, for which he or she has limited experience and life skills. Thus, the return of seizures due to failed surgery may represent a welcome return to the previous situation'.

The Epilepsy Society of Australia was established in 1986, and Bladin was its first president. In 1989, aided by Dreifuss, the society became the Australian chapter of the ILAE. Development of lay organisations in Australia occurred first in Melbourne, with the founding of the Victorian Epilepsy Bureau in 1964[178] (which changed its name to the Epilepsy Foundation of Victoria in 1978).[179] Thereafter, clinical services for epilepsy progressed apace in Melbourne and

---

[176] Bladin has described the early development of epilepsy in Australia in his papers: Bladin, 'Reflections on a life'; Bladin, *Prejudice and Progress*. Both have been the source of detail in this account.

[177] Wilson, Bladin and Saling, 'The "burden of normality"'.

[178] As has been, and remains, almost always the case, the lay organisations were formed as the result of lobbying and fundraising by committed individuals with a close personal interest in epilepsy – Mary Davis and Greg Hirsch in the case of the Victoria Epilepsy Bureau.

[179] Other states followed suit. In 1983 the National Epilepsy Association of Australia (NEA) was formed, with the intention of having a national rather than a state-based organisation. However, the NEA later split into factions, and different state organisations were formed.

Sydney, and subsequently in other Australian centres. Research also flowered, and Australia came to rank highly in epilepsy clinical work and research. A series of gifted figures emerged performing innovative work in, amongst others, epilepsy genetics, experimental epilepsy, MRI imaging, chronic invasive EEG and seizure prediction.

Epilepsy in India

From the seventeenth century until independence in 1948, mainline Indian medicine was the product of the colonial administration. The East India Company was the first to install doctors in the country, but they were in very short supply and primarily responsible for the health of the military and the European colonists. After the British government took over control of the country from the East India Company in 1858, hospitals began to be built, often relying on philanthropic support, to serve the population. In parallel, a large number of dispensaries were created, which were preferred by many Indians who were suspicious of hospitals with their associations with foreign power. By the early twentieth century, the colonial government had established a system of general hospitals, mental hospitals and medical schools. But there were no neurologists in the country, and epilepsy treatment, if any, was carried out in asylums by psychiatrists often out of touch with contemporary Western developments (although not always, see p.171). Private Western-trained doctors treated the educated and the wealthy, but most of the population relied on traditional healers and Ayurvedic medicines. Only a very small percentage of persons with epilepsy had access to any western medicine.[180] Epilepsy seems not to have been the topic of any academic study, and, as elsewhere, patients' voices went almost completely unrecorded.

As in Australia, the profile of epilepsy within medicine in India began to change in the 1940s and 1950s with the establishment of neurology in the country's major cities.[181] In this fledgling specialty, epilepsy was recognised immediately to be the most common condition and a potentially treatable one, and all the early Indian neurologists focused on the topic. In the absence of any formal neurological training in India, those learning the speciality spent periods

For a time, the idea of a nationwide lay epilepsy movement was lost (it has, however, more recently been resuscitated).

[180] One East Indian Company doctor, William O'Shaughnessy, experimented with Indian hemp (cannabis) for various ailments and published his findings in the *Provincial Medical Journal*, where it excited much interest. Almost immediately John Reynolds found it effective in epilepsy, and called it 'one of the most valuable medicines we possess' (Pain, 'High times'). Other East India company doctors collected herbs for use in epilepsy.

[181] Srinivas, *Indian Epilepsy Association*. This book is the source of much of the information in the text.

of time abroad, usually in Britain or North America. EEG was just emerging as an exciting and promising technology, which further encouraged interest in epilepsy. India's first neurosurgeon, Jacob Chandy, and the neurologists Baldev Singh, B. Ramamurthi, S. T. Narasimhan, Eddie Bharucha and T. K. Ghosh all spent time in the United States, Canada and Britain, and came back to India well aware of Western neurological thought. Between 1949 and 1954, departments of neurology were set up first in Vellore (Chandy and Singh), Madras (Ramamurthi and Narasimhan), Delhi (Singh), Bombay (Bharucha) and Calcutta (Ghosh). In 1951, Singh, Chandy, Ramamurthi and Narasimhan created the first professional organisation – the Neurological Society of India (NSI) – and in the 1960s an epilepsy section was formed within this organisation.

A particular landmark in the story of epilepsy in India was the founding in 1970 of the Indian Epilepsy Association (IEA), which worked in conjunction with the NSI epilepsy section. The IEA was remarkable for the extent to which lay persons and doctors worked together in the charitable field, and in this sense was an example to the world. The IEA became an IBE member and led what was to become a special emphasis on the social aspects of epilepsy in India.[182] Within two years chapters had formed in Bombay, Madras, Delhi and Bangalore and the IEA had applied to the ILAE for membership. However, the poor relations between the ILAE and the IBE at an international level had resulted in a rule that no national organisation could be a member of both, and official membership of India in the ILAE thus had to wait until 1997, when a separate professional organisation, the Indian Epilepsy Society, was formed and became the ILAE chapter, whilst the Indian Epilepsy Association remained affiliated to the IBE. Making a distinction between lay and professional organisations in India, as in many other countries especially in the developing world, was senseless, not least because the lay organisations were usually run by doctors. Few patients would dare to challenge a doctor or would want to do so, and in general the neurologists in India were more engaged in voluntary work in epilepsy, and took a more synoptic and less exclusively medical view of epilepsy, than those in Europe or North America. India's lack of membership in the ILAE notwithstanding, the 18th International Epilepsy Congress of the ILAE and IBE was held in New Delhi in 1989, and was the first of the ILAE international congresses to feature heavily on its programme the problems of epilepsy in developing countries. The Indian neurologists also played an important role in the World Federation of Neurology. Noshir Wadia, who established the second department of neurology in Bombay in 1957, and Eddie

---

[182] The leading figures in the formation of the Indian Epilepsy Association were B. Singh, B. Ramamurthi, T. K. Ghosh, E. P. Bharucha, A. D. Desai, N. H. Wadia, K. V. Mathai, K. S. Mani and Mrs R. H. Dastur. All were to become leading figures in Indian neurology and Indian epilepsy. All had a deep interest in epilepsy.

Bharucha both served as vice presidents.[183] As a result of the link with the international organisations, India became the leading representative of neurology and epilepsy in the region.

Epilepsy was a highly stigmatised condition in India. The IEA became very active in attempts to alleviate stigma, and set up a number of programmes which distinguished it from Western models. It ran monthly camps for patients, gave awareness lectures in school and colleges, conducted seminars aimed at primary care physicians and ran regular counselling services, self-help groups, yoga classes and holiday camps for children.[184] In few other countries was the lay organisation so active on the ground, and many neurologists and psychiatrists gave freely of their time in supporting and promoting these activities.

One sign of the burden of having epilepsy in India were the eugenical laws – the Hindu Marriage Act of 1955, and the Special Marriage Act of 1954, which specifically stated that if either party suffered from epilepsy or insanity, a marriage could be annulled. Between 1987 and 1996, K. S. Mani and Eddie Bharucha, on behalf of the Indian Epilepsy Association, petitioned prime ministers and parliament to change the law, and in 1996 the association successfully filed a public interest litigation before the supreme court. The clause was finally removed in 1999. Another campaign led by Bharucha succeeded in removing the law which classed those with epilepsy as insane.

Mani[185] led the Bangalore chapter of the Indian Epilepsy Association for many years. He had founded the Department of Neurology at the All India Institute of Mental Health and Sciences in 1957, and was appointed professor and head of the department in 1969. He was indefatigable in his advocacy for patients, and a great showman, famous for his imitations of epileptic seizures on the conference stage. He arranged enormous meetings for his patients and their families, and I remember speaking at one in which more than 1,000 persons were present. The IBE honoured Mani with the Award for Social Accomplishment in 1997 and the ILAE with the Lifetime Achievement Award in 2001 – posthumously, for he died after a short illness before he could attend the ceremony (George Burden is the only other person to have received both awards).

---

[183] See Bharucha, Katrak and Singham, 'In memoriam: Noshir H Wadia'; Shah and Seshia, 'Dr. Eddie Phiroz Bharucha'. Eddie Bharucha was trained in neurology at the National Hospital in London. He returned in 1952 as a founding father of neurology in India. He also served as President of the Neurological Society of India in 1956 and was President of the XIV World Congress of Neurology in Delhi in 1989. He had a huge neurology practice in Bombay and was renowned for his kindness and compassion.

[184] The holiday camps for epileptic children were especially innovative. Doctors ran the camps, parents were excluded, and the children played games, were read stories and gained confidence in their abilities.

[185] See Meinardi, 'K. S. Mani'.

Clinical research in epilepsy in India began to develop after 1980. Research initially focused on epidemiology (not least the Yelandur epilepsy control study, which involved Mani and others; and epidemiological studies amongst the poor in Mumbai and Pune); studies of attitudes and practice of epilepsy in rural populations; the specific causes of epilepsy in India (for instance neurocysticercosis); and specific types of epilepsy (the studies from NINHAMS in Bangalore on hot-water epilepsy are a notable example). The international contacts of many individual neurologists were important for epilepsy in India, as was the support of the pharmaceutical industry, which saw great financial opportunity in the vast population of the subcontinent.

The examples of Australia and India are illuminating in a number of different ways, and have interesting parallels. Both had a colonial history, and in both a reasonable colonial medical structure existed with an imported Western-style medical education and medical practice. However, epilepsy was largely neglected until the specialty of neurology developed after the Second World War. Where institutional care was needed, it was provided largely in lunatic asylums (or prisons) until well into the twentieth century. In neither country were epilepsy colonies well developed, but in the second half of the twentieth century, with the development of specialisation, neurological and neurosurgical units were established in which epilepsy featured strongly. In both countries, exceptional individuals exerted strong personal influence on emerging epilepsy services. These epilepsy facilities were based entirely on Western models, and leading physicians and surgeons spent periods of training in Britain, other European countries or in North America, which ensured the hegemony of Western scientific medicine, as did contacts with the international epilepsy movement through the IBE and the ILAE. The pannational pharmaceutical industry also ensured that therapy followed Western lines. Despite their reliance on Western models, in both countries leading practitioners were particularly interested in local social and societal perspectives, although in Australia epilepsy in the indigenous aboriginal populations seems to have been largely ignored. The lay and professional organisations were important and contributed greatly to the strides epilepsy made in both countries. Studies of traditional systems of belief about and attitudes to epilepsy, or of its treatment, were not a primary concern in Australia, but were carried out in India and widely elsewhere.

Epilepsy in Zimbabwe

Sub-Saharan Africa was one of the areas of the world which was a focus for the ILAE and its Global Campaign Against Epilepsy (pp. 575–581). Data from Zimbabwe illustrates the extent to which such external campaigns can and cannot achieve change, as well as the extent of the need for basic care and the dependency on technology. The facilities for epilepsy have been described by Gifte Ngwande, one of the only two full-time neurologists in the country in 2020,[186] and are typical of many countries in the region. Neurology and neurosurgery in Zimbabwe had got off to a good start, with inspired leadership from Prof Laurence Levy, neurosurgeon, and Prof Jens Mielke, neurologist. Levy was a British national who settled in Southern Rhodesia (now Zimbabwe) in 1956. He was said to be the first neurosurgeon in Africa. He was deeply interested in epilepsy, and his seventh epilepsy surgery patient, Nicholas George, founded the Nicholas George Epilepsy Centre and Epilepsy clinic in Harare (previously Salisbury). Mielke was a German national who moved to Zimbabwe aged twelve, trained in medicine in South Africa and neurology in Britain and returned to Zimbabwe aged thirty-three in 1993. He quickly developed a reputation for his work, and he was commissioned to carry out a demonstration project for the Global Campaign Against Epilepsy on the topic of improving epilepsy care in rural areas of Africa. He travelled monthly to Botswana, where there were no neurologists at all, and sadly his life was cut short in a plane crash at the age of forty-seven. Services in the country had always been stretched by the massive political upheavals in the country: first a unilateral declaration of independence (UDI) from Great Britain in 1965, a long civil war, the long and disastrous autocratic dictatorship of Robert Mugabe (1980–2017) and then the military coup in 2017. Inflation, corruption and political killings marred a beautiful country. Despite the egregious effect of political corruption and mismanagement of the medical services and then a huge HIV epidemic (in 1998 the prevalence of HIV/AIDS in the population was 40%, and it was still 14% by 2020), the physicians and surgeons battled on. By 2020, in addition to the two neurologists, there were 15 psychiatrists, 80 physicians, and 12 neurosurgeons in the country, with its population of 16.5 million and 500,000 persons with epilepsy. There was a single weekly clinic dedicated to epilepsy, but technology was in very short supply: there were 4 EEG machines in the public hospitals in the country (in 2020, all were broken) and 3 in private hospitals; for radiology there were 6 CT and 1 MRI scanners in the public sector and 11 CT and 6 MRI scanners in the private sector, but no dedicated radiologist in the public sector. Medical services were provided in 8 provincial hospitals, 63 district hospitals (with 3–5 doctors) and over 9,000 local clinics run by nurses or GPs. There was no neurology training in the country; young doctors had to do this in South Africa or abroad. The only antiepileptic drug widely available was phenobarbitone, and the only drugs available in the public sector were phenobarbitone, phenytoin, carbamazepine and valproate. The treatment gap was measured at over 85% and the stigma of epilepsy was profound, with many patients believing the cause to be

[186] Lecture to ILAE British Branch, July 2021; Sen et al., 'A neurological letter from Zimbabwe'

possession by demons or evil spirits, other supernatural or God-given punishments, or contagion. Traditional healers were (and remain) the first port of call to help eject the demons, and treatment in the form of ceremony, herbals or many other, often religiously inspired, alternative remedies. In tandem with the Global Campaign, the ILAE and IBE did form professional links for the epilepsy doctors in Zimbabwe, providing moral support and international recognition, if not much else. For patients, cost of treatment was a prime limitation. The average cost of one the newer drugs in the private sector was equivalent to an entire annual salary, or more.[187] A similar gloomy picture was probably repeated in many countries in the developing world.

Epilepsy in Other Countries

Excepting Japan and South Africa, before the 1970s scholarly studies in epilepsy from other countries in Asia or Africa hardly existed. Little research was prosecuted and little was known about the way epilepsy was perceived or treated. This is not to say that the condition did not exist. In fact, the reverse was the case, as the prevalence of epilepsy in the developing world was almost certainly higher than in the Western world, linked as it is to such aspects as neonatal care, nutrition, infectious disease and demographic differences. Where medical studies were performed, they almost always originated in Europe or the United States, sometimes in collaboration with local medical centres, and were firmly in the Western medical tradition.

From the 1970s onwards, as part of the trend to globalisation, the ILAE began to take a particular interest in epilepsy in developing countries. The league then had no chapters in Africa and only a few in Asia. A meeting was planned for Kampala but was cancelled in the wake of Idi Amin's coup d'état. In its place the ILAE arranged a travelling seminar on epilepsy which visited seven African countries in 1972. In 1973, Meinardi called for the establishment of an ILAE commission on developing countries, which in fact was only realised in 1986 when Meinardi was elected ILAE secretary-general. The commission stimulated much activity, and in subsequent decades the problems of epilepsy in developing countries rose in prominence.[188]

---

[187] In 2020, a typical salary of a teacher or mid-range civil servant is equivalent to around US$200/mn. The cost of a CT scan in the private sector was $215 and in the public sector $40; of an MRI $250–300 in the private sector and $100 in the public sector; and of an EEG $100–150 in the private sector and $20 in the public sector (data from G. Ngwande, lecture to ILAE British Branch, 2021).

[188] The concept of the epilepsy treatment gap was one result of this focus.

In some countries, attention began to turn to traditional views about epilepsy. The similarities and differences in cultural beliefs and societal attitudes about epilepsy would, it was hoped, put Western dogma into perspective. The earliest studies of epilepsy in the developing world came from the fields of social anthropology and ethnology, and a leading figure was Arthur Kleinman, trained both as a physician and anthropologist. He favoured the 'illness narrative'[189] as a method of exploring the ethnographic aspects of diseases such as epilepsy. Two books of the period exemplify this approach.

Call Mama Doctor: African Notes of a Young Woman Doctor (1979), is an account written by a Norwegian doctor, Louise Jilek-Aall, working amongst the Wapogoro tribe in Tanganyika in the early 1960s. In this region, epilepsy was common (known in Swahili as *kifafa*, meaning 'the little death'). Owing to the tortured expression of the sufferer, convulsions were believed to be the product of possession by a powerful spirit. Onlookers moved away when seizures occurred in the belief that the spirit might jump to any person in contact with the sufferer's saliva or excrement. The afflicted were ostracised, even by their family members, and led a miserable life of humiliation and fear. Children were forbidden to attend school or gain employment, and their families were shunned:

> *Kifafa* is looked upon not only with fear but also with shame. It is a disgrace to the entire family and is believed to be caused by witchcraft or to be the punishment for certain misdeeds of the afflicted himself or of his kin. The parents' quarrel might lead to *kifafa* in their child, or if a mother is unfaithful during the time of pregnancy, she or her child might become epileptic. Breaking the taboos, alcohol abuse, laziness or other vices incur ancestors' wrath. They might punish the family by sending the evil spirit of *kifafa* (pp. 191–2).

Sometimes the young persons with epilepsy were left to fend for themselves in huts in the bush. Jilek-Aall tells the story of one child who became a helper in her clinic. When he developed epilepsy, his parents told him

> never to touch another person; his food was prepared in separate dishes and he had to fetch his own water from a waterhole far away. Even at night he had to stay away from the others and sleep alone close to the door. With growing grief he realized how everybody, even his mother, avoided his company ... [T]he parents finally decided that he had to leave the home. His father knew of an old abandoned hut in the forest. That was where he would have to live ... The boy remembered how desperately frightened he was when he found himself abandoned there in the forest. In the beginning

[189] Kleinman defined the illness narrative as 'a story the patient tells, and significant others retell, to give coherence to the distinctive events and long-term course of suffering' (Kleinman, *Illness Narratives*, p. 49).

> he would run home when fear overwhelmed him, but each time he turned
> up at home his parents became increasingly annoyed and took him back to
> his lonely abode. His father warned him not to come close to the village.
> Anyone knowing that he was an epileptic possessed by evil spirits could
> stone him, chase him away or even kill him (p. 189).

Many of the epilepsy patients Jilek-Aall came across were malnourished, frightened and rejected. Some died from burns when falling into the domestic fire or drowning when fetching water or fishing in the river, or simply from marasmus and intercurrent illness. In 1960 she founded the Mahenge Epilepsy Clinic, which provided care for the local people with epilepsy including treatment with phenobarbital, phenytoin and primidone. In the first two years, she treated 200 cases and, despite repeated difficulties, continued the clinic for many years. Jilek-Aall did not hesitate in choosing Western medicine over what she considered primitive superstition, although she was intensely sympathetic to her patients. She did not question the assumptions underpinning Western allopathic medicine, nor did she acknowledge the fact that it has a distinct and hermetic culture which defines our understanding of disease, its pathogenesis and its symptoms, and dictates the approach to treatment.

This was not the case in *The Spirit Catches You and You Fall Down* (1997),[190] an extraordinary book by Anne Fadiman, who provides a meticulously researched illness narrative of epilepsy in a Laotian Hmong patient, then a refugee in California, which highlights the cultural divide between American and Laotian medicine. Fadiman, who is not a physician but an editor and essayist, tells the story of Lia, a young epileptic girl, and her parents, who believe her disorder to be due to possession by an evil spirit, a dab (*qaug dab peg* – 'the spirit catches you and you fall down'). The illness results in the loss of one of Lia's spirits that was responsible for health and happiness. The spirit was frightened away when Lia's sister slammed the door shut and Lia was captured by a *dab*. Lia's parents felt she should be treated by a shaman, who could negotiate with the spirit world. They were also proud of Lia as they believed that those with epilepsy often became *txiv neeb* (shamans or spiritual healers) when they grew up. The family came up against Western medicine, and a mutual total lack of understanding ensued. Lia underwent many visits to the emergency room and admissions to hospital, where a range of antiepileptic drugs were tried (including phenytoin, phenobarbital, carbamazepine and valproate). Her parents often failed to administer the antiepileptics, which they believed were harmful and made the condition worse. Instead, they sacrificed chickens and pigs to appease the *dab* and sought the help of a *txiv neeb* to find Lia's lost spirit and entice it to return. At one stage the girl was removed by the local child services into foster care for non-compliance. However, Western medicine failed, and the girl suffered severe brain damage

---

[190] Fadiman, *Spirit Catches You.*

due to a bungled diagnosis of sepsis and status epilepticus. When death was believed to be imminent, the Lees were permitted to take Lia home. Two years later, she was still alive and being lovingly cared for by her parents. They had removed all Western medical life support and were hoping to reunite her soul with her body, arranging for a Hmong shaman to perform a healing ceremony with the sacrifice of a live pig in their flat. Lia lived a further twenty-five years in a persistent vegetative state.

The book emphasised various other aspects of cross-cultural misunderstanding. For example, the *txiv neeb* spent many hours with the ill person, at their home, never asking rude or intimate questions, never undressing the patient and treating the soul as well as the body; the Western doctors did the reverse. The doctors were also prone to taking repeated blood samples which horrified the Hmong, who considered the removal of blood to be extremely harmful. The Hmong also shunned anaesthesia, believing that people's souls wander when they are unconscious, as well as surgery, which led to imbalance and disfigurement in the next life. For sanitary reasons, doctors and nurses routinely cut 'spirit-strings' from people's wrists or neck rings, which the Hmong believe held the 'life-souls' of infants. When asked their opinion of medical care, some amongst the Hmong thought that allowing doctors to examine your body was required in order to stay in the United States and that they would be sent to prison if they refused surgery. Doctors also insulted families by directly addressing an Americanised teenager rather than her non-English-speaking father, trying to maintain friendly eye contact, touching an adult on the head without permission and beckoning with a crooked finger. They could lose patients' respect by not acting like authority figures, as young residents did when wearing jeans under their coats, carrying their medical charts in backpacks or introducing themselves by their first names. It was a common belief that a baby's beauty was not to be commented on lest a *dab* overhear and try to snatch the baby's soul, another hazard in Western hospitals. Nevertheless, most Hmong women took the risk of going to the hospital to give birth, as they erroneously believed that babies born at home would not become US citizens. What counts as knowledge was demonstrated by Fadiman to be utterly different in the two cultures. She was clearly on the side of the Hmong, and intensely sympathetic to their views, although she also believed fundamentally in the curative power of Western medicine. The book was widely praised in liberal Western circles; to some in the Hmong community, however, it was perceived as colonialist and racist.

Both these books emphasise the cultural relativity of epilepsy, and of medicine in general, and that is their point. It is also clear that incorporating some of the traditional beliefs into Western methods of treating epilepsy would no doubt add depth and meaning to treatment for patients, a lesson also brought home in ICEBERG and other investigations of epilepsy in non-Western populations.

THE EXPERIENCE OF HAVING EPILEPSY: THE 'INSIDER'S VIEW'

The more progressive societal attitudes and practices towards epilepsy that had appeared in the early post-war years grew stronger throughout the century. Possibly for the first time in history, the voice of many persons with epilepsy began to be clearly heard. There were many reasons for this change, including the rise of science, more effective and less toxic treatments, better education, the perception of epilepsy as a neurological and not a mental disorder, the new liberalism, anti-authoritarianism, and renewed respect for individual rights and those of disabled people. Levels of hostility and stigma encountered by patients greatly diminished. In my view, this fundamental attitudinal change proved of far greater importance to the generality of people with epilepsy than any medical advance.

The formation of the IBE in 1961 was both a consequence of these changing social attitudes and also a stimulus for moving that agenda along. The IBE provided a powerful platform for those acting on behalf of people with epilepsy. Over the next few decades, this shift began to have an impact on medical practice. More respect for the patient's viewpoint took hold, and 'partnership' between doctor and patient gradually became the keyword in practice style. No longer were orders or directions pronounced by the neurologist; rather, the doctor's role was to suggest options and to explain pros and cons. In other words, treatment choice was now left to the patient, with the doctor as adviser. In parallel, the paternalism and elitism of previous generations of neurologists diminished. In the medical centres of Europe, top hats, striped trousers and black jackets (still de rigeur in the 1940s) had disappeared, to be replaced by lounge suits, and later still by jeans, with white coats discarded and a less formal consultation style. These changes, reflected both greater egalitarianism and also the growing power of consumers in all aspects of late-twentieth-century medicine.

The Sociology and Stigma of Epilepsy

It was in this period too that epilepsy attracted the attention of academic sociologists. The distinction between an 'illness' and a 'disease' had been articulated by Talcot Parsons, who described illness as a deviant behaviour because it rendered people unable to fully engage in social roles such as employment or family life.[191] This lead to the study of illness behaviour and the sufferer's experience of illness – the 'insider's view'. An impressive early study was that of Schneider and Conrad, who examined the insider's view by in-depth interviews with eighty individuals from the midwest and east coasts of America between 1976 and 1979.[192] They were interested in how people saw

---

[191] Parsons, *The Social System*
[192] Contained in their book, published in 1981, *Having Epilepsy*.

their epilepsy, and particularly how they negotiated the 'stigma' of epilepsy: 'We cannot understand illness experience by studying disease alone, for disease refers merely to undesirable changes in the body. Illness however is primarily about social meanings, experiences, relationships, and conduct' (p. 205). This was, in a sense, the first move away from the medicalisation of the concept and meaning of epilepsy which then largely pertained. They explored how individuals managed uncertainty, their treatment regimens, the need to acquire knowledge and reduce dependency, the importance of taking control and avoiding parental overprotection, concealment and strategies for conducting relationships with friends and family:

> Illness is a moral experience. When we are sick we soon face new definitions of who we are, what we are capable of, and how others will see us. This is particularly notable for chronic conditions because of their permanence ... Some illnesses, such as epilepsy, are also stigmatised. They carry associated meanings of disgrace and shame beyond the general undesirability of illness itself ... These negative social meanings were often more difficult to contend with than the disease itself. (p. 220)

Schneider and Conrad had a number of suggestions for change: the public image should be normalised by education and legislation; the doctor–patient relationship should change into a partnership; individuals should 'own' their epilepsy, take control and realise their self. And for this openness rather than concealment was a prerequisite. Their call for action was in many ways heeded, and the blueprint for change outlined in their remarkable book has to a large extent remained valid up to the present.

Schneider and Conrad's work was followed by a systematic study of the stigma of epilepsy, published in 1989, by Graham Scambler. He introduced a 'hidden distress model' which he developed out of the earlier work of Erving Goffman.[193] Goffman maintained that societal reactions to epilepsy lower the sufferer's self-esteem, creating the inner sense of being discredited or discreditable, and that over time this injury compromises the sense of identity.[194] Scambler pointed out that stigma is not only external and due to '"normal" people who, ignorant and apprehensive about what epilepsy is, tend to maintain social distance through discriminatory practices',[195] but is also generated internally, is dependant on the perception of the sufferer and is related to personality factors, self-confidence and other psychological attributes. He drew a distinction between 'enacted stigma' and 'felt stigma', the former referring to actual instances of discrimination and the latter to personal feelings

---

[193] Scambler, *Epilepsy*, p. 57.
[194] Goffman, *Stigma*. Canadian born, Goffman's career was mainly in America, where he was appointed Chair in Sociology and Anthropology at the University of Pennsylvania.
[195] Scambler and Hopkins, 'Generating a model'.

of inferiority and unacceptability and fear of encountering stigma.[196] He conducted sociologically structured interviews with ninety-eight persons with epilepsy in London, and found that although nine out of every ten people interviewed admitted to suffering intermittently from felt stigma, only a third could recall having encountered enacted stigma in any of their roles or life activities (even in the form of casual ridicule). He determined that people with epilepsy characteristically adopt a 'special view of the world' in which the fear of enacted stigma predominates. This special view leads the individual to attempt to conceal the condition, and its medical label, and to try to pass as normal. One important consequence of this finding was that felt stigma had a more disruptive effect on people's lives than enacted stigma. A key question in Scambler's view – and one that remains partly unanswered – is to what extent felt stigma is justified. The idea has been extended with the concept of 'self-stigma' which encompassed, for instance, feelings of inadequacy, that I am damaged, I am incompetent, I am not normal, I am a burden, I will trouble others, I will make others feel uncomfortable or embarrassed, I will never be able to make relationships, epilepsy ruins me and so on.

As the long twentieth century drew to a close, in Western societies at least, evidence clearly pointed to a decrease in both felt and enacted stigma as well as self-stigma.[197] Indeed, in a 1994 study of felt versus enacted stigma in Britain, Ann Jacoby found remarkably low levels of enacted stigma and (importantly) little evidence of felt stigma in patients whose epilepsy had gone into remission, suggesting that remediation was possible.[198] Similar findings were reported by others. These trends in the West were encouraging, but in many developing countries both felt and enacted stigma remained strong and exerted powerful influences, adding a heavy burden of stigma to the equally dire oppressive effects of poverty and deprivation. In many ways, the situation in this regard was similar to that in Europe at the end of the nineteenth century, perhaps itself a sign of how deeply engrained these prejudices were; one overall conclusion to draw is that attitudinal change is difficult and slow.

Within a family, epilepsy was (and to a lesser extent still is) often seen as a 'family secret' and felt and self-stigma was exacerbated by parental instruction to deny or conceal the condition. In an interesting study by Scambler and Hopkins, published in 1986, only half of brothers and sisters knew of a sibling's diagnosis, and only one-fifth of children knew of an epilepsy diagnosis in a parent.[199] Similarly, marriage partners were often kept in the dark about the condition. Overprotection of a child was another very common situation, resulting in social isolation and development

[196] Scambler, *Epilepsy*, p. 56.
[197] See, for instance, Caveness and Gallup Jr, 'Thirty years'; Ryan, 'Stigma of epilepsy'; Jacoby, 'Felt versus enacted stigma'.
[198] Jacoby, 'Felt versus enacted stigma'.   [199] Scambler and Hopkins, 'Being epileptic'.

of an insecure, overly dependent and emotionally immature adult. Another central issue for many with epilepsy revolved around employment. Even in 1986, in the advanced economies, more than half of fully employed persons with epilepsy had not disclosed their condition to their employers,[200] despite the fact that repeated studies had shown those with epilepsy to be more likely to value their job and to take less time off with illness than their peers without epilepsy. Similarly, in various studies, around half of employed persons with epilepsy reported having been discriminated against at work, although it is not clear how much this reflected felt or enacted stigma. Lack of ambition was another common problem encountered in clinical practice, as a response to the many hurdles that 'being epileptic' seemed to erect.

Anthropologists and ethnologists also became interested in this area. Arthur Kleinman, for instance, introduced the concept of epilepsy's 'social course':[201]

> The social course of epilepsy indicates that epilepsy develops in a local context where economic, moral and social institutional factors powerfully affect the lived experience of seizures, treatment and their social consequences. The social course of epilepsy, furthermore, is plural, heterogeneous and changing. It is as distinctive as are different local worlds, different social networks, different social histories ... To understand that lived experience we also suggest that the suffering associated with epilepsy has to be viewed as occupying an interpersonal space, a world of local *social experience* that connects moral status with bodily status, perhaps even social networks with neural networks. (p. 1328)

Kleinman suggests that the social course of epilepsy depends not only on stigma or a 'spoiled personal identity', but also on factors inherent in the social experience, 'such as deprivation and delegitimation' (p. 1328). Social experience connects the 'moral status' of the person with the bodily illness, with attendant effects on relationships, employment and social relationships. Any attempt at treatment must consider both factors. This now seems obvious, but the lived experience of a person had been largely ignored in medical descriptions of the disease.

Medicine, always seduced by figures, has attempted to quantify stigma by questionnaires, typically taking the form of knowledge, attitude and practice studies.[202] Since 1980 such studies have been conducted in many developing countries, based on a methodology which did not have the depth or richness of sociological models of stigma. A note of caution is needed in interpreting all these studies, as beliefs and attitudes do not necessarily dictate behaviour, and

---

[200] Scambler and Hopkins, 'Social class'.   [201] Kleinman et al., 'Social course of epilepsy'.
[202] The ICBERG series of studies from Kenya and Ecuador are good examples of these. See Shorvon et al., *Management of Epilepsy*. A fictionalised account of these is found in Farmer, *Snakes and Ladders*.

the relationship between actions and expressed attitudes can be frankly tenuous. This problem is exacerbated by the nature of survey instruments in many studies which were superficial and poorly designed.

Epilepsy in Film, Television and Literature

Epilepsy appeared not infrequently in film and television in this period, trumping literature in the immediacy of its impact. Visual imagery may be more powerful initially than the written word, but the effect of novels is longer-lasting, and creative fiction has proved generally to be more nuanced and more effective in conveying shades of opinion and meaning about epilepsy than film or television. Still, all three media proved capable of conveying public attitudes more strongly and in more depth than any questionnaire or survey.

Two important provisos, however, limit their value for cultural analysis. First, all good creative fiction operates on a variety of levels and is open to different interpretations; ambiguity and nuance defy compartmentalisation, and good literature creates a blur and a vacuum which modern science abhors. Second, attitudes and mores differ widely amongst individuals in a culture at any given time. There are *all sorts and conditions of man* and generalisations have only limited value. Nevertheless, a selective look at post-war films, television and novels does give a broad sense of social attitudes towards epilepsy and how these had evolved. There was in general much more openness and discussion about epilepsy, but there were exceptions. Several major novelists of the period – for instance, Laurie Lee – strove to conceal their epilepsy, in much the same way as did John Cowper Powys a few decades and Edward Lear a century earlier. Like Lear, who kept his 'terrible demon' entirely out of his works, Lee, whose frequent seizures were a central feature of his life and personality, wrote nothing on the topic despite 'his entire opus consisting of fragments of autobiography'.[203]

In the post-war years, in film and fiction, the antagonism and prejudice which were predominant themes of the eugenic age had largely disappeared. By the 1970s, no leading creative work addressed the deleterious effects of epilepsy on civilisation or Western culture in the way that was commonplace in the 1920s and 1930s, nor was an epileptic seizure the butt of comedy or satire as was the case in the days of silent film. Epileptic rage and violence continued to function as a dramatic device, especially in more popular and less intellectual work, and fear of epilepsy and isolation remained prominent themes. In the early post-war years the condition was still often treated in a patronising and infantilising manner, but this too diminished in later decades. As time passed, films and novels began to paint a more naturalistic and generally more

---

[203] Grove, *Laurie Lee*, p. 563.

sympathetic and adult view of epilepsy than did earlier efforts. Although a period of transition, there were nevertheless still notable exceptions to the generally more positive stance. The theme of the family shame of epilepsy, so commonly portrayed in the earlier eugenic era, was still depicted, for instance in Masha Norman's play *Night Mother* (1982; adapted into a film in 1986), which won the 1983 Pulitzer Prize for drama, in which the old subtexts of degeneration and the psychopathic family rear their heads. The lead character, Jessie, has epilepsy and planned to commit suicide (with her father's gun) – she sees herself as ugly, was divorced and epileptic, dependent on cigarettes, with a son who was a thief and drug addict and an inadequate, lonely mother. She had been told by her mother that the epilepsy was due to trauma, but in the last day of her life it transpired that her father had epilepsy, that it was hereditary – a family curse kept secret from all.

In both film and fiction epilepsy sometimes functioned as a device to move the story along or to change the direction of the narrative, rather than as a basis for exploring character or attitude, as it had always done. Although film was generally not nearly as prejudicial towards epilepsy, nor as damaging, as it had been in the past, old stereotypes were not infrequently repeated, potent symbols of how slowly attitudes change. In her analysis of sixty-two films featuring epilepsy as a theme,[204] Sallie Baxendale noted that the idea of epilepsy as an inherent flaw persisted in several films and novels. *La Storia* (1986) is an example. Based on the 1974 novel by Elsa Morante, it tells the story of a woman, Ida, who was raped by a German soldier during an epileptic seizure and whose child, conceived during the attack, also had epilepsy. The child, named Giuseppe, turned into a sensitive and gentle boy, open and innocent, much like Myshkin in *The Idiot*, but he, too, died during an epileptic seizure. In her grief, Ida ends up in a lunatic asylum. Baxendale also noted that even in these post-war years, epileptic characters were often still depicted as disturbed, violent or as having degenerate personalities – although it has to be said that the depictions are far less venomous than previously. Examples include *I Pugni in Tasca* (*Fists in the Pocket*, 1965), *La Vie de Jésus* (*Life of Jesus*, 1997), *The Bone Collector* (1999, based on the book by Jeffery Deaver), and *'night Mother* (1986; based on the play by Marsha Norman). The theme of concealment of epilepsy also persisted, as in *The Andromeda Strain* (book by Michael Crichton 1969; film 1971), and *The Lost Prince* (2003), a historical movie about Prince John. Baxendale notes that in earlier films, epilepsy was concealed from the audience – for instance in *A Matter of Life and Death* (1946) or *Snow White and the Seven Dwarfs* (1937) – whereas the audience is 'let into the secret' in films made after 1960. Indeed, in later films a prominent theme is the struggle of

---

[204] Baxendale, 'Epilepsy at the movies', which followed a lecture at the 2012 International Congress of Epilepsy in which Baxendale showed extracts of films depicting epilepsy and seizures.

persons who are open about epilepsy. Baxendale also observes that '[t]here is a strong gender bias in the ways in which epilepsy is portrayed. Male characters with idiopathic epilepsy tend to be mad, bad, and are commonly dangerous, whereas the same disorder in their female counterparts evokes exotic intrigue and vulnerability' (p. 769).

In other work, various new ideas emerged albeit mixed with old stereotypes. Crichton's sci-fi thriller *Terminal Man* (1972),[205] turned into a film in 1974, depicts the link between epilepsy, crime and loss of responsibility with an imaginative commentary on attempts to alter personality by neurosurgical means. The central character, Harold Franklin Benson, has epileptic fits following a head injury in a car accident: 'These blackouts ... were often preceded by the sensation of peculiar, unpleasant odors' (p. 14). They then evolved, 'becoming more frequent and lasting longer ... He often regained consciousness to find himself in unfamiliar surroundings ... [H]e never remembered what occurred during the blackout periods' (p. 14). During these periods, Franklin carried out violent assaults (pp. 15–18). He was diagnosed as having 'Acute Disinhibitory Lesion syndrome' and submitted himself to an electronic brain implant in his amygdala to control the seizures. The treatment was planned to work as follows: as soon as a seizure started, the electrodes would pick it up and send an electrical stimulation to the same area (the amygdala) (pp. 21–3). However, the stimulation had the opposite effect causing a state of increased violence and sexual pleasure, and after the operation Franklin learned how to deliberately increase the rate of seizures. That in turn led to an orgy of violence, including the attempted rape of the (sympathetic) junior doctor looking after him. Of course, the story is a mixture of fact and a great deal of fantasy. Disinhibition can be caused by traumatic brain injury, and stereotactic destruction of the amygdala was a recognised (though by then largely abandoned) therapy. Temporal lobe seizures were also known to occasionally cause intermittent violence, but Crichton's fiction attributed prolonged and planned rape and other extremely violent behaviours to epileptic seizures. This depiction is highly inaccurate, and the treatment largely invention. All the same, the portrayal of epileptic seizures as extremely violent and beyond control is an archetype embedded deep within contemporary cultural consciousness. Crichton was medically qualified, although he never acquired a licence to practice, and his disillusionment with medicine and with human misuse of technology resulting in catastrophe were common themes in much of his work (*Jurassic Park*, 1990, is another example). The control of human behaviour by computers was a subsidiary theme of the book and a device typical of Crichton's oeuvre. The fictional extrapolation of epilepsy provided an ideal dramatic example, but also added to the stigma and distress of

---

[205] *The Terminal Man* was actually first published in a different version in *Playboy* magazine.

people with real epilepsy. So much so, in fact, that the American Epilepsy Foundation complained that it was 'unjust to epileptics'[206] and Crichton had to publish a rejoinder in later editions of his book. In another of his novels, *The Andromeda Strain* (book, 1969; film, 1971; TV mini-series, 2008), Crichton depicts epilepsy as a danger to civilisation. Dr Leavitt (male in the novel, female in the film; and whose name was changed to Dr Chou in the mini-series), one of a small team of scientific researchers, hides the fact that he/she has epilepsy but then has a seizure at a crucial time. The event caused the team to lose the opportunity of neutralising a microbe (the Andromeda Strain) that menaced the world. Had she/he not had epilepsy, the disaster would potentially have been avoided – although in the end, all ends happily as the microbe mutates to become harmless. As in *Terminal Man*, epilepsy was utterly wrongly portrayed as a potentially dangerous disease that threatens others – a theme harking back to late-nineteenth-century criminology.

In their analysis of 242 films, the Kersons see seizures being used in different ways.[207] These include driving the narrative and 'genre enhancement', for instance making a comedy funnier, as in the 1921 film *Leap Year*, or more violent, as in the *Curse of the Living Corpse* from 1964 (p. 327). Crichton's book can be viewed as one such example. Images of seizures persist at one level because they are dramatic and visually interesting, and these types of literary narrative devices are in some ways entirely legitimate.

However, Kerson and Kerson note that seizures are also used to evoke a specific emotional reaction, such as compassion or disgust, and to support behavioural traits, such as violence, vulnerability and fragility or voyeurism (as in the 1953 film *Cleopatra*, whose heroine watches Caesar have a seizure through a spyhole). The use of seizures in these ways is prejudicial and stigmatising, and should be recognised as such. But the dividing line between a legitimate and a prejudicial narrative device is difficult to draw. They suggest

> that writers and directors create interesting, positive, forceful, and well-drawn continuing characters who manage epilepsy as a part of their healthy and successful lives ... [and] find new opportunities to counter [stigma] with examples reflecting contemporary scientific understanding. Why not have the advocates for those with epilepsy control the gaze? Have the world see epilepsy as we would like it to be seen! (p. 334)

Sadly, this was, and is still, not the case.

As pointed out by Irma Ozer,[208] herself a disabled person, this was a period, when novels, film and TV did often portray people with epilepsy as 'normal' and 'that there are human beings who have epilepsy (rather than who are epileptics). These human beings are simply part of the continuum of what we

---

[206] Cromie, 'Bestseller unjust to epileptics?'   [207] Kerson and Kerson, 'Truly enthralling'.
[208] Ozer, 'Images of epilepsy'.

know as normal: no more and no less than merely human'. Examples of the fictionalised characters she cites were the heroine Daphne in Rona Jaffe's novel *After the Reunion* (1985); Daniel Cooper, the central character in Richard Pollaks' 1987 novel *The Episode*; Zora in Terry McMillan's 1989 novel *Disappearing Acts*; and Geoffrey, the child of the heroine Diana in the 1990 novel *Dearly Beloved* by Mary Jo Putney.[209] She also notes that in this period, many novels, television and films overtly and consciously 'advocate' for epilepsy.

Snakes and Ladders[210] (1993) is a fictional account of the real-life ICBERG epidemiological studies in Ecuador and Kenya (the ERGO studies in the book!). The book was unusual in focusing not on the findings but the process of the research project, and how it was entangled with, and dependent on, the complicated emotional lives of the researchers. At the centre of the story is a charismatic Canadian drug executive, Carter Jacoman, whose global pharma company had bankrolled the projects and whose commercial interest was in studying untapped markets for epilepsy drugs in Third World countries. Carter though, was more interested in science and epilepsy than in the Swiss company's bottom line, and so were the neurologist David and his wife Anna – indeed, in actual fact, it was from this study that the concept of the treatment gap emerged, and other findings related to the prognosis of untreated epilepsy and the success of treatment amongst the rural poor. Buffeted also by personal and domestic crises, Carter brought his Boston manners and energies to the uncomprehending – and, to him, incomprehensible – rustic settings (the epilepsy equivalent of the east coast executive Macintyre in the 1983 film *Local Hero*), and the story tells of how the complicated running of such studies are universes away from the boardrooms of New York, London or Basel. Anna – the central protagonist of the novel and a medical anthropologist – interviews those with epilepsy and their community leaders and reveals a full range of beliefs and attitudes (these were not fictional but based on real data). The social implications of epilepsy amongst the uneducated and the poverty stricken are faithfully described. In Kenya, for instance, *Lead Informant #12*, a local pastor says: 'My community thinks it [epilepsy] can be caused by witchcraft. I too think it might be. I think those people are dangerous to the community, and I would not like my son or daughter to marry one of them' (p. 235). Her subjects with epilepsy have a range of beliefs: for instance, that 'kifafa' (epilepsy) is caused by a lizard in the head, by breaking a taboo or by the patient's mother breaking a taboo, is a curse from ancestors, is transmitted by touch, causes headaches/stomach aches/depression and so on. The focus of the book, however, is not on the results of the

---

[209] The point is emphasised in a 'note about epilepsy' at the end of the novel in which she writes: 'Even now, epilepsy is a little understood condition that can arouse fear and prejudice. Nonetheless, in the past as well as the present, many people with epilepsy lived reasonably normal lives.' She also records that '[In] Great Britain the terms "seizure" and "fit" are both used, and that usage is reflected in this book. However, I would like to note that in the United States, the preferred term is "seizure."' (p. 354)

[210] Farmer, 'Snakes and ladders'.

studies, but on how the private internal lives of the personalities colour the research work, and how circumstances conspire to cause complex and tangled diversions which often threaten to derail the collection or analysis of data. Side-swipes are taken at the pharmaceutical industry, as well as local doctors, whose agendas and prejudices and jealousies ('internal torments', as the Ecuadorian neurologist puts it) nearly destroy the projects. Reading the book reminds one that the outcome of epidemiological research depends on the weakest link in a chain, which might often be, as Kleinman once put it, the village night-watchman. The ladders in the title are career paths in global pharma, and the snakes the consequencies of misdirected attempts at healing. There is no other fiction which portrays the reality of the research process so well, with its dependence on personalities, grievances, and hidden agenda, none of which appear in the dry output of scientific journals. Nothing better reveals the relativity of science, as Andrew Clifford put it in his *New Scientist* book review (20 March 1993):

> Farmer has offered what seems like a surprisingly easy path through the art/science divide. Crammed with theories, statistics, definitions (maybe not high science, but certainly a good deal of hard, factual stuff) as the book is, nothing is lost or diminished in any way by being integrated into a gripping, ever melodramatic tale of relationships and personalities. Instead, the reader receives a panoramic human picture of science.

THE INTERNATIONAL LEAGUE AGAINST EPILEPSY AND THE INTERNATIONAL BUREAU FOR EPILEPSY

International organisations in many fields of medicine, including epilepsy, flourished in the post-war years and grew larger in size and influence. And, despite their internal arguments, this was such a period of faltering expansion for both the ILAE and IBE.

The Rise and Fall of Epilepsy International

Following the failure of attempts in the 1960s to develop a closer relationship between the ILAE and the IBE, new leaders and a seemingly more progressive professional climate reignited the possibility of joint action in the early 1970s. The suggestion was made that the two organisations should form an 'International Epilepsy Foundation' on the basis, quite obvious, that both shared similar goals, that competition was corrosive and that shared resources would bring efficiencies.[211] Over the next eight years this proposal lumbered along, consuming energy and engendering bitterness and contention. Ultimately, like previous efforts, it failed.

---

[211] This section borrows extensively from Weiss and Shorvon, 'International League Against Epilepsy', pp. 76–7, 77, 78–9.

The project started brightly. In 1973 the executive committees of the ILAE and the IBE agreed to make the president and secretary-general of each organisation ex officio members of the other's executive. In 1974, Penry told the League's executive committee that the presidents and secretaries-general of both had met in Bethesda in June and formulated 'long-range plans of more intimate cooperation [that] will be discussed later'. At the same meeting, Ellen Grass, president of the IBE, cited questions she heard regularly in soliciting funds: 'Isn't there more than one organisation? . . . What do they do that you don't do? Are you quarrelling with one another? . . . Just what is it all about? We're confused'.[212] The December 1974 issue of the IBE's newsletter carried the first public notice of the proposal (a declaration of intent signed by David Daly and Penry for the ILAE and Grass and George Burden for the IBE), laying out the principles of cooperative action. An organisation named Epilepsy International was created, with the aim of combining appropriate programmes, a newsletter and fundraising activities through a shared office and administrative staff. Epilepsy International was to be an umbrella organisation, within which both the ILAE and the IBE would retain their separate identities, although an aspiration remained, if all went well in the future, at some point to merge the two into a single entity. The proposals were overly optimistic, and soon relationships began to sour. By 1977 little progress had been made, and petty arguments delayed movement. Originally, Epilepsy International was run from the IBE office in London and an office in Washington. But political pressure resulted in the setting up of a single office in Geneva – Switzerland being considered 'a neutral country'. Nonetheless, there were ongoing wrangles about finance, and the resignation of executive director (Richard Gibbs). The office then moved to Milan, where an honorary executive director (Patsy McCall-Castellano) was appointed. During this time, the congresses of the ILAE and the IBE were badged as Epilepsy International events, which in reality meant very little. In 1981 the ILAE and the IBE consulted their member countries about a merger. Although the IBE Assembly had accepted the proposal, the motion was voted down in the ILAE General Assembly by twenty-eight votes against and fifteen in favour, with four abstentions. ILAE president Mogens Dam had supported the proposal. In an editorial in *Epilepsia* in 1982[213] after the vote, he reiterated his belief that it was 'much more effective to have one organisation' and blamed the hitherto ineffectiveness of Epilepsy International on a lack of resources and changes in personnel. He had wished to strengthen the organisation and hoped that the ILAE vote to reject the proposal was due to 'too little information available about the ideas behind Epilepsy International'. He made a plea for a single organisation at the international

---

[212] Weiss and Shorvon, 'International League Against Epilepsy'.
[213] Dam, 'Message from the President'. Dam was ILAE president between 1981 and 1985.

level, even if both ILAE and IBE chapters were to remain at a local level, but the ILAE leadership was split with some dedicated behind the scenes to undermining Dam, and he received only lukewarm support. After limping on for another two years, Epilepsy International was finally dismantled in 1984. It was a bruising encounter. At the heart of the conflict were personality clashes, petty jealousies and a feeling in the ILAE that the IBE benefitted more. Underlying all this was the turf battle between doctors and patients – a recurring theme in twentieth-century Western cultures.

The failure of Epilepsy International meant that the joint annual symposia were no longer held, and the IBE and ILAE went their separate ways. However, both executive committees continued to include the presidents and secretaries-general of the other as ex officio members facilitating communication, and both organisations continued to be joint organisers of the quadrennial scientific meetings.

The ILAE after Gastaut: Kiffin Penry and Fritz Dreifuss

Penry's life and academic work are briefly sketched out elsewhere in this volume, and here is outlined his time as the crucial post-Gastaut leader of the ILAE. His initial involvement was as secretary of the League's first Commission on Antiepileptic Drugs. He became secretary-general in 1973, and president in 1977. He joined the executive at a turbulent time. In 1973, Gastaut's preferred candidate as vice-president had been turned down (the first time the General Assembly had rejected the executive's proposed candidate), and relations between Gastaut – who viewed this as a personal insult – and the League became strained. Otto Magnus had also resigned over what he perceived to be slander, innuendo and mistreatment by the executive, and the ILAE changed guard in an atmosphere of bitter rancour. Penry managed to overcome these ominous beginnings. Despite his focus on NIH and on US epileptology, he was a keen internationalist who supported efforts to expand ILAE activities into developing countries and encouraged European developments. He took a personal interest in those colleagues with whom he came into contact, charming all with his enthusiasm and drive. The ILAE had set up a pharmacological advisory committee in 1969. This committee first met in Scottsville, Arizona, in September 1971, during the aforementioned workshop of the NIH Epilepsy Branch (planning publication of the first edition of *Antiepileptic Drugs*). Penry was a key figure in both. In 1973 the committee evolved into the ILAE Commission on Antiepileptic Drugs, which held its first symposium on the topic during the 12th International Congress in Barcelona in 1973. By 1974 the commission had published its own guidelines for the clinical testing of drugs, and had made recommendations about antiepileptic drugs and laboratories for measuring drug levels. In all of these activities, Penry's organisational vision and genius were much in evidence. His achievement in joining together NIH and ILAE activities in basic and clinical research and practice in relation to antiepileptic drugs did much to stimulate activity in this field. He expanded the ILAE's membership and fostered relationships between the League and the pharmaceutical industry. He was a keen advocate of Epilepsy International, and its demise represented one of the few projects that he failed to successfully prosecute.

When Penry's term as ILAE president came to a close in 1981, his friend and colleague Fritz ('Fred') Dreifuss was appointed secretary-general.[214] Dreifuss was born in Dresden in 1926 and as a Jew was forced to flee with his family, first to South Africa and then to New Zealand. He received his medical degree from the University of Otago, and underwent postgraduate training at the National Hospital in London, before moving in 1959 to the University of Virginia in Charlottesville. There, he indulged his growing interest in seizure disorders. In the 1960s he and Penry became collaborators and close friends. Under the aegis of NIH, Dreifuss developed the Comprehensive Epilepsy Program in Virginia, described earlier, which became a model for projects worldwide. He also carried out studies of EEG treatment in petit mal epilepsy, and published a definitive description of the automatisms of absence seizures and of the effectiveness and side effects of valproic acid. He installed radiotelemetry at the University of Virginia and made landmark studies of the 24-hour pattern of spike–wave discharges. He served on the ILAE's Commission on Classification and Terminology from 1977 until his death in 1997, and for most of that time was its chair. At the conclusion of his term as ILAE secretary-general in 1985, he was elected as the League's president. He organised symposia and lectured extensively, and was a brilliant teacher. Dreifuss was famous for his refreshing plain-spokenness and was a master of the mot juste, an attribute as rare as it was useful in navigating the hostile political waters of the international epilepsy movement. Despite his fame he was utterly modest and fully dedicated to even the most deprived patients, who adored him. He died of lung cancer in 1997 at the age of seventy-one, at the height of his powers.

By then, the ILAE had become the premier international professional association in the field of epilepsy, and its executive committee, voted in by the chapters every four years, automatically became a prominent voice in epilepsy matters worldwide. In the years following Gastaut, Penry and Dreifuss, one American (David Daly), and two Europeans (Mogens Dam from Denmark and Harry Meinardi from Holland) held the presidency. Meinardi was born in France in 1932 but moved as a young child to the

---

[214] Porter, 'In memoriam: Fritz E. Dreifuss'.

Dutch East Indies.[215] During the course of the Second World War he was interned in a labour camp and separated from his parents, whom he never saw again. This experience had a deep and wounding influence on his life and philosophy. He trained in medicine at Leyden, and after a period of research in New York moved to the Instituut voor Epilepsiebestrijding at Heemstede, the leading epilepsy colony in Holland, where he worked from 1966 to 1992. He was also appointed Professor of Epileptology at the Catholic University of Nijmegen. In the great tradition of Dutch epileptology, he was interested as much in the social aspects of epilepsy as in the scientific aspects, and he worked tirelessly on behalf of persons with epilepsy. Meinardi was an inspiring leader. In addition to serving as President of the ILAE (1989–93), he earlier had served as President of the IBE (1977–81) – the only person so to do – and in both roles he spearheaded action in the underdeveloped world, not least by establishing the ILAE Commission on Developing Countries. Under Meinardi's presidency, the number of ILAE commissions more than doubled to twelve, as he was keen to involve a much greater number of people from around the world, thus greatly expanding the reach of the League. Later in life he developed an interest in the history of epilepsy and was instrumental in salvaging the ILAE archive, which he indexed and arranged. He died in 2013, choosing euthanasia as he faced the onset of dementia.

The ILAE made good progress during these years, moving, as Dreifuss put it, from 'a saltatory to a more continuous activity'.[216] With money pouring into congresses, the League's chapter numbers doubled and its finances burgeoned, from assets of around $4,000 and 20 national branches in 1970 to more than $1,300,000 and 48 chapters in 1995.[217] *Epilepsia* became established as the premiere epilepsy journal under the successive editorships of Arthur Ward, Jim Cereghino and Tim Pedley. Successful international congresses were held, for a period annually. The Vancouver meeting in 1978 was the first stand-alone meeting held by the ILAE and the IBE, which no longer needed the congress framework provided by other organisations. In total, 350 fifty papers were presented, representing around 600 authors, in a pattern of plenary and parallel sessions which would provide the format for all subsequent meetings.[218] This congress had no commercial sponsorship, but that was soon to change. The first

[215] See Perucca and Reynolds, 'In memoriam: Harry Meinardi'.

[216] Weiss and Shorvon, 'International League Against Epilepsy'.

[217] The term 'branch' was changed to 'chapter' in 1973. The reasons are unclear, and it is a pity, as 'branch' evoked Lennox's image of the ILAE as a tree, growing and expanding – perhaps the tree of knowledge. Only the British branch resisted this change in terminology (a particular preference of its then president Tim Betts) and still retains its original title (for a few years in the early 2000s the term 'branch' was changed to 'chapter', in line with other countries, but then the term 'branch' was reinstated).

[218] The 350 papers and abstracts were published as a book: Wada and Penry, *Advances in Epileptology*.

satellite symposium was held at the 1982 London congress. By 1995, around 2,000 delegates were attending the congresses, which lasted 5 days and featured up to 8 satellites in addition to the main programmes – as a raft of new drugs entered the arena and the pharmaceutical industry ploughed money into advertising and sponsorship. In these few years, epilepsy had become a global commercial product, bringing in its wake an unexpected windfall for the ILAE.

After the refounding of the ILAE in 1935, national congresses also began to be held, albeit taking different forms in different countries. The British branch provides an example of how one such chapter developed. The inaugural meeting was held in 1936 with thirty-five founding members present and seven scientific papers given. A second meeting was held in 1937, before the war interrupted the series. The third meeting took place in 1945, and thenceforward they were held annually. Up until the 1980s these meetings were half-day affairs, polite and quiet, with usually one keynote or international speaker followed by a series of research papers. The meetings all took place at the National Hospital, Queen Square without sponsors or pharmaceutical industry involvement. The only extravagances were cups of tea and plain biscuits, the cost of which was met by the minimal registration fee. The 1984 bylaws stated that the 'meeting should be held in one day, with a morning session, lunch and an afternoon session if there was sufficient work. Each talk was 15 minutes or less and with discussion time limited for 5 minutes. No reporters were allowed to be present and no account of the meeting was to be transmitted to the National newspapers'![219] Then everything began to change, fuelled, as were the international meetings, by sponsorship from the pharmaceutical industry. In 1997 the first annual scientific meeting outside London was held in Oxford, and thereafter the annual general meetings moved around the United Kingdom. The programmes were expanded to include more didactic lectures and invited reviews. Poster sessions were introduced, along with increasingly large commercial exhibitions and satellites. The branch has also held semi-regular meetings with other national and international groups, the first being in Dunblane in 1968 with the Scottish Epilepsy Association. Of particular interest were the joint meetings of the British–Danish and Dutch branches of the ILAE, the first of which was in 1981 in Heeze in Holland, with the fortunate accompanying persons being treated to a tour of a wooden shoe factory and a folklore evening. The third meeting, held in York in 1986, was the 50th anniversary of the British branch and its biggest meeting to that date. Spread over 3.5 days, the event attracted more than 500 delegates and featured a large exhibition with 12 commercial firms and 122 posters. In 1990, the meeting expanded into the Northern European Epilepsy Symposium, held in Aalborg

[219] British Branch of the ILAE, *Bylaws*.

in Denmark. This grouping and these symposia ceased when the ILAE developed its own regional European congresses, the first being in 1994.

Throughout the earlier part of this period, the agenda of the League's executive remained infuriatingly inward-looking, with changes to its constitution, manoeuvring around voting and infighting over finance dominating their meetings. External activity was restricted to clinical topics, and the rapid growth in laboratory science had, it seemed, passed largely unnoticed. This was to change, however, with the establishment of more commissions, and in 1991 of the first workshop in neurobiology (the so-called WONOEP) by Jerome Engel. The WONOEP series of conference workshops has continued and basic science thereafter acquired greater visibility and prominence in ILAE activities. In 1991, too, for the first time the abstracts of talks and posters (more than 500 in total) at the ILAE congress were published as a supplement of *Epilepsia*, putting the programme into the public arena. What was absent up to this point was any major public initiative by the ILAE on behalf of people with epilepsy – and this was to be remedied in 1993 with the start of planning for the Global Campaign Against Epilepsy.

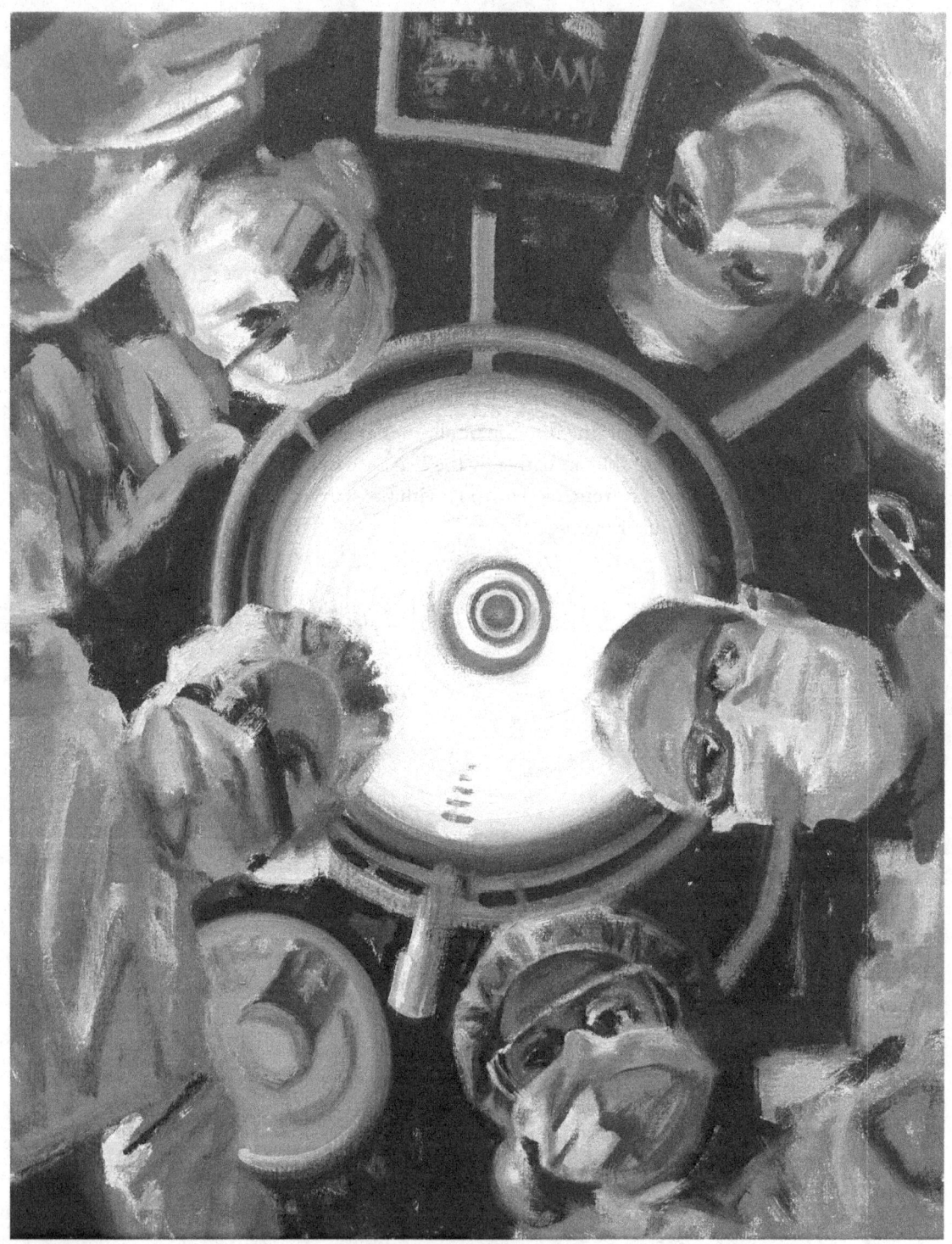

37. **'What must it be like to undergo an open craniotomy?'** (A painting by David Cobley, 2021).

FIVE

1995–2020: THE EPILEPSY FLOODS ARE TOO RECENT

HISTORY IS MERCURIAL. ITS SHAPE, DEPENDENT ON CONTEXT, changes as time passes. Scale is important – a 200-year view of world history might highlight the impact of industrialisation, but a 500-year view the rise of the European empires. Not long ago, it was common to view the twentieth century as 'short', framed by the Russian revolutions of 1917 and the fall of the Soviet Union in 1991. Now this view seems almost irrelevant in the wake of global capitalism and the inexorable rise of China. If the nineteenth century was England's century, and the twentieth America's, the twenty-first century may well be China's – a possibility scarcely contemplated in the 1990s.

It goes without saying that the appearance of this last quarter-century of *Epilepsy's* voyage is likely to be very different today to the shape it will take in the future. It is also obvious that the floods are too recent to guess the final topology of the epilepsy landscape, or which of the myriad waves then carving it will have an enduring impact. Foolhardy indeed are those who think they can predict the future of epilepsy, dependent as it is on the rapidly changing narratives of science, medicine and society.

It is with these provisos that this chapter proceeds. Because of the recency of this period, and despite the fact that much has happened, this chapter is necessarily briefer and more tentative than its predecessors. Here, only a few selected topics are addressed, chosen as those that seem to the author to best define the direction of *Epilepsy's* travel. Another limitation – as explained at the start of this book – is that no attempt is made to adjudge the contributions of *living persons.* Although this undoubtedly weakens the history, and is unfair to some, it is a decision made, surely correctly, in the knowledge that assessing the ultimate impact of individuals on the tide of history is not possible while the flood is still in progress.

During the twentieth century science elbowed out all opposition to become the predominant conceptual framework of medicine. This process was initially rather slow and tentative, but by the dawn of the twenty-first century, the triumph of science was absolute.[1] In my fifty years of practice I have witnessed this profound transformation, and its implications and ramifications have been great. The scientific paradigms of epilepsy prevailed to the exclusion of other perspectives. Sociological and psychological explanations of epilepsy were essentially relegated to the periphery. Non-scientific theories extensively explored in the past, such as psychoanalytical and Marxist interpretations, were hardly ever referred to, and models of disease which focused on such concepts had virtually disappeared from mainstream debate. Everywhere, hard science replaced other ways of thinking. The idea took root that epilepsy could be fully explained by neurochemistry and neurophysiology, molecular genetics and anatomy. The authority of science dominated despite the obvious fact that science has no moral compass and yet medicine, an art as well as a science, requires strong moral guidance.[2]

It was the basic sciences in particular that made the greatest strides. At no time in history had the laboratory proved so important or decisive in epilepsy. Strangely, though, the laboratory topic which had had throughout this history the most impact was that which had had the greatest entanglement with sociological and political theory – the science of *genetics*. There was massive interest in laboratory genetics, with research output and funding growing exponentially. To what extent genetics will make any large positive effect in the clinic is too early to say, but its risks and downsides were also hardly considered. The second area in which both clinical and basic sciences had their greatest impact was in pharmacological treatment; by the end of this period, a range of new therapies had been licensed and, perhaps more importantly, paradigms of drug discovery had changed considerably, with great promise for the future. The purely clinical science of epilepsy lagged somewhat behind, and most disappointing was the endless and wasteful tinkering with classification and terminology.

---

[1] As this book goes to press, the Covid-19 epidemic had proved a paradigmatic example of the rise of science. It demonstrated the central position of science in society and politics and, perhaps for the first time, public attention was heavily focused on science. This may prove to be the virus's lasting legacy.

[2] It is an illusion to think that science is a body of knowledge that sits away from politics – as the history of epilepsy in the long twentieth century has demonstrated.

The supremacy of science was matched by the rise of a more muscular form of capitalism. The fall of the Soviet Union in 1991 had led to widespread disillusionment with centrally planned economic policies. Neoliberal political and economic policies emphasising the individual over collective choice began to take their place at least in the West; in China and the 'tiger' economies of South-East Asia the population were fed stories of 'Asian values' by their leaders to keep a stranglehold on power. Even in one of the most centralised healthcare systems in the world – Britain's National Health Service – an internal market was created to engender competition and, it was hoped, efficiency and effectiveness. Market-driven societies also saw the inevitable rise of consumerism and this had profound effects on the practice of medicine. The role of the doctor, and the doctor–patient relationship, changed accordingly with medical advice increasingly seen as a commodity and a commercial transaction.

In part as a reaction to this, there was also an extraordinary flowering of epilepsy as a topic in the creative arts – wherein it was treated in a more subtle, less hostile and altogether more sympathetic manner than ever before. Epilepsy became more public and more open. Many memoirs and autobiographies of those with epilepsy were published, and it seemed that, at last, epilepsy was not something that had to be concealed or denied. Underpinning all was a lessening of stigma and a greater respect for people with epilepsy, and this was perhaps the most gratifying of all the major changes engulfing epilepsy. However, by the end of this period, the tenets of social democracy, which had ruled in prior decades, were becoming somewhat battered, and its demise was widely trailed. These had been good for persons with epilepsy, and any retreat would be keenly felt.

EPILEPSY HEALTHCARE AND STYLE OF PRACTICE

By the end of the twentieth century, healthcare featured high in government agendas in most Western countries, on a par with defence and education, another extraordinary transformation. In contrast to earlier years, when health was considered essentially a private matter for citizens, most governments were now being held to account on health matters; in many Western countries in the twenty-first century, in the absence of war, it was in fact the major political narrative. For people with epilepsy, incorporating healthcare into government policy had had many benefits. Barriers to access for those with epilepsy fell, and specialist facilities for epilepsy, now firmly in the domain of neurology, flourished everywhere. Nevertheless, in all Western countries, these gains came at the cost of increasing anonymity within a system of healthcare dominated by politics, managerialism and finance. Some with epilepsy claimed this worsened the feeling of isolation and dismissal of their suffering.

Translated into practical healthcare, scientific discoveries are almost always expensive, sometimes considerably so, and often with only small incremental benefits. Since the 1960s, in all countries where governments subsidised or owned healthcare, continued attempts had been made to restrain expenditure and rein in the potential of new science by limiting rising costs.[3] These efforts had proved largely politically impossible, and health expenditures continued to grow. In North America and Europe in 1980, 5–9% of GDP was spent on health; by 2018 this figure had risen to 9–17% (with, furthermore, huge increases in GDP in many countries). In the OECD countries, costs were lower in publicly funded systems than in private ones. For instance, in 1999 about $4,500 per person was spent annually on health in the United States, and between $1,000 and $2,500 in Europe, Australasia and Japan. In low- and middle-income countries, however, not only were the amounts available to spend on health much lower – around $200 per capita per year in much of Asia and Africa – but costs were generally borne by the patient (>80% in India, for instance)[4] and not the state. What became clear everywhere was that costs seemed to have no ceiling. In the latter years of the twentieth century, public debate about health increasingly tended to revolve around finance (or lack of it) – a remarkable shift of emphasis from earlier times, when cost was seldom discussed. Healthcare expenditure rose because inflation in healthcare products was greater than general inflation, populations were becoming older, scientific discovery was creating more and more therapies and diagnostic tools, individuals required increasingly intense care and large corporations had moved into healthcare with a primary goal of profit. Increasing numbers of personnel were involved in healthcare.[5]

In Western countries, however, there were (and remain) wide variations in the underlying priorities of the health system. In Britain and Canada, health systems were built on principles of equity of access and treatment, with a high degree of governmental regulation and cost control. In other countries, such as the United States, principles of equity hardly exist, and the relatively unregulated practice of medicine led to wide disparities, with substandard healthcare

---

[3] The impact of scientific medicine was greatest in infectious diseases and cancer. Moreover, because of better health and nutrition, longevity and life expectancy had risen to remarkable levels, and continue to rise (global life expectancy in 1950 was forty-six years; as of 2020, it was seventy-three years).

[4] Costs in purchasing power parity dollars. According to *OECD Health Data 2000*, the proportion spent in 1999 by government, private insurance or individual patients, respectively, was 84%, 5% and 11% in the United Kingdom; 45%, 37% and 18% in the United States; and 1%, 2% and 85% in India.

[5] By 2020 in Britain, for example, around one in every twenty employed persons in the country worked for the NHS.

for some and world-beating, cutting-edge facilities for those who could pay. New drugs, introduced after 1990, cost up to 500 times more than traditional drugs despite the lack of *any evidence* that they were, at least in population terms, more efficacious. Care, especially of the handicapped, became hugely expensive, as did increasingly complex technologies such as magnetic resonance imaging and invasive electroencephalography. Because epilepsy is, in a significant number of cases, a chronic condition, most individuals required ongoing long-term care, which further magnified the growing expense. Indeed, the 'cost of epilepsy' became a topic for academic research.[6] Also important was the fact that patient and professional groups lobbied hard for better services, access and facilities, and to a large extent they were successful.

Consumerism in the healthcare of epilepsy drove up standards and quality, but at a price. It changed the nature of the doctor–patient relationship and the sociology of epilepsy. On the positive side, there was a consolidation of the partnership model of consultation in which the role of the doctor was to advise, not to dictate, and the paternalism and elitism which had characterised medicine in previous decades largely disappeared. Patients were more respected and their power increased, lay organisations became more vocal, exclusional laws were struck out, and the rights of the disabled and equality of access became political priorities. The patient lobby raised the profile of epilepsy, and it is surely true to say that never before had epilepsy been treated with more equality and fairness. Treating medicine as a commodity though had drawbacks, not the least of which was a loss of trust, and the consequential rise in complaint and litigation.

Medicine in middle-income countries had evolved at a great rate. In the rising economies of many such countries, patients who could afford it were offered, for the first time in their countries' history, levels of healthcare for epilepsy that were similar to those of Western Europe or North America, although provided mainly privately and not by the state. Access, dependent on wealth, was not universal, and in those countries adopting the capitalist model, inequality grew rapidly, with great variation in epilepsy care. Brazil can be taken as an example. In that country of 180 million persons there were, in 2008, around 1,200 neurologists (1 per 150,000 of the population) and the Brazilian Epilepsy Society had 477 members. Fifty-two per cent of neurologists practised exclusively in the private sector, with only 23% in hospitals and only

---

[6] See Cockerell and Shorvon, 'Economic cost of epilepsy', for the difficulties in estimating costs and the limitations of these analyses. Costs were noted to depend on perspective, country and type of epilepsy, and varied wildly. In 1994, in Britain, the direct medical costs of active epilepsy were found to be around £4,000 per patient per year. What was clear, however, was that the indirect costs of epilepsy – for instance, loss of employment, loss of life, benefits and so on – hugely exceeded these medical costs.

3% in the federal health system. In the poorer regions there were 0.1–0.9 neurologists per 100,000 people and phenobarbital was the only widely available epilepsy medication. Centres for rehabilitation of people with epilepsy were (and remain) few, and (as of 2008) only eight centres were accredited to perform epilepsy surgery. Like many such countries, professional and lay organisations played a crucial role in education and information.[7] In India, too, the voluntary sector provided a great deal of epilepsy support through camps run by the Lions or Rotary Clubs or lay chapters of the International Bureau for Epilepsy, with physicians providing time and expertise without payment, and through educational and public health campaigns.

Treatment of epilepsy in low-income countries, where the majority of people with epilepsy in the world resided, was for the poorest no better than 100 years previously. As an example, Senegal, with its 12 million inhabitants, had 17 neurologists in 2007, all situated in the capital city Dakar and all in private practice. Eleven CT scanners were available (6 in the public sector and 5 in the private sector), and there were 2 MRI scanners in the private sector and 4 EEG machines. Epilepsy care was provided for the great majority of the population by non-medical personnel in primary healthcare centres in which only phenobarbital, phenytoin and intravenous diazepam were generally available.[8]

In the West, one response to the economic and societal pressures was for epilepsy healthcare to become progressively more protocol driven and thus more uniform (as in many other areas of medicine). More than ever before, treatment was forced down so-called pathways of care, in a guideline culture that focused on the disease and not any idiosyncrasies or vagaries of an individual patient. Doctors became more technocratic and more sophisticated scientifically, but the medicine they practised was confined by increasingly narrow parameters.

Regulatory hurdles also grew. Antiepileptic drugs were subjected to a lengthy regulatory process (too cautious and too long, in the view of many in the pharmaceutical industry). Even when licensed, reimbursement of the costs of drugs and the more complex diagnostic technologies became subject to bureaucratic limitations in many countries. In practice, availability was limited by competition for funding with other therapies in other areas, or by government priorities or insurance company terms.

Surprisingly, though, none of the expensive high-end epilepsy surgical procedures or investigations (invasive EEG or multimodel epilepsy surgery planning) had been subject to anything but a rudimentary evaluation, either regulatory or even by health technology assessment or cost-effectiveness appraisal. In many cases, it is difficult to see how these represented value for money, or were even of proven clinical effectiveness, but in market-driven health economies they were heavily promoted.

[7] Guerreiro, 'Brazil'.   [8] Gallo Diop and Ndiae, 'Senegal'.

LABORATORY-BASED SCIENCE OF EPILEPSY

By 2020, more scientists and clinicians around the world were working in the field of epilepsy than ever before, and their endeavours were stimulated and interconnected by the revolution in communication technologies. Just as economic capitalism had become globalised, so too had medical science. Research in basic epilepsy expanded in Asia and Australasia, as well as in Europe and North America, and by 2020 especially in China. The work was based in universities, in research institutes and in industry. Never before had the diverse aspects of the underpinning science of epilepsy been studied so widely. Paradigm shifts were few, but the soil of Kuhn's 'normal science' was being intensively farmed. Here only a few examples of this explosion of science can be given, but they give a flavour of the times.

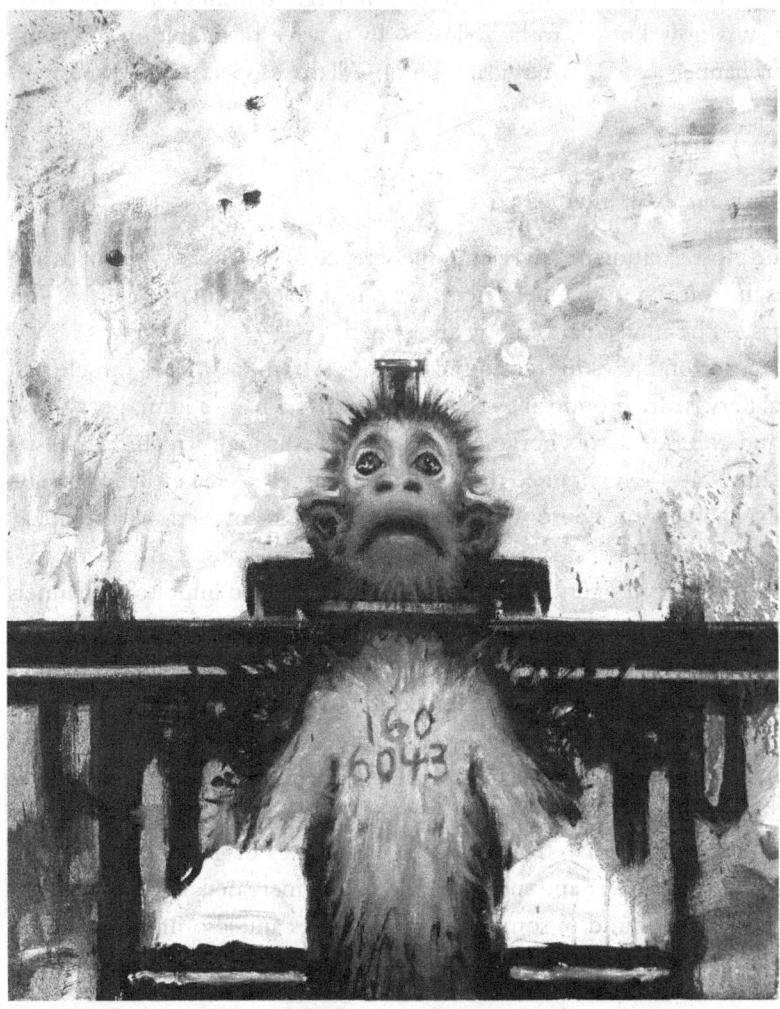

38. **'The experimental model'.** (A painting by David Cobley, 2021).

Mechanisms of Epileptogenesis

The term 'epileptogenesis' was coined by David Prince in 1978 to refer to the abnormal cerebral mechanisms that produce the state of epilepsy. These occur at many different levels, and in the period 1995–2020 enormous progress in understanding these processes was made. Animal models of epilepsy played a major role in the past, but by the turn of the twenty-first century human tissue removed during surgery was also increasingly used, as were other in-vitro laboratory techniques and molecular genetic technologies in a field which previously had largely depended on neurophysiology and neuropathology. The paroxysmal depolarisation shift (PDS) was a key electrical signature studied at the level of the individual neurone and also in neural networks. The effect of a variety of molecular parameters on the PDS became a major line of research. It was recognised that the PDS was generated by the concerted activity of ion channels and glutaminergic transmission. Moreover, activation was now known to be followed by a wave of inhibition involving potassium channels and GABAergic inhibition. All these aspects were extensively studied.

Ion Channels and Neurotransmitters

One of the most exciting discoveries in the science of epilepsy in the 1990s and 2000s was the role of ion channel defects as a causal mechanism of epilepsy. This charge was led by molecular biology and genetics.

The electrical impulses in the central nervous system (as well as muscle and peripheral nerves) are produced by the flow of ions such as sodium, potassium, calcium and chloride across nerve cell membranes through structures known as ion channels. It was recognised that such ion channels were key determinants of the excitability of neurons and the generation of action potentials. Neurotransmitter release at synapses by binding to the post-synaptic neurotransmitter receptors triggers the opening of excitatory and inhibitory channels and the resulting ionic flows underpin the transmission of signals between neurons. Genetic mutations leading to dysfunction of the ion channels were found to affect the excitability of cells (i.e. their ability to transmit electrical currents). Because the epileptic seizure is a state of abnormal neuronal excitability, such mutations in ion channels and neurotransmitter receptors were suspected immediately to be prime suspects in the search for a genetic cause of epilepsy. And so they proved to be. As technologies of genetic sequencing developed, and the power and speed of sequencing increased, abnormalities in various genes were found in some human epilepsies and also in other central and peripheral nervous system disorders. These discoveries stimulated further scientific studies of gene function in animal models of epilepsy and in in vitro preparations.

The first identification of a mutation in a human ion channel gene causing epilepsy was made in 1995 and was followed over the next decade by the detection of other genetic variants in other ion channels and receptors. Using voltage-clamp and current-clamp techniques, the physiological changes brought about by manipulating ion channel and receptor function through genetic mutation or pharmacological means were rapidly identified. The discovery of a mutation of the *SCN1A* gene in human Dravet disease (a rare form of epilepsy) in 2001 led to a focus on the sodium channel. Not unexpectedly, it was first recognised that genes caused loss-of-function defects in inhibitory processes, thus resulting in hyperexcitability (in effect, much as Hughlings Jackson had postulated 150 years earlier). These defects were observed, for instance, in different sub-units of the post-synaptic $GABA_A$ receptor and in presynaptic defects of the sodium channel Nav1.1 in inhibitory interneurons, or dysfunction of axon initial segments, where action potentials were generated and in which many channels are localised (for example, Nav1.2 sodium and Kv7 potassium channels). Perhaps more surprisingly, some gain-of-function mutations were also identified in inhibitory receptors, emphasising the complexity of the system. Similar studies were subsequently carried out on a range of other genetic changes in potassium, calcium, acetylcholine and HCN (hyperpolarisation-activated cyclic nucleotide–gated) channels, and the various subtypes of GABA and glutamate receptors.

Receptor and channel function was investigated by a range of new genetic techniques, such as cloning, inserting channels into oocytes and gene editing, and by the use of selective receptor agonists and antagonists. The work was carried out in the laboratories of leading universities and pharmaceutical companies. Interestingly, much of this work was fuelled by findings from genetic studies of human epilepsy, and it was uniquely in the field of genetics that human discovery led laboratory and animal experimentation.

In the 1980s and 1990s, neuronal pathways in the brain were understood to be served by specific receptor types, and molecular studies showed that the four principal categories of glutamate receptors existed in a number of distinctive sub-units. The diversity of responses elicited by glutamate was found to be related to the different combinations of sub-units making up the receptor, and similar findings were made in relation to the GABA receptor. One major consequence to epilepsy of the explosion of knowledge in the fields of molecular biology and molecular genetics was renewed interest in epilepsy in the pharmaceutical industry, especially in relation to ion channel function and glutamate and GABAergic conduction. Numerous compounds were developed and studied in the hope of influencing channel and receptor function.

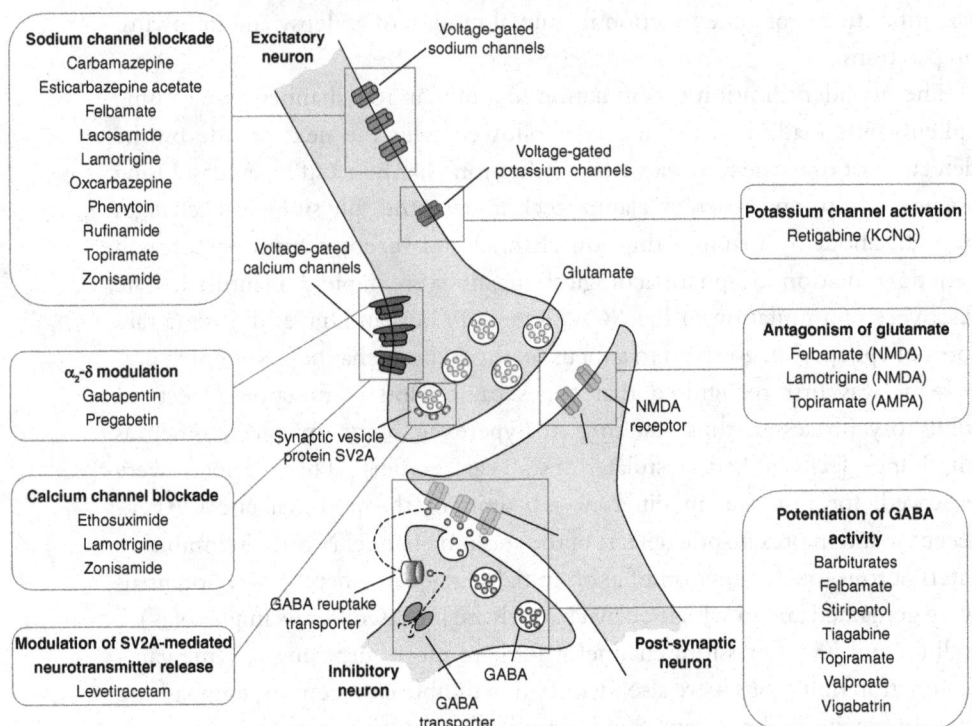

39. Diagram of structures involved in drug action and their sites on the neuron and synapse. (From: Perucca and Mula, 'Antiepileptic drug effects on mood and behavior').

These depended on receptor and channel cloning in the late 1980s and 1990s, the identification of their crystalline structure in the 1990s, and of their genetic codes from 1990 onwards.

Huge sums of money and time were ploughed into this area, seen as it was to provide a rational basis for drug discovery. In practice, though, the results of this targeted approach, in epilepsy at least, proved somewhat disappointing (at least by 2020). Despite the intense focus on the glutamate receptor, only one antiepileptic based on it was commercialised: the selective non-competitive AMPA receptor antagonist perampanel, licensed for human use in 2012. Similarly, only one antiepileptic, retigabine, was licensed which was designed specifically to enhance the activity of an ion channel (the newly studied neuronal potassium channel), mutations of which had been found to be associated with early-onset epilepsy. Retigabine subsequently failed in clinical practice, largely due to side effects, prompting its manufacturer, GlaxoSmithKline, to leave the field of epilepsy altogether due to the expense and difficulty of research in this area. Similarly, the three drugs developed as a result of the earlier GABA wave – vigabatrin, progabide and tiagabine – also failed, due to lack of clinical effect or side effects. Disappointing as it was that the massive amount of molecular work had not resulted in more products to control seizures or epileptogenesis, the genie had been let out of the bottle and work continues, hopefully to bear fruit in the future. As will be described later, it turned out that the most successful pharmacological discoveries of the period were still at least partly made more by luck than design.

Networks and Systems

Although alteration in excitability of individual neurons is a fundamental requirement for epileptogenesis, discharges from a single neuron alone will not cause a seizure. Synchronisation of a larger mass of hyperexcitable neurons is needed. Epilepsy, therefore, can be seen as not only a disease of individual neurons but also, and more importantly, as a disease of a system (a 'neural network'). A system in this sense was defined as 'a construct or collection of different elements that together produce results not obtainable by the elements alone ... The value added by the system as a whole, beyond that contributed independently by the parts, is primarily created by the relationship among the parts: that is, how they are interconnected'.[9] The molecular biology of systems became a line of intensive research.

An intrinsic bursting property – inherent excitability which might explain the generation of epileptic seizures – was first demonstrated in 1989 in some of the neurons in a deep layer (layer V) of the cerebral cortex of the rat (known as 'intrinsically bursting neurons').[10] These neurons were subsequently shown to have axons that were connected via synapses to a large number of neighbouring neurons. Their bursting was found to be primarily dependent on currents generated by the sodium channel, and also influenced by calcium and potassium channel activity. By 2010 it was clear that these neurons might be central to the synchronisation of epileptic discharges, and that genetic or acquired changes to their sodium channel function might play a crucial role in recruiting the critical mass of neighbouring neurons required to create an epileptogenic area.

Then, in the hippocampus, some CA3 neurons were also identified which had intrinsic bursting properties, and these showed greater dependence on calcium channel currents. These neurons were extensively connected to CA1 neurons to form part of a circuit involving wider areas of the hippocampus (the dentate gyrus and entorhinal cortex), and thence other limbic structures. Of critical importance was the realisation that in focal epilepsy it was the inter-action of neurons in such multiple locations that underpinned the epileptic seizure. In other words, seizures were not the product of a single, highly

---

[9] Rechtin, *Why Eagles Can't Swim*, cited in Avanzini and Franceschetti, 'Mechanisms of epileptogenesis', p.46
[10] Chagnac-Amitai and Connors, 'Synchronized excitation and inhibition'.

localised focus. The invalidity, in many epilepsies, of the cherished concept of the 'epileptic focus' was a paradigm shift, and might explain the lack of success of localised surgery in such cases. The network most intensively studied is the limbic system, through large intact slice preparations involving principal components of this circuit. Other networks of importance in epilepsy had been identified, including the thalamocortical loop in absence seizures (the same system is also involved in the control of vigilance) and those underpinning juvenile myoclonic epilepsies, benign childhood epilepsy with centrotemporal spikes and West syndrome.[11]

Networks were found to have additional properties, perhaps the most important of which from the epilepsy point of view was their plasticity (i.e. their ability to change over time). Following the observation in 1969 that seizures changed networks – by kindling – in experimental models of epilepsy, it was realised that this plasticity might induce permanent changes in the human epilepsy networks and be the basis of epileptogenesis.

Networks were also studied from the perspective of neurochemistry and genetics. It was found that a single gene mutation can affect the expression of multiple other genes, especially in neurodevelopment. One such neural pathway, which was to attract considerable interest in the 2010s, was the mTOR (mammalian target of rapamycin) pathway.[12] mTOR function was found to be altered in conditions causing epilepsy such as tuberose sclerosis complex, cortical dysplasia, brain tumours, neurodegenerative disorders and traumatic brain injury. An antiseizure action of mTOR inhibitors had been suggested by the observation of a decrease in seizure frequency in tuberose sclerosis treated with rapamycin (which was in use to treat cancer and prevent transplant rejection), and subsequently confirmed in animal models of epilepsy. Experimental evidence of a role in adult hippocampal neurogenesis, synaptogenesis and dendritic growth was also uncovered, suggesting that mTOR inhibitors might be anti-epileptogenic.[13] Despite this, it was recognised that epileptogenesis was neither a unitary nor a simple process, and no method of prevention or treatment that would prove to be universally effective was found.

Cellular Damage Due to Seizures

Following Meldrum's demonstration in the 1970s of brain damage from prolonged seizure activity, the investigation of changes induced by epileptic

---

[11] Avanzini et al., 'System epilepsies'.

[12] mTOR is a widely distributed protein kinase, a cellular molecule which had been found to be central to a range of biological processes such as cell survival, growth, proliferation and metabolism, as well as synaptic plasticity and cortical development.

[13] See Avanzini and Franceschetti, 'Mechanisms of epileptogenesis'.

seizures themselves, and the idea that this seizure-induced damage might be part of the process of epileptogenesis, continued. This thinking recapitulated the concept, introduced by Gowers in 1880, that 'seizures beget seizures'. Plastic changes to the excitability of membrane ion channels and in receptors were reported, and so too were changes in brain circuitry, reducing sensitivity to antiepileptic drug treatment. One example of a potential mechanism was the development of 'mossy fibre sprouting' seen in experimental models after kindling even in the absence of any other sign of cellular damage, as well as in pathological specimens in human epilepsy. Sprouting mossy fibres make synaptic contacts in new locations and thus might provide an excitatory feedback circuit. It was postulated, therefore, that both in experimental animals and in humans, an initial episode of persisting epileptic activity can set in motion a series of events which could explain not only the tendency of temporal lobe epilepsy to became unresponsive to antiepileptic drugs, but also the latent interval often seen between the initial event and the development of chronicity.

Other studies showed that the development and maintenance of epilepsy depended not only on neuronal connectivity but also on other mechanisms, including changes to glia, the blood–brain barrier, the influence of inflammation and generation of reactive oxygen species. In the 2010s, research was initiated to determine to what extent changes in gene expression explained the temporal aspects of this process, but no significant findings were made, emphasising that epileptogenesis was likely to prove a complex and difficult area of study.

The recognition that seizure-induced changes evolved progressively over time also raised the possibility that giving 'neuroprotectants' after the initial brain insult might prevent the development of these changes. A range of compounds were studied, although by 2020 none were shown to be efficacious.

What did become clear from the laboratory studies was the complexity and variability of epileptic activity in the human brain – there was neither a simple explanation nor a single mechanism. This should not have been surprisingly, but nevertheless it was disappointing to many, and the finding of a universal panacea for epilepsy remained a distant dream.

GENETICS OF HUMAN EPILEPSY

Human genetics was the clinical area in epilepsy that attracted the greatest academic interest throughout the first two decades of the new century. Huge sums of research money were poured into the genetics of human epilepsy, and this topic garnered wide publicity. The result has been mixed. Striking discoveries and great advances were made in relation to basic mechanisms (as outlined in the previous section) and clinically in relation to rare epilepsies, especially those of infantile or early childhood onset. The clinical application of genetics to the generality of persons with epilepsy, however, proved much more limited.

The earliest clinical discoveries were the identification, by classical linkage methodology, of ion channel mutations in rare familial epilepsies. The first mutations, discovered in 1995, were in a gene that encoded nicotinic acetylcholine receptors in the newly described syndrome of autosomal dominant nocturnal frontal lobe epilepsy (ADNFLE; affected genes: *CHRNA4*, *CHRNB2*). In 1998 mutations in potassium channel genes were identified in benign familial neonatal seizures (BFNS; affected genes: *KCNQ2*, *KCNQ3*). Then, in 2000, the newly described syndrome of generalised epilepsy with febrile seizures plus (GEFS+) was found to be due to mutations in sub-units of the voltage-gated sodium channel or the GABA A receptor (affected genes: *SCN1B*, *SCN1A*, *GABRG2*). Conditions due to mutations in ion channel genes became known as 'channelopathies', and by 2001 the idea was put about that all idiopathic epilepsies might turn out to be channelopathies (this proved not to be the case). The electrophysiological changes induced by these mutations, including effects on the PDS, were quickly identified, and the potential for targeting treatment was postulated.[14]

This was an exciting time. The pace of discovery in epilepsy genetics accelerated, much as that in MRI had done in the 1980s and 1990s. As with MRI, it was technological improvements that provided the opportunity. Advancing technology increased the power of genetic sequencing, making it possible in the late 1990s to use candidate gene approaches to identify new (de novo) pathogenic mutations in 'sporadic' cases (i.e. in which only one member of a family is affected). The most prominent early clinical finding was that of *SCN1A* mutations in Dravet syndrome, first identified in 2001.[15] The most sought-after prize in epilepsy, though, was not in these rare conditions, but was the possibility of discovering the genetic basis of the common idiopathic epilepsies of late childhood and adult life – the syndromes of idiopathic generalised epilepsy (IGE) and of idiopathic focal epilepsy. Perhaps inevitably, expectations were raised to unrealistic levels, but the quest failed. A large number of genome-wide association studies (GWAS) were undertaken but none found a gene with any strong influence. Then, after around 2010, even more powerful sequencing methods (the so-called 'next generation sequencing') permitted whole exome and whole genome searches for genetic causes

[14] The original discoveries were made by Scheffer et al., 'Distinct clinical disorder', Biervert and Steinlein, 'Benign familial neonatal convulsions' and Escayg et al., 'Mutations of SCN1A'. The situation in 2001 was well summarised in Lerche, Jurkat-Rott and Lehmann-Horn, 'Ion channels and epilepsy'.

[15] Claes et al., 'Myoclonic epilepsy of infancy'.

of all the common epilepsies. Mutations were found in many diverse genes, but as the genome of a healthy person has 3.2 billion base pairs, it also has thousands of genetic variants, and the finding of any one does not mean it is pathogenic. Consequently, some of the new genetic variants claimed for epilepsy had to be retracted.[16] Huge sums of public money were expended, but the results of these studies (at least by 2020) had proved disappointing.

As the smoke cleared, it became clear that the 'epilepsy genes' which had the greatest human impact were those that acted alone - ie causing the monogenic or single gene epilepsies. The rare infantile epileptic encephalopathies had relatively high pick-up rates for single gene mutations, and were all found to de novo mutations – in other words, not inherited. The other epilepsies which turned out to have a relatively high rate of monogenic defects (or other clear-cut genetic mechanisms) were those associated with inborn errors of metabolism, cortical dysplasias, and the rare progressive myoclonic epilepsies. But it soon became apparent that the common idiopathic epilepsies only rarely resulted from mutations in any one causative gene. There were similar failures to identify single genetic causes in other common neuropsychiatric diseases, and so this should perhaps not have been surprising – not least as any common serious genetic disease would surely be selected out by evolution.

The concept then grew up of 'susceptibility' genes, and of 'complex inheritance' where variants within specific genes contribute a small amount to the population occurrence of a disease. Several models of complex inheritance were postulated. The oligogenic model is one in which a small number of variants with strong effects combine to cause disease – these variants of large effect are postulated to be rarely present in the population. The other model proposed was that many common variants of small effect (perhaps hundreds) combine in an individual to cause epilepsy. By 2020, debate about which model was more likely to be important in genetic epilepsy raged, with advocates on both sides, but neither model delivered findings of any real clinical significance. It had also become clear that most common 'idiopathic' epilepsies were not exclusively the result of genetic variants but were also caused by strong non-genetic environmental and developmental influences. In this regard, epilepsy (and other common neuropsychiatric disorders) are like other developmental attributes such as intelligence, height and weight.[17] Indeed, a '4th law of behavioural genetics' had been postulated which holds

[16] Examples include variants in the *SCN9A*, *CACNA11H*, *MAG12* and *EFHC1* genes.
[17] The obvious analogies are with height and weight, for which a range of susceptibility genes have been discovered; but their effect is superseded by nutrition and eating habits, by hormones in milk consumed in childhood and the addictive properties of some foods, such as chocolate.

that 'a typical human behaviour is associated with very many genetic variants each of which accounts for a very small percentage of the behavioural variability'.[18] Some then have questioned whether there is any point in identifying individual changes in genes which by themselves were likely to have only very minor relevance (colourfully described as MAGOTS – many assorted genes of tiny significance). MAGOTS do indeed infest epilepsy genetics, as they do most human attributes.

By 2017, mutations in 693 genes had been found in which the symptoms of the disease included epilepsy.[19] These were made up largely of genes causing cortical dysplasias and other structural anomalies of cortical development, and – by far the largest group – genes causing inborn errors of metabolism in which epileptic seizures are usually only one of many abnormal phenotypic features.

As genetic knowledge increased, it was also clear that mutations (or single nucleotide polymorphisms) were not the only genetic abnormality that could result in epilepsy; rather, some conditions were due to abnormal 'repeats' in the genetic sequence or to deletions, duplications or mal-arrangement of whole stretches of the chromosome (these duplications and deletions are known as copy number variants; CNVs). These were detected by microarray analysis, and could be missed by genome or exome sequencing. Another important mechanism that was recognised to be of importance was genetic mosaicism. Here, the genetic mutation occurs as cells divide and therefore is present only in a portion of the cells of the body. An early epilepsy example was in the condition known as RIng Chromosome 20, in which it was also shown that the severity of the epilepsy is related to the proportion of cells affected.

The genetics of congenital structural diseases of the brain causing epilepsy – for instance, focal cortical dysplasia, polymicrogyria, double cortex syndrome and subependymal heterotopia – became the subject of much fruitful study. Many of these structural abnormalities were only identified in the MRI era and their importance in epilepsy had been entirely unexpected. But as soon as MRI identified these lesions and genetic study became possible, a range of genes were identified causing these conditions, many related to brain scaffolding and neuronal migration. In some the genetic defects were due to a mosaicism, one example being hemimegalencephaly due to mosaicism in the *AKT3* gene.

It is very likely that epigenetic factors are of particular importance in the production of epilepsy. These are factors which switch on and switch off genes over time – in other words, they are one of the mechanisms underlying *brain development*. By 2020, the methylation of genes, a major mechanism of

---

[18] Chabris et al., 'The fourth law'.   [19] Wang et al., 'Epilepsy-associated genes'.

epigenetics, was beginning to be studied in epilepsy, with notable successes in the field of brain tumours and cortical dysplasia. Identifying epigenetic factors may well turn out to be more important than identifying individual genes, and DNA methylation profiling, for instance, proved reliable as a marker of specific types of dysplasia (and might well turn out in the future to be a useful criteria for classification – getting closer to Jackson's botanist rather than gardener type of classification).[20]

In parallel, the many genetic variants causing inborn errors of metabolism were also unravelled. Most were rare, and some extremely rare, occurring in only a handful of families (sometimes single families) in the world. These discoveries did make it possible to identify metabolic pathways resulting in epilepsy, and as a result, targeted therapies to replace defective proteins or even defective genes were sought and were slowly becoming available.

Another consequence of the advancing genetic research was the recognition that a similar clinical effect could be due to mutations in differing genes. In the syndrome of infantile spasms, for instance, mutations in at least thirty-five genes had been found to cause an identical clinical picture. In Dravet syndrome, although mutations in the *SCN1A* gene were the most common, identical cases with mutations in other genes had been uncovered. A similar picture was identified in the syndrome of epilepsy with migrating focal seizures, where mutations in the *KCNT1* gene accounted for about a third of cases, and mutations in twenty other genes for some of the remaining cases; and in a sizeable number there was no genetic mutation found at all.

Intriguingly, mutations in many of the involved genes were found to have widely differing clinical effects (the 'phenotype'), emphasising the importance of developmental, epigenetic and environmental factors. An example was the *SCN2A* gene, where gain-of-function mutations in different positions caused an early-onset epileptic encephalopathy or benign familial neonatal seizures and loss-of-function mutations were associated with autism and intellectual disability.

As mentioned earlier, the early-onset epileptic encephalopathies were often found to be due to genetic defects. This was hardly surprisingly, as severe diseases presenting in infancy are often of genetic origin. Moreover, the earlier the onset of the epilepsy, the more likely a genetic cause was to be found.[21] Because of this, these rare conditions became the subject of intense research. An epileptic encephalopathy was defined by the ILAE as a condition in which 'the

---

[20] See Kobow and Blümcke, 'DNA methylation in epileptogenesis'. Katja Kobow won the 2021 Michael Prize for her work on DNA methylation.

[21] By 2020, panels of 120 genes were used routinely in neonatal units in Britain, for instance, in all cases of early-onset epilepsy. If the panels produced negative results, whole exome and genome sequencing was carried out by NHS laboratories organised on a regional basis.

epileptiform EEG abnormalities themselves were believed to contribute to a progressive disturbance in cerebral function', but it had been always obvious that the brain damage was probably as much due to the effects of the underlying genetic defect on brain development as to the continuous epilepsy. As a result, the more appropriate term 'developmental and epileptic encephalopathies' (DEE) had become current by 2020. By then, mutations in more than sixty genes had been identified which could result in an early-onset encephalopathy. These genes were involved in numerous cellular mechanisms, including ion channels and processes such as cell migration, synaptogenesis, apoptosis, neurite formation, adhesion, myelination, vesicle cycling, cell growth, synapse formation and mTor pathway regulation. The genetic defects were found usually to be due to new mutations and not inherited, but in some cases the parents were genetically mosaic. Dravet disease, the commonest early childhood genetic epilepsy, is one example.

By 2020, uncovering the genetic aetiology had not led to much in the way of new therapy, but there was optimism that this, too, might change, not least with the promise of wholly novel approaches such as viral vector single-dose genetic therapies and the use of antisense oligonucleotides.[22] The diagnosis of an inherited monogenic disorder could be of potential help in counselling. In the common epilepsies which are not monogenic, however, counselling was not based on any sophisticated genetic assessment but more simply on estimates of familial risk (which had been known for years) and uninfluenced by the presence of minor susceptibility genes.

The enormous complexity of genetic influences seemed daunting, but the number of cases of epilepsy found to have a clear-cut and predominant genetic cause was relatively small. By 2020, monogenic causes of epilepsy amounted probably to less than 5% of the total number of patients with epilepsy, although higher rates are found in those with early-onset epilepsies and those with learning disabilities. Despite enormous fanfare, the practical utility of the advancing genetic knowledge for the common epilepsies had proved relatively limited.

One final consequence of the genetic work in epilepsy was its effect on epilepsy classification. As different genes could cause a similar phenotype and as mutations in the same gene could cause a different phenotype, it became clear that classification schemes based on clinical descriptions make little scientific sense. Nor did dividing epilepsy and its syndromes into focal and generalised categories. Genetic studies have also blurred the distinction between idiopathic and symptomatic epilepsy. In part, as a result, epilepsy classification entered a period of turmoil.

---

[22] Rinaldi and Wood, 'Antisense oligonucleotides'.

DEFINITION, TERMINOLOGY AND CLASSIFICATION

History tends to travel in circles, and sometimes in fruitless directions. There are no better examples of this than the constant tinkering with the definitions of epilepsy, and its twin shadows: classification and terminology. Throughout the twentieth century, these proved to be minefields in the epilepsy theatres of war.

After the controversies of the 1970s and 1980s, the world of epilepsy nosology and classification had seemed to settle down. Gastaut's definition and the 1981 classification of seizure types were widely accepted as, albeit with less enthusiasm, was the 1989 classification of epilepsy and its syndromes. But this period of consolidation was to be short lived.

In 1997, the International League Against Epilepsy established a new task force on classification and terminology to re-examine the issue, In 2001, Jerome (Pete) Engel, on behalf of the task force, published a significant report[23] stating wisely that it was, at the time, not yet possible to replace the current international classification with another that would be universally accepted and that would meet all the clinical and research needs such a formal organisational system would be expected to provide. Rather, the task force proposed that the ILAE should focus on 'a diagnostic scheme' and define seizure types in a way that could be used as diagnostic entities. This scheme suggested descriptors to define a patient's epilepsy, under five 'axes': ictal phenomenology, seizure type, syndrome, aetiology and impairment. The conception of axes was based on similar work in the field of psychiatry, and was indeed an appropriate plan, although it must be said that a similar concept, albeit under other names, was also found in the 1964, 1969/1970, 1981 and 1989 classification schemes. The crucial difference in 2001 was that no attempt was made to force these axes into the straitjacket of a single framework (a single classification scheme); rather, it was decided to produce simple lists within each axis – a wise decision, in the opinion of the author – and the report did include useful lists of syndromes and seizure types.

At the same time, the task force published a glossary of terms – shorter and more succinct than Gastaut's 1973 dictionary. Therein, epilepsy was defined as '[a] chronic neurologic condition characterised by recurrent epileptic seizures' and epileptic seizures as '[m]anifestation(s) of epileptic (excessive and/or hypersynchronous), usually self-limited activity of neurons in the brain'.[24] Both definitions were based on those of Jackson made nearly 150 years earlier, and avoided reference to any of the wider issues inherent in the concept of epilepsy.

---

[23] Engel, 'Proposed diagnostic scheme'.
[24] Blume et al., 'Glossary of descriptive terminology'.

In 2005, a new ILAE task force and a new ILAE executive felt it again necessary to produce updated definitions, claiming that there was 'little common agreement' on the definitions of epilepsy and seizures, although it is not clear why this was thought. It was also stated that the 2001 glossary definition was 'preliminary', although there was nothing in the 2001 publication to suggest this either. Epilepsy was then newly defined as '[a] disease characterized by an enduring predisposition to generate epileptic seizures and by the neurobiological, cognitive, psychological, and social consequences of this condition'.[25]

This widened the definition of epilepsy beyond that of seizures, and in this sense returned to the definitions widely accepted in the early 1900s at which time these extra features were considered inherent to epilepsy. An example was the definition by Turner in 1907 (see pp. 80–1) which was strikingly similar to the 2005 formulation (the one important difference was that, in 1907, only idiopathic epilepsy was considered 'genuine epilepsy').[26] In 2005, the definition of an epileptic seizure was also left virtually unchanged from that of Jackson (see pp.64–5): 'An epileptic seizure is a transient occurrence of signs and/ or symptoms due to abnormal excessive or synchronous neuronal activity in the brain'.

In 2006, the next incursion into classification was made when the Core Group of the ILAE task force published a report describing its discussions regarding 'the feasibility of creating a paradigm shift in our concept of classifications in the field of epilepsy, based on the establishment of measurable objective criteria for recognising epileptic seizure types and epilepsy syndromes as unique diagnostic entities or natural classes that can be reproducibly distinguished from all other diagnostic entities or natural classes'.[27] The task force produced listings of seizures and epilepsy syndromes that differed in interesting ways from, and were generally less comprehensive than, the listings in the 2001 paper, and again cautioned that this should not be interpreted as a classification scheme. The group also considered that the 1981 classification of epileptic seizure types and the 1989 classification of epilepsy syndromes and epilepsies were generally accepted and workable, and need not be discarded.

The ILAE executive then changed again, and the new executive replaced the existing task force with a new Commission on Classification and Terminology, which in 2010 published a further report reiterating the opinion of the 2001 task force and the 2006 Core Group that a new classification was not yet possible. In its place, the new commission saw it necessary to provide new 'terminology and concepts that better reflect the current understanding of these

---

[25] Fisher et al., 'Epileptic seizures and epilepsy'.   [26] Turner, *Epilepsy*, p. 1.
[27] Engel, 'Report'.

issues'.[28] In 2014, the Commission published a further paper which labelled the 2005 definition as 'a conceptual' definition, although it was not so named at the time, and proposed that a new 'practical' (operational) definition of epilepsy was needed – namely:

1. At least two unprovoked (or reflex) seizures occurring >24 h apart
2. One unprovoked (or reflex) seizure and a probability of further seizures similar to the general recurrence risk (at least 60%) after two unprovoked seizures, occurring over the next 10 years
3. Diagnosis of an epilepsy syndrome

> Epilepsy is considered to be resolved for individuals who had an age-dependent epilepsy syndrome but are now past the applicable age or those who have remained seizure-free for the last 10 years, with no seizure medicines for the last 5 years.[29]

The thinking behind the 'practical definition' was that the earlier definition was not specific enough to be used in clinical practice. This was indeed the case, but an unfortunate consequence was that two definitions now existed. To the world outside epilepsy, and to many within, this dual scheme was confusing and unnecessary. What the Commission did not attempt, surely a missed opportunity, was to rethink the whole question of whether epilepsy really was a unitary condition (a 'disease') at all, especially in the era when more and more genetic factors and underlying causal diseases were being identified.

Three aspects of the changing definition are worth emphasising. First was the fact that epilepsy was described as a disorder in 2005 but as a disease in 2014. The main reason for the change appears to have been the insistence of fundraisers, and the pharmaceutical industry, that providing money for a disease was easier than for a disorder – a sad reflection on the level to which ILAE was by then dependent on the industry. Although much was made of this change, nowhere was the distinction between disorder and disease made clear, and, as argued earlier, the terms are actually to a large extent synonymous.[30] The second important aspect of the new definition was the inclusion of the statement that epilepsy can be considered as resolved when individuals 'have remained seizure-free for the last 10 years, with no seizure medicines for the last 5 years'.[31] The word *cure* was avoided, but this was the first time that a definition of the end of epilepsy had been formalised. Previously, epilepsy was considered to have truly ceased only when the last seizure had occurred, which

[28] Berg et al., 'Revised terminology and concepts'.
[29] Fisher et al., 'Practical clinical definition'.
[30] The stated reason was as follows: 'The term disorder implies a functional disturbance, not necessarily lasting; whereas, the term disease may (but not always) convey a more lasting derangement of normal function' (Fisher et al., 'Practical clinical definition').
[31] Fisher et al., 'Practical clinical definition'.

although clearly accurate is something which can only be known retrospectively. Of course, there were exceptions to the new rule in clinical practice, but an attempt to define the end of epilepsy did at least address the unfairness of the thought that 'once an epileptic, always an epileptic' which pervaded the older literature. Finally, and crucially, the 2005 definition had reverted to the concept that epilepsy was 'more than just seizures' and had inherent biological and psychological components. But the 2014 definition reversed this and referred again only to seizures, blurring the distinction between epilepsy and seizures. The question of whether 'epilepsy' and 'epileptic seizures' are distinct or coterminous concepts is a fundamental issue, debated in the last pages of this book.

The commission also made changes to terminology, replacing 'idiopathic', 'symptomatic' and 'cryptogenic' with 'genetic', 'structural/metabolic' and 'unknown'. These changes were, in the opinion of many, a most egregious example of unnecessary tampering.[32] The substitution of 'genetic' for 'idiopathic' was a particularly flagrant and misleading example. The genetic basis of the great majority of idiopathic epilepsies was (and is) unknown. As mentioned earlier, these epilepsies are likely to have multifactorial causal influences that encompass environmental, developmental, provoking and genetic factors, and it was a gross simplification to label them merely 'genetic'. It implied, reductio ad absurdum, that everything about us is genetic (including physical characteristics such as height and weight, and intelligence and behaviour), thus rendering valueless its meaning in medicine. The term 'idiopathic' implied a wider and more complex scope that incorporated genetic factors, epigenetic factors, epistatic factors, the influence of the temporal aspects of cerebral development and the (probably great) influence of chance – and was thus a better choice.

Similarly, the substitution of 'unknown' for 'cryptogenic' created no new concept but appeared wholly to be a change for change's sake. Replacing 'symptomatic' – a universally understood term used throughout medicine – with 'structural/metabolic' was linguistically clumsy. It also ignored the many symptomatic epilepsies that involve no macroscopic structural or measurable metabolic change, such as those resulting from immunological, inflammatory, degenerative, toxic or biochemical causes (these omissions were in fact corrected in later publications from the commission).

In 2017, the ILAE produced another 'classification of epilepsy' – this time with no discussion about the principles of classification and also ignoring Engel's warning that a new classification was not yet possible. The new palimpsest established three 'levels of diagnosis' – seizure type, epilepsy type

---

[32] The name of the syndrome 'idiopathic generalized epilepsy' was changed to 'genetic generalized epilepsy'. This decision was subsequently reversed following widespread disapproval.

and epilepsy syndrome – with comorbidities and aetiology running in parallel. Whether this hierarchy had any advantage over (or, indeed, was in any essential way different from) the five axes proposed in 2001 is doubtful. In fact, the scheme in reality was a diagnostic manual in the Engel sense, not a classification, and to mislabel it confused the distinction.

In that same year, the ILAE also set up a 'seizure type classification task force'. This task force aimed simply to rename the seizure types. One important step was to change 'partial' to 'focal'. The taskforce seemed unaware that Gastaut had deliberately chosen the term 'partial', rather than 'focal', to emphasise that these seizures were often network phenomena and not localised to any discrete focus. Changing back to 'focal' lost this insight and flew in the face of much of the experimental work into epilepsy systems. Other changes were made for no good reason. For example, the terms 'simple' and 'complex partial seizures' were changed to the ungrammatical and ugly terms – 'focal aware' and 'focal unaware' seizures – finally destroying the *poésie* which had anyway been damaged by the replacement of 'grand mal' by 'tonic–clonic'. All these changes in definition, terminology and classification were seemingly unnecessary and aroused considerable controversy at the time. The ILAE response was to advertise and promote the changes, turning what should have been a scientifically based debate into a propaganda circus.

Of more intellectual interest than tampering with classification was the fact that by 2014 the concept of epilepsy had widened to include what became known as 'comorbidities'. This term had arisen in the late 1980s, and the old idea that there was more to epilepsy than just having seizures began to creep back into the medical literature. Because attention was focused mainly on the psychiatric conditions that often occurred in epilepsy, it was not a big step to declare that these conditions were not 'add-ons' but in fact an integral part of the condition. This view had begun to gain force in the early 2000s. One stimulus was the finding that several copy number variants (CNVs) occurred not only in epilepsy but also in other psychiatric syndromes,[33] raising the possibility that similar mechanisms were the cause of both. This had some similarities to the late nineteenth century concept of the neurological trait, and the then prevalent view that psychiatric disorders were an inherent part of the

---

[33] Until around 2010, the twenty-three pairs of chromosomes were thought to remain largely unchanged as they were passed from generation to generation. It then became apparent that deletion or duplication of various stretches of DNA, usually incorporating a number of genes, occurs frequently throughout the genome in healthy subjects, but only some are pathogenic. The 15q13.3 microdeletion was first found in patients with learning disability. Later, it emerged that it also occurs more often also in those with schizophrenia, autism and epilepsy. Similarly, CNVs affecting 15q11 and 16p13 have been found to cause epilepsy, autism and other psychiatric disturbances; and account for about 10% of those with both epilepsy and autism, and 5–10% of all DEEs.

condition. Although reflecting advancing knowledge, these changes also encouraged the categorization of epilepsy as a 'mental disorder', as it had been in the past, with its attendant potential for stigma and social exclusion.

NEUROLOGY OF EPILEPSY

Before 1950, epilepsy research was conducted in a relatively small number of locations, but thereafter this was rapidly to change. By the end of the century, thriving epilepsy research and training centres had been established, within neurological settings, in many cities around the world.

In parallel to this expansion was one of the most striking changes to epilepsy practice in the later decades of the twentieth century: the enormous increase in numbers of scientific and clinical papers published in the medical literature. The latter can be appreciated from a scrutiny of Pubmed, the indexing system developed by the National Library of Medicine.[34] This is an online index of all articles published since 1950 in those medical journals which meet certain minimal standards, as well as articles from the major journals published earlier (most between 1945–50, and less comprehensive indexes from earlier years). On PubMed, from 1860–2020, 157,188 articles were indexed on the topic of epilepsy (less than 1% were published before 1945 and the rest after this date), and of the 156,842 papers published between 1945 and 2020, 8% were published between 1946 and 1970, 21% in 1971–95 and 71% in 1996–2020. In Table 5.1, the numbers of papers by topics and the proportion published since 1996 is shown.

A parallel phenomenon was the growth in the number of conferences and presentations made at these conferences, but, despite this expansion, the type of topic within epilepsy at these congresses have changed relatively little. The topics of all nine lectures in the 1969 ILAE conference [35] might easily have been found in any of the international congresses up to 2020.

Disappointingly, this massive burgeoning of medical literature and research activity did not reflect or result in an equivalent improvement in epilepsy practice, which changed only incrementally throughout this quarter-century. That is not to say that there were no advances: there were especially in basic

---

[34] Pubmed is an online system that developed from the existing listings known as *Index Medicus*, which, since 1879, has consisted of a paper-based monthly index of new medical articles.

[35] Classification of the Epilepsies; The Clinico-electrographic Differentiation of Minor Seizures; The Differentiation between Absence Status and Temporal Lobe Status; Reticulo-cortical Epilepsy; Stereo-encephalography in Minor Seizures; NIH Collaborative Study of Absence Attacks; The Evolution and Prognosis of Minor Seizures; EEG Telemetry and Behaviour; Patterns of Development in Children with Minor Cerebral Seizures.

TABLE 5.1 *Number and classification of journal articles in the field of epilepsy 1946–2020*

Topic	Total number of papers published 1946–2020	% Published between 1996–2020
EEG	42,922	65%
Antiepileptic drugs	38,350	70%
Genetics	21,494	85%
MRI	18,393	92%
Surgery	23,229	79%
Paediatric epilepsy	19,220	92%
Epidemiology	15,412	86%
Status Epilepticus	14,148	83%
Classification	6,093	80%

(Devised by author from MedLine listings using keywords)

science, clinical genetics and pharmacological treatment – and these three areas are covered elsewhere in this chapter. There were also developments in: epidemiology, especially in relation to global comparisons of disease burden and the mortality of epilepsy; status epilepticus and its treatment; and the study of 'aetiology', especially in relation to the rare causes of epilepsy. The use of 'big data' was another trend developing after 2010. These topics are surveyed briefly here, not in a comprehensive fashion but to give a flavour of the time. Nevertheless, there was (and remains) a massive degree of reiteration in the literature and redundancy of research – a point taken up in the Epilogue.

Epidemiology, and the Mortality of Epilepsy and SUDEP

The epidemiology of epilepsy was studied in many different regions, countries and locations, with findings that demonstrated epilepsy to be a universal condition, occurring in all nationalities, social classes and races, but also one that was commoner in low-/middle-income countries (LMICs) than in high-income countries (HIC). The reasons were found to be complex, but included such factors as the younger age of LMIC populations, their lower nutritional and health standards and higher rates of infection and head injury. A meta-analysis of incidence studies found an overall incidence rate of epilepsy was 61.4 per 100,000 person-years; 139.0 in LMIC and 48.9 in HIC. The overall lifetime prevalence of epilepsy was 7.60 per 1,000; 8.75 in LMIC and 5.18 in HIC.[36] In 2016, epilepsy was estimated to be present in around 46 million people in the

---

[36] Fiest et al., 'Prevalence and incidence of epilepsy'.

world, of whom 80% were in LMIC. Of particular interest, and novel to this period, were the epidemiological studies of the *burden of disease*. This was a term coined to reflect the impact epilepsy had in terms of disability, premature mortality and cost. A commonly used measure of impact was the so-called DALY (disability-adjusted life year), a measure which combined the number of years of life lost due to premature mortality (YLLs) and years of life lost due to time lived in states of less than full health or disability (YLDs). The DALY proved an effective tool for comparing the impact of diseases and for ascertaining what value to put on interventions and where health resources should be directed. Epilepsy accounted for >13 million DALYs globally, and was responsible for 0.5% of the burden of all diseases. In terms of DALYS, it ranked between positions 2 to 8 amongst neurological diseases, depending on the geographical region.[37]

Mortality rates were also reported, with the Standardized Mortality Ratio (SMR) ranging from 1.6 to 3.0 in HIC and 19.8 in LMIC.[38] SUDEP (sudden unexpected death in epilepsy – see Chapter 4) continued to be a topic which excited considerable interest, and was found in one large study to occur in 1.2 per 1,000 person-years in epilepsy populations. In 1997, a supplement on SUDEP was published in *Epilepsia*, in which Nashef proposed a definition of SUDEP which became universally accepted,[39] and by then most of the demographic and clinic features had been established. But a veritable torrent of papers followed (between 1945–2020, 14,148 journal articles were published on SUDEP of which 90% dated from 1996–2020, and which largely reinforced what was already known. Some of the emphasis has switched to prevention – and a whole issue of the journal *Epilepsy and Behavior* was devoted to preventing unavoidable deaths.[40]

One reason for the rapid escalation of interest in the topic had been the involvement of a British patient support group, Epilepsy Bereaved, started in 1992 by Jane Hanna, a lawyer whose partner died of SUDEP. This group worked indefatigably and gained international traction. There is no better example in the modern consumer age of the power of a lay group with effective leadership, exactly as was the case in the 1940s with the example of Lennox and the American Epilepsy League. Partly at the instigation of Epilepsy Bereaved, the first international workshop on SUDEP was held in 1996, and its

[37] GBD 2016 Neurology Collaborators, 'Global burden of disease study 2016'.

[38] Thurman et al., 'The burden of premature mortality'.

[39] *Epilepsia*, 38 (1997) Supplement 11. Nashef's definition was: 'Sudden, unexpected, witnessed or unwitnessed, nontraumatic and nondrowning death in patients with epilepsy, with or without evidence for a seizure and excluding documented status epilepticus, in which postmortem examination does not reveal a toxicologic or anatomic cause for death.' Nashef, 'Sudden unexpected death', p. S6.

[40] Kerr, Sen and Hanna, 'Time to listen'.

proceedings published as a supplement in *Epilepsia*.. SUDEP began to appear on the agenda of many large epilepsy meetings, including the 1997 International Epilepsy Congress in Dublin and the 2013 Presidential Symposium of the Epilepsy International Congress in Montreal.

At the urging of Epilepsy Bereaved, modern epilepsy practice also changed, with most neurologists in Europe and the United States being instructed to discuss the possibility of SUDEP with all patients early after diagnosis. Several high-profile court cases were publicised, in which neurologists were taken to task for not doing so. With further lobbying from Epilepsy Bereaved, in 2002 the UK government held a national audit, concluding that about 40% of SUDEP deaths could have been avoided. Two leading American epilepsy specialists published an editorial in *The Lancet* stating that the results of the audit should be a wake-up call to the medical profession prompting a targeted campaign to improve care for people with epilepsy. Epidemiological data were collected over the next decade from many countries, and SUDEP registries and surveillance programmes were set up in Ireland, the United States, Canada and France, as well as Britain. In 2018 a SUDEP Action Day was declared, and eighty-four organisations from nine countries were represented through social media activities.

The campaigns around SUDEP adopted a propagandist approach to science, a feature of this period in which health issues increasingly became the topic of mainline media interest and public concern. Treating the narrative as much politically as scientifically turned out to be a highly effective strategy in the societal context of the twenty-first century.

Status Epilepticus

The field of status epilepticus also moved forward in this period – and especially in relation to its basic science. It had been known since 1984 that GABA receptors move from the surface of a cell into its interior, a process known as trafficking or internalisation.[41] A key discovery in the field of status epilepticus was that this process of internalisation greatly increased during prolonged seizure activity.[42] The falling density of receptors reduces GABAergic transmission and was seen as one reason for the cardinal feature of status epilepticus: a failure of the seizures to cease spontaneously. In addition, it was demonstrated that excitatory NMDA receptors were trafficked onto the surface of the synaptic membrane exacerbating the problem. The falling effectiveness of GABAergic drugs in status epilepticus had been earlier explored by Jaideep Kapur and Robert MacDonald, who demonstrated, in a classic

---

[41] Wilkinson, Jacobson and Wilkinson, 'Brain slices'.
[42] The group of Wasterlain in California pioneered this work: Naylor, Liu and Wasterlain, 'Trafficking of GABA(A) receptors'; Goodkin, Yeh and Kapur, 'Status epilepticus'.

experiment, that the dose of diazepam needed to control a seizure lasting 45 minutes was 10 times the dose needed to control a seizure lasting 10 minutes.[43] The trafficking of receptors was considered the cause of this loss of effect. The process also emphasised the importance of the phrase 'time is brain', coined for the treatment of stroke but applicable equally to the treatment of status epilepticus.

Receptor trafficking was a novel discovery and provided an explanation for the persistence of seizure activity in status epilepticus. This mattered enormously as it was also found that it was the excessive *prolongation* of seizure activity that caused cerebral damage in status. In the 1970s, in baboon and rat models, Meldrum and his team found that cell death and atrophy developed only after a seizure had been prolonged beyond around 30–60 minutes – and that shorter seizures did not result in damage. Meldrum postulated that the cellular damage was due to calcium entry into the cell as a result of glutaminergic receptor activity, and to his credit, even 50 years later, this has remained the orthodox explanation.[44]

Thus, by 2000 it had dawned upon the clinical community that the key both to successful treatment in status epilepticus and to the prevention of cerebral damage was to control the seizures as soon as possible. This shift in thinking led to the early use of anaesthesia and the transfer of in-hospital care to an Intensive Therapy Unit (ITU) setting, and crucially also to efforts to start initial emergency drug treatment outside hospital. Practice changed, and buccal and intranasal drugs were permitted to be administered out of hospital by non-medical personnel – for instance parents, carers and teachers – or by ambulance staff. Several formulations of buccal midazolam were licensed, and its use revolutionised treatment. After many decades of inaction, these were perhaps the most important public health developments in epilepsy in the whole of this period.

Between 2007 and 2019, a series of seven biannual international congresses on status epilepticus were held (the London–Innsbruck Colloquia on Status Epilepticus), and their proceedings were published. These events had the effect of bringing together scientists and clinicians from around the world and also stimulating interest in the condition. One pressing issue in the field of status epilepticus was the lack of controlled or scientifically rigorous clinical trials. Following discussions at the first colloquium, a series of important trials were carried out after 2010 which improved the scientific basis of treatment. The novel concept of a stage of super-refractory status epilepticus[45] was conceived

---

[43] Kapur and Macdonald, 'GABAA receptors'; Kapur and Macdonald, 'Status epilepticus'. In this chapter by Kapur and Macdonald, the reduction of GABAergic function was attributed to other mechanisms that did not involve receptor internalisation – and it is possible that various mechanisms contribute to the loss of function.

[44] Meldrum and Horton, 'Status epilepticus in primates'; Meldrum, Vigouroux and Brierley, 'Epileptic brain damage'.

[45] Shorvon and Ferlisi, 'Super-refractory status epilepticus'; Ferlisi and Shorvon, 'Outcome of therapies'.

at a later colloquium. A range of epidemiological studies and a series of new therapies were also widely debated.[46] Interest in status epilepticus was certainly growing and in the period 2007–20, nearly 8,000 publications had been indexed on PubMed – nearly twice the number in the previous 100 years.

Aetiology of Epilepsy: MRI, Genetics and Rare Causes

In 1940, Kinnier Wilson had written that listing all the causes of epilepsy would be an 'act of supererogation',[47] an *ipse dixit* true at the time when at least two-thirds of epilepsy cases were designated 'cryptogenic' and without the diagnostic technologies developed later in the century. This was to change, especially after the 1980s, as the technological advances in imaging, clinical biochemistry and genetics increasingly moved the focus of clinical studies back again to the question of aetiology, and this indeed proved a rich seam to mine. The first book to focus exclusively on epilepsy aetiology was published in 2011 (second edition in 2019) and therein were listed several thousand different conditions in which epileptic seizures were present (Table 5.2).[48]

As before, it was novel investigatory techniques that stimulated research. The first was of course MRI. Throughout the 1990s and 2000s, technological innovation in magnets, computers and software improved the quality of images. The earlier magnets were less powerful, but by 1997 1.5-Tesla scanners and by 2005 3-Tesla scanners were standard imaging hardware. Software developments brought new techniques into clinical practice, including MR spectroscopy, functional MRI, diffusion and perfusion scanning, MR angiography, tractography, automated analysis and the co-registration of fMRI with other modalities such as invasive EEG and positron emission tomography. By 2020, 7-Tesla scanners were installed in research units but had not entered routine clinical practice.

Since the first publication in 1987, more than 15,000 articles had been published on MRI and epilepsy by 2020.[49] From the outset, MRI made two key contributions to epilepsy: identifying the structural aetiologies in symptomatic epilepsy and enabling epilepsy surgery. With fair confidence, by 2020 all conditions causing structural brain changes of greater than 2 mm in size

---

[46] Shorvon, Trinka and Walker, 'London–Innsbruck Colloquium'.
[47] Wilson and Bruce, *Neurology*.
[48] Shorvon, Andermann and Guerrini, *Causes of Epilepsy*. A second edition in 2019 identified further causes and proposed a new classification: Shorvon et al., *Common and Uncommon Causes*.
[49] MRI in epilepsy has certainly spawned a publishing frenzy. The first PubMed entries that listed epilepsy and MR scanning appeared in 1987 – in which year there were 20 entries; by the end of 2007 there were 6,212 entries. See Shorvon, 'History of neuroimaging'.

TABLE 5.2 *The causes of epilepsy in 2019 (categories and examples)*

Main category	Subcategory	Some examples[1]
Idiopathic Epilepsy	Pure epilepsies in which there is no clear single gene defect and which are likely to have a complex epistatic, epigenetic or developmental origin	Idiopathic generalised epilepsy (and its subtypes, for instance: childhood absence epilepsy, juvenile myoclonic epilepsy, epilepsy with seizures only on awakening) Idiopathic partial epilepsies of childhood (and its subtypes, for instance: benign rolandic epilepsy, benign occipital lobe epilepsy)
Symptomatic Epilepsy of Genetic or Developmental Origin	Pure epilepsies due to single gene disorders	Autosomal dominant nocturnal frontal lobe epilepsy; benign familial neonatal convulsions; familial lateral temporal lobe epilepsy; genetic epilepsy with febrile seizures plus
	Epilepsies with a mitochondrial genetic basis (including defects of nuclear genes affecting mitochondrial function)	MEGDEL; Leigh syndrome; MELAS; MERFF; NARP; POLG-related syndromes; mitochondrial deletion disorders
	Epileptic encephalopathies and severe epilepsy syndromes[3]	Dravet syndrome; early infantile encephalopathies (and its various subtypes); early myoclonic encephalopathies, Landau–Kleffner Syndrome (some cases)[2]; Lennox–Gastaut Syndrome (some cases)[2]; West syndrome (some cases)[2]
	Progressive myoclonic epilepsies	Dentato-rubro-pallido-luysian atrophy; Lafora body disease; mitochondrial cytopathy; neuronal ceroid lipofuscinoses; sialidosis; Unverricht–Lundborg disease
	Neurocutaneous syndromes	Neurofibromatosis; Sturge–Weber syndrome; tuberose sclerosis
	Inborn errors of metabolism and other single gene disorders	Angelman syndrome; disorders of creatine metabolism; CGD; Fatty-acid oxidation syndromes; GLUT1 deficiency; lysosomal disorders; Menkes' disease; neuroacanthocytosis; organic acidurias; PCHD19 syndrome; peroxisomal disorders; porphyria; pyridoxine-dependent epilepsy; Rett syndrome; CDKL5 encephalopathy; urea cycle disorders; Wilson's disease
	Disorders of chromosome function and copy number variations	Down syndrome; fragile X syndrome; inverted duplicated chromosome 15; ring chromosome 20; ring chromosome 14 and other ring chromosomal disorders; Wolf Hirschhorn syndrome; X128 dup syndrome

(continued)

TABLE 5.2 *(continued)*

Main category	Subcategory	Some examples[1]
	Developmental anomalies of cerebral structure[3]	Agyria-pachygyria-band spectrum; agenesis of the corpus callosum; Arachnoid cysts; focal cortical dysplasia; hemimegalencephaly; tubulinopathies and mTOR pathway disorders; microcephaly; periventricular nodular heterotopia; polymicrogyria and schizencephaly
Symptomatic Epilepsy of Acquired Origin	Hippocampal sclerosis	Sometimes divided into subtypes
	Cerebral trauma	Open head injury; closed head injury; neurosurgery; non-accidental head injury in infants
	Cerebral tumour	Glioma; ganglioglioma and hamatoma; DNET; hypothalamic hamartoma; meningioma; secondary tumours
	Cerebral infection	Viral meningitis and encephalitis; bacterial meningitis and abscess; malaria; neurocysticercosis; parasitic disorders; tuberculosis; HIV
	Cerebrovascular disorders	Arteriovenous malformation; cavernous haemangioma; cerebral haemorrhage; cerebral infarction
	Cerebral immunological disorders	Auto-antibody auto-immune encephalitic disorders; Rasmussen encephalitis; SLE and collagen vascular disorders
	Degenerative and other neurological conditions	Alzheimer disease and other dementing disorders; eclampsia; multiple sclerosis and demyelinating disorders; hydrocephalus; posterior reversible encephalopathy syndrome; vaccination and immunisation
	Perinatal and infantile causes	Neonatal seizures (various causes); cerebral palsy; post-vaccination
Provoked Epilepsy	Reflex epilepsies	Auditory-induced epilepsy; eating epilepsy; hot-water epilepsy; photosensitive epilepsies; reading epilepsy; reflex epilepsies associated with higher-level processing; startle-induced epilepsies
	Provoking factors	Alcohol and toxin-induced seizures; drug-induced seizures; fever; menstrual cycle and catamenial epilepsy; metabolic and endocrine-induced seizures; sleep-wake cycle; stress
Cryptogenic Epilepsy		

[1] This listing of examples is representative but not exhaustive.
[2] These epilepsy syndromes can also have acquired causes.
[3] Although included here, many cases have no known cause and others are caused by external (environmental) insults. (From Shorvon 'The concept of causation in epilepsy').

could reliably be detected. MRI had in effect replaced morbid anatomy and refined it to a hitherto unprecedented level. It was said to provide 'in vivo pathology', and to an extent this was true. But MRI could not detect either microscopic changes at the level of neuronal organisation, for instance, nor biochemical changes. These were to be the challenges for the future.

All the significant parameters of the use of MRI in epilepsy were established by the end of the 1990s. Since then, progress had been relatively incremental at best. Research into new techniques was justified as having potential importance in the 'localisation' of the focus, but such tests had seldom been validated, and their sensitivity, specificity and predictive value were not robustly established. The diagnostic yield from some techniques has been small, for example in the field of fMRI or spectroscopy which showed very little clinical usefulness in the diagnosis of epilepsy, even after a quarter-century of research. As in all medical fields, the initially steep curve of progress flattens over time. This happened in epilepsy earlier with EEG and with TDM, and by 2020, in MRI the curve was almost horizontal.

The second group of technologies which had transformed the detection of aetiologies was of course those in the field of epilepsy genetics, described earlier. The genetic causes of a multitude of rare diseases, either structural dysplasias of the brain or biochemical defects (inborn errors), or both, were identified. These were commonest in infancy or early childhood, and so the field of epilepsy paediatrics became swamped with the new genetics. Knowing the genetic aetiology of most of these conditions though had only a small impact on treatment. Most of these conditions were untreatable prior to the new genetics and most remained so even when their bases were identified and the biochemical or structural defects uncovered. This has been disappointing.

'Big Data'

One interesting development in the 2010s was a growing interest in the potential for collecting vast numbers of data points and conducting complex mathematical analysis, just to see what emerges and without any real hypothesis. Many conservative scientists were appalled as the importance of an *a priori* hypothesis had been (and remains) a cornerstone of all science. Of course, such analyses depended on the development of powerful computing technologies.[50] It was around 2009 that 'big data' first made its appearance in epilepsy, and since then massive datasets have been increasingly used in the collection of long-term EEG data, imaging data, genetic data, and clinical data in electronic patient records.

[50] The first examples were probably the Collossus Machines, developed by code-breakers in 1943–5 for military purposes, which were used, amongst others, by Turing for his cryptanalysis of the German ENIGMA machines.

Perhaps the most fruitful findings were in relation to seizure prediction, based on prolonged (for months) recording of EEG.[51] Big data also spurred multicentre collaboration, especially in the fields of genetics (for instance, the Epi25, Epi4 K, EpiPEX consortia) and in imaging (for instance, the sententiously named ENIGMA project). The main advantage of vast numbers is the opportunity for detailed sub-analyses, but the disadvantage is that the quality of the data is often substandard ('garbage in, garbage out') and this is especially true of subjective data where the trade-off is uncertain. The Human Brain Project, which had been applied to epilepsy but without any real findings, proved, at least up to 2020, a paradigmatic example of this.

TREATING EPILEPSY

The Pharmaceutical Industry

In the 1980s and 1990s, the pharmaceutical market had grown at double-digit rates and became dominated by giant global conglomerates. Mergers and acquisitions were the order of the day in the 1990s. Of importance to epilepsy were the mergers of Glaxo and Wellcome in 1995 to form GlaxoWellcome, which then amalgamated in 2000 with SmithKline Beecham to form GlaxoSmithKline. Ciba and Geigy, which had already merged to become Ciba-Geigy in 1970, did so again with Sandoz in 1996, becoming Novartis. Hoechst aligned with Roussel and Marion Merrell Dow in 1997 to become Hoechst Marion Roussel, and then Aventis in 1999. In 2004 Aventis was taken over by Sanofi.[52] Indeed, so successful financially was the industry that by 1999, eight of the world's twenty-five largest corporations were pharmaceutical companies (an astounding record considering their small size in the early twentieth century). Profits were huge, but dark clouds gathered on the horizon. Although the industry was heavily research and development driven, the number of new game-changing drugs successfully being licensed in this period began to fall.[53] Part of the reason was the increased expense of bringing a drug to market due to the interconnected escalation in the costs of research and regulation. It was claimed that the overall cost of R&D for each new product rose from $110 million in 1976 to $6,000 million in 1997. The time taken from initial discovery to licensing had also risen to 10–15 years, as regulatory procedures and the required amount of testing increased. A striking contrast

---

[51] See Cook, 'Advancing seizure forecasting'.

[52] Another stimulus to acquisition was the fact that by 1995 the top twenty-five companies accounted for about 50% of production, but none had more than 6.5% of total sales.

[53] Spending by the pharmaceutical industry on R&D increased from $5.4 billion in 1981 to more than $40 billion in 1998, amounting in 1999 to 18% of annual sales. Despite this, the number of licensed new molecular entities (a commonly used categorization for a 'new' drug) in all medical areas fell from 60 in 1987 to 37 in 1997.

to the less than two years taken from the first trials of phenytoin to its licensing in 1940 – still one of the world's most-prescribed antiepileptics. Other factors compounded the difficulties. Many potential drugs failed to make it through the process to licensing,[54] and by 2000 a large number of conventional drugs were falling out of patent. Litigation had also boomeranged: between company and company, usually over patent or intellectual property rights; by governments over regulatory matters; and by individuals over side effects. Legislative changes also played a role, leading to rapid growth in the number of generic manufacturers. These were often based in developing and middle-income countries with a lower cost base.

The major companies at the time were either American or European. Of the new molecular entities launched in 1997, 75% of products came from the United States, Switzerland, Germany and Britain. Access to drugs was also highly unequal. In 1999, for example, 80% of world production was sold in only fifteen industrialised countries (America accounting for most), with drugs often in very short supply in the developing world. This inequality resulted in large-scale public campaigns to force the companies to supply the developing world without making large profits, not least during 'epidemics' such as AIDS in the 1990s and Covid in 2020.

Overshadowing all this was the demonisation of the industry in the public mind. Public hostility was mainly directed at the industry's controversial marketing methods, relating, for instance, to the biased conduct and reporting of clinical trials, fraudulent practice and excessive profiteering. Criticism was also levelled at the extent of 'gifts' to health professionals, sponsorship of journals and conferences, funding of lay groups, lobbying, and of flawed research. Disease mongering[55] (and the 'medicalisation' of behaviours, an endemic problem by then in psychiatry) had also been considered to explain in part the growing number of people identified to have epilepsy and of 'epilepsy syndromes', thus increasing the size of the pharmaceutical market. The claim that the medical and pharmaceutical industries lacked transparency led in the United States to the passage of the 'Physicians' Payment Sunshine Act' of 2010, which required the pharmaceutical industry to make public their financial payments to physicians and hospitals.

---

[54] A number of drugs advanced almost to the end of the development pathway in these years, only to be discontinued because of side effects or lack of effectiveness in humans. Such drugs included, by 2010: remacemide, denzinamide, nafimidone, ralitoline, loreclezole, losigamone, carisbamate, seletracetam, valrocemide, propylisopropyl acetamide, fluorofelbamate, huperzine A, talampanel and tonabersat.

[55] See Healy, *Pharmageddon*.

Despite the downsides, the value of the antiepileptic drug market had increased dramatically. The total sales of antiepileptic drugs in the United States, for instance, rose from $400 million in 1990 to $3 billion in 2000. In 2001 the total world market for epilepsy was valued at around $5 billion, with some 42 million people diagnosed with epilepsy globally and around 3.5 million new cases each year.[56] The potential profits had attracted the largest pharmaceutical companies and by 2009, five of the six largest pharmaceutical companies were marketing antiepileptic drugs and accounted for approximately 75% of the global antiepileptic market in monetary terms. The success of the newer antiepileptics was all the more remarkable given that, in epilepsy, none had proven to be, in controlled clinical trials, any more efficacious than the older, much cheaper drugs, nor were they free of side effects.

One major attraction of this market was the fact that the drugs, once licensed for epilepsy, also then tended to be used in other conditions – notably for pain, bipolar disease and other psychiatric disorders, which were even more lucrative markets. Up to June 2004, for instance, around one-third of Pfizer's total sales were due to Neurontin, which had been licensed first for epilepsy in 1994 but then became very much more widely used to treat pain.

The lure of large profits and the lack of clear-cut scientific evidence to justify the costs were one reason for the enormous rise in marketing budgets within the pharmaceutical industry. The recognition that 'a brand is simply a perception' led the industry to spend large sums of money on changing perceptions. In the early post-war years, marketing was limited and restrained, but from the 1980s the mood changed. Marketing became increasingly sophisticated, and powerful methods were used to target doctors.[57] Details are often difficult to uncover, but two examples in the public domain deserve mention. The first was the filing, in 1996, by David Franklin, an American microbiologist employed by Parke-Davis, of a whistle-blower lawsuit alleging illegal promotion of Neurontin (the antiepileptic gabapentin). In 2004, Pfizer (which had acquired Warner Lambert in 2000; Warner Lambert had acquired Parke-Davis in 1976) pleaded guilty to the charges and paid over $400 million in fines.

[56] The difference in price between the traditional drugs (long off patent) and the new antiepileptics was staggeringly high. In 2009, based on 2008 figures from the British National Formulary, a year's supply of phenobarbital (the cheapest drug) in the United Kingdom at a standard dose range (60–180 mg/day) cost the NHS £9.12–27.36 (in 60 mg tabs). This compared with a cost of £1,255 and £4,852 for a standard-dose range of levetiracetam (1,000 mg/day in 500 mg tablets to 4,000 mg/day in 1,000 mg tablets), a 138–177-fold difference (Cockerell and Shorvon, 'Economic cost of epilepsy', p. 115).

[57] Patient organisations also began to receive financial support from the pharmaceutical industry and were often more naïve about the terms than the medical organisations. In some countries, notably America, direct marketing to patients was also permitted, resulting in heavy advertising in public and social media – a practice prohibited in Europe.

Because of the legal proceedings, details of the marketing budget and marketing strategy were made public, including the epilepsy-related activities, and the documents analysed in detail in a seminal article from which all the following information is taken.[58] In 1998, the draft total advertising and promotion budget of gabapentin by Parke-Davis, the manufacturer, was $40 million. Several strategies were employed by the company, including the use of advisory boards in cultivate relationships and the sponsorship of education, publication and research. Nineteen million dollars was spent on professional education arranged by Parke-Davis directly or indirectly through medical communication companies. Doctors, both speakers and delegates were paid to attend conferences, sometimes in fashionable resorts, or teleconferences, and one physician speaker requested or was allocated over $175,000 for participation in activities over a five year period. The company contracted with medical education companies to expand the literature on gabapentin by developing reviews and original articles and letters – paying up to $18,000 per article – signed off by leading physicians. Some were ghost-written and some failed to acknowledge sponsorship. Parke-Davis also sponsored an uncontrolled open-label study (the STEPs study) in which more than 700 physicians were each paid $300 per enrolled patient. Under the guise of research, the papers show that this was considered a 'seeding study' by the company. Some authors of the resulting publications – names well known in the field of epilepsy – had substantial financial relationships with Parke-Davis and six were claimed to have participated in a total of 263 activities sponsored by the company between 1993 and 1997, with requested or allocated payments of up to $69,000 per author.[59]

A second example of the sophistication of marketing techniques was the 'integrated segmentation' strategy of UCB's campaign to promote Keppra (levetiracetam). Keppra proved to be a highly successful compound, with sales amounting to more than $1 billion dollars in 2006, and this single drug propelled UCB, then a relatively small Belgian pharmaceutical company, into the big league. The integrated segmentation model showed the subtlety and detail with which pharmaceutical companies made their pitch to the medical profession (their customers).[60] Instead of targeting physicians on the basis of the volume of prescriptions they wrote, which had been the traditional model, the integrated segmentation model was an analysis of individual prescribing behaviours, demographics and psychographics (attitudes, beliefs and values) to fine-tune sales targets. For a particular product, for example, one segment might consist of price-sensitive physicians, another might include

---

[58] Steinman et al., 'Promotion of gabapentin'.
[59] Details of all these allegations are taken from Steinman et al., 'Promotion of gabapentin'.
[60] Brand and Kumar, 'Detailing gets personal'.

doctors loyal to a given manufacturer's brand, and a third might include those unfriendly towards reps.

The *Franklin* v. *Parke-Davis* case spawned further claims and encouraged a wave of litigation from other companies involving antiepileptic drugs. Abbott paid $1.5 billion in 2012 to resolve clinical and civil investigations of off-label promotion of Depakote.[61] In the same year, GSK agreed to pay $2 billion to resolve its civil liabilities with the US federal government as well as the individual states, for a range of drugs, including the antiepileptic Lamictal.[62] In 2004, UCB paid $34 million to resolve criminal and civil charges for mis-selling Keppra. These are just some examples. In a 24-year period up to 2020, it is said that 373 settlements for marketing fraud were made by pharmaceutical companies, amounting to $35.7 billion.[63]

Marketing practices were often at the heart of these claims, relating to off-label marketing, and activities in research, publication and medical education (as 'Medical Education drives the market').[64] Most of the lawsuits originated in the United States, but the European Union and China had, by 2020, also entered the fray. For instance, in 2015, more than 700 generic drugs, including common antiepileptics, were recommended for suspension by the European regulators because of data manipulation in studies conducted by the Indian research company GVK.[65] It was partly as a result of these claims that the pharmaceutical industry was voted in 2019 as the most poorly regarded industry in the eyes of the American public.[66]

By 2000 pressure to introduce new business models was growing, and the pharmaceutical landscape began to change. Major pharmaceutical multinationals increasingly outsourced fundamental research to smaller biotechnology companies, often with single biotechnology-produced products targeted at novel biochemical processes. If the product was successful, these small companies were then acquired. This was an effective model because although there were thousands of small and medium-sized companies, only the largest companies could afford to bring a drug success-fully to market. The mode of drug discovery had also evolved after 2000. New animal and in-vitro models, and new computing and biological tech-nologies, changed the way drugs were discovered and screened, and research was targeted at known biochemical processes. But, disappointingly, only a

---

[61] 'Abbott Labs to pay'.   [62] 'GlaxoSmithKline to plead guilty'.
[63] Compton, 'Big pharma'. Although big sums, the total global revenue of pharmaceutical companies in 2014 was over $1 trillion, and profits from prescription drugs were expected to reach $610 billion by 2021.
[64] Steinman et al., 'Promotion of gabapentin'.
[65] Pharmaceutical company activities are tracked by a number of individuals and organisations, including the website FiercePharma.com.
[66] McCarthy, 'Big pharma sinks'.

handful of new antiepileptics using these approaches were successfully licensed; chance, random screening and the minor structural manipulation of known antiepileptics still predominated.

With the lack of success in finding effective pharmaceuticals using traditional models, the emphasis on drugs for the common forms of epilepsy was replaced in the 2010s by a growth in innovative drugs for rarer diseases and orphan and genetic disorders, many of which cause seizures. These new classes of medicines were directed at novel molecular targets and exploited the rash of molecular genetic discoveries. For rare metabolic epilepsies, such medicines were sometimes the only effective treatment, a monopoly position that allowed breathtakingly high prices to be charged. In 2017, for instance, the agent cerliponase alfa was licensed for a rare condition[67] – infantile neuronal ceroid lipofuscinosis type 2, which results in devastating epilepsy – at a cost of more than $700,000 annually per patient and the need for lifelong therapy. The median price of novel drugs by 2015 had risen to an annual cost of more than $100,000 per patient, as companies saw the opportunity for high profits. Suddenly, too, events and conferences were being organised and papers written on the topic of rare diseases, often stimulated behind the scenes by industry strategists.

Large numbers of smaller biotech companies sprang up, producing totally novel compounds such as monoclonal antibodies and gene therapies. By the 2010s the industry was in the grip of change as great as that of the 1960s, with implications for epilepsy that were (and still are) entirely unpredictable.

New Antiepileptics

Despite the industry turmoil and the numerous hurdles to drug licensing, between 1995 and 2020 thirteen new drugs were approved for use primarily in epilepsy (tagged as third-generation antiepileptics by inventive pharmaceutical marketeers) – albeit, for the first time, some for specific epilepsy syndromes only (Table 5.3).

Perhaps surprisingly, chance and random screening rather than design still played a major role in the discovery of most of these agents. The two most successful drugs were developed for another indication, and their antiepileptic potential was found later by random screening. Topiramate (licensed in 1995) is a monosaccharide derived from fructose, and was initially developed as an antidiabetic drug. Levetiracetam, licensed in 1999 in the United States and in 2000 in Europe, was developed as a 'cognitive enhancer' but was shown in its

---

[67] For instance, there were thought in 2020 to be 3–6 new cases in the United Kingdom each year and 30–50 existing cases (from a national population of more than 60 million persons).

TABLE 5.3 *Antiepileptic drugs licensed in Europe and the United States, 1995–2020*

Year of first licence	Proprietary name	Country in which first licensed	Manufacturer
1995	Topiramate	UK	Johnson and Johnson
1996	Tiagabine	France	Novo-Nordisk
1999	Levetiracetam	USA	UCB Pharma
2000	Zonisamide*	USA	Elan pharmaceuticals
2004	Pregabalin	Europe	Pfizer
2007	Stiripentol	Europe	Laboratoires Biocodex
2007	Rufinamide	Europe	Eisei
2008	Lacosamide	Europe	UCB Pharma
2009	Eslicarbazepine acetate	Europe	Bial
2010	Retigabine	USA	GSK
2012	Perampanel	Europe	Eisai
2016	Brivaracetam	Europe and USA	UCB Pharma
2018	Cannabidiol	USA	GW Pharma

* Zonisamide had been licensed in 1989 in Japan and South Korea.

first trials to have little effect in this indication. The mode of action of both drugs was obscure at the time of licensing.[68]

Other 'designer drugs' were deliberately constructed to attack a specific mechanism, but were found to be of little utility in clinical practice or to have an alternative mode of action. Tiagabine, a selective GABA-reuptake inhibitor, was licensed first in 1996 in Europe, but was found to be relatively ineffective and its use then petered out. Retigabine (licensed in 2012) was a truly novel drug which acted directly at the voltage-gated potassium channels that conduct the M-type potassium current. However, patients taking it developed blue colouration of the face and hands, and the drug was discontinued. Gabapentin (licensed in 1993) was designed as a GABA analogue, but its mode of action[69] turned out to have nothing to do with GABA-ergic transmission, and it anyway turned out to have only limited value in epilepsy. Perhaps only one new antiepileptic, perampanel, a drug designed to block the AMPA receptor, seemed to make the grade as a rationally designed and effective drug.

[68] In 2004 the levetiracetam binding site in the brain was found to be a synaptic vesicle protein (SV2A) involved in synaptic vesicle exocytosis and presynaptic neurotransmitter release. But how binding confers antiepileptic action is unknown.

[69] It has been found to act by binding to the $\alpha 2\delta$ sub-unit of the neuronal voltage-gated calcium channel, reducing calcium influx into the nerve terminals and, in turn, a decrease in glutamate release.

Other drugs were derivatives of existing drugs, with very slight differences in structure, including eslicarbazepine acetate (licensed in 2009), a derivative of carbamazepine and oxcarbazepine, and brivaracetam (licensed in 2016) a close relation of levetiracetam. The major success story of this type was pregabalin (licensed in 2004 in Europe and 2005 in the United States), which was discovered in 1989 by medicinal chemist Richard Silverman, working at Northwestern University. Pregabalin is a derivative of gabapentin but binds much more tightly than gabapentin to its molecular receptor. Its success, though, was not so much as an antiepileptic, as its effect in epilepsy proved rather modest, but as a drug to control neuropathic pain, and in this indication it brought in $1.2 billion in sales. Interestingly, both Silverman and Northwestern accrued huge sums from the royalties, and pregabalin raised the university from 71st to 11th in the league of US universities' industrial earnings. Another drug, lacosamide (licensed in 2009), was designed to block sodium channels, as did conventional drugs such as carbamazepine, phenytoin and lamotrigine, although acting mainly on the so-called slow component of the channel (Table 5.4).

Other 'new' drugs had a more tortuous and long-drawn-out history. Zonisamide was discovered in 1972, and was approved for licensing in Japan and South Korea in 1989. An attempt to license the drug in Europe and the United States failed due to its perceived toxicity and lack of effect. But, following a new series of randomised clinical trials in the United States, it was approved there for prescribing in 2000, in the United Kingdom and Germany in 2005, and subsequently in many other countries. The drug had, in the meantime, proved popular in Japan, where by 2016 it was said to account for about 15% of the Japanese antiepileptic drug market. Stiripentol was identified as an antiepileptic in 1978, but its initial trials in adults with partial epilepsy were relatively disappointing. It was then found to have a seemingly specific action in severe myoclonic epilepsy in infancy (Dravet syndrome) and was licensed in 2007 under the newly created orphan drug scheme of the European Medicines Agency for use only in conjunction with clobazam and valproate, and only in patients with this rare condition. This was the first antiepileptic drug to be licensed for a rare disease and with such a narrow indication. It was quickly followed by rufinamide, a drug initially trialled in adults with partial epilepsy with rather disappointing results, but later licensed in children with Lennox–Gastaut syndrome under the same European scheme.

Another newcomer was cannabidiol, essentially an herbal derived from the cannabis plant. Cannabis had been recommended for epilepsy for centuries, but drug abuse laws in most countries of the world prohibited its sale and use (legislation in the more punitive countries carried the death sentence). Nonetheless, it continued to be widely illegally available and used. Increasingly, families of children with severe epilepsy campaigned for the licensing of cannabis derivatives and governments worldwide faced mounting public criticism for their position. When GW, a small British pharmaceutical company, was able to purify cannabidiol

TABLE 5.4 *How the antiepileptic effects of contemporary therapy were discovered*

Drug	Antiepileptic action found by:	Comments
Carbamazepine	Manipulation of existing structure and random screening	Found by chance in an attempt to develop drugs for bipolar disease
Benzodiazepines	Random screening initially and then manipulation of existing structures	
Brivaracetam	Manipulation of existing structure	
Cannabidiol	Purification of a natural product	Natural compound known to have antiepileptic properties
Eslicarbazepine	Manipulation of existing structure	
Ethosuximide	Manipulation of existing structure	
Felbamate	Random screening	
Gabapentin	Attempted rational design, but wrong mechanism	Designed as a GABAergic drug, but mechanism is actually non-GABAergic
Lacosamide	Manipulation of existing structure	
Lamotrigine	Attempted rational design, but wrong mechanism	Found in a screen of anti-folate drugs, on the erroneous assumption that antiepileptic action could be due to anti-folate properties
Levetiracetam	Manipulation of existing structure	
Oxcarbazepine	Manipulation of existing structure	
Phenobarbital	Pure chance	Observation that phenobarbital given as a human sedative also controlled seizures
Phenytoin	Random screening	
Piracetam	Pure chance	Observation that piracetam given as a cognitive enhancer also controlled myoclonus
Pregabalin	Attempted rational design, but wrong mechanism	Designed as a GABAergic drug, but mechanism is actually non-GABAergic
Retigabine	Rational design	Designed to be an allosteric modulator of cerebral potassium channels
Rufinamide	Random screening	Designed for partial seizures, bu failed and then screened in Lennox–Gastaut syndrome
Stiripentol	Random screening	Designed for partial seizures, but failed then screened in Dravet syndrome

(continued)

TABLE 5.4 *(continued)*

Drug	Antiepileptic action found by:	Comments
Tiagabine	Attempted rational design, but wrong mechanism	Designed as a GABAergic drug, but mechanism is actually non-GABAergic
Topiramate	Random screening	Designed initially as an antidiabetic drug
Valproate	Pure chance	
Vigabatrin	Rational design	Designed to be a GABA agonist

(one of the alkaloids from cannabis and one said not to have the psychotropic action of cannabis itself) and to show that it had antiepileptic action, pressure intensified. Resistance cracked, and the GW drug was licensed for use in the United States and Europe under the orphan drug scheme in 2017/18 for Lennox–Gastaut or Dravet syndrome, but only in combination with clobazam. Other drugs aimed at the mechanisms of specific inborn errors of metabolism, rather than at seizures per se, still seemed to improve epilepsy in these conditions. The abovementioned cerliponase alfa, which corrects the enzyme defect in Neuronal Ceroid Lipofuscinosis type 2, was the leading example.

The overall impact of his raft of new drugs though proved disappointing. None proved to be a magic bullet in the common epilepsies and none were shown in any randomised or blinded trial to be superior to the older conventional drugs such as carbamazepine or valproate. Furthermore, the wilder promises of the molecular age, such as personalised medicine, pharmacogenetically determined therapy, stem cell therapy and gene therapy, remained almost entirely unfulfilled.

Specialisation and Clinical Guidelines

An indirect result of the increasing range of potential therapies was a change in the pattern of clinical practice. As the number of drugs multiplied, so did sub-specialism. General neurologists increasingly felt out of date with the new drug introductions, and there was an increasing tendency for some individuals to restrict their practice and to specialise in epilepsy. For similar reasons, sub-specialism occurred in other fields, for instance in movement disorders and multiple sclerosis, and as hospitals expanded their neurological departments, neurologists began to be appointed with narrow fields of interest. The sub-specialty of 'epileptology' flourished as never before. Whether this was a good thing or not is arguable, not least as such sub-specialism carried the great risk of isolating epilepsy from the mainstream of neurology, deskilling its practitioners in other areas. As specialists became more and more involved in single diseases, and applied their technical knowledge, patients complained that the holistic aspects of medicine were increasingly ignored.

Clinical guidelines, which had increased dramatically in number since 1995, were another new fashion and very much a curate's egg. Authoritative advice was helpful to all clinicians, but the extraordinary proliferation of epilepsy guidelines has been described as an avalanche that 'risks burying the clinician in a white snow of double-talk and humbug'.[70] This is no exaggeration: up until 1980, a PubMed search for 'epilepsy guidelines' turned up only 191 hits; by 2020, there were 35,000.[71] By the 2010s, guidelines on the clinical management of epilepsy were produced by governments, hospitals groups, professional and lay bodies, groups sponsored by industry and individuals. Monthly journals of guidelines were published, sponsored by the pharmaceutical industry. Most of these guidelines are based on the same data sets and, on the face of it, represent a large-scale and wasteful duplication of effort.

Even where guidelines were based on the same clinical trial data they did not necessarily come up with the same conclusions or recommendations. The only explanation is that they could not have been scientifically objective. And indeed many were not, for the committees producing guidelines were almost invariably subject to political pressures and commercial interference. Objectivity proved a fragile edifice. It had been repeatedly shown that commercially funded reviews were prone to bias in favour of the sponsor, and there could be no doubt that, under the cover of such guidelines, evidence could be massaged or reinterpreted. Some companies played a long game by funding studies with low scientific value whose goal was primarily to influence opinion, and then to use the studies in the production of guidelines. The same applied to guidelines promoted by professional organisations and government bodies, where deeply engrained prejudices often played a key role.

Guidelines raised another issue at the heart of ethical medical practice. Before the guideline culture became embedded in medicine, doctors were able to exercise freedom to prescribe any drug licensed for the purpose and to form their own independent judgement about a medicine's utility in any individual patient. The guideline culture turned medicine into a more and more protocol-driven process, and in doing so inevitably eroded the principle of clinical freedom. There were also legal ramifications. Guidelines were not generally intended to be regulations but were nevertheless often treated as such, and were, for instance, increasingly used as evidence in medical litigation. The best clinical guidelines provided a framework for the clinician who needed to

[70] Shorvon, 'Clinical guideline'.
[71] Some have argued that the guideline culture benefits authors more than patients, as a doctor's name on a guideline publication increases his or her visibility and citation index.

weigh the advice and adapt it to the personal needs of an individual patient. This was the initial purpose, but increasingly, through a subtle transition, the guideline became a rulebook.

Epilepsy Surgery

By 1995, epilepsy surgery was well into its second century. Over the first hundred years, the fashion for surgery had fluctuated remarkably. Operations largely ceased in the early twentieth century, and increased again briefly in the 1950s, but interest then waned, both because of better medical treatment and because the long-term outcome of surgery was not as good as had been hoped. Then in 1986, the first Palm Desert conference on the surgical treatment of the epilepsies[72] was held, and, with strong support from high-profile figures in the epilepsy world, it served to rekindle interest in the topic. ILAE president Jerome Engel was the leading advocate, expressing in 2009 the view that '[s]urgical treatment for epilepsy is arguably the most underutilized of all accepted therapeutic interventions in the entire field of medicine', and that 'the uncontested cost-effectiveness of surgical treatment ... must be contrasted not only with the monetary cost of a lifetime of disability, but also with the human cost of premature death, morbidity and social and psychological compromise'.[73] The comment on cost-effectiveness was a reference to a randomised trial (conducted in Western Ontario by a future ILAE president, Sam Wiebe[74]) which found that a year after surgery 64% of operated patients were free of disabling seizures, compared with 8% who continued medical therapy alone. What was often not appreciated was that this study was of a highly selected group, and the cost-effectiveness of surgery applied only to a narrow band of subjects. Nevertheless, this was the only randomised and controlled study of epilepsy surgery and therefore a landmark in the field. In 2003 the American Academy of Neurology issued a report, authored by Engel, Wiebe and others, concluding that surgery was the treatment of choice for medically intractable temporal lobe epilepsy.[75]

The long-term studies of temporal lobe surgery (the commonest operation) do indeed show that more than 50% of operated patients are rendered free of disabling seizures (but not minor episodes). Not reported, however, were the opportunity costs − and these deserve consideration (a topic taken up in the Epilogue) − nor the vital fact that in a private health system, such as in the United States, the hospitals (and surgeons) saw in epilepsy surgery the

---

[72] Published by Engel as *Surgical Treatment of the Epilepsies*, first in 1987. A second edition appeared in 1993. The first conference was deliberately scheduled to be held on the centenary of the first modern epilepsy surgery by Horsley in 1886.

[73] Engel, 'Surgical treatment of epilepsy', p. 743.

[74] Wiebe et al., 'Surgery for temporal-lobe epilepsy'.   [75] Engel Jr et al., 'Practice parameter'.

prospect for financial profits. For some programmes, financial gain was a primary motivation.

The temporal lobectomy resects about 15% of brain tissue, and the adverse consequences of surgery were another pressing medical issue. Numerous case reports attested to a variety of psychological and behavioural disturbances following epilepsy surgery, affecting sexuality and libido, anxiety, depression, aggression, obsessionality, empathy and emotional warmth, memory and psychosis. However, the standard of evidence was entirely anecdotal. Neither the overall frequency nor severity of these side effects were known. Ever since Pearce Bailey opined in the 1950s that epilepsy surgery was not psychosurgery pains were taken to differentiate the two, but there was no doubt that psychological deficits can be a consequence and that there is a significant overlap. Another concern was the effect of resective surgery on 'cerebral reserve', a concept increasingly recognised – not least in legal proceedings – as important in deciding the risk of later dementia. Despite the long history of surgery, these aspects remained untested.

One field which became increasingly technologically based was the assessment of people for surgery. Assessment aimed at identifying the 'epileptogenic zone' (a concept first described by Horsley), defined as the area of brain necessary and sufficient for initiating seizures and whose removal or disconnection was necessary for their abolition. This is a circular definition based on the result of surgery which it purports to predict, and as such is impervious to proof, but this did not stop its widespread adoption. The major developments in this period had focused on the application of technologies to identify this zone, rather than the type of surgery carried out. Prolonged invasive EEG recordings and frameless MRI stereotaxy were introduced, requiring complicated technologies and analysis. A new sub-specialty grew up within clinical neurophysiology. How much this all added to surgical outcome was (and remains) completely unknown, but many in the field were hypnotised by the complexity and elegance of the recordings. Increasingly, these recordings were integrated with MRI and PET scanning and post-processing to identify the 'focus'. The added value of each investigation was never assessed, and the field remains one where practice varies considerably, and where clinical and financial interests are intimately entangled. Strikingly absent during this period was any sort of independent technology assessment.

With the advent of MRI-directed stereotaxy, neurostimulation was resuscitated and underwent one of its periodic resurgences after around 2005. A number of high-technology systems were produced. The largest study was the SANTE trial of deep brain stimulation (DBS; published in 2015)[76] of the

---

[76] Salanova et al., 'Long-term efficacy and safety of thalamic stimulation'.

anterior nucleus of the thalamus, which found a 29% decrease in seizure frequency over a three-month period, and which reached statistical significance (although note that one person with a large increase was excluded from the analysis as an 'outlier'). The improvement was said to be sustained on long-term follow up. There was also an RCT of responsive stimulation reported in 2014 (the Neuro-Pace trial[77]) – that is, stimulation to the epileptic 'focus' triggered by a developing epileptic seizure (this method requires continuous monitoring of the EEG by implanted electrodes in addition to stimulation technology). This found a reduced seizure frequency of 24.9%, results which were not really different from those of VNS (albeit in different populations). The FDA has approved both methods, and the financial gains for the manufacturers were gratifying, but whether any of the stimulation methods will provide long-lasting or worthwhile improvement in seizures in routine practice is totally unclear – and the long past history of cerebral stimulation for epilepsy does not give grounds for optimism. The technique was heavily promoted in many medical fora by opinion leaders sponsored by the device manufacturers, much as had been the pattern in the pharmaceutical arena (indeed, sometimes the same persons have promoted both devices and drugs). One notable difference is that regulations controlling the marketing of devices are generally far less restricting than those for pharmaceuticals.

THE EXPERIENCE OF HAVING EPILEPSY

This was a period when general attitudes towards epilepsy improved significantly. In consequence, the experience of having epilepsy was less ringed with hostility or rejection. This was a trend which in liberal democratic societies had started in the post-war decades and gathered momentum throughout the century.

Changing Public Attitudes and Stigma

The practice, begun after the war in America and then Europe, of surveying public opinion on epilepsy had by the 1990s expanded to many corners of the world. And, as in the original surveys, the focus was on negative attitudes, which formed the basis for enacted stigma.

In the Western economies, consumerist at heart, these surveys were often conducted by voluntary agencies for the purpose of lobbying, and some (though not all) were more propagandist than scientific in nature. An example was the statement of the Epilepsy Foundation of America, which proclaimed in

---

[77] Heck et al., 'Responsive neurostimulation'.

its survey of November 2001 of 20,000 adolescents that 'about 50% of adolescents were not sure whether epilepsy was contagious or not and only 31% said they would "date" a person with epilepsy'.[78] In fact, most had indicated they did not know the cause of epilepsy, only 4% actually said they thought epilepsy was contagious and only 11% said they would not date a person with epilepsy. Nonetheless, the survey painted a considerably more positive picture than had surveys of a few decades earlier. What was also revealed, perhaps not surprisingly, was that knowledge about, and familiarity with, epilepsy was relatively sparse. As a result, a ten-year campaign was launched between 2003 and 2013 to raise awareness, using traditional and social media. Whether these efforts changed perceptions and stigma is not reported.

Jacoby carried out a survey of 1,694 individuals from a randomly selected cohort in Britain in 2011.[79] This study found that the public were relatively well informed about epilepsy and that attitudes to epilepsy were generally more favourable than previously. Around 90% thought that people with epilepsy are as intelligent as everyone else; children with epilepsy should be allowed to play with other children; people with epilepsy can be as successful as anyone else in their chosen careers; and people with epilepsy can lead a normal life. However, more than half of the informants agreed that people with epilepsy are treated differently by society. Exclusion, restriction and non-normality were commonly cited as reasons for this perception, and epilepsy was ranked highly as a condition of great concern to respondents if they had to work with someone affected by the disease. Jacoby took this finding as confirmation of Goffman's concepts of non-normality and differentness. She concluded that public attitudes towards epilepsy had shifted considerably since the street surveys of the 1980s, and that '"the full force of past and contemporary social prejudice and misunderstanding" [a quote from Trostle, 1997] may finally be diminishing' (p. 1412). This seems correct.

One explanation for the lessening of stigma, at least in Western cultures, had, in Jacoby's words, been the trend to 'value rather than reject human differences and to redefine as normal conditions of being (including health conditions and disabilities) previously viewed as abnormal'.[80] She made the interesting and thoughtful point that although the medical model had generally reinforced the classification of ill and disabled people as abnormal, this transformation in the case of epilepsy from the moral to the medical domain, and from badness to sickness, had almost certainly contributed to its decreasing stigma and had done much to lessen the private grief of people with epilepsy about their condition.

---

[78] Austin, Shafer and Deering 'A survey of adolescents'.

[79] Jacoby et al., 'Public knowledge, private grief'; Trostle 'Social aspects, stigma'.

[80] In the liberal democratic social ethos that prevailed, similar improvements were seen in all stigmatised groups, for instance towards homosexual individuals and racial minorities.

Geography matters, and in general, in countries in the developing world cultural attitudes had not changed much, with as many as 90% of people with epilepsy and 75% of their family members reporting felt stigma. An interesting study from China[81] showed epilepsy to be perceived as a 'terrible' condition, with very few considering people with epilepsy as being the same as those without. And, because seizures are considered to be unpredictable, the affected person was seen as 'out of control'. Epilepsy was considered incurable and often inherited. As one community leader put it:

> No psycho disease can be radically cured. [The patient] has to take medicine for the long-term. It impacts on daily life seriously, increasing the burden for the family. They can maintain things well if they persist with taking medicine, but cannot be radically cured and will have seizures easily when being anxious, angry and tired. It is therefore a heavy economic burden and a psychological pressure to the patient and the family.

Others considered it 'impossible for some to marry and have children', and some neurologists and traditional practitioners thought that those with epilepsy were likely to have an 'epileptic' character. These attitudes were strongest in rural areas. Concealment was commonly driven by the need for work and prospects for marriage. Numerous other studies in other parts of the developing world reported similar findings.

Many other aspects of the stigma of epilepsy were studied in this period, emphasising its complexity and its effect on social identity.[82] The importance of religious belief was emphasised in a study from Saudi Arabia, regarding both the cause of the condition (God's will) and its treatment, with 93% of respondents believing that religious treatment rituals should be used in parallel with orthodox medical treatment methods. This study also emphasised the importance of the family in supporting and approving treatments, and the need for physicians to understand the family dynamic and to recommend treatments that accord with it.[83]

Explanations of stigma by sociologists were generally more convincing and less superficial than the medical theories, but all acknowledged that stigma was the result of a complex mix of societal and personal experience, preconceptions and expectations. Identified cultural factors included: education, disability legislation, attitudes towards equal opportunity, cultural norms of behaviour, public and social media messages, parental reaction to the diagnosis (shame, concealment or, alternatively, overprotection), stereotypic expectations, life experiences, the severity of epilepsy, the personality of the individual and

---

[81] Yang et al., 'Epilepsy in China'.

[82] See, for instance, Jacoby, Snape and Baker, 'Epilepsy and social identity'.

[83] Alkhamees, Selai and Shorvon, 'Beliefs among patients'.

victimhood. In many Western countries, the lay organisations carried out campaigns to improve attitudes with varying success. Possibly it was the complexity of these factors that rendered well-meaning but naïve attempts to combat stigma futile, and most individual campaigns made little difference. Nevertheless, the sum total of all these efforts must have contributed to the improving attitudes.

Labels and terminology are another source of stigma. In the 1970s campaigns were launched to replace the term 'epileptic' by 'people with epilepsy', an effort that was largely successful. In the first decades of the twenty-first century, attention shifted to pejorative meanings of the word 'epilepsy' in some Eastern languages. Successful campaigns were launched to change the name in Korea, where the traditional name has associations with madness, and Hong Kong, where the word has associations with animals and madness. In Japan, too, it has been pointed out that the word used for epilepsy – *tenkan* – carries connotations of 'to become mad' and to have 'a violent temperament that is apt to be infatuated', and the word itself was taken as evidence of the deep roots of discrimination and stigmatisation.[84] Similar linguistic associations existed in other countries, especially in Africa and other Asian languages.

The Changing Experience of Epilepsy in Films, Novels and Memoirs

How epilepsy is dealt with in the creative arts has always been, and will always be, kalaidoscopic in scope and nature. But despite this, the general thrust of the depiction of epilepsy in this period underwent a remarkable change. The old eugenical theme of the person with epilepsy as weak, impaired and worthless largely disappeared and was replaced by the portrayal of characters with epilepsy as brave, strong and more emotionally mature than those around them. The old characterisations of the person with epilepsy as insane, degenerate, amoral, feeble-minded or possessed vanished as the focus of much creative work switched to describing how individuals overcame epilepsy, or at least accommodated it. Quite remarkably too, for the first time many memoirs and autobiographic writings of authors with epilepsy were published in which epilepsy was a central theme. Prior to 1985, only a handful of such books were published (Margiad Evan's *Ray of Darkness*, for instance) but since then a whole genre has appeared.[85] Gone, it seems, were the days when the imperative was to deny or conceal the condition.

As the century drew to a close, epilepsy also became an ever more familiar theme in cinema and television. In her review of 192 non-documentary films

---

[84] Kuramochi et al., 'Self-stigma of patients'.

[85] A host of such books were produced in the 2010s, often with titles to do with electricity: *Short Circuit: An Epileptic Journey* (Alyssa D'Amico, 2017), 'Brain storm: an electrifying journey' (Kate Recore, 2019), 'Electrogirl: living a symbiotic existence with epilepsy '(Lainie Chait, 2017), 'Sailing through the storms of seizures' (Jon Sadler 2018).

and TV series which included epilepsy between 1900 and 2005, Toba Kerson found that more than two-thirds were released between 1990 and 2005, with 64% being categorised as dramas, but also comedies (17%), horror and science fiction (7%).[86] Similarly, epilepsy featured in numerous TV 'soaps', both medical and non-medical.[87] This coincided with a public appetite for medical stories in general, but it also seems likely that the campaigns to bring epilepsy 'out of the shadows' had borne fruit.[88]

Linked to this was a new realism in the depiction of seizures themselves. In increasing numbers of films and TV shows of this period, the convulsive epileptic seizure was vividly portrayed, in a true-to-life way which would simply not have been acceptable in the past. Examples include Sari's seizures in the Finnish film *Year of the Wolf* (2007) and in the British film *Control* (2007). *Control* was about the life of Ian Curtis, an English singer-songwriter who had epilepsy in real life and who in the film had a seizure onstage. In the case of both films, neurologists advised on the phenomenology of epilepsy, and the seizures were staged with a nod to accuracy. This reflected the trend in many societies to view epilepsy more as a genuine disease and naturalistic phenomenon and less in terms of the negative social metaphors of epilepsy. Epilepsy had been in some senses reinvented as a medical not a moral phenomenon.

An example of this trend was the novel *Electricity*, by Ray Robinson (2006), which depicts epilepsy in unprocessed unemotional realism and which was turned into a film, directed by Bryn Higgins, in 2014. The book has a number of epilepsy themes not covered in the film, but both make for uncompromising reading/viewing. The central character, Lily Jane, was born into an abusive working-class family in northern England and developed epilepsy after being thrown downstairs by her inadequate, wretched mother. Lily Jane experienced a deprived, loveless upbringing and was teased at school by her classmates, who nickname her 'FIT-TASTIC SPASTIC' (p. 13). However, stunningly beautiful, loyal and intelligent, Lily Jane was to be admired far more than most of the human wreckage she was surrounded by – and the central message of the story is that it is possible to transcend your illness and to be, in all essential ways, a better human being than others. She was an edgy, strong character ('Lily Jane, tall as a crane'; p. 23) and the book is essentially about her determination not to let herself be defined by epilepsy. Nonetheless, she did have plenty of seizures,

---

[86] Kerson and Kerson, 'Implacable images'.

[87] For instance, in the United Kingdom and the United States: *Coronation Street, East Enders, The Young and the Restless, Casualty, Chicago Hope, Grey's Anatomy, House* and *ER*. These are just a sampling; epilepsy has featured almost certainly in many others.

[88] Despite this, Ian Bone, in his review of epilepsy in the arts 'Sacred lives' p.155) considered that the depiction of epilepsy remains 'unacceptably negative' and that the movie industry should be lobbied to prevent this. However, the goal of creative cinema is not necessarily to be educative. Nevertheless, it is true that the depictions on film play an important part in both mirroring and moulding social attitude.

and the film opens with her recovering consciousness after a seizure, being stared at by uncaring onlookers far uglier and more stupid than she. The unpredictability of the seizures, their intensity and the resulting bruises and grazes were graphically described without sentimentality or pity. Doctors were shown to be well intentioned but focused on medical science – EEG, 'localisation' and medication – and therefore completely uncomprehending of her feelings or suffering. In fact, the doctors were in most important senses quite irrelevant to her life. At one point, she decided to give up all medication and, whilst clubbing, has a very severe seizure which nearly killed her (as she murmurs, 'I'm not going to die again, I've done that'). The story (and the film) are told in the first person, with the reader/viewer being taken through what it was like to have seizures. The story is based on Robinson's own childhood observation of his cousin, who lived in his household and who had daily convulsive and partial seizures. It is one of the few serious attempts to share the experience of seizures, much as Dostoyevsky did. But, unlike Dostoyevsky's, this depiction is raw, unflattering and without symbolism: epilepsy as it really is, without any signification, other meaning or metaphor.

There were exceptions to the improving portrayal of epilepsy especially in mainstream, as opposed to independent, cinema. The dramatic, sudden and arresting image of a seizure and loss of consciousness, as in earlier periods, continued to be used as a narrative device to move a story along even if epilepsy was not an essential theme of the film. Although the seizure as such could be neutral, in practice it often carried negative connotations, sometime subtle and sometimes rather obvious – for instance, in the linking of seizures with demonic possession. An example of the latter is the use of a seizure in *The Exorcist*, a film version of the 1971 horror novel by William Peter Blatty. The film (1973/2000) depicted seizures not as naturalistic convulsions but rather as overdramatised flurries of jerking and rhythmical movements which served to reinforce the ancient view of epilepsy as possession. The chief character of *The Exorcist*, the priest and psychiatrist Damien Karras, compared the human body to an ocean liner, with the brain cells as the crew. When the crew revolts (as Hughlings Jackson put it, became 'bastard cells') the body became possessed – an interesting analogy for epilepsy. Although not about epilepsy, the story carried strongly negative messages about epilepsy in which the drama hinged on a battle between good and evil, with the epileptic fit the visible sign of the presence of malignancy. Other examples of this trope were the depictions of epilepsy in the *Exorcism of Mary Rose* (2004) and in *Gods and Monsters* (2004).[89] In a minority of films, seizures were used as narrative devices to engender sympathy and respect for the person with epilepsy, even if the sense of 'otherness' and 'being different' was

[89] The director of *Gods and Monsters*, Tony Robinson, has explicitly said the film demonstrates the belief that epilepsy is possession, although in the film version (but not the TV version) epilepsy is not explicitly mentioned: 'Demonic possession?'.

never very far from the surface – for example Sam's seizures, enacted by Natalie Portman, in *Garden State* (2004) and the Reverend Smith's seizures in the TV series *Deadwood* (2004–6).

The idea that the epileptic seizure brought with it danger also persisted. The curious analogy of epilepsy as a 'wolf' ready to attack at any time is implied in the title of at least two films (*Moon of the Wolf* and *Year of the Wolf*). In a documentary film, *What's the Time Mr Wolf?*, director Sal Anderson explained that he saw 'a seizure as like a Wolf creeping up on you, ready to pounce'.[90] Enardo Baldini's prize-winning novel, *Come Il Lupo*, is another example. The metaphor also has obvious connotations of danger, aggression, violence and predation.

Epilepsy was sometimes shown in a touching or sentimental light. It featured as a major theme in several love stories: for instance, *Garden State* (2004) and the Chinese film *You Only Alone* (2020). The latter film, without much subtlety, illustrated a number of other aspects – the person with epilepsy as an outsider and the loneliness of a life with epilepsy (a central theme, as its title implies). Chi Li has epilepsy and was rejected and shunned because of it. She had opted for a life alone and marginalised, and its hardship and emotional trauma were pitilessly exposed. Chi Li yearned for her previous life as a dancer, but only had a job in a local cinema named (without irony) 'Perfect Life'. Her stance softened when she fell in love with a sympathetic man, but the hurdles of social prejudice and the perception that she was unmarriageable prove insurmountable. The film is heart-breaking and poignantly explores the rigid and intolerant culture of North China, rarely shown before, and the rather primitive nature of the stigma in that society, at a level not unlike that of pre-war Europe. Chi Li showed extraordinary fortitude and bravery in the face of brutality, but the story ends ambiguously. Epileptic seizures were vividly portrayed and play a central role. This was possibly the first and only Chinese film to be produced in which epilepsy was a topic.

Whilst Lily Jane in *Electricity* struggled with epilepsy, *Electricity* was not about overcoming seizures, but about not being defined by them. Overcoming epilepsy was, however, a major trend in other works. A prominent example is the memoir, based on diaries and recordings made through his life, by *New York Times* journalist Kurt Eichenwald.[91] Indeed, the publication of a rash of memoires and biographies of people with epilepsy represented a new literary phenomenon at the end of the long twentieth century,[92] and a great contrast to

---

[90] Cited in 'Epilepsy in movies and television'.

[91] Eichenwald, *A Mind Unraveled*. The book was a finalist for the Pulitzer prize.

[92] Among other perhaps less literary but still passionate examples of this new genre are *Electro Girl: Living a Symbiotic Existence with Epilepsy* (Lainie Chat, 2017); *Brain Storm: An Electrifying Journey* (Kate Recore, 2019); *Short Circuit: An Epileptic Journey* (Alyssa D'Amico, 2017); *All*

the almost complete absence of biographical exposure in the earlier years[93]. By 2000, it seemed, the disease had indeed begun to emerge into the light of publicity. Eichenwald's memoir makes this explicit. He was advised by his first neurologist never to mention epilepsy, as making it public would ruin his life. In fact, his rejection of this advice and the consequences of 'coming out', and his ultimate success in overcoming prejudice, are leitmotifs central to his story.

Eichenwald's account is preceded by a health warning to doctors and patients alike, and a sign of the changing times:

> If you have epilepsy, this book does not foretell your future, Everyone's experiences differ, and many of mine occurred because of my own bad decisions … I was told fictions about epilepsy that damaged me, and some doctors made mistakes that an educated patient never would have allowed … Do not judge doctors – particularly neurologists – by the arrogant incompetent ones who treated me in the earliest years … [Now] perhaps most important … is the growing recognition of the failures by neurologists in the past to understand the psychosocial difficulties faced by people with this condition and the role the medical community can play in helping to address them. (p. xiv)

His early treatment really was a disaster, not assisted by the denial of the epilepsy by his doctor father, who could not mention the word 'epilepsy', and who was childishly obsequious to a neurologist whose main activity was research not clinical practice, who made elemental clinical mistakes and whose treatment was utterly incompetent. He was not the only incompetent doctor Eichenwald met – there were many. And although he has unreserved praise for his good doctors, the medical profession comes across poorly in this book. Interestingly, strongly and repeatedly stated was the attribute Eichenwald considered to be most important in his doctors: humility and their ability to say they 'don't know' – a feature not often associated with neurologists in the past. Although the narrative is a salutary lesson for all aspiring physicians, the main interest of the book is not neurological incompetence, but rather the reaction Eichenwald's epilepsy caused and his own response to it. He was sent to a disastrous liberal arts college, where he struggled against prejudice, and which illegally tried to expel him. He fought his ground and eventually won, being allowed to complete his education – his first, and defining, tussle against prejudice and marginalisation. He was treated appallingly by early employers

---

Eyes on Me: Epilepsy 'You Are Not Alone' (L. Brandon Magoni, 2019); *The Potter's Wheel: How Epilepsy Changed My Life* (Reverend George L. Choyce, 2017); *Seizure Mama and Rose: An Epilepsy Memoir* (Flower Roberts, 2020). Many of these books describe the struggle epilepsy caused and how the author overcame it, laced with criticisms of the medical profession.

[93] The first and perhaps only major exception seems to be the work of Margiad Evans, discussed in Chapter 4.

and was constantly side-lined and rejected. After one seizure he awoke to find that he had been brutally anally raped. The message of his story is that people must not let seizures govern their life: if that happens, you might live, but you also die. Seizures should not be hidden, and with grit and determination a person can succeed despite the seizures. It is, of course, not a subtle theme. But its simplicity and readers' obvious admiration for the author ensured its success. The book was avidly taken up by the epilepsy charities (appearing on their websites) and its royalties were shared with some of them. Similar sentiments were expressed about his own son's epilepsy in a book by the clinical neurologist Dr Ian Bone.[94]

Another aspect of the kaleidoscopic depictions of epilepsy is the affectionate and altogether more subtle exploration of the illness in the form of biography in *The Music Room* (2009) by William Fiennes. The author's brother, Richard, had epilepsy. Fiennes painted a sympathetic and moving portrait of the life of Richard, who neither accommodated nor overcame his epilepsy, and in the end succumbed to it. The theft of control was an important element, as was the effect of the condition on family life as well as on the individual. Richard comes across as a charming and interesting person at times, at others a bore, and at yet others frighteningly aggressive when he flies into rages or engages in terrifying rampages (which he forgets instantly). As he tried to progress in his life, these rages end up causing his expulsion from the Chalfont Centre for Epilepsy (where he had been a long-stay patient), involvement with police and multiple drug side effects. Fiennes wrote that the doctors attributed the behaviour to frontal lobe damage, caused by an episode of status epilepticus, but that 'I couldn't think of Richard's personality as a set of symptoms; I couldn't think of his character as a manifestation of disease. That would have implied the existence of an ideal healthy Richard my brother was an imperfection of, a dream-Richard this actual person couldn't measure up against. But there wasn't any other Richard' (p. 97). The book is a tender yet accurate portrayal of someone with severe epilepsy and behavioural disturbances, but, as *Guardian* critic John Burnside wrote, 'it is, at its heart, an inquiry into how fundamentally we are defined by the duties of care that we assume or inherit: care of the land, care of a house, care of ourselves, or care of a difficult and sometimes dangerous son and brother'.[95] In this sense, *The Music Room* is a uniquely interesting and touching, as well as beautifully written, book. The description of the author's parents, who look after Richard, is equally touching, as Burnside observed: 'patient, stoical, perplexed, quietly heroic, they get on with things, only rarely allowing their pain and bewilderment to show through'.

The link between religious belief and epilepsy was also re-explored in several novels and books, perhaps most successfully in *Lying Awake* (2001) by Mark

---

[94] Bone, *Sacred Lives*, pp. 313–34.   [95] Burnside, 'Voyage around my brother'.

Salzman. This is an unusual book which, on one level, is a poetic meditation on the spiritual nature of epilepsy. Sister John of the Cross, a contemplative nun in a strict Carmelite monastery on the outskirts of Los Angeles, had entered the monastery years earlier. She assumed her name after the sixteenth-century mystic and author of the poem '*The Dark Night*, which described the soul's crucifying but purifying journey away from self and toward God' (p. 97). For thirteen years, life in the monastery had been spiritually sterile, a desert (as that chapter of the book is titled) in which 'her heart felt squeezed dry. God thirsted, but she had nothing to offer. The Gregorian melodies, sung without harmony, sounded like dirges' (p. 95). But then came rain from heaven (the title of the next chapter), and she began to have extraordinary visions of the grace of God:

> Every movement, every breath was poetry. She had passed through her dark night of the soul, and understood now how the light in one's heart – the light of faith – could shine brighter than the midday sun. When the bell rung for private prayer, she went to the scriptorium to get a notebook. She brought it back to her cell, closed the door, and watched in amazement and joy as light poured out of her onto the pages. (p. 116)

She turned her visions into a book of poems, which became a bestseller, and she was transfigured:

> Pure awareness stripped her of everything. She became an ember carried upward by the heat of an invisible flame. Higher and higher she rose, away from all she knew. Powerless to save herself, she drifted up toward infinity until the vacuum sucked the feeble light out of her ... More luminous than any sun, transcending visibility, the flare consumed everything, it lit up all of existence. In this radiance she could see forever, and everywhere she looked, she saw God's love. As soon as she could move again, she opened her notebook and began writing. (p. 6)

Ominously, though, her visions began to be accompanied by headaches, and Sister John reluctantly sought medical attention from a neurologist named Dr Sheppard (an ironic reference to the good shepherd?). A temporal lobe meningioma is diagnosed. Her transfigurations were taken as symptoms of hyperreligiosity and hypergraphia; the doctor informed her that her visions were in fact epileptic seizures. From 'materials' he gave her, she not only learned that Dostoevsky had similar experiences in his own epilepsy (p. 120),[96] but also that

---

[96] Dostoevsky's seizures bore a striking resemblance to those of Sister John, and she quotes him from *The Possessed*: 'There are moments ... and it is only a matter of five or six seconds, when you feel the presence of the eternal harmony ... a terrible thing is the frightful clearness with which it manifests itself and the rapture with which it fills you. If this state were to last more than five seconds, the soul could not endure it and would have to disappear. During these five seconds I live a whole human existence, and for that I would give my whole life and not think that I was paying too dearly' (p. 120).

St Teresa of Avila (later a doctor of the church) had epilepsy and shared Sister John's fear and uncertainty:

> No-one agonized more than she [St. Theresa] over the question of how to tell the difference between genuine spiritual experiences and false ones. At one point she even feared for her own sanity, but after being assured by Saint Peter of Alcantara that her spiritual favors were from God, she never again lost confidence in her visions, even after being denounced to the Inquisition. (p. 121)

Sister John prevaricated when Dr Sheppard urged her to seek a cure through resective surgery, and she sought the opinion of her own priest about whether or not to proceed. The story then moved to a chapter titled 'Surrender', in which she consents to surgery and the visions were abolished. The operation was deemed a success, and the doctor explained:

> Don't worry about it if you feel a bit washed out. Almost all patients experience some postsurgical depression, especially after this kind of surgery. Life without seizures may seem a bit dull at first, but that's a normal adjustment ... A normal adjustment? For three astonishing years she had lived and prayed from the inside of a kaleidoscope. Everything fit into a design of feeling, a pattern linking all souls and minds together. She felt God's presence in the design, and nothing seemed out of place. Every person was like a piece of glass in a giant rose window. (p. 159)

The book raises many fascinating issues, framed in a misty and impressionistic atmosphere of poetry and devotion. Can thoughts due to seizures be as 'true' as conscious reasoning? Sister John realised that her visions were symptoms of a physical neurological illness, and this challenged her spiritual beliefs and, indeed, her own existence and identity: '*If what you have shown me these past three years has all been a mirage, then I am worse off now than I ever was. If I lose my sense of you, I lose everything*' (p. 122, italics in original); 'In religious life ... if you lose confidence in your personal experience, it's hard to keep from doubting everything'[97] (p. 159). Were her visions, and therefore God's love, fraudulent or somehow fake, simply manifestations of a neurologic dysfunction? Ultimately, she considered that their origins were irrelevant, as to her the message of the visions was authentic, and how the visions were conceptualised came down to a matter of belief. Sister John shares with Martin Luther, as depicted in John Osborn's play *Luther* (1963), the idea that seizures provide divine revelation. The book also asks what makes up the 'self', and here Salzman was quite clear: Sister John's epilepsy was part of her, and was what enlivened and enriched her. Her poetry, too, was not a neurological defect (hypergraphia or hyper-religiosity), but a gift and a mode of spiritual

---

[97] Salzman gives a playful reply to her question. He had nearly 'quit medicine' as he realised he had gone into it 'for the wrong reasons'. But he was glad he 'had stuck with it', having found out that '*everybody* gets into medicine for the wrong reasons' (p. 159).

communication – and how, she asked, 'do you talk about infused contemplation with a neurologist?' (p. 47). By restoring her to a state without epilepsy, medicine had damaged her sense of self, a thought which seemed not to occur to her neurologist. But in the end her compassion and the memory of ecstasy remained, and in this sense the self to Sister John is more than just a collection of neurons. Alasdair Coles, both a neurologist and ordained minister, made a similar point when he emphasised that the ecstatic visions of temporal lobe epilepsy have significance and importance for the person long after the seizure has ended.[98]

Sister John retained her belief in God despite accepting that her ecstasy was 'epileptic'. This was not the conclusion reached by another nun–turned–prolific writer, Karen Armstrong, who rejected her trust in conventional religion when she realised that she had temporal lobe epilepsy, misdiagnosed for years.[99] A linked notion, frequently surfacing in literature and film was that epilepsy confers the gift of special prophecy – an idea stretching back to biblical times. One example, in Salman Rushdie's *Midnight's Children*, was that of the gnarled soothsayer who had an epileptic seizure as she foretold the future of an unborn child, and another was that of the beautiful peasant orphan girl, Ayesha, in Rushdie's *Satanic Verses*, who was granted prophesies, this time by the archangel Gabreel.

The mystical and positive elements of epilepsy were also the theme of the remarkable music video accompanying the song 'Epilepsy is Dancing' by Antony and the Johnsons. The song depicts a girl's epileptic seizure, in which a bleak and lonely journey was suddenly and temporarily changed by a seizure into an oneiric world, much like that of Shakespeare's *A Midsummer Night's Dream*, with a sense of orgasm and euphoric loss of control. The association of a seizure with an orgasm is an echo of Galen's aphorism 'Coitus brevis epilepsia est', but poetically transformed in this video into pleasure and beauty in a way that, in reality, even orgasmic seizures rarely are. This surely must be one of the most poetic and enriching depictions of epilepsy. In 2007, Sallie Baxendale published a survey of depictions of epilepsy in popular music, and it is perhaps surprising how often epilepsy appears. Is this because the younger generation were less tied to the old mythologies of epilepsy? Whatever the reason, most depictions were, however, far from positive, and Antony and the Johnson's music video, emphasising life-enhancing qualities, was very much an outlier. More typical perhaps was the rap artist Cage, cited by Baxendale, whose girlfriend (previously 'the hottest bitch') contracted meningitis and now had seizures during sex: 'Tried to give me a

---

[98] Coles, 'Temporal lobe epilepsy'.

[99] 'Is it possible that the feeling I have had all my life that something – God perhaps? – is just over the horizon, something unimaginable but almost tangibly present, is simply the result of an electrical irregularity in my brain? It is a question that can't yet be answered, unless it be that God, if He exists, could have created us with that capacity in for him, glimpsed at only when the brain is convulsed'; Armstrong, *Beginning the World*, p. 23.

kiss / Before I tasted her lips, she dislocated her hips' – and he had since become known as 'the creep who is into zombies'. Baxendale notes that epilepsy is often likened to madness and retardation, and to sex and dance.[100]

'Education' of the public, embedded within a drama, was another fashionable trend, especially in TV series, producing worthy, if rather earnest, depictions of epilepsy. The lobby of lay organisations to move epilepsy into the open had been instrumental in exploiting this trend. The TV soap *The Young and The Restless* (2006), for instance, was a collaboration between CBS Television and the Epilepsy Foundation of America. The main character (Victor) had post-traumatic epilepsy, perhaps a deliberate shying away from the more stigmatising 'inherited' epilepsy.[101] However, the series still disappointingly reiterated old tropes. Victor not only had epilepsy but also underwent a personality change, becoming violent and murderous, hearing voices, and was admitted to a psychiatric hospital. Education was sometimes served up with a ladle and lost any subtlety, even if clothed in a good story. An example is a film originally made for television, *First Do No Harm* (1997), a paean to the ketogenic diet which saved Robbie, a young child, from a life of intractable seizures, incompetent doctors, destructive neurosurgery and from being taken out of the custody of his brave mother (played by Meryl Streep, who was nominated for several awards for the role). The film was directed and produced by Jim Abrahams, whose son Charlie had epilepsy and for whom the ketogenic diet was a salvation. Abrahams also set up the Charlie Foundation to promote the diet and research into it.

Finally, an interesting, and most unusual, book, which deals with many epileptic themes, is *Lying: A Metaphorical Memoir*.[102] The book takes the form of an autobiography in which Lauren Slater (the authoress) purports to suffer from epilepsy. But as the story develops, it becomes unclear whether this claim is genuine or fictitious. She described her epilepsy surgery, only later to assert that it did not happen, and admitted that she faked all her illness (the first chapter comprises only two words: 'I exaggerate'; p. 3). She distinguished between factual truth and emotional truth, and what she calls narrative truth and historical truth.[103] She also reminded us that memory is unreliable, and, as with truth, she distinguished between her emotional and factual memories: 'The neural mechanism that undergirds the lie is the same neural mechanism that helps us make narrative. Thus all stories ... are at least physiologically linked to deception' (p.164). The book is divided into sections reflecting the

---

[100] Baxendale, 'Epilepsy in popular music'.

[101] In contrast to the many earlier examples, for instance *The Black Stork* and *Dr Kildare's Crisis*.

[102] The book was published in London by Methuen, with a revised title: *Spasm: A Memoir With Lies* (2000).

[103] The similar relativity of science, one of the themes of this book, is a similar distinction (although, exaggerated and more flagrant in Slater's fiction!).

stages of an epileptic fit (onset, rigid, convulsive, recovery). In 'Onset', she described her relationship with her mother. The initial seizures were seen as a reaction to living with this appalling woman:

> I have epilepsy. Or I feel I have epilepsy. Or I wish I had epilepsy, so I could find a way of explaining the dirty, spastic glittering place I had in my mother's heart. Epilepsy is a fascinating disease because some epileptics are liars, exaggerators, makers of myths and high-flying stories … My epilepsy started with a smell of jasmine, and that smell moved into my mouth. And when I opened my mouth after that, all my words seemed colored, and I don't know where this is my mother or where this is my illness, or whether, like her, I am just confusing fact with fiction, and there is no epilepsy, just a clenched metaphor, a way of telling you what I have to tell you: my tale. (pp. 5–6)

In the 'rigid' stage, Slater was sent to a school for children with epilepsy where she had to learn how to fall without injuring herself. Both her mother and the nuns running the school told her to conquer her illness. But falling represented to her an acceptance of the epilepsy, and for some time she refused to fall. Then, at a funeral, she fell deliberately into an open grave, although she admitted later that she did not actually fall but just thought about it. She hated her mother and her climbing out of the grave was depicted as a rebirth. She developed a crush on Dr Neu, her neurosurgeon. When he suggested that he might be able to cure her, she faked seizures, thereby requiring admission to multiple hospitals. She describes her corpus callosotomy, and the fifth chapter of the book purports to be a reprint of Neu's case report of Slater ('LJS') in a medical journal which he had entitled the 'Biopsychosocial Consequences of a Corpus Callosotomy in the Pediatric Patient'. This splitting of the left from the right brain can be seen as a metaphor for the other severings in the book: between literal and figurative truths, reality and imagination, mind and brain. Describing her condition before and after surgery, in the abstract Dr Neu was purported to have written:

> Sixty per cent of patients with temporal lobe epilepsy display dysfunction, psychological profiles that include emotional lability; mythomania with all its attendant exaggerations and untruths; tendency to hypergraphia and hyperreligiosity. This paper addresses the degree to which a successful surgical intervention that reduces or eliminates tonoclonic seizures can concomitantly reduce or eliminate the epileptic's dysfunctional personality style. (p. 98)

This is, of course, medical nonsense, and Slater revels in the hypocrisy and deceit.

In the 'convulsive' chapters, during which much time is spent having sex with a famous author, sexual and epileptic imagery fuse. At one point Slater was told that there is no Dr Neu and that in fact she did not undergo surgery. She still felt the scar and was certain that she did. The night before the operation she mused that the surgery is removing her soul. She remembered a priest who told her that sin was the refusal of responsibility, and that she later apprenticed herself to him. In a chapter titled 'How to Market This Book', she queried the degree to which the story was true, but in doing so insisted that it is no less true than many contemporary biographies. She asks the publisher to market the book as nonfiction. In the section titled 'Recovery', she found herself in an Alcoholics Anonymous meeting and noted similarities between her counting the days without seizures to counting the days without a drink. She was urged to discuss her condition in a group meeting. But when she told the group that she suffered not from alcoholism, but from a mental illness, they considered her to be in denial. The book demonstrates that it is impossible to tell the complete truth about life, and that a writer needs to embroider and embellish. To Slater, diagnoses such as epilepsy are cultural constructs: she pointed out that in the past she would have been accused of demonic possession, and not a disease in the medical model. She makes the point that much of diagnosis is fake news and irrelevant to lived experience. She concludes that if you read the book as a true account, then she feels she will have failed:

> I record *my life*, sifting and trying to separate what is real from what I've dreamed. I have decided not to tell you what is fact versus what is unfact primarily because (a) I am giving you a portrait of the essence of me, and (b) because, living where I do, living in the chasm that cuts through thought, it is lonely. (p. 163, italics in original)

This is a caution that to some extent applies to all works, fictional or medical/scientific.

MEDICAL COMMUNICATION AND EDUCATION

Of all the technological changes in the quarter-century from 1995 to 2020, perhaps none had more social impact on epilepsy than that of the rise of the Internet and of electronic communication generally. The electronic information structures provided a system for the rapid dissemination of medical and research information to an extent unimagined in previous generations and although this was of enormous benefit to epilepsy, there were downsides too. The effects, both positive and negative, are outlined briefly here, at least as far as they had evolved by 2020. This though is unfinished business; and the ultimate impact cannot be even broadly predicted.

Medical Journals

This electronic revolution, in very short order, transformed academic publishing. First, journal numbers enjoyed enormous growth in these years. By 2015, there were estimated to be 5,000–10,000 journal publishers in the field of science, medicine and technology; around 35,000 peer-reviewed scholarly journals (of which 82% were English language); and 2.5 million articles a year.[104] In epilepsy, as in other fields, since 2000 (when *Epilepsia* went digital) the whole publishing process, including manuscript submission, review, revision, proofing and publishing, had become entirely electronic. Except where they remained a compulsory feature of society subscriptions,[105] print editions became virtually extinct. This migration of journals to digital format was extremely profitable for publishers,[106] not least as the published articles were provided at no cost (and in some journals were even charged for), peer review was carried out de bono, and digital production and distribution, via online platforms, was mechanised and remarkably cheap.

Digitisation also affected how journals were used. While some print journal copies were still be read cover to cover, most scientists and clinicians searched online for specific articles, ignoring the context in which the article was placed. The discovered articles were then read either in digital form[107] (e.g. on computer screens, cell phones or other mobile devices) or after printing a PDF. *Epilepsia*, for instance, had more than a million such downloads by 2008. There was also no limit on the size of a journal digitally: there was, for instance, a fourfold increase in the number of published pages in *Epilepsia* between 1988 and 2008.

Until 1985, *Epilepsia* was the only specialist international journal devoted specifically to epilepsy. But over the next fifteen years, five other international journals were launched; by 2020, there were at least twenty (and epilepsy articles also appeared in vast numbers of other journals with a wider scope). The success of any journal depended on search engines identifying the epilepsy content of a paper. The leading medical search engine was PubMed, but general search engines such as Google proved easier to navigate and became more widely used. By 2020, Google handled more than 5 billion searches per day, with quite extraordinary speed and accuracy. The online indexes and search engines replaced the paper-based indexes such as the *Epilepsy Abstracts* which ceased publication in the early 1990s as the Internet rendered it redundant. As search engines such as PubMed and Google are free to use, research discovery and clinical advances became almost instantly available to everyone: potentially all doctors and all patients around the world – a remarkable achievement. Never before had information from medical journals been so plentiful and so accessible.

[104] Ware and Mabe, *STM Report*.
[105] For instance, the American Epilepsy Society membership included a print edition of *Epilepsia*; the British Medical Association included a print edition of the *British Medical Journal*.
[106] In 2005, Reed Elsevier's annual profit was 20% of turnover. It was the unseemly profits of such publishers that led to the Open Access movement.
[107] For the journal *Epilepsy and Behavior*, for instance, in 2020 less than thirty paper copies annually were routinely printed.

In the field of clinical epilepsy, *Epilepsia* remained the leading journal, but with varying roles over the years. It has had a complex publishing history, being produced in four series (Series I, 1909–14/15; Series II, 1937–50; Series III, 1952–5; and Series IV, 1959/60 to the present day - see Appendix 13). The first series was primarily a scientific enterprise, but reports of ILAE activities and critical abstracts of epilepsy publications elsewhere were also included. Series II acted primarily as a record of ILAE activity, with a focus on social care but with abstracts of the scientific literature from elsewhere. This model was not a success, and publication limped on until 1950 when it was terminated, to no one's disappointment. When the ILAE executive discussed restarting publication, opinion was split between those who wished for a scientific journal and those who wished it to be in effect a newsletter for the League. When the third series was inaugurated in 1952 the goal was not to publish original articles, but instead to concentrate on critical reviews and also reports from all the ILAE branches. The resulting annual volumes were an unsatisfactory mix of science and non-science; and publication was again abandoned in 1955. In 1959/60, the journal was relaunched, this time as an organ 'for informed, original and critical studies' covering all fields of epilepsy research.[108] The aim to publish original basic and clinical research papers coincided with the post-war rise in research activity and this 'fourth series' flourished. The publishing philosophy remained unchanged over ensuing years, with research articles still at its heart, although space was given to more general ILAE activities when *Epilepsia* launched its 'Gray Matters' section in 2007. Despite the influx of new epilepsy journals in the decades since 1990, and the changing publishing landscape, it was with that hybrid model that *Epilepsia* has held its position at the front of the epilepsy publishing pack. As journals expanded in number, ILAE, in 2013, acquired *Epileptic Disorders* to be dedicated primarily to education, and in 2017 launched *Epilepsia Open* as an outlet for more general papers. It was by responding thus to the changing publishing environment, that *Epilepsia* had flourished.

The success of the medical journal system, however, had come with significant drawbacks. The rapid increase in journal numbers outpaced advances in research and this jeopardised the quality of published output. In the year 2019, more than 8,000 epilepsy papers were listed on PubMed, compared with 2,000 in 1995 and 306 in 1970,[109] and it is no exaggeration to say that any paper, no matter how bad, was likely to find publication somewhere – a galling thought is that a reader would need to read more than 150 articles a week to have a complete view of the literature. The published

---

[108] Walshe, 'Editorial note'.
[109] Figures derived from a search for the word 'epilepsy' in the title or abstract.

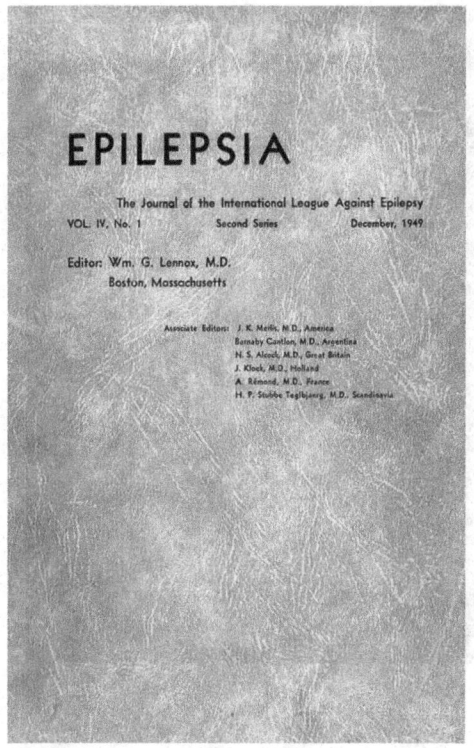

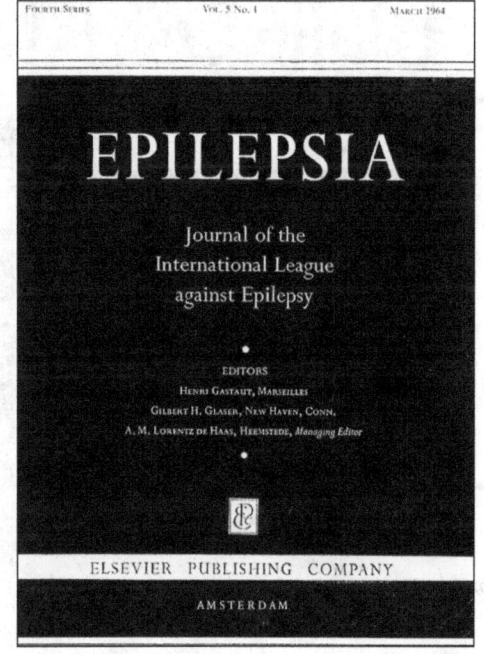

40. The changing covers of Epilepsia. The first cover of 1909, and covers from series II (1949), III (1952) and series IV (1964, 1974. 1995, 2005 and 2019).

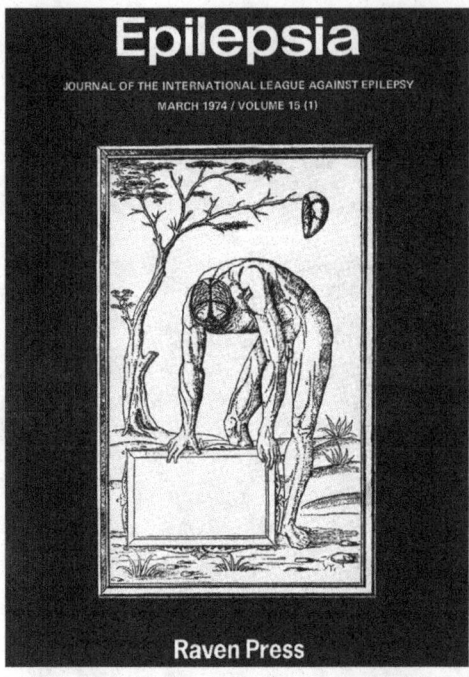

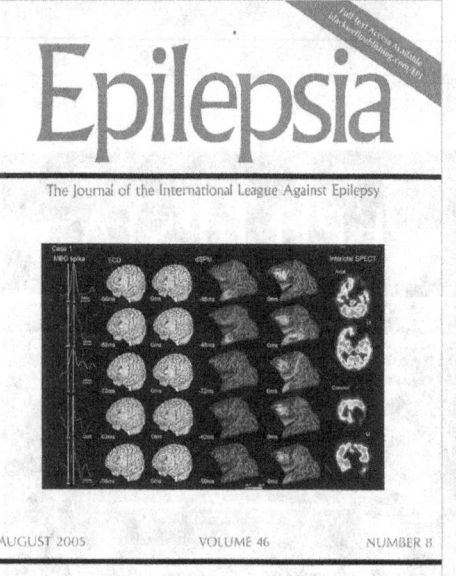

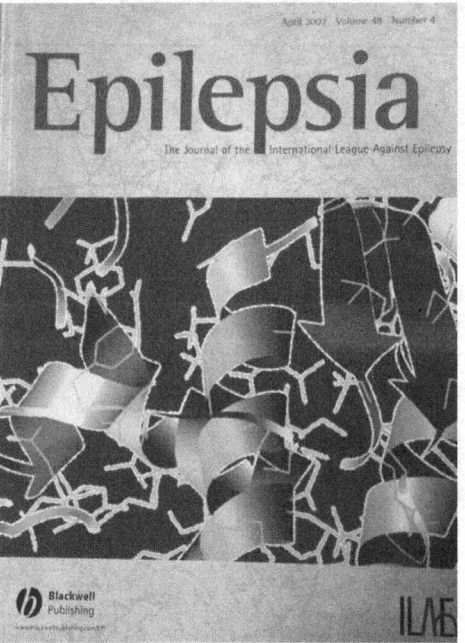

40. (cont.)

medical literature became (and remains) littered with papers demonstrating flawed methodology and biased reporting, and bulged with a mass of low-value reports. Obviously, no single person could possibly keep up with all publications, and the sheer volume of white noise risked obscuring papers of better value. The enduring value of clinical research publications in epilepsy (a surrogate sign of quality) had been measured by a scrutiny of a random selection of 300 papers published in 1981, 1991 and 2001, which were then assessed for their value 10 or more years later. Of those papers, 71% were categorised as having 'no enduring value', and only 4% as having high enduring value.[110] This problem was exacerbated by the trend for academics to be graded on the basis of the number of papers they have published, which encouraged gaming the system, for instance, by 'salami slicing' research so that only a part was reported in any one paper, republishing the same findings, and publishing reviews of other people's research ('parasitic' publications, as they were sometimes known). Another practice that developed was the adding of a name to a paper's authorship with the primary purpose of enhancing a curriculum vitae (to the extent that some papers a few pages long might list the names of several hundred authors).[111] The motivation of authors was studied, showing that furthering career and maximising future funding were common and important drivers of publication, and sometimes more so than advancing medical science.

Perhaps not surprisingly, the quality of the published medical research literature had became the subject of scrutiny. Its truthfulness and honesty became a crucial issue. In 2005, John Ioannidis published a devastating criticism of the statistical and methodological basis of published research.[112] 'There is', he concluded, 'increasing concern that in modern research, false findings may be the majority or even the vast majority of published research.' Factors which rendered a study 'less likely to be true' included a small number of subjects; a small effect size; less preselection of tested factors; greater flexibility in design, definition, outcome or analytical methods; greater financial and other interests and prejudices; and the 'hotter' the scientific field. In epilepsy all these points applied, and particularly in the twenty-first century in the fields of clinical genetics and therapeutics. This criticism was followed by further papers in

---

[110] Gregoris and Shorvon, 'Enduring value'.

[111] 'Authorship' became a taxing issue. The major publishers tried to agree guidelines for who should have their names on papers, but these are widely ignored. A study of hyperprolific authors, defined as those publishing more than a paper every five days, demonstrates the ludicrous nature of this system: Ioannidis, Klavans and Boyack, 'Thousands of scientists publish'.

[112] Ioannidis, 'Published research findings'. John Ioannidis is professor of health research and policy at Stanford. This paper became the most downloaded technical paper from *PLoS Medicine*.

which Ioannidis noted the prevalence of bias and spin, the latter defined as 'the infusion of unwarranted optimism in presenting and interpreting the results of a study or a systematic review. Spin can take many forms, and its manifestations represent a blending of chosen language, statistical support, and (lack of) balance. Eventually, it boils down to overselling the results and their meaning and implications.'[113] He also pointed out that most systematic reviews, with or without spin, had nothing to do with clinical utility, and when they did, this 'may be the most serious type of spin' (p. 864). Ioannidis railed against the proliferation of systematic reviews and meta-analyses, noting these 'ha[ve] skyrocketed across disciplines'.[114] More than a quarter of a million medical systematic reviews, and over 1,500 in epilepsy, had been published, but only a very few were novel or unique, let alone well done and useful. Overlap, redundancy and duplication escalated and continue to do so. In a article titled 'Why most clinical research is not useful', Ioannidis summarised his opinion that: 'In general, not only are most research findings false, but even worse, most of the findings that are true are not useful.'[115]

What he concluded about utility and truthfulness was certainly relevant to epilepsy. Many published papers were indeed of little utility, and there was also, in the field a spectrum of inaccuracy and dissemblance. Some fallacious findings were the result of unconscious bias, not deliberate fraud – in other words, poor science rather than dishonesty. Others were due to conscious data massaging, such as ignoring outliers or results which do not conform, and others to over-interpretation or over-enthusiasm with no malicious intent. Ignoring experimental data that do not support a hypothesis was perhaps the commonest type of scientific misconduct, sometimes justified by the belief that 'my theory must be right'.

The elephant in the room though was deliberate fraud. Flagrant deception was probably quite rare in the field of epilepsy, but its detection was difficult and some believed it to be more widespread. I am certainly aware of several senior epilepsy researchers whose findings were repeatedly never reproduced. Money was often at the root of the problem. Research funding involved huge sums and as a result of the intense competition for grants and the pressure to 'publish or perish' medical researchers were under intense pressure to perform. Furthermore, the burden of oppressive and sometimes unnecessary regulations, bureaucracy and management demands had increased the tendency to take shortcuts. Falsifying results was a particular problem where big data was involved, for instance in the field of epilepsy genetics, but was not confined to these types of research. A detailed survey reported in the journal *Nature* (of

[113] Ioannidis, 'Spin, bias, and clinical utility'.
[114] Siontis and Ioannidis, 'Replication, duplication, and waste'.
[115] Ioannidis, 'Not useful'.

medical research in general, not specifically epilepsy) found that 0.3% of researchers falsified data, 6% failed to present data that contradicted their results, 13% overlooked questionable interpretation or flawed data and 16% changed their study methodology in response to funding-source pressure.[116] It was also estimated that approximately 10–20% of all research and development funds are spent on studies characterised by misrepresentation of data, inaccurate reporting and fabrication of experimental results. One well publicised example of deliberate fraud in epilepsy was the publication of findings which claimed that four common subtypes of an inherited form of epilepsy were associated with three different mutations in a single gene coding for a chloride-gated ion channel. The data was entirely made up and an admission of fraud was published six years later. The worrying extent of alleged commercial interference in the publishing process was another problem compromising the value and quality of much of the medical literature.[117]

As Ioannides demonstrated, it seems likely that massive misinformation existed (and continues to exist) in the domain of scientific research in many areas of medicine.[118] This induced a large degree of scepticism amongst seasoned researchers, but the public media was more gullible, with news report after news report pumping out flawed science purporting to be a 'breakthrough'. There were many such examples in the field of epilepsy genetics, therapeutics and surgery.

Medical Conferences

Another phenomenon worthy of comment was the proliferation and changing nature of medical conferences. As will have been clear from Chapter 1, these were not a new phenomenon, and by the late nineteenth century very large gatherings were held that fulfilled both a medical and a social role. However, after the 1960s, the number and size of conferences progressively increased. By 2019, the eMedEvents website, for example, listed 29,000 conferences, including 1,157 in the field of neurology.[119] ILAE conferences were a signal example of this trend (see Appendix 1). By 1990, its international congresses lasted 5 days and boasted between 2,000 and 5,000 delegates.[120] Then, in addition to their

---

[116] Martinson, Anderson and De Vries, 'Scientists behaving badly'.

[117] Vedula et al., 'Neurontin litigation'.

[118] An early study of this was Broad and Wade's, *Betrayers of the Truth: Feud and Deceit in the Halls of Science*.

[119] This list includes only the most prominent national and international congresses listed on the website; many other congresses will have also taken place.

[120] The 2005 conference in Paris was held over 5 days with 350 lectures by over 250 speakers and 1,372 poster presentations.

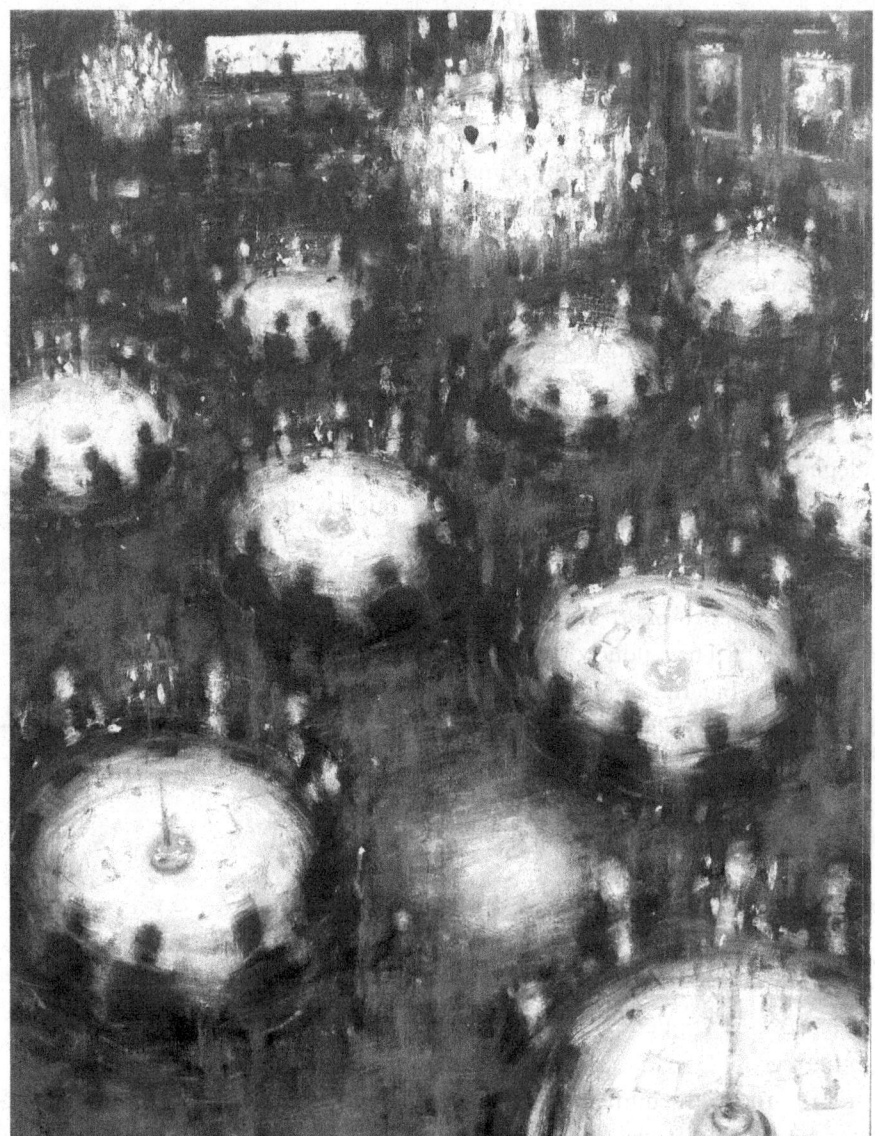

41. 'Banquet'. The highlight of the epilepsy conference circuit (A painting by David Cobley, 2021).

international congresses, regional ILAE congresses were also established, first in Europe in 1994 and then Asia in 1996, South America in 2000 and Africa in 2013. The European congresses became larger than any others, and for example, the 2012 congress in London[121] was held over 5 days, with 4,000

[121] The congresses by now were complex events which offered additional features to promote the ILAE. In London in 2012, novelties included a Nobel Prize winner's lecture (by Peter Mansfield) and a lecture by the Fields medallist (Tim Gowers), a historical exhibit on epilepsy in London 1860–1910, a teaching course on the causes of epilepsy, a session on documentary films about epilepsy, a series of workshops on

delegates, up to 7 parallel sessions, more than 300 presentations, around 900 posters from 48 different countries and 8 satellite sessions, as well as a commercial exhibition.[122] In addition, a number of stand-alone congresses, not run by either the ILAE or larger associations, were also established on specialised topics within epilepsy, such as the 15 biannual Eilat Conferences on Antiepileptic Drugs and the 8 biannual Colloquia on Status Epilepticus.[123]

A major stimulus for the growth of ILAE congresses was their commercial potential to the pharmaceutical industry, which resulted in a change in their nature and culture. Funds flowed in from the industry, and for organisations such as the ILAE this was transformative. Conferences which had previously been a drain on resources soon became a major source of revenue and profit.[124] Satellite symposia were industry-sponsored and organised sessions within the main congress, and these were particular money-spinners. By 2016 some pharmaceutical companies were paying over $100,000 for a package which included advertising in programmes, having a stand in the commercial exhibition and a satellite symposium. These symposia were separate sessions, usually consisting of two or three lectures, added to the conference programme but organised by the company, which paid expenses to key delegates and an honorarium to the lecturers, as well as the large sum to the ILAE. The content of most satellite symposia was entirely ethical, with very little commercial interference, but the advertising and marketing surrounding them ensued commercial success.

Perhaps inevitably, too, by the turn of the new century supporting doctors to attend conferences had itself became a political issue and a source of adverse public comment. In response to this, after 2000, increasingly stringent national and regional regulations about what was permissible were put in place in Western countries.

Although the whole system, with its commercial underpinnings, was open to abuse, most marketing efforts were ethical and, without the financial input of

specialised topics decided in advanced by delegates, and – as the Olympic Games had taken place a few months earlier in London (with some indoor games at the conference venue) – there was also an 'Epilepsy Olympiad', with national teams competing against each other in an epilepsy quiz (won by Ireland).

[122] There was one significant drawback to the growth of ILAE conferences, and this was its effect in reducing the epilepsy content of the general neurology and psychiatry congresses which were also rapidly expanding. This was the inevitable effect of sub-specialisation, and as a result neurologists not specializing in epilepsy become less well informed about the condition.

[123] The proceedings of both conference series were published (the Eilat congresses in *Epilepsy Research* and the status epilepticus colloquia in *Epilepsy and Behavior* and *Epilepsia*).

[124] The costs of the international ILAE conferences exceeded income right up to 1986. Since then, the surplus has been steadily growing (see appendix 4 in Shorvon et al., *ILAE Centenary History*).

industry, much of the postgraduate education provided by the conference circuit would have been lost, as neither hospitals nor universities were prepared to fill the educational vacuum. It was also deemed that organising a conference without sponsorship was unworkable – although it must be pointed out that until the 1980s, such sponsorship hardly existed and the costs were met by the delegates and the professional organisations.

Industry involvement had other effects. A glitzy and commercial atmosphere replaced the previously more sombre academic tenor of the congresses. This represented an enormous cultural change. More important than atmosphere, though, was the direct and indirect influence the commercial companies could exert on the congress programmes. From the companies' marketing perspective, conferences were to a large extent seen as advertising events and opportunities to influence opinion leaders and delegates. It was through such event that industry partly set the agenda of epilepsy itself and the very framework within which epilepsy was viewed.

From the early 1990s, tensions were voiced among ILAE executive committee members about the need to strike a balance between the financial benefits of the involvement of industry and the loss of academic independence. In 1996, guidelines were drawn up that covered the general responsibilities of companies in relation to the satellites, entertainment and travel of delegates. These were, by modern standards, relatively unrestrictive, but still caused much controversy. In many countries, the industry regulators drew up their own codes of practice, which became progressively more stringent and more restrictive, establishing levels of control that were higher in the arena of health than in many other industries. Nevertheless, in this period, the medical conference circuit ensured that the communication of epilepsy research and teaching had been transformed into a big and lucrative business.

The impact of the 'information revolution' on the lay public and people with epilepsy

It was of course not only in professional and medical circles that the methods for the delivery of information, and its quality, had changed. In 2000, Krauss and colleagues published an analysis of stories about epilepsy in English-language newspapers,[125] and found many 'errors' such as 'descriptions of seizures that use demonic or deathly imagery, portrayals of typical seizures as life-threatening and epilepsy depicted as socially crippling' – and attributed this to the need for the press to heighten the drama. They encountered headlines such as 'Epileptic son begged her to kill him' and 'Raging demons that lurk in the mind'. The authors wondered whether such 'otherworldly imagery might convey the

---

[125] Krauss et al., 'The Scarlet E'.

experience of epilepsy in a way that is emotionally valid', but what was clear was that much of the press (and this is hardly unsurprising) sacrificed truth at the altar of malevolence in epilepsy as in much else, for this sold copy. Responsible reporting can be very influential, but was in short supply in relation to epilepsy.

On the Internet, information about health had also rapidly expanded. By 2017, there were said to be 70,000 health-related websites, and 7% of all searches were health-related. In the developing world the Internet was proving to be a particularly important source of information. In a study from China, 40% of 780 epilepsy patients surveyed had Internet access (55% of urban and 19% of rural patients); of these, about three-quarters had searched for general information on epilepsy and two-thirds for treatment information.[126] In this study, 30% of patients used the information gathered to prepare for hospital visits, 12% to communicate with other patients and 5% for purchasing epilepsy products. The commercial potential of the technology was also obvious, and by 2020 virtually all epilepsy businesses worldwide had websites, with many making unsubstantiated claims and some selling unregulated products.

The professional and lay organisations developed a strong Internet presence. In 1996 the ILAE formulated plans for its first website. After considering and rejecting the idea of having a joint website with the IBE (in retrospect, this seemed a missed opportunity) and after abortive discussions with various website developers, the ILAE website went live in 2001. By then, major sites had been developed by other organisations including, for instance, the Epilepsy Foundation and Epilepsy Action. The ILAE also set up the ILAE Virtual Epilepsy Academy (which evolved from the pre-existing European Virepa distance-learning programme) with the aim of providing a competency-based educational curriculum for epileptology. In addition to its tutored courses, a series of interactive self-paced e-learning course were available, including the epilepsy sections of *eBrain*, a comprehensive neurology training resource produced by the British Joint Neurosciences Council, an epilepsy imaging course and a series of case reports. In addition, the ILAE provided various multimedia materials, including a video-EEG database, a series of published seminars in epileptology and histopathology tutorials.

A new hurricane then began to whip up the seas of both medical and public communication: social media. Starting around 2010, by 2018 this new medium had become the dominant form of short discourse, characterised by ubiquity and immediacy. Uniquely in the history of the world, this meant

---

[126] Liu et al., 'Internet usage'.

that information – and disinformation – could be distributed to more people faster than ever before. By 2017, Facebook was found to have 640 pages related to epilepsy, with over 3 million 'likes', and Twitter 137 pages and 327,917 followers – with a nearly 100% increase in the numbers of users between 2012 and 2016.[127] Most represented charitable groups or patients, but around 1 in 10 involved epilepsy medical centres or commercial businesses. Initially, most provided information or support, but fairly quickly there developed an increasing tendency to present research or medical knowledge without peer review or any other accuracy filter.

Social media provided the first ever readily available outlet for the ordinary person with epilepsy to voice his or her opinions and concerns. Personal stories of seizures accounted for around a third of all such traffic, and this was truly transformative for the lives of many. Conversely, unregulated as it was, social media also became a source of malicious and stigmatising content. In 2012, an analysis of messages about epilepsy on Twitter over a 7-day period found 41% to be derogatory in nature, and 9% took the form of ridicule or jokes. The researchers concluded that although Twitter could be used, and had been used, to disseminate accurate information on seizures, it commonly glorified negative and hostile attitudes.[128] This might have been over-pessimistic as social media also had many outstanding qualities, but the ease of misuse was, and remains, a deep concern. Video media too might seem ideal for depicting epilepsy, and a study in 2013 concluded, rather optimistically, that these may lessen stigma.[129] Much of what became available, though, was misleading, and in a straw poll of contemporary *YouTube* videos at least one-third of examples purporting to be epileptic seizures seemed more likely to be psychogenic non-epileptic attacks. Social media also presented an obvious opportunity for academic study of public and patient attitudes to epilepsy, but by 2020 this was an area which remained largely unexplored.

Books

Whilst social media celebrated immediacy, at the other end of the spectrum was the traditional source of information: the medical textbook. The intersecting network of journals, conferences, Internet sites and social media had challenged the need for such books, and their demise had been frequently discussed. But in fact, and perhaps counter-intuitively, the medical book not only survived but actually flourished. Their success was

[127] Meng et al., 'Social media in epilepsy'.
[128] McNeil, Brna and Gordon, 'Epilepsy in the Twitter era'.
[129] Wong et al., 'Epilepsy in YouTube videos'.

partly facilitated by the same processes that led to the escalating numbers of journals: electronic word-processing and computing facilities, automated production methods and online marketing. A whole slew of medical textbooks on epilepsy were published – more, in fact, in this period than in any earlier time.[130] However, unlike previous periods, almost no books were written by a single author; 'monographs', which were the standard format until around 1960, had become a rare species.[131] The majority of epilepsy textbooks were composed of chapters written by individuals and collected together by the editor of the book (who sometimes had done little or no editing at all). These types of textbook are in effect not dissimilar from journals, comprising collections of review articles brought together under a single cover. The first multi-authored epilepsy textbook was probably Woodbury et al.'s *Antiepileptic Drugs*, which was first published in 1972 and ran to five editions, the last in 2002. There have since then been numerous other examples,[132] ever more voluminous and increasingly with little editing or oversight. In addition, there had been several series of epilepsy books,[133] epilepsy volumes in more general series,[134] and individual one-off smaller books on specific topics in epilepsy – all multi-authored. The only utility of such books, and their advantage over journal articles, was (and remains) that they condense information into one space and the authorship tends to be highly selected. All these books still found a place on professional

---

[130] Yokio Fukuyama published his *Epilepsy Bibliography* of books published since 1945 on eight occasions between 1945 and 2003. In 1975, 137 books were listed and by 2004, 1,349.

[131] Examples of monographs published in the period 1995–2020 included O'Donohoe, *Epilepsies of Childhood*; Panayiotopoulos, *The Epilepsies*; Engel, *Seizures and Epilepsy* and Shorvon, *Status Epilepticus*.

[132] Just some examples of multi-authored textbooks published in the English language since 1970 include the following: Richens and Laidlaw, *A Textbook of Epilepsy*, two editions: 1976, 1982; Roger et al., *Epileptic Syndromes in Infancy, Childhood and Adolescence*, two editions: 1984, 1992; Aicardi, *Epilepsy in Children*, two editions: 1986, 2003; Engel, *Surgical Treatment of Epilepsy*, two editions: 1986, 1993; Hopkins, *Epilepsy*, two editions: 1987, 1995; Dam and Gram, *Comprehensive Epileptology*, 1991; Pellock et al., *Pediatric Epilepsy: Diagnosis and Therapy*, four editions: 1993, 2001, 2008, 2016; Wyllie, *Treatment of Epilepsy*, seven editions: 1993, 1997, 2001, 2005, 2010, 2015, 2020; Wolf, *Epileptic Seizures and Symptoms*, 1994; Engel and Pedley, *Epilepsy: A Comprehensive Textbook* (this is probably the largest, with the second edition containing 307 chapters and representing nearly 600 authors), two editions: 1998, 2008; Shorvon et al., *Treatment of Epilepsy*, four editions: 1996, 2005, 2009, 2016; Lüders and Comair, *Epilepsy Surgery*, 2001; Wallace and Farrell, *Epilepsy in Children*, 2004; Lüders, *Textbook of Epilepsy Surgery*, 2008; Shorvon et al., *Causes of Epilepsy*, 2011, 2019; Alarcon, *Introduction to Epilepsy*, 2012; Shorvon et al., *Oxford Textbook of Epilepsy and Epileptic Seizures*, 2013; Lhatoo et al., *Invasive Studies of the Human Epileptic Brain*, 2019.

[133] Examples include the series edited by Pedley and Engel, *Recent Advances in Epilepsy*, six volumes between 1983 and 1995; and *Progress in Epileptic Disorders*, 14 volumes between 2005 and 2017.

[134] In such series as Handbook of Neurology, Advances in Neurology and Handbook of Experimental Pharmacology.

bookshelves and in libraries, although shelf space in the latter was, by 2020, in the throes of massive reduction.

Medical Education

Finally, a word about epilepsy education. Despite its importance, epilepsy barely featured in the crowded curricula of medical students in any country. The average student might have received a day or two's tuition on the topic, but almost all training and teaching on epilepsy in the twenty-first century was carried out in other arena. Much was in-service learning following the apprenticeship model or formal learning for postgraduate examinations. Ad hoc teaching courses were run in many countries, some by professional organisations such as the local ILAE chapters, some by universities and many by pharmaceutical companies. Since 2000, this type of instruction had increasingly gone online, and a huge number of resources had become available. Few young doctors-in-training did not carry around a smartphone or computer linked to the Internet in their day-to-day work, allowing them instant access to epilepsy information. There were numerous reputable sites. The effects of these profound changes in the way in which information was provided and accessed has not been formally assessed, but there seems little doubt that doctors in this period could be better informed about epilepsy, as well as other topics in medicine, than at any time in the past.

THE INTERNATIONAL LEAGUE AGAINST EPILEPSY

The ILAE grew from 48 national chapters in 1995 to 98 in 2007 and 123 in 2020 – another sign of how interconnected the world had become in the digital age. Epilepsy had become the global village, wished for by Lennox and to a significant extent brought about by the ILAE. Some national chapters comprised very few individual members, but others were large. By 2020, national chapters claimed more than 25,000 members worldwide, and the ILAE had further consolidated its position as the primary association for those interested in epilepsy. For most of its early history, without paid staff, and the administration was conducted entirely by its voluntary officers; but, as the League grew, this situation became unsustainable. In 1993, secretarial support was first paid for in the offices of the president and secretary-general; in 1997, a professional administration was established in Hartford, Connecticut; and in 2001, a second office was opened in Brussels (and closed later, due to escalating costs and inadequate supervision). From 1999, the ILAE also set up and contracted with a conference organising company (Chancel Ltd) to arrange its international and regional congresses. But in the face of increasing concern and financial criticism, this arrangement was dissolved in 2020 and the ILAE decided to bring conference organising in-house again. For most of its existence, the ILAE had been run on a modest monetary basis; but, as pharmaceutical sponsorship of conferences and journals grew, so too did the ILAE coffers. In 1939, its annual income was £105 (with assets of £91), rising to $22,000 by 1985. At this stage, income came almost entirely from the dues of the national chapter, but by 1995 the annual income of $600,000 (and assets of around $1 million) was derived largely from the international conferences and royalties from *Epilepsia*, with chapter dues amounting only to $29,000. By 2006, the ILAE's central administration had an annual income of around $3 million and accumulated bank holdings of $9 million. By 2020, the assets amounted to around $20 million.[135]

This massive rise in income was derived from the pharmaceutical industry, directly or indirectly through monies paid to the League conferences, via registration fees, the exhibition and satellite sessions, or to *Epilepsia* as advertising revenue. The finances of the national chapters had always been outside of the control of the central administration and these, too, were heavily subsidised by the pharmaceutical industry. The exact extent of pharmaceutical companies' financial support of the ILAE is impossible to ascertain, but by 2009, estimates of around 80% were made and are probably not far off the mark. Once the professional administration was in place, its costs increased rapidly from around $150,000 in 1994 to more than $1.7 million by 1998. This aroused concern and the administration was overhauled in the years after 2016. Another contentious policy was the decision in the 1990s to accumulate a $20 million surplus in order to endow the League's administration.

From its inception, the major activities of the ILAE were the holding of scientific congresses and the publication of the journal *Epilepsia*, although early in its history it also lobbied for the establishment of epilepsy colonies and the collection of national statistics on epilepsy. At its restitution in 1935, as in 1912, congresses and *Epilepsia* remained its main activities. Colonies, however, were no longer mentioned, and membership was now largely devolved to the national branches, with the stated objective of the League being 'to coordinate the activities of those who are interested in the better care and treatment of epileptics, and to stimulate interest in the social and scientific aspects of the disease'.[136] By 1973 the ILAE's objectives were listed as 'advancing and disseminating knowledge; encouraging research; promoting prevention,

---

[135] This is an approximate figure, as the ILAE did not respond to repeated requests for information in 2020 about its income and expenses, which after 2009 remained outside the public domain. (See Shorvon et al., 'The International League Against Epilepsy 1909–2009', appendix 4, for financial details of earlier years.)

[136] Shorvon and Weiss, 'International League Against Epilepsy', p. 292. This was the first written constitution of the revived League, and different in many ways from that of 1912 (pp. 291–2).

diagnosis, treatment and care; [and] improving education and training in the field of the epilepsies'.[137] In 2009, the ILAE celebrated its centenary with an International Congress in Budapest, the city in which it was founded, a historical display and the publication of a detailed centenary history.[138]

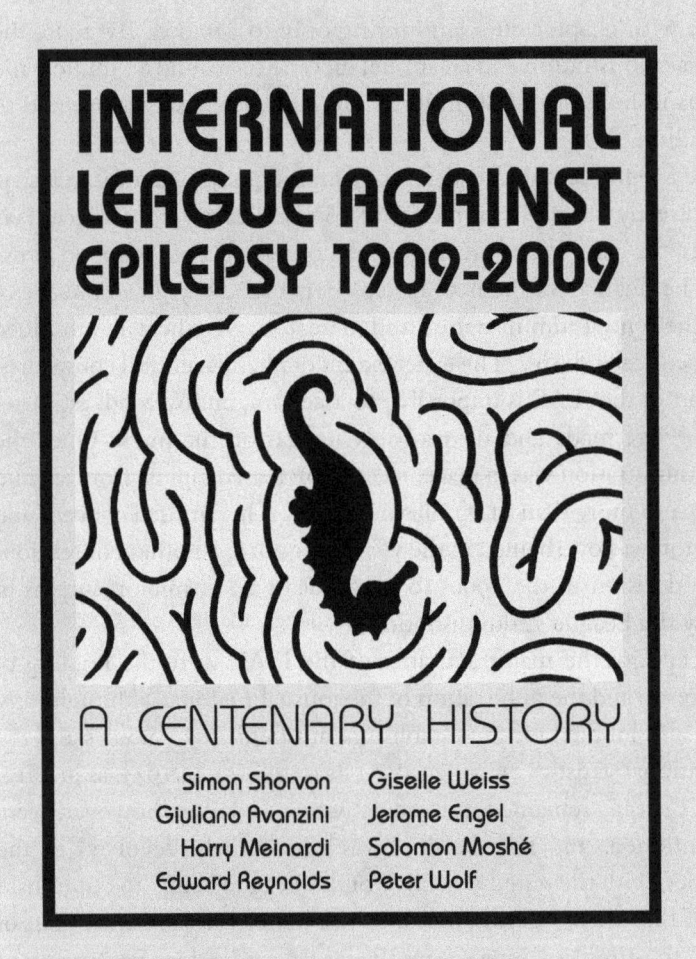

42. The ILAE centenary history book. The cover design is entitled 'The hippocampus' and was drawn by David Cobley (2009).

[137] Shorvon *et al.*, *International League Against Epilepsy*, p. 295. A similar set of objectives had been adopted in 1953, but without the fourth aim of improving training and education (p. 293).

[138] The display panels and book are on the ILAE website, along with the history and archives and details of the ILAE Centenary Film Festival (www.ilae.org/about-ilae/history-and-archives).

As it emerged into its second century, the congresses and journal remained its core activities and its enduring contribution, but it had also begun to engage more actively in policymaking and political lobbying on behalf of epilepsy. For this purpose, the ILAE's links with the IBE proved of great importance, as in the consumerist political environment, the combined professional and patient lobby carried great power. The first example of this trend was the lead Lennox took with the American branch of the League, in jointly lobbying the American government with the lay organisation, the American Layman's League. Other examples had followed over the years, but were never a prominent feature of the ILAE's ventures, engaged as it was largely with its congresses, *Epilepsia* and its own internal squabbles. This was to change completely with what turned out to be the most successful and far-reaching of all its external undertakings: the Global Campaign Against Epilepsy.

The Treatment Gap and the Global Campaign Against Epilepsy

In 1988 a new statistic emerged in the field of epilepsy. The 'epilepsy treatment gap' was defined as the proportion of patients with active epilepsy who were, at any one time, not taking antiepileptic drug medication.[139] Using data on drug supply to a country, the figure was calculated by working out the proportion of prevalent active cases on any one day who could have been treated with antiepileptic drugs even assuming a low drug dose, monotherapy and no drug wastage. The first studies were conducted in Pakistan, the Philippines and Ecuador (Table 5.5). The results indicated that, in the three developing countries studied, on any one day, only 6–20% of patients with active epilepsy

TABLE 5.5 *The first reported treatment gap figures (1988)*

Country	Estimated numbers of people with active epilepsy*	Estimate number of people receiving treatment**	Treatment gap***
Pakistan	450,000	22,000	94%
Philippines	270,000	14,000	94%
Ecuador	55,000	11,000	80%

* Based on a prevalence of active epilepsy of 0.5%
** Based on drug supply figures, minimum standard doses, monotherapy
*** The percentage of people not receiving therapy at any one time
(Derived from: Shorvon and Farmer, 'Epilepsy in developing countries')

[139] The term and concept were first proposed, and figures given, in Shorvon and Farmer, 'Epilepsy in developing countries' (1988 and 18988b). See also Ellison et al., 'Programme of transcultural studies' (1989).

could have been taking antiepileptic medication, even at the low doses. In other words, in these three countries there was a treatment gap of between 80–94%. These figures were truly shocking, and then similar findings were made in subsequent prospective surveys by the same authors in Kenya, Ecuador and Pakistan, using real patient data from community surveys. In all countries, a rural/urban divide reflected the dire state of medical services in poor rural areas (for instance, in Pakistan only 2% of rural and 27% of urban dwellers with epilepsy were found to be receiving antiepileptic drugs). The earliest studies were conducted as part of the work of the ICBERG group,[140] with its treatment gap studies sponsored by Ciba-Geigy, which obviously stood to gain from increasing markets but which nevertheless were keen to pursue rigorous science. Numerous studies were then reported from different countries, all finding large treatment gaps; this was a genie now very much out of the bottle. The first studies were carried out independently of governments, but twenty years later, in China, a government-sponsored WHO/ILAE/IBE door-to-door survey among 55,000 people was carried out which found a treatment gap of 63%.[141] The root causes of the large treatment gaps were an often complex mix of cost,[142] cultural beliefs, lack of drug supply, inadequate capacity and inequitable distribution, poor access to health facilities, alternative traditional treatment and inadequately skilled personnel.

The treatment gap studies had a major impact and became the topic of much debate at ILAE conferences. The concept was also taken up in the ILAE and IBE's recently inaugurated joint Commission on Developing Countries as an ideal hook on which to hang policy. Then, in 1993, the WHO, together with the IBE and ILAE, embarked on a joint campaign initiated by the ILAE's then president, Ted Reynolds, titled the Global Campaign Against Epilepsy. The treatment gap was a major element of the campaign.

The fact that the ILAE was prepared to co-operate in such a venture with the lay organisation, and thereby cede influence, deserves comment. It was symptomatic of changing social values, the diminishing paternalism of medicine and the stronger voice of the patient as customer. Such cooperation

---

[140] International Community Based Epilepsy Research Group (ICBERG) was an initiative founded in 1986 with the aim of studying and improving epilepsy in rural areas of developing countries. In 1991, it published the first primary care manual for the management of epilepsy in developing countries (Shorvon et al., *Management of Epilepsy in Developing Countries*.

[141] Wang et al., 'Prevalence and treatment gap'.

[142] At the time, WHO published (and still does) a *Model List of Essential Medicines* that includes four antiepileptics: phenobarbital, phenytoin, carbamazepine and valproate. All were very inexpensive. For instance, the cost of phenobarbital was in the region of only $5 per year. Although higher prices were often charged on the ground, cost was generally not an overriding obstacle.

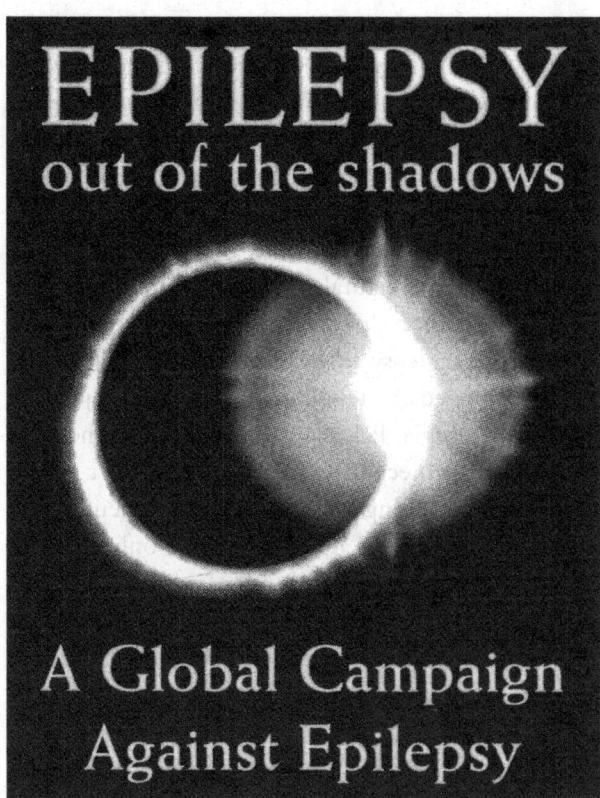

43. The logo of the WHO/ILAE/IBE Global Campaign Against Epilepsy, 'Out of the Shadows'.

between the ILAE and the IBE had failed spectacularly two decades earlier, in the Epilepsy International debacle, but this time joint action was to prove extremely successful. The joined-up effort of this triumvirate was to achieve an enormous amount in the field of epilepsy – much more than any of the partner organisations could have managed alone.

The Global Campaign Against Epilepsy was the ILAE's most important public health initiative, unequalled either before or since. Its primary intentions initially were to raise 'epilepsy to a new plane of acceptability in the public domain',[143] improve education, identify needs and encourage governments to address these needs. The campaign motto was 'Out of the shadows', and a logo showed an eclipse of the sun.[144] Planning took place between 1995 and 1997. The Global Campaign was first announced at the ILAE European and Asian and Oceanian congresses in 1996 and was launched at the WHO headquarters

[143] Reynolds, 'Epilepsy in the world'.
[144] The name and logo were conceived by Ted Reynolds in 1996. This may have been inspired by a solar eclipse that occurred over Europe in 1993. Similar images appeared in the national newspapers of the time.

in Geneva on 19 June 1997. A conference was held in Dublin, and details of the campaign were written up in a special supplement of *Epilepsia*[145] and in other articles.[146] Excellent support was provided by then WHO director-general Gro Harlem Brundtland. A major conference on the treatment gap was organised in Marrakech in May 1999. The concept proved to be a powerful lever and could be used as a long-term measure of the success of any epilepsy intervention. The campaign was awarded 'cabinet level' status within the WHO in 1999 and a second phase was launched in 2001. The inaugural address by Brundtland on 12 February 2001 was, in Reynolds's opinion, 'perhaps the most important and influential political statement about epilepsy made during the whole of the ILAE history'.[147] The campaign spawned a series of 'demonstration projects' in Argentina, Bolivia, Brazil, China, Georgia, Pakistan, Senegal, East Timor and Zimbabwe.[148] The aforementioned project in China was a product of the campaign, and was the most successful. Using methods and instruments based on the earlier studies in Ecuador, researchers determined not only that the treatment gap was 63% but also that the disease burden was 2.08 DALYs (disability-adjusted life-years) per 1,000 persons. The study demonstrated that trained primary healthcare physicians could successfully diagnose and treat people with epilepsy, and a 13% reduction in the treatment gap was said to have been achieved.[149]

Healthcare provision for epilepsy has always varied widely around the world. In 2005 the WHO, on behalf of the Global Campaign Against Epilepsy, published an atlas of epilepsy and epilepsy care.[150] Large inequalities were found across regions and income groups, with low-income countries having extremely meagre resources. The work concluded that, globally, about 50 million persons suffered from epilepsy, with 80% of the burden of epilepsy in

---

[145] Reynolds, 'Epilepsy in the world'.
[146] Reynolds, 'The ILAE/IBE/WHO Global Campaign "Out of the Shadows": bringing epilepsy "out of the shadows"'; Reynolds, 'ILAE/IBE/WHO global campaign "out of the shadows": global and regional developments'.
[147] The speech is reproduced as an appendix in Reynolds, 'Global and regional developments'.
[148] The stated objectives of these projects were to reduce the treatment gap and the physical and social burden of people with epilepsy by intervention at a community level; to train and educate health professionals; to dispel stigma and to promote a positive attitude toward people with epilepsy in the community; to identify and assess the potential for prevention of epilepsy; and to develop models for promotion of epilepsy control worldwide and for its integration in the health systems of participating countries. These were lofty objectives, and some projects were more successful than others. The most widely conducted project was carried out in China and guided by Li Shichuo, the leading Chinese figure in the field of epilepsy. He had formerly worked with the WHO and the Chinese government for much of his professional life. He was the founder and president of the Chinese Association Against Epilepsy, the Chinese chapter of the ILAE, established in 2006. He was awarded the ILAE Lifetime Achievement Award in 2021.
[149] *Epilepsy Management at Primary Health Level in Rural China.*
[150] *Atlas, Epilepsy Care in the World.*

low- and middle-income countries, and that epilepsy accounted for 1% of the global burden of disease. Although the atlas was mainly a propaganda tool and contained a great many inaccuracies,[151] its figures on such aspects as resources and epidemiological measures were acceptable as rough estimates.

In 2011, the WHO Region of the Americas approved a strategy and plan of action on epilepsy for 2012–21, and the European Parliament approved the written declaration on epilepsy. A WHO programme titled Reducing the Epilepsy Treatment Gap was set up in 2012, and pilot initiatives were initiated in Ghana, Mozambique, Myanmar and Vietnam. In 2014, WHO listed action in seven areas that it considered were most needed to make progress in improving epilepsy care globally.[152] Epilepsy was also included as a priority condition in the WHO Mental Health Gap Action Programme. A key part of this programme was to develop guidelines for primary healthcare in the developing world – a goal explicitly and repeatedly identified since the 1970s, but one that still needed to be articulated. In 2015 the World Health Assembly reviewed the progress of its work in epilepsy, and took the further step of adopting a resolution on the global burden of epilepsy and the need for coordinated action. The resolution urged the 194 WHO member states to strengthen leadership, governance and policies in epilepsy, and to make financial, human and other resources available. In 2020, at the World Health Assembly, epilepsy again was specifically mentioned in a resolution urging 'appropriate support to WHO to develop the Intersectoral Global Action Plan on Epilepsy and Other Neurological Disorders'.[153] This request was based on the recognition that despite the low cost of effective interventions for epilepsy (estimated at less than US\$ 5/per person/year), the current treatment gap was more than 75% in most low-income countries and 50% in the majority of middle-income countries; and also that lack of access to medicines and other effective interventions and specialist consultations, coupled with discrimination and stigma associated with this condition, were resulting in avoidable disability, mortality, social exclusion, economic disadvantage and negative mental health outcomes in people living with epilepsy. And noting further that addressing epilepsy was widely considered to be a public health

---

[151] Nine years later, the WHO published figures showing that epilepsy accounted for 0.5% of the global burden of disease. Quite why the figure should have halved over this period is a mystery, and certainly does not reflect reality. See *Global Burden of Epilepsy*.

[152] The seven recommended actions were to strengthen effective leadership and governance; improve provision of epilepsy care; integrate epilepsy management into primary health care; increase access to medicines; support strategies for prevention of epilepsy; increase public awareness and education; and strengthen health information and surveillance systems (*Global Burden of Epilepsy*, p. 3).

[153] Resolution 73.10 – Global Actions on Epilepsy and Other Neurological Disorders. www.ibe-epilepsy.org/wp-content/uploads/2021/05/WHA73.10.pdf

imperative, as had been concluded in the WHO/ILAE/IBE Global Report on Epilepsy.[154]

Thus, from its original conception twenty years earlier, the Global Campaign Against Epilepsy had resulted in a very significant rise in the profile and awareness of epilepsy globally, as was its original intention, and had diverted considerable resources to epilepsy. It is difficult to measure the difference the Global Campaign made on the ground to individuals with epilepsy, but an impact must surely have been felt in many countries. There certainly was much more engagement of governments – and it was they who held the epilepsy healthcare purse strings. As a result of these efforts, it seems likely that attitudes, knowledge and practice in epilepsy did make significant strides. It is instructive to note that the WHO work was based solidly on Western medical concepts, and it was in some quarters criticised as neocolonialism. Globalisation confirmed the hegemony of Western medical practices and structures, and the assumption that these were superior to any that existed elsewhere. And even though the campaigns paid lip service to incorporating local customs and traditions, this proved a vague aspiration and a gesture made with the understanding that it would facilitate implementation of the Western model.

Following the Global Campaign, the European ILAE chapters joined with the sister IBE chapters to lobby for the European Union's white paper on epilepsy in 2003. The aim of this effort was to lessen stigma. The EU's publicity material referred to a woman in the Netherlands in 1996 who was whipped and put into isolation because her seizures were believed to result from magic, and the case of Congressman Tony Coelho, 'barred not so many years ago by the Vatican from becoming a Jesuit Priest because a person with epilepsy was still under Canon Law deemed to be possessed by devils – a designation dating from the 4th century'.[155] These perhaps slightly over-egged the facts, but by then propaganda was the stuff of publicity. The campaign also cited the estimate that in Europe, the direct and indirect health and care costs of epilepsy amounted to €20 billion. It was followed up by a written declaration on epilepsy by the European Parliament in 2011, a European forum on epilepsy research and commitments for research funding.[156] Then, after a further lobbying campaign by the ILAE, in 2015 a Resolution on Epilepsy was approved at the World Health Assembly. Although the extent to which the actions were heeded varied around the world, the ILAE was indubitably making a real and direct impact on the lives of people with epilepsy.

---

[154] 'Global actions on epilepsy', pp. 2, 4.
[155] Tony Coelho, a former US Congressman with epilepsy, gave an interesting interview about stigma on the A11y Rules podcast ('Interview with Tony Coelho').
[156] Baulac et al., 'Epilepsy priorities in Europe'.

In 2000, the ILAE established a strategic planning process and plans were periodically approved, although seldom did events turn out to closely follow the plan (in fact the plans were regularly updated to incorporate what had already actually happened). The last of these in this period was in 2009, which had four priority areas for ILAE action: (1) to serve as a premiere international resource for epilepsy knowledge; (2) to serve as a leader for optimal, comprehensive epilepsy care; (3) to ensure the organisational and financial viability of the League; (4) to implement thought-provoking and innovative concepts that advance the League's vision and mission. Emilio Perucca was ILAE President from 2013–17, and devoted enormous energies to the ILAE. In his valedatory report of his tenure, he described the achievements of the ILAE in meeting these key priorities in those years. The first objective was contributed to by commission reports, and especially work on classification (described earlier) and guidelines. The second objective relied on politicking, and on this the league devoted much effort. The 2015 WHO approval of a Resolution on Epilepsy was the gratifying culmination of this work. The ILAE also encouraged research, but as it was not a funding body, these exhortations were largely platitudinous. The third objective was successfully achieved and the ILAE gathered together a nest egg of $20 million, with most derived directly or indirectly from the pharmaceutical industry. This was used to endow the Executive Committee activities and the ILAE administration. However, as the ILAE accounts in these years were never published, the details of exactly how the money was accounted for were not made publically accessible.

It is clear from this report that the ILAE was engaging more with the wider world than it had for many decades. Lobbying and propaganda became part of its daily work. In the world of consumerism and soundbites, truth and reasonable balance were casualties – a problem which plagued organisations representing many other diseases in the politicised healthcare environment of the twenty-first century. One voice was missing altogether though from ILAE activities – that of the patient. Links with the IBE were more cordial than often previously, but renewed attempts to join forces were no longer on the agenda.[157]

---

[157] Attested, for instance, in the 'ILAE Strategy 2030', in which the IBE is briefly mentioned only once; www.ilae.org/files/dmfile/APPROVED-ILAE-STRATEGY-2030-as-of-2021-08.pdf (accessed in December 2021).

SECTION 3

EPILEPSY: THE PARADIGM OF THE
SUFFERING OF BOTH BODY AND SOUL
IN DISEASE

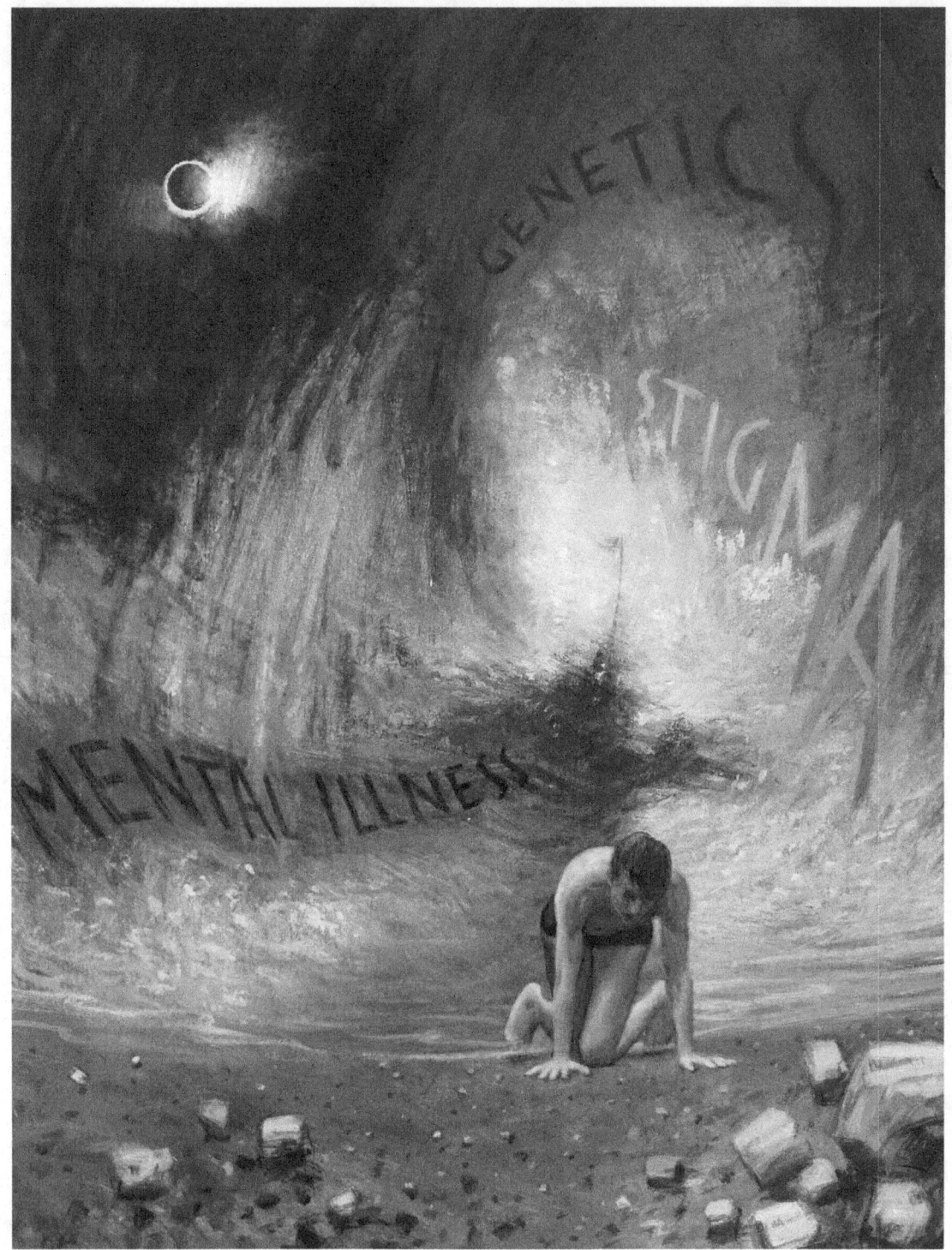

44. **'I've survived'.** (A painting by David Cobley, 2021).

EPILOGUE

THE SEPARATION OF THE WHEAT FROM THE CHAFF

IN TELLING TO STORY OF EPILEPSY, THROUGH THE LONG TWENTIETH century, the approach taken in this book has been to paint a broad canvas, on the example of Burton, drawing on more than just the medical aspects of epilepsy. It is an approach summed up neatly by Walt Whitman: 'Of physiology from top to toe I sing, / Not physiognomy alone, nor brain alone, is worthy for the Muse –, I say / the complete is worthier far'.[1] Beyond 'brain alone', the wider societal and personal issues, 'the form complete', help provide context and meaning to *Epilepsy's* long and erratic voyage. Not limiting the story entirely to the narrow horizons of medicine, although this would have been easy to do, has hopefully given at least a sense of the *why* as well as the *what* of epilepsy.

Even if fascinating in its own right, any history of epilepsy can be useful only if it helps make sense of the reality of epilepsy today.[2] In his 1999 novel *Timeline*, Michael Crichton, the doctor-novelist interested in epilepsy, addressed the question of why we should bother with history. The novel's

---

[1] 'One's-self I sing', in Murphy (ed.), *Walt Whitman: Complete Poems*, p. 37. Whitman's brother Edward suffered from epilepsy and Whitman's poem, 'Faces', makes a celebrated reference to the condition.

[2] It has often been said that the purpose of studying history is to draw parallels with current facts or events so as, for instance, to prevent the repetition of mistakes. But history can only stimulate new thinking about the present, and it is a mistake to think that events are homologous. Hannah Arendt put it well: 'To look at the past in order to find analogies by which to solve our present problems is, in my opinion, a mythological error' (Hill, *Hannah Arendt*, p. 14).

main character quotes his professor as saying that 'if you didn't know history, you didn't know anything. You were a leaf that didn't know it was part of a tree.'[3] The history of epilepsy very much proves this point. Yet, all too often to contemporary eyes, the leaf is all there is.

Not only that, for history moves on. Ideas, like leaves, seeming strong and vigorous at one time, wither and fall with a transience and an insignificance unthinkable at the time. But the tree also has a trunk and branches, permanent structures that slowly grow and enlarge. So it has been with epilepsy, where, superimposed on evanescent and transitory theories and practices, there has been an expanding core of enduring knowledge. To make sense of its history, the process of winnowing, separating the wheat of epilepsy from its chaff, is necessary and it is to this task that this last chapter is directed, with two primary aims.

Aim 1: The first aim is to summarise how epilepsy changed between 1860 and 2020 to identify *which were developments over the long twentieth century that have endured*. The earlier chapters, in section 2, are concerned as much with the leaves as with the trunk, describing events and theories which came and went; here the focus is on the trunk and its branches – the parts of the journey which solidified and became permanent. This risks over-repetition of points already made in earlier chapters, but such iteration seems necessary in the winnowing process. Despite the fact that *Epilepsy* has commonly taken blind alleys and not infrequently travelled back on herself, a substantial body of knowledge has been accrued[4] and progress has been made – at times remarkable progress, and sometimes in surprising directions. This Epilogue celebrates and takes stock of that knowledge.

Aim 2: The second aim is more controversial – to identify where epilepsy seems *now* to be taking wrong turnings, and to highlight *current concepts* which are likely to wither away, as have others in the past. Here, the spotlight is on criticisms of, and on reservations about, current knowledge, attitude and practice; and in a few examples, on the 'dark side' of epilepsy where ideas are not only wrong but damaging or detrimental.[5] It is in relation to this second endeavour that the book here departs from any pretence of objectivity and becomes inevitably a personal view in which the author's standpoint and prejudices are fully exposed.

A rough balance sheet of the positive and negative has been drawn up in Appendix 1. All is not positive, but overall the conditions for those with epilepsy are indubitably far better in 2020 than they had been at any time earlier, despite the many storms that had to be confronted.

---

[3] Crichton, *Timeline*, p. 73.

[4] Illustrating the truth of the aphorism 'history teaches, but it has no pupils' (attributed to Antonio Gramsci). In epilepsy (and medicine in general) the historical development of topics is often ignored.

[5] The dark side is also explored in Schmidt and Shorvon, *The End of Epilepsy*.

As indicated at the start, perspective is crucial. The story of epilepsy over the long 20th century will have appeared quite different to the scientist, the doctor, society and the person with epilepsy. History encourages many ways of thinking critically about a topic such as epilepsy, and an attempt has been made here to accommodate these four points of view, thus broadening the scope of the story beyond that of a simple medical narrative. It has certainly been easier to chart the evolution of the medical and scientific perspectives on epilepsy than the others, not least because of the objectified nature of science and the linear traces left by papers in scientific and medical journals and books. Social influences are more complex and more subject to varied interpretation, but most difficult of all has been the exploration of the patient's perspective. In this respect much reliance has been placed on memoirs and what has been revealed in creative fiction and film, albeit whilst recognising their subjectivity.

Within this framework, it is hardly surprising that *Epilepsy* has failed to steer a straight course. But, it is perhaps not too great a generalisation to state that the two strongest currents which have most dictated the direction of travel, as of much else in the twentieth century, have been, first, the hegemony of capitalism, particularly in its twentieth century manifestations as social liberalism and liberal democracy, and, second, the rise of science.

And it is with these thoughts in mind that this chapter will embark on the winnowing: to summarise what has endured and to air misgivings about some directions currently being taken.

SOCIETY AND EPILEPSY

Making generalisations about societal influences is fraught with bias and error, and inevitably over-simplifies often complex issues. Within any democratic society, at any time, a whole range of attitudes and opinions prevail, often contradictory and inconsistent: the antivivisectionists and the basic laboratory scientist will never see eye to eye, nor will the eugenicist and the ethicist, nor the socialist and the neoliberal. Nonetheless, broad trends in any contemporary zeitgeist can be discerned, and *Epilepsy's* main direction of travel can be best interpreted only within the context of the prevalent sociocultural–political forces. From the mass of information and data available to anyone writing about the history of medicine, selection is inevitable, and my choice of material will not suit everyone (or anyone) but there it has to be. It seems to me that of all the societal influences, those of national politics and economics, legislation and social attitude, the nature of healthcare systems, and of the pharmaceutical industry are the most powerful. The professional organisations and the explosion of communication technologies also have had large effects, as has the globalisation of medicine.

The Political and Economic Context

At the start of our history in the late nineteenth century, in Europe and the United States at least, a classically liberal laissez-faire ideology held sway, more or less. At the risk of extreme generalisation, the attitude of the state towards epilepsy (and most of medicine) was essentially non-interventional. Epilepsy was considered to be a private affair and not the business of government. Action was resisted on the grounds that it would reduce the responsibility of individuals to provide for themselves, undermine free enterprise and hamper growth. Compassion and philanthropy were lauded, but were a moral choice for individuals and not the state. The impact of the state in relation to epilepsy, then viewed as a mental disorder, was largely restricted to its role in confining those with excessive mental disturbance in asylum settings.

As time passed, and especially after 1917, when revolutionary communism replaced capitalism in Russia, the fear of revolution and the influence of socialism and communism stimulated more state intervention. In the interwar years, Western governments slowly became more entangled in healthcare and in financing health. In parallel, society itself was often viewed in biological terms, and considered 'sick', some felt terminally so. Eugenic theory seemed to offer a solution, within which epilepsy became ensnared. The Second World War was a watershed. In Europe, health rapidly became a central feature of governmental policies and a central political priority. In the post-war period, the ideals of a 'welfare state' quickly became established. Social democracy became a predominant political narrative which would, it was hoped, remove inequality and promote social justice, security and prosperity – and healthcare became a central pillar of these policies. For those with epilepsy this was a boon. Medical care in Western countries became rapidly available at levels never previously attained. In parallel, the emphasis on the rights of the disabled from the 1960s was to provide unprecedented equality for those with epilepsy. In America, the European ideals of social democracy and the welfare state were always (and unfairly) tarred with the brush of communism, and competitive market-driven policies were a stronger influence. There a free market in medicine flourished, and so did the glossy technologies of epilepsy for those who could afford them, excluding a significant proportion who could not. Even in America, though, the right to health of all citizens with illnesses, including epilepsy, had by 2020 risen up the agenda and forced a significant degree of state intervention.

Famously, Francis Fukuyama saw liberal democracy as a 'final form of human government'.[6] His belief that its triumph signalled the endpoint of humanity's sociocultural evolution is highly arguable, but there is no doubt that this political ideology facilitated many of the beneficial developments, both

---

[6] Fukuyama, *The End of History*, p. xi.

social and medical, in epilepsy in the post–Second World War years. Liberal democracy provided an environment in which the social position of persons with epilepsy could greatly improve. In all advanced societies, it facilitated wide access to good healthcare through its emphasis on individual rights. At the level of laboratory and clinical science, it provided an infrastructure in which science could flourish through a system of relative intellectual freedom and access to funding. It was through funding that the state could, and did, further influence the course of epilepsy. At the industrial level, the post-war social democratic policies fuelled the rise of the pharmaceutical industry and the production of the technologies of medicine (EEG, imaging, surgery, drugs). Governments exerted influence here too by regulation and oversight of licensing, advertisement and marketing.

In the early post-war years, modern medicine – clothed in the armour of science and technology and weaponised by pharmaceuticals and modern investigatory paraphernalia – wielded new power and influence, and doctors assumed new authority. Their numbers rapidly increased, specialisations developed and in parallel health became a staple of the news of the day. Governments began to devote more and more resources, but as science advanced and made possible new investigations and treatments, costs grew precipitously.

The fall of communism in 1989–92 allowed a rawer form of capitalism to flourish, and the post-war social contract emphasising equity of access to health care was increasingly challenged by a resurgence of neoliberal policies focused on transferring costs from state to individuals and downgrading ideals of equality. Consumerist policies and market forces were increasingly prominent. With the inflation in healthcare costs, by the end of the century the willingness of the state to provide all that medicine could offer was being reeled back. Nevertheless, by 2020, in Western Europe, relatively easy and affordable access to publicly funded health care was still preserved for the majority of the population including those with epilepsy.

Paradoxically, it was in the countries of the world with the lowest incomes and where health needs were greatest, that governments spent least on healthcare. In many countries by 2020, although health facilities on the Western model did exist in the large cities for those who could pay, there were few such services in the rural areas, and the care available for most persons with epilepsy had in effect changed little since pre-modern times. Japan was the first Asian country to become a big player on the global scene and steered a course between the European and American trends when it came to health. By 2020, China, nominally a communist power, had adopted severely oppressive authoritarian control over its population and neoliberal economic policies, but even there in the 2010s attention was being paid by the state specifically to epilepsy, in the form of large-scale epidemiological surveys undertaken to explore the extent and effects of epilepsy and the value of epilepsy treatment facilities.

The WHO was an important influence on the agendas of government, and its Global Campaign Against Epilepsy, 'Out of the Shadows' produced many policy changes – and continues to do so. Political forces can change rapidly, but at the time of writing, they seemed largely on epilepsy's side.

Legislation and Social Attitude

In democratic countries, legislation can be seen roughly to reflect majority social norms, albeit with a lag and often shaded by conservatism. In the early years, legislation in relation to epilepsy was, in most countries, limited to the administration of asylum care. Laws were enacted for the provision of asylums and colonies where persons would be separated from normal society. These tended to make no distinction between those with epilepsy and those with mental impairment, insanity, mental illness and dementia; with all these conditions lumped together.

In the early years of the twentieth century, due in no small part to the effects of the eugenics lobby, cultural attitudes hardened, and epilepsy became weighed down by hostility and social oppression. Legislation became mainly concerned with methods for containment, control and segregation. As the eugenics movement grew stronger, in many countries laws were passed mandating segregation, prohibition of marriage and in some locations involuntary sterilisation (the most extreme action, the euthanasia of the Nazi regime, however, was carried out surreptitiously and never enacted in law). After the war, and in part a reaction to previous abuses, Western societies adopted more sympathetic public attitudes. Other factors, too, were important, including better understanding of, and treatments for, epilepsy and the increasing power of the lobby of patient groups in the consumerist world. Legislation followed, and in the late twentieth century levels of protection never previously attained were afforded to those with disabilities in equal rights legislation. This gave individuals, including most of those with epilepsy, the ability to determine their own care to a greater extent than ever before. Legislation was passed in relation to the protection of employment, education and domestic matters. Laws regulating clinical experimentation and also research (especially genetic research) were enacted in many countries, including antivivisection legislation which extended rights to animals and limited the actions of researchers.[7] Legislation affecting epilepsy infiltrated into other diverse areas, including for instance driving licensing, for instance, where laws tried to balance public safety with individual freedom.

---

[7] For instance the EU directives, and in Britain the Animals (Scientific Procedures) Act (1986; and its later amendments). Similar legislation was passed in many other countries.

How transient these freedoms and protection will be for people with epilepsy is a question for the future, but the example of early-twentieth-century history does not give grounds for untrammelled optimism. Perhaps the greatest threat arises now, as it did in the past, from the potential of new genetic practices to facilitate a new wave of eugenic activity albeit under the guise of new terminology.

In other cultures, no such changes occurred or were less far-reaching. In China and much of the Far East and South-East Asia, more authoritarian laws and more repressive social norms were retained. The last vestiges of the eugenic measures were removed from the statute books slowly, although laws against marriage of those with epilepsy remained in force in several countries, including India, until the early years of the twenty-first century, and naïve eugenic policies (love-boat cruises and the like) were encouraged in places such as Singapore.[8]

The delivery of Epilepsy Healthcare

One of the greatest transformations in the treatment of epilepsy between 1860 and 2020 was in the delivery of healthcare.

It is easy to forget how little medical attention was paid to those with epilepsy at the beginning of this period. In the Western world, in the nineteenth and early twentieth centuries, the average person with epilepsy living in the community, and keeping the condition as hidden as possible, did not to access any medical care except for occasional visits to the local family doctor. Those who could afford it consulted private physicians or psychiatrists, but for most this was not an option. Diagnosis was rudimentary, there were no investigations and treatment was largely ineffective. Epilepsy – considered a mental disorder – was not in the main treated in general hospitals, except in emergency situations. Where inpatient care was needed it was most often provided by psychiatrists in asylums or colonies. The colony movement was a reaction against the abuses of asylums and the overdue recognition that those with epilepsy should not be bundled together with those with other mental disorders. It was initially strongly supported by almost all those committed to the better medical care of patients with epilepsy, and for instance the promotion of epilepsy colonies was the primary goal of the ILAE at its foundation. Originally conceived to provide compassionate and philanthropic care (and, for children, education), and then taken into state control, these institutions grew in strength throughout the early twentieth century, but with the demise of asylums after the 1960s, colonies too either closed their doors or adapted their role, some changing into 'special centres'.

[8] Chan, 'Eugenics in Singapore'.

The pattern of care (or, rather, non-care) that existed in these earlier years had been utterly transformed by 2020. In all Western countries, at least, epilepsy was now a condition diagnosed and treated largely by neurologists and not generalists, and in a hospital outpatient setting. In 1860, psychiatry was the specialty in charge of epilepsy and so it remained well into the twentieth century, until slowly and progressively this role was ceded to neurology, at least in Western countries, and epilepsy became no longer a 'mental disorder'. Although in last decades of our history, a growing irredentist trend has developed, as psychiatry has assumed the clothes of molecular science and the distinction between psychiatry and neurology has become less absolute. In the decades following the second World War, sub-specialism within neurology grew up. Epilepsy was one of the first diseases in which subspecialisation occurred, and with the discipline of epileptology came a more technological and more scientific and forensic approach. Epilepsy units and centres sprang up widely within neurological settings. Asylums closed down and long-term institutionalisation became rare. Diagnosis was still based essentially on the clinical history and examination, but now supplemented by EEG to refine seizure type and syndrome, and imaging and biochemical tests to establish the cause.[9] A large range of medical and surgical therapies became available.

These developments were almost wholly advantageous and, from the medical point of view, at no time in history had specialist management and treatment been so accessible for those with epilepsy and so potentially effective. Furthermore, the input of science acted to demystify the condition and to distance it from superstition and irrationality. In the last decades of this history, as neoliberal policies eroded the Welfare State, health care was again under relative threat; but even then, by 2020, those with epilepsy, at least in the Western world, had probably never been better served by the state.

Criticisms of the healthcare available for epilepsy by 2020 were however being levelled in three particular areas. First, was the view that the modern system of medical care – with its emphasis on super-specialism and technology, guidelines, protocols and finance – depersonalised both the doctor and the patient. Especially when squeezed financially, as an institution, medicine had come to be seen by many, fairly or unfairly, as increasingly inhuman. Although whether this had really changed appreciably from the equally out-of-touch doctors in the nineteenth century or the authoritarian medicine of the first half of the twentieth century is unclear. Medicine's defence was that it should act scientifically and engage only in areas which have a high-quality evidence base. But individual concerns are just exactly that, and not susceptible to controlled study.

---

[9] The principles of epilepsy diagnosis have changed little in 150 years. The process is two-stage: first, to decide whether a seizure is 'epileptic' in nature and, second, to establish its cause. Even today, they depend to a large extent on the clinical history and examination, and generally more so than on any one investigatory test.

A second criticism was that, in the consumerist and market-driven societies of 2020, trust in the medical process had become eroded, as it had been in many late-twentieth- and early twenty-first-century institutions. Such society, as John Berger wrote, 'wastes and, by the slow draining process of enforced hypocrisy, empties most of the lives which it does not destroy.'[10] The more holistic approach of 1900 provided far more inexact diagnoses and far less effective treatment, but it at least attended to the parts of the patient experience which modern medicine had somewhat discarded.

The third, and perhaps most important criticism of epilepsy healthcare in 2020 was that still in much of the developing world, the delivery of medical care to people with epilepsy had hardly evolved. In the rural areas of many low-income countries, healthcare resembled that in Europe in the late nineteenth century – with most patients in the community still untreated, with no access to orthodox medicine, and where persons with epilepsy were hidden or rejected. When incarceration could not be avoided, this meant only the lunatic asylum. In the larger cities, Western-style facilities existed in most countries but access was very limited. The Global Campaign Against Epilepsy produced data from many low- and middle-income countries, demonstrating large treatment gaps and lack of access to medical care. In such places, traditional healers and non-allopathic medicine played an important role and social norms were a significant influence on treatment. In conservative and religious societies, such as Saudi Arabia, the family and religious faith played a prominent role. In all countries, treatment was assumed to be most successful when allopathic medical guidelines were adapted that incorporated local cultural and social attitudes, but that had always proved difficult in practice.

The Pharmaceutical Industry

Medical treatment, by 2020, had become dominated by pharmaceuticals – with both marked benefit and some downsides. At the beginning of our history, the pharmaceutical industry played little part in the daily lives of the sufferers from epilepsy or their doctors. The most effective antiepileptic drugs were the bromides, which were prepared and formulated largely by local pharmacists from raw chemicals. It was only in the mid-twentieth century that the pharmaceutical companies had emerged as powerful industrial complexes, mainly in the USA, Germany, Switzerland, Britain and France, and then, as time passed, in many other countries. In the decades following World War Two, the power and influence of 'big pharma' gathered considerable momentum, drugs swept aside other forms of therapy and the pharmaceutical industry became central to the whole business of the medicine of epilepsy and of its

---

[10] Berger, *A Fortunate Man*, p. 167.

science. By the end of the century, the industry had become a paradigmatic example of late twentieth century capitalism – with massive mergers and acquisitions, wrangles over patent rights, huge swathes of litigation, sophisticated marketing, lobbying and the garnering of political influence. Very large sums were spent on research and development of new drugs[11] – but it was nevertheless through their marketing and sponsorship activities that the companies exerted much of their influence on the diagnosis and treatment of epilepsy, as well as on the institutions of the epilepsy world. It was within the bewildering world of high finance and pharmaceutical company boardrooms that many priorities of the epilepsy world and much of the epilepsy agenda were decided, and to a large extent this was totally opaque. Industry was able to wield it power because of its massive financial clout which oiled the wheels of epilepsy through lobbying and direct payment to professional bodies and 'key opinion leaders'. Its influence acted at the multiple levels of government.

In the last three decades of the century, the industry became truly globalised. By 2014 sales for pharmaceuticals exceeded $1 trillion globally, and by 2021 profits were expected to top $600 billion. By 2020, more was spent on promotion/lobbying and advertising than on basic research. In America, for instance, there were more than 1,378 paid lobbyists in 2020, and between 1998 and 2016 'Big Pharma' had spent $3.5 billion on lobbying expenses – more than any other industry.[12] The industries benefitted hugely from government funding of healthcare and did themselves contribute much to national economic growth. But there was a dark side, for as the power and financial muscle of big pharma grew, so did the perception that it was the pursuit of profit had led to unethical behaviours. Trust towards the pharmaceutical industry, in large sections of the public, became eroded. There has grown up a prevalent view that the industry routinely manipulated markets, doctors and the professional organisations (such as the ILAE) through sponsorship and skilful marketing. Similarly, governments and regulatory agencies struggled against the pharmaceutical lobbies in their attempts to make drugs safer and their effects more transparent. Major calamities, such as the thalidomide disaster and a host of smaller scandals, resulted in the phenomenal growth of lawsuits, which spread into the world of epilepsy therapeutics and further fuelled the suspicion and hostility that the industry engendered.

Of course, the benefit of drug therapy should not be underestimated – without modern drugs, the medical treatment of epilepsy would be

---

[11] Indeed, by 1971 American pharmaceutical companies were spending more on research and development than any other area, bar aerospace and communication industries: Swann, 'Evolution of the American Pharmaceutical Industry'.

[12] Figures from Compton, 'Big pharma', *Drugwatch*.

rudimentary, and uncontrolled seizures would be a fact of life for many more people. It is indeed an extraordinary paradox that the industry which had contributed so much to global health should be held in such disdain. But attention to more scrupulous and truthful behaviour would have done much to restore its image. Perhaps, just as this history is reaching its end, the arrival of the Covid-19 pandemic might prove a turning point. If the industry succeeds in vaccine and treatment development to control the epidemic, and if it does so in a transparent and proportionate way without exploitation or profiteering, it has the opportunity again to regain the high ground and the respect and gratitude of the public, and a rise in trust to levels not seen since the 1940s. Although Covid-19 has little effect on epilepsy per se, a positive change in the public perception of pharmaceuticals could well be of future benefit to epilepsy.

The ILAE and Other Epilepsy Bureaucracies

The first professional association dedicated to epilepsy was the ILAE, founded in 1909. It was initially a small club, which in 1914 had fewer than 100 members but large ambitions. Then the First World War abruptly terminated all activity. The League was revived in 1935, and again put to sleep by the Second World War. It was revived yet again in 1945 and, in the last decades of the century, had rapidly expanded. By 2020, the ILAE had changed beyond all recognition, with 25,000 members and chapters in 123 countries. Its success in maintaining the professional leadership of epilepsy was due largely to the holding of international and national congresses and the publication of what became, and has remained, the premier epilepsy journal, *Epilepsia*. In these ways, the ILAE provided an indispensable forum for postgraduate education and presentation of research – a singular achievement worthy of celebration. Two other activities deserve special mention, and proved key to putting the ILAE at the top of the epilepsy pyramid: the formulation of the International Classification of Epileptic Seizures in the 1960s, which placed the ILAE for the first time at the centre of the professional epilepsy spotlight, and the Global Campaign Against Epilepsy, in partnership with the IBE and the World Health Organization, which raised the profile of epilepsy and promised to make a potentially huge difference to sufferers in the developing world. Without the ILAE, the epilepsy world would have been less prominent and less connected, and the dissemination of Western medical practice in epilepsy less rapid and less complete. Other professional organisations have arisen in the fields of neurology which have epilepsy divisions, but the ILAE remained the only major professional organisation dedicated solely to epilepsy and to leading the epilepsy portfolio worldwide. In parallel, the IBE, a lay organisation, was established in the 1960s, and it too had grown to include 135 chapters in 104 countries by 2020, was leading efforts to increase the power of the patient lobby and had become instrumental in injecting the patient's voice into epilepsy decision-making.

By 2020, the ILAE had become open to criticism on several fronts. First, had been the fact that since the late 1980s the ILAE had become almost entirely dependent on funds originating directly or indirectly from the pharmaceutical industry. Although excellent procedures had been put in place to keep the overt commercial influence at arm's length, and indeed industry itself had been constrained by increasingly strict national and international regulatory limitations, the reliance to this degree on industrial sponsorship posed, and continues to pose, a hazard to the values and culture of the organisation. Second had been the tendency of the ILAE to be inward looking. Internal politics always loomed large in the machinations of the organisation, and at times had proved disastrous, and much depended on the wisdom and skill of its leadership the quality of which had varied. Also, in the view of many, too great a proportion of its funds had been diverted to support internal processes rather than its mission. By 2020 the ILAE had accumulated a nest egg of more than $20 million to endow its own administration, which might well have been better spent on its goals. The organisation's authority had also been weakened by the repeated tinkering with its constitution, often for short-term political purposes, and also the classifications and terminologies of epilepsy.

Arguably, though, the ILAE's greatest failure had been the lost opportunity to form closer links with the IBE. Attempts were made in the 1970s to federate the ILAE and IBE under the umbrella of 'Epilepsy International', but this floundered and then failed largely due to personality differences amongst the leadership and a lack of synoptical vision. A less formal partnership of the IBE and the ILAE was resuscitated in the 1990s and was key to the recruitment of the WHO and the success of the Global Campaign and other recent lobbying efforts. A more coordinated organisational structure might have exerted more influence and have further benefitted the position of those with epilepsy.

Information and Communication

Before World War One, most medical instruction in epilepsy took place via books, with scientific journals, less numerous and less influential, playing a subsidiary role. Books were usually by single authors and provided a forum for presenting research as well as current practice. At conferences, too, the major lectures were important and authoritative events – providing new data and new ideas. As the century moved on, though, these time-honoured staples of academe were to be modified. After World War Two, the publication of original medical research was increasingly restricted to journals. By the last few decades of the century, the major books on epilepsy typically took the form of collections of reviews by a multiplicity of authors, and had a mainly pedagogical not research role. This evolution was partly a response to the transfiguration of scientific knowledge, its quantity and nature, the compulsion to establish precedence and the burgeoning specialisation. And perhaps only the bibliophil would regret this transition. The role of congresses changed too, as with less new information to be presented, they became more educative in nature.

In the last few decades of our history, a further series of profound changes in medical informatics occurred: the advent of computerisation and digitisation, then the establishment of the Internet as the primary source of medical information, then the wholesale move of medical journals into an online format, and finally the explosion of social media as a means of conveying information. The distribution and dissemination of knowledge and opinion about epilepsy was ramped up to a previously unimagined level. In 2000 *Epilepsia* went online and became a largely digital publication, and by 2020 there were hundreds of additional online journals and other outlets for medical communications in epilepsy. So much information became available that indexing became crucial, and extraordinarily powerful 'search engines' and digital indexing systems, such as Medline and Google, developed. It became easy for all persons around the world to obtain information, often free of charge. Consequently, electronic communication not only globalised information but became an important levelling influence, enabling almost anyone – whatever their location or personal circumstances – to access knowledge about epilepsy. This applied not only to doctors, but also to their patients, and as a result both became far better informed than at any previous time; this too contributed to the changing of the doctor–patient relationship. Social media gave epilepsy an even wider platform, providing people with epilepsy, and not just their doctors and scientists, a means of easily expressing their own opinions, ideas and concerns.

The globalisation of communication, twinned with the successes of free-market capitalism and liberal academic policies (an example being the free availability worldwide of Medline), facilitated the hegemony of the Western medical model and of its transaction in the English language. Guidelines produced in New York or London were applied in Chennai or Beijing. There is no doubt that modern systems of communication improved access to information and knowledge about epilepsy, but the extent to which these developments raised the quality of life for the generality of those with epilepsy is quite unknown – but surely they must have done so.

Perhaps inevitably, there have been challenges. Even by 2020, regulation of social media and the internet was rudimentary, and a significant proportion of the available information about epilepsy was inaccurate or biased – with social media in particular more suited to kite-flying than reasoned argument. Even more problematic had been the disregard for truth, a trend in society encouraged and seemingly sanctioned by its leaders – the examples of Russian,

American and Chinese autocrats spring to mind. By 2020, the disdain for factual honesty was endemic, and undermined the value of the information revolution. Truth has been both a victor and a casualty in epilepsy as in all other areas of modern life – but, given the unique vulnerability of those with epilepsy, dishonesty, propaganda and prejudice remain threats to its future.

The Globalisation of Epilepsy Research and Medicine

Another striking phenomenon of the long twentieth century was the increasingly global nature of epilepsy knowledge and practice. In 1860, epilepsy research and innovation was generated largely from a few countries in Western Europe. By 1900, epilepsy research activity had also developed in North America. It was then only in the second half of the century that advanced clinical and research facilities began to spread to the rest of the world, and by 2020 leading centres existed in many countries, challenging the traditional hegemony of Western Europe and America. Linked to the information and communication revolution, this surely has assisted many patients with epilepsy. The lower income countries still lagged behind and the levelling up of care remains a most pressing issue for epilepsy medicine in future years,

THE SCIENCE OF EPILEPSY

Science has been a pre-eminent and growing influence on the course of epilepsy in the long twentieth century. As the century progressed, scientific discovery flooded the epilepsy landscape, and its impact became all-pervading. Science bought benefits to epilepsy (as to much of medicine), delivering better understanding of pathophysiology, better diagnostic methods and better treatment, but there were downsides. The agnosticism of science has been (and remains) its Achilles' heel. Science has no intrinsic interest in distinguishing right from wrong, and throughout the twentieth century this has caused harm and distress to many with epilepsy, for instance through eugenics, false theories of aetiology, dangerous investigations, pharmaceutical calamities and failed and inappropriate surgery – examples are listed in Appendix 2. The balance, though, is surely positive. There is no doubt that, because of science, epilepsy became better understood and better managed and treated by 2020 than ever before. Science and its technologies have led to greater prosperity and opportunities for people with epilepsy, and today, because of science, surely few with epilepsy would opt for an earlier time. It is, however, a reflection of the power of science that latterly society has had to put in place constraints on its lack of moral compass, by the rise of regulation, medical ethics, the recognition of the rights of the disabled and by democratic social oversight.

In 1860, scientific research in epilepsy hardly existed, and where it did it was conducted in an essentially amateur fashion, by a small number of clinicians, based in hospitals, universities or research institutes,[13] but not industry. It seldom had specific funding, and was almost all based in Europe. The most important landmark in the science of the brain at this time was the development of the theory of cortical localisation – and the study of epileptic seizures was central to this work.

In the early years of the twentieth century, fundamental discoveries were made in the basic life sciences of neurophysiology, pathology and neurochemistry, but this was not focused on epilepsy and had little impact in the clinic at that time. The applied technology which had the greatest impact on the course of epilepsy in the mid-century was electroencephalography (EEG). Although interestingly this was developed scientifically for other purposes, with its application to epilepsy being rather an afterthought. In the later decades of the twentieth century there was a rapid expansion in the power and scope of science. The focus of neurological research moved to molecular genetics, neurochemistry and neurophysiology, and epilepsy was in the mix of much of this basic work. By 2020, partly stimulated by a number of new animal models and new laboratory techniques, a succession of research findings in the previous four decades had resulted in a detailed understanding of the basic chemical and physiological mechanisms of neuronal transmission which were the nuts and bolts of seizure generation. Cellular defects that could predispose to seizures were identified in ion conductance, neurotransmitter release, inhibitory and excitatory synaptic and receptor function, and wide neuronal systems. As neurochemical concepts of neurotransmitters and receptors began to dominate scientific thought, the mechanisms of drug action, unknown up until the 1980s, were elucidated and the potential for new treatments stimulated activity in basic neuropharmacology, which began to dictate the direction of clinical treatment.

In the post-war period, a quick succession of extraordinary discoveries were also made in the field of basic genetics which were to transform the entire life sciences landscape and which, culminating in the Human Genome Project, were amongst the greatest scientific discoveries of the twentieth century. After 1995, the application of new genetic technologies provided the key to many advances in understanding the causes of epilepsy and its pathophysiology.

The benefits of the behavioural sciences to epilepsy were less clear cut. In the early twentieth century, flawed psychological theories in relation to mental handicap, and the inevitability of progress to 'epileptic dementia' and to the

---

[13] Victor Horsley, for instance, was appointed as professor superintendent of the Brown Institute, where much of his research was carried out.

'epileptic personality', caused immense harm to people with epilepsy, and were anyway later discredited. The same applied to psychoanalysis. Attitudes to epilepsy also became entangled in the many battles between neurology and psychiatry in this period.

Physics, electronics, computing and engineering became vital ingredients of post-war medicine. Perhaps the most significant product of these physical sciences was the development of magnetic resonance imaging which provided detailed images of morbid anatomy and pathology and dramatically advanced an understanding of the underlying conditions causing seizures, with clinical implications which were as great, or perhaps greater, than those of electroencephalography.

The geography of epilepsy science also underwent dramatic changes. By 2020, basic laboratory research into epilepsy was being undertaken in many different countries and continents, and a huge number of individuals had become involved. Scientific research flourished as governments, research charities and especially industry allocated enormous funds. Increasingly, too, professional scientists had taken the reins of much basic research out of the hands of clinicians. Scientific research became more rigorous and specialised, and more regulated. Behind all this has been the underpinning notion (first recognised in post-war America) that science in medicine had an enormous commercial potential. It was this simple and fundamental fact that above all drove the endeavours – and in this sense science can be seen a triumph of the capitalist model. Traditionally university based, much of the basic research in epilepsy was by the later post-war years conducted in the laboratories of pharmaceutical and biotechnology companies, searching for commercial opportunities and shifting fundamentally the ethics and processes of science.

But despite its multitudinous benefits, the wheat of epilepsy science was mixed with chaff, and the undoubted successes of scientific medicine had been tempered by problems and pitfalls, some with deep ramification. In 1978, Colin Dollery, in an interesting intellectual game, formulated a 'charge sheet' against medical science, and then, acting as judge, rejected each of the charges.[14] As a leading clinical pharmacologist, Dollery was hardly an unbiased adjudicator, and although he dismissed the charges, they succinctly summarised the anxieties of the time about the course of medical science and even by 2020 four of his seven critiques remained worth considering, namely: that science is a conspiracy against the public, a charge brought by Ivan Illich; that it shows a callous lack of concern, a charge by Maurice Pappworth; that medical science is an irrelevance to health, a charge by Thomas McKeown; and that society has

---

[14] Dollery, *End of an Age of Optimism*; Illich, *Limits to Medicine*; Pappworth, *Human Guinea Pigs*; McKeown, *Role of Medicine*; Cochrane, *Effectiveness and Efficiency*.

a too-credulous acceptance of new procedures and drugs, a charge by Archibald Cochrane.

Illich's view that 'The medical establishment has become a major threat to health' is obviously polemical, but it still contains a kernel of truth. Medicine had done harm in epilepsy as to other conditions, in his words, by its transition from enhancing the healing effects of nature to 'engineering the dreams of reason'.[15] However, an advance of basic scientific understanding is needed for any rational therapy, and technological solutions had by any yardstick clearly helped many patients. His parallel opinion that the medical care system is a doctor-inspired conspiracy also had an element of truth. However, by 2020, the power wielded by epilepsy doctors over their patients was much more constrained than it had been in the earlier years, not least by much ramped up regulation of clinical practice and the many platforms made available for the patient voice. Dollery rejected Illich's criticism, but my view is that, although exaggerated, strands of his criticism require constant vigilance.

Pappworth's opinion that the medical profession engaged in unethical experimentation and callous practice carried much less weight in the field of epilepsy by 2020 than it did when he published *Human Guinea Pigs*. There however remained two specific areas in which there was a worrying lack of oversight: the use of invasive devices and the trialling of new surgical approaches. In both, regulation was far less than in the area of drug therapies, and more vigilance surely was, and continues to be, needed. He was concerned with human experimentation, but the antivivisection movement which first surfaced in the mid-nineteenth century gained much traction after the 1970s due to the vast numbers of animals used in research and its dubious ethical basis.[16]

McKeown's criticism was that much of medical practice was irrelevant to health. He based his analysis on life expectancy, and it is undeniably true that, in the field of epilepsy as elsewhere, the money spent on treatment could have been more usefully spent on other non-medical projects that would have improved overall life expectancy to a greater extent, especially in the developing world. His criticism does not, however, account for the fact that medical science has improved the quality of life of patients with epilepsy, even if not their life expectancy – and, as Dollery himself put it, death is not the only end point. It has been the case, though, that swathes of science – both basic and clinical – have had little or no impact and are quickly forgotten; such research is

---

[15] By social historians as well by novelists and writers: see, for instance, Feinstein, *Clinical Judgment*, David B., *Epileptic*.

[16] The antivivisection movement was empowered by books such as Peter Singer's *Animal Liberation* and the regular exposés of distressing activities in the laboratories of the pharmaceutical companies and universities. Epilepsy researchers were in the midst of the resulting turmoil.

effectively just Brownian motion. The level of redundancy has been huge. Indeed, whole areas of medical research in epilepsy have resulted in little of lasting benefit to patients, and wasted time, talent and money. At the time of writing functional brain imaging (fMRI) and pharmacogenetics are examples [17] that might potentially suffer the same fate as earlier practices and theories such as psychoanalysis or autointoxication.

Redundancy was (and is) exacerbated by the poor conduct of science. As Ioannides pointed out, much published clinical research suffered from sloppy data collection, lack of statistical significance, lack of defined objectives (and data mining), lack of oversight, and the curse of assuming an association is causal. Even when well conducted, much research has no practical utility. The massive change in medical publishing following the introduction of digital technologies facilitated this by making it possible to publish almost any paper, however poor its science, in some scientific journal or other. Other negative consequences identified by Ioannides were the flood of repetitious papers, unnecessary reviews ('parasitic publications'), the 'salami slicing' of research, and the misuse of scientific journals for marketing purposes by industry. Given that there was a limit to what could usefully be read, the academic of 2020 was in serious danger of being swamped simply by the volume of poor quality published research.

Cochrane's censure was widely accepted and, as a result of public and governmental pressure, much more stringent testing of pharmaceutical products was put in place. Perhaps though the pendulum had swung too far and the cost involved and time taken to assess potential new medicines had inhibited growth. What was (and still is) undoubtedly a concern, though, was that new diagnostic technologies, new medical devices used in treatment and new surgical procedures were not subject to the same interrogation.

Other more generic criticisms of science are also worth commenting upon, as these too had an impact on epilepsy. First was, and is, the belief, not least amongst scientists themselves, that science is in some way an inherently superior way of viewing a condition like epilepsy *because of its objectivity*. According to this view, science occupied the high ground, seeking fundamental truths on a plain above messy political or social agendas. To some extent this narrative is justified in rarefied elements of university-based pure science; but, for the more mundane clinical sciences, in such fields as epilepsy this was clearly not the case. The medical science of epilepsy was, and remains, at one level a social science and at another a moral science, entangled in politics and economics and swayed by cultural norms. It is conducted via practices framed by social forces, by scientists imbued with strong value systems, and funded by corporate, military

---

[17] See for instance Tallis, *Aping Mankind*. Tallis refers to these as neuromania and Darwinitis, and provides a withering attack on both.

or governmental sources. The economic and political influences on medicine are extraordinarily powerful, as governments struggle to take control of agendas of medicine often in clownish and improvident ways. This is an old problem – for instance, Galileo and Darwin were both enmeshed in politics – but in the twentieth century the integration of science into the pursuit of profit and power had dictated its direction perhaps more than at any time in history. It may be reassuring to think of science as an ivory tower, a body of knowledge which sits quite apart from politics or societal trends, but this is a dangerous illusion. Yet it is also true that the interaction of society and science has worked in both directions, and science has transformed public discourse and 'revolutionized the rules by which the intellect operates'[18] – and generally for the better. This applied particularly to a condition such as epilepsy, where science has been instrumental in diminishing the hostile archetypes and damaging mysticism.

Another fissure has been the difficulty of translating scientific research into clinical practice in epilepsy. Few basic science developments, even if good science, altered clinical practice in any substantive way. This seems a lost opportunity. In epilepsy, the most successful scientific translation was in the production of diagnostic technologies, for instance in EEG, MRI and genetic sequencing; however, most of these were generic and not specific to epilepsy. By 2020, although basic molecular pharmacology had made great progress, drug development still had to cross what had become known as the 'valley of death' between the basic laboratory and late-stage clinical trials. It remains the case that 80–90% of compounds fail even to make it into early-stage clinical trials, and 50% fail in Phase 3 clinical trials. Indeed, it has been estimated that only around 0.1% of new drug candidates make it to the clinic; this is a high attrition rate, and one wonders if the hurdles are not now too onerous.

Finally are two other dark undersides to the glossy surface of science which, by 2020, had become prominent and urgent problems – fraud and hyperbole. Some well-publicised examples of fraud involving epilepsy are described in the previous chapter. These may be just the tip of the iceberg. Hyperbole – the communication of distorted fact (truth decay) – is a modern plague and exaggerated pronouncements no longer seem to be subject to the same moral sanction or punishment as was the case in the past. The modern history of epilepsy genetics is an example, described as a 'history of [unrealised] promises'[19] and in relation to epilepsy, the promised benefits were spun and exaggerated to such an extent that the true situation, like chasing the end of the rainbow, seems always within sight but never attainable. There is a danger that the public will weary of this, damaging the name of science. This has already

[18] Levi-Strauss and Eribon, *Conversations with Levi-Strauss*, p. 119.
[19] Comfort, *Science of Human Perfection*, p. ix.

happened to some extent, especially in relation to the pharmaceutical industry, where there is widespread cynicism and mistrust; a tragedy of its own making.

THE MEDICINE OF EPILEPSY

I have made previous reference to the lecture 'The Present and Future of Neurology', given by Francis Walshe at the 50th Anniversary of the Neurological Institute of New York in 1959. Walshe noted how much physiology had advanced in the first half of the twentieth century, but how little it had contributed to 'those age-old burning problems of the etiology, pathogenesis, and treatment of the many chronic, disabling, and killing affections of the nervous system'. His venom was particularly directed at clinical electroencephalography. This was the discovery of greatest import to epilepsy, and it certainly changed the concept of epilepsy and its nosology, but he was correct in seeing that, on clearing away the haze of hyperbole, its contribution to aetiology, pathogenesis and treatment had been relatively small. To Walshe this was a waste of resources and the future lay in neurochemistry and physics, as he put it: 'I was born too soon to see from the Pisgah heights of modern chemistry and physics what fair perspectives of fruitful and healing research now lie spread before the younger generation.' This was a prescient thought.

The massive development of molecular neuroscience and pharmacology, and of neuroimaging, surely justified his regret. However, the 'age-old burning problems of the etiology, pathogenesis, and treatment' are indeed still at the centre of epilepsy, and I will consider each in turn, but first a brief word on description and classification.

Clinical Description and Classification

When Walshe started out in clinical neurology, the specialty was concerned with descriptions of the complex phenomenon of neurological diseases and their classification. As he wrote: 'If you turn back to the pages of the neurological journals of the opening decade of the present century [the twentieth century] you cannot but admire the minuteness of observation and recording which characterized clinical neurology at the time.'[20] This certainly applied to epilepsy. Almost all of the clinical features of epilepsy had been fully described by then – most, indeed, before the end of the nineteenth century – and little of fundamental note has been described since. Where description did advance was in the integration of information from new technologies, especially EEG and based on this the grouping into the epilepsy syndromes.

---

[20] Walshe '*Future of neurology*'.

Although the clinical descriptions hardly changed, classification and terminology have been throughout this period something of a battlefield. An ideal classification would be based on scientific principles – for instance, on physiology or pathology. Instead, the most popular classifications have been based on clinical descriptions – especially of seizure type – which, as Hughlings Jackson famously commented, is like classifying plants by their value as food or ornament rather than being a botanical or scientific taxonomy. He called the former a 'gardeners' classification and the latter a 'proper' classification 'as might a botanist attempt'. A proper classification should provide, as he put it, for 'the better organization of existing knowledge, and for discovering the relations of new facts; its principles are methodical guides to further investigation'.[21] Over the years, the classification schemes of epilepsy were subject to a number of revisions, but all have been gardener's schemes, and whether there is really any advantage to the schemes of 2020 over those of 1860 is highly arguable. The disconnect between the clinical classification schemes and the insights from science, especially molecular science, is a loss of opportunity. This matters, for, as Jackson realised, a classification scheme sets the framework for research, which a poor scheme may well inhibit or retard.

In a similar vein, changing terminology is only worthwhile if it advances the conceptual base of a science. As recent history showed this point has been ignored. Change for its own sake has had many downsides, not least the confusion caused in the wider medical community, and the consequences in non-medical arenas such as the courts, the press and social services. Guidelines, regulatory definitions and case law, using old terminology, were rendered redundant for no real advantage. There are social consequences too, as shown for instance in the labelling of some epilepsies as 'genetic' even in the absence of any known genetic mechanism (a point further discussed below).[22]

Aetiology

The first of Walshe's age-old burning issues was aetiology. It was true that by 1959, when he spoke, only limited progress in this regard had been made. Cobb could identify sixty causes of epilepsy in 1941 and most cases of epilepsy were still of unknown cause – a situation not much different from that in 1860 although advances in basic clinical chemistry, bacteriology and radiology had

[21] Jackson, 'On classification', pp. 191–2 (originally published in the *Medical Press and Circular* between 14 October 1874 and 13 December 1876).

[22] One is reminded of the warning of Confucius: 'If names be not correct, language is not in accordance with the truth of things. If language be not in accordance with the truth of things, affairs cannot be carried on to success'; *Chinese Classics*, pp. 263–4.

had some impact. It was, however, to be the development of magnetic resonance imaging, then molecular chemistry and molecular genetics that were to be transformative. With these technologies, a very large number of underlying aetiologies were identified and by 2011, when the first textbook devoted to the cause of epilepsy was published, several thousand causes were known and the number continued to grow, especially in the field of genetics.[23]

But with this emphasis on aetiology came also the realisation that assigning cause in epilepsy was not at all straightforward.[24] There are essentially three reasons for this:

Epilepsy is multifactorial in nature: The cause of an epilepsy may often be the result of several interacting factors. These can be genetic influences, acquired influences and provoking factors. In this situation, assignment to any single aetiology is to an extent arbitrary. One cause may be overwhelming or predominant in some cases, but in others several aetiologies may contribute significantly. In the latter situation, individual aetiologies are best considered as 'causal factors' ('susceptibilities') rather than as absolute 'causes' and handled statistically by the use of odds ratios.

The multifactorial nature of epilepsy was well recognised in 1860, where causes were often differentiated into *predisposing* and *exciting* categories. The analogy of gunpowder and the match was often used (including by Jackson), in which the combustibility of gunpowder was the predisposing factor and the spark from the match the exciting cause. In 1960, Lennox emphasised the multifactorial nature of epilepsy by his famous analogy of the river, reservoir and dam, and this contributed too to the idea that there was a 'seizure threshold' (an amalgam of predisposing and exciting factors) which set the level at which seizures would occur (see Figure 26). Despite this, the idea had then grown up that the exciting factors are not really causes in the same way as the predisposing factors. But logically this does not make sense. An example would be the person with Idiopathic Generalised Epilepsy who only has seizures when sleep deprived. There seems to me no cogent reason for not considering both the genetic basis and sleep deprivation as equally causative.

The 'level' of causation: The importance of 'level' was recognised by Hughlings Jackson, who made a distinction between a 'remote' cause and a 'proximate' cause. Take the case, for instance, of a cerebral haemorrhage resulting in epilepsy. To Jackson, haemorrhage was the 'remote' cause but the real cause of the seizures was the cellular molecular changes in the cortical cells from which the epileptic discharges were originating (the proximate cause). Jackson considered

---

[23] Shorvon et al. 'Causes of epilepsy'.
[24] Discussed further in Shorvon, 'The concept of causation in epilepsy'.

these to be nutritional abnormalities, and today we could call these molecular or biochemical abnormalities, but they amount to the same thing. In other words, it is the *mechanisms of epileptogenesis* which Jackson considered most 'causal', and surely this is correct. We look forward to a time when the mechanisms are well understood, and indeed when an aetiological classification is possible that is based on proximate molecular mechanisms as well remote categories.

Epilepsy is a process which changes over time: In the late nineteenth and early twentieth centuries, it was fully recognised that, in many individuals, what caused the first seizure was not necessarily the cause of continuing epilepsy – an insight that became somewhat lost over the course of the century. In recent times, numerous molecular and system changes have been recognised which develop progressively after the onset of epilepsy and which may well contribute to the ongoing processes in epilepsy ('epileptogenesis'). That such changes occur can be inferred clinically by the resistance to drug therapy of chronic epilepsy when compared to new onset epilepsy, and by the evolution of EEG changes over time, and by the late development of symptoms such as psychosis. Epileptogenic processes might indeed precede any seizures, as for instance in symptomatic epilepsies in which there is a 'latent' period which can extend for months or even years after the causal cerebral damage and before the onset of seizures. However, the nature of these processes is entirely unknown.

Pathogenesis

This brings us to pathogenesis. Not much was known of these processes in the early part of the long twentieth century, but spectacular progress was then made largely since the 1970s. Earlier in the century, a variety of erroneous theories came and went, and many theories became widely accepted only later to be discredited. Such scientific blind alleys included ideas of degeneration, autointoxication, reflex mechanisms, vascular theories, ideas of acid-base disturbance, eugenics, and theories of acetylcholinergic mechanisms. By 2020, though, the underlying physiochemical mechanisms of seizures and causal mechanisms had been explained in some detail and advances in this area were amongst the most striking in epilepsy. Much of the evolution of knowledge in the field of aetiology and pathophysiology has been due to the impact of science and it is here that science has been at its most imperious.

Heredity

One category of aetiology and pathogenesis requires special consideration, given its impact on epilepsy, and this is the science of heredity. The extent to which it is an inherited/genetic disorder has been central to the concept of epilepsy. More than any other aetiology or pathogenic factor, heredity has proved a uniquely sensitive – and, at times, uniquely damaging – concept to individuals with epilepsy. Viewed as 'the essence' of a person, genetic make-up was, and is, closely linked to personal identity and self-image. The societal implications of the 'labels 'inherited' or 'genetic' throughout this period have extended far beyond being a medical or scientific issue. Genetic differences assign individuals to groupings – in effect, underclasses – thus rendering them vulnerable to social exclusion or other more severe measures. Repeatedly over the long twentieth century, genetic findings led to curtailment of rights, limitation of freedoms, and, when epilepsy was the focus of the eugenics movement, even more restrictive and coercive measures.

In 1860 and for most of the early twentieth century, there was a widespread belief that epilepsy was in large part inherited and was due to defective and degenerative germ plasm. Anxiety about inherited degeneration became a predominant societal fin-de-siècle concern. Also widely accepted was the flawed demographic assumption that, as those with defective germ plasm reproduced, the number of degenerates in the population would rapidly increase.[25] Epilepsy was at the centre of this whirlpool. Eugenics became a central feature of public policy in many countries, and eugenic solutions were enacted against those with epilepsy. Poor science was transformed into massive social injustice in what was one of the darkest moments in the history of twentieth century epilepsy, and there is no greater example of the moral and physical harm which scientific medicine can inflict. The willing participation of doctors, in particular psychiatrists and neurologists, was one of its greatest ethical abnegations.

In part as a reaction against this, eugenics disappeared as a topic of social discourse after the Second World War, and in epilepsy genetic research largely disappeared. However, the basic sciences of genetics made spectacular progress in the second half of the century, unlinked to social policy or to epilepsy. It was only again in the 1990s that epilepsy research turned towards genetics, and by 2020 it was again centre stage. In the fertile seas of epilepsy, fishing for genes had become a favourite medical pastime.

The way genes cause a susceptibility to epilepsy is by no means simple, and a variety of complex mechanisms were discovered. It is perhaps partly this complexity and its intellectual challenge that has contributed to the medical enthusiasm for epilepsy genetics which by 2020 was not dissimilar to that for heredity in the early twentieth century – and, perhaps more worrying, with

---

[25] Disproved by the Hardy-Weinberg principle, enunciated in 1908 but ignored by most eugenicists.

a similar level of hyperbole. Exaggerated claims about new genetic discoveries in epilepsy flooded the medical and lay press, and continue to do so. While it is clear that, as is the case in all human characteristics, epilepsy will have genetic influences, it is only in a relatively few cases – perhaps 5% of the total – that a genetic variant has to date been found to be a 'predominant cause'; and these are mainly (but not exclusively) in epilepsies developing in the neonatal or early childhood years. This should not be surprising as a genetic variant with a marked tendency to cause epilepsy would have been subject to strong negative selection pressures.

In my view, and contrary to current ILAE policy, it would be far better to restrict the term 'genetic epilepsy' to those few cases in which there are strong genetic influences – the majority being the monogenic disorders of early childhood – and not to conditions where the genetic influence may be only slight.

Does the label 'genetic' still matter? It may well do. In the shadow of history, 'eugenics' has become a highly disparaged term, but many practices of contemporary genetic science, for instance gene editing, prenatal diagnosis, pre-implantation selection, have the same objectives – to improve the human condition, 'cleanse the germ plasm' and to produce healthy offspring. One important difference today is that the individual has the freedom to choose whether or not to engage with such practices (albeit within legal frameworks) and these are not decisions delegated to others to make. However, soft coercion by medical and social agencies is common.

The politics of genetics in the early twentieth and early twenty-first centuries share certain striking similarities: a contradictory attitude to the disabled; the power of doctors, through their specialised knowledge, to decide how genetics is incorporated into clinical decisions; the idea that scientific and technical knowledge is 'neutral'; and the idea that the accruing of scientific knowledge is progress.[26] These issues are all ethically and philosophically complex. However, in the real world, casual decisions which take into account none of these niceties are commonplace, and is not difficult to see how eugenic measures might be extended further in the future. Indeed, in some countries compulsory measures have already been instituted. An example is China's 1994 Eugenic and Health Protection Law, a name changed in short order to the Maternal and Infant Health Care Law and passed into legislation in 1995. In Singapore, the government organised dating parties for high achievers in the misconstrued hope that they might marry and have high achieving offspring.

The current lazy and fashionable emphasis on genetics in epilepsy has developed with little debate or nuance. This situation is wholly unsatisfactory. Science is not morally neutral, and scientists and clinicians have a weighty

---

[26] Kerr and Shakespeare, *Genetic Politics*.

responsibility in this area – a fact worthy of emphasis as practice becomes more and more scientific, and increasingly oriented towards the disease not the individual with the disease.

Another regrettable aspect has been the tendency to hyperbole. The journalist David Dobbs has published an analysis of the hyperbole around the topic of medical genetics, pointing out that in 2000, Francis Collins, the leader of the Human Genome Project, predicted that the genomic revolution could reduce cancer to zero and would make gene-tailored personalised medicine common by 2010.[27] This resulted in the expenditure of billions of dollars but, as Dobbs put it, the genetics of most common conditions are infected by MAGOTS (many assorted genes of tiny significance), resulting in the identification of 'a mass of barely significant genes explaining little'. The same MAGOTs are found in the epilepsy world, and perhaps if similar amounts of research money, time and talent had been spent on the environmental or developmental determinants of epilepsy, advances of greater practical utility might have been made.

The keeping of a balanced perspective is vital in all medical affairs, but in genetics this is especially so. Perhaps I am wrong, and perhaps the pathogenesis and aetiology of epilepsy will become widely explicable in genetic terms and treatment widely tailored to an individual's genetic make-up – but I feel this is unlikely. Whatever else, the power of the new genetic science must not be allowed to dilute or distort societal values or ethics – for epilepsy is, and has always been, uniquely vulnerable to this danger.

Drug Treatment of Epilepsy

The third of Walshe's age-old burning issues was treatment – and of all the neurological conditions, epilepsy has been the one in which drug treatment has been most available throughout the long twentieth century; treatment has occupied a central place in the medicine of epilepsy in a way which hardly applied to any other neurological condition for most of the period.

The key transition in the early years was from herbals to manufactured chemicals. The paradigmatic example was that of bromide. This compound, found by chance on the basis that damping down sexual excitement could reduce hysterical seizures, proved to be by far the most effective drug remedy for epilepsy discovered up until then, and was soon rapidly disseminated around the world. Other medicaments, largely herbals, were available, but most had minimal pharmacological effect and after millennia of usage herbals faded away, becoming historical footnotes by the mid-twentieth century. As

[27] Dobbs, 'What is your DNA worth?'

William Lennox had written of treatment prior to bromide, perhaps with only slight exaggeration, 'it is doubtful whether the epileptic who consulted the faculty members of the medical department of Harvard University was better off than the one who appealed to Hippocrates'.[28] Although an improvement (on nothing!), bromides were only partially efficacious and also burdened with side effects. They were far from a perfect solution.

In 1912, the serendipitous discovery of the antiepileptic effects of phenobarbitone transformed therapy again, as did that of phenytoin in the 1940s and then a clutch of drugs – notably carbamazepine, valproate and benzodiazepines – in the 1960s. Around the same time, technologies for measuring the blood level of drugs in the body were introduced which proved a boon to more rational drug use. As a result, in the 1970s and 1980s, monotherapy with antiepileptic drugs became the standard. By then, the general principles of the approach to the treatment of epilepsy had assumed the form which continued to apply right up to 2020. The number of drugs licensed for use in clinical practice also began to increase, and by 2020 there were at least fifteen first- or second-line antiepileptic drugs widely available throughout the world, as well as a range of more esoteric compounds.

Pharmaceuticals increasingly dominated in the arena of epilepsy therapy in the post-World War two period, and this was a radical change. The emphasis on hygienic measures which had remained central right up to the 1940s was then relegated to only brief mention in any of the leading textbooks. The Western pharmaceutical model of treatment had achieved complete hegemony by 2020. Whether this was a good or bad thing in overall terms was difficult to say. There remain a significant number of patients in whom drugs fail to control seizures, and others burdened with side effects. Patients in western countries frequently felt dissatisfied enough to seek the help of alternative practitioners, and in developing countries many patients continued to have more faith in traditional healers.

Many factors were responsible for the dominance of drug treatment in epilepsy in the post war years. First, the basic sciences of neurochemistry and of pharmaceutical medicine had made tremendous advances: for instance, in the development of effective methods of laboratory identification and differentiation of potential antiepileptics, and in elucidating the nature of neural transmission, the molecular biology of epilepsy and the mechanisms of action of drugs. By 2020, the new molecular knowledge was being translated into novel therapies aimed at modifying a range of molecular targets. Second, the clinical testing of drugs had become much more rigorous, notably with the introduction of the randomised controlled trial (RCT; the first usage in epilepsy being in 1975). These developments put treatment in the clinic on a much firmer

---

[28] Lennox, *Epilepsy and Related Disorders*, pp. 31–2.

scientific footing. Third, the potential for commercial exploitation and profit contributed to the extraordinary rise in the power of the pharmaceutical industry, with marketing playing a central role. In the vortex of more rigorous and scientific medicine and aggressive commercialisation, holistic approaches and attention to lifestyle issues largely disappeared from mainstream epileptology. The pharmaceutical industry has been accused of creating diseases ('disease mongering') so that it can sell its drugs to treat the disease, especially in the field of mental disorder. Whether this has happened in epilepsy is a moot point, but certainly there have been a plethora of new syndromes and new classifications of seizures which have increased the range of drug indications, and the size of the pharmaceutical market in epilepsy seems to increase year on year.

As drugs became more powerful, so did the regulatory hurdles to be overcome; partly as a result of this, the cost of development of drugs has risen sharply, as has the time taken to bring a new compound to market. Some argue against the regulatory hurdles, saying they inhibit innovation. Furthermore, the increased regulation has not entirely prevented the licensing of dangerous drugs. Even after 1990, at least three antiepileptics introduced into clinical practice had to be rapidly withdrawn due to the development of toxic effects not detected prior to licensing. Regulation has meant, however, that huge investment is now required to develop a new drug and only the largest and richest companies are in a position to deliver drugs to the clinic. In the pre-regulation days, such compounds as phenytoin and phenobarbitone were introduced into clinical practice after only a short period of evaluation and at minimal cost, to the great benefit of millions of people with epilepsy (albeit with many suffering side effects). Weighing the benefits of such stringent regulation against the disadvantages in terms of cost and time is a political choice. Common sense is needed to strike the correct balance – and how this is struck is a matter of public opinion and policy. Whether the whole regulatory framework is now in need of radical correction is an arguable point.

The obvious question to be resolved before the value of medicinal therapy can be properly assessed is the extent to which treatment with new drugs does improve the prognosis of epilepsy or the quality of life of those with the condition. Surprisingly, this question remains largely unanswered. There is surely no doubt that the introduction of phenobarbital, phenytoin, carbamazepine, valproate and benzodiazepines did have a significant impact in stopping seizures, but none of the subsequent drug therapies had been shown to be strikingly more efficacious than these older drugs. Different individuals respond differently to different drugs, and, consequently, the greater the range, the more likely seizure control is to be achieved or side effects avoided; but the extent of the improvement in population terms has not been established. One influential set of studies suggested that if two drugs did not control seizures, then no others will – but this is palpably false as many persons achieve full control of their epilepsy once the correct drug at the appropriate dose is arrived at. Furthermore, even partial control can make a huge difference to the life of those with epilepsy. Nevertheless, even by 2020, drugs fail to control seizures to an appropriate level in 10–30% of all persons developing epilepsy. These are the persons with epilepsy who are in the greatest need – and it is for these 'drug-resistant' patients that new therapies are urgently needed.

By 2020, two other unsatisfactory aspects of treatment should be highlighted. First, and regrettably, in many countries a huge *epilepsy treatment gap* remains. In the developing world, the gap has only slightly narrowed since the first descriptions in the 1980s, and this despite the heavy focus of public health campaigns. Cost remains a crucial factor, but it is not the only reason. Inadequacies, inefficiencies and corruption in drug distribution, as well as the power of traditional beliefs, also play a part. Much could be improved and practical and logistical hurdles which impede progress could be easily overcome. The other disappointing area in the field of epilepsy therapeutics has been the lack of impact of pharmacogenomics (sometimes labelled 'personalised medicine' – a triumph of marketing hyperbole). This is the idea that specific genetic variants underlie drug response, and thus that therapy can be tailored according to a person's genetic make-up. However, no such variants have been identified which predict the response to treatment in any of the common epilepsies, and to date this is a research area in which enormous resources have been wasted.[29] The postulation that drug resistance is uniquely genetically determined is overly simplistic, as many non-genetic factors have an obvious influence on the effectiveness of drug treatment.[30] The head of research at Glaxo informed British neurologists in 2000 that 'pharmacogenomics in epilepsy will be widely practiced within 5 years', but sadly this has turned out to be very widely off the mark.[31]

Specialist and subspecialist care undoubtedly have led to a more scientific approach to drug treatment, and the seismic shift to specialisation in epilepsy medicine has been beneficial to many patients. There are some downsides, not least the frequent public complaint that the broader aspects of therapy have been undermined. Certainly, in the past there was a much

---

[29] Not least due to misleading publicity and hyperbole about its 'promise'.

[30] These include the aetiology of the epilepsy, the position in the brain of the epileptic focus, its size and severity, lifestyle factors such as stress and alcohol, liver enzyme induction and even drug dose.

[31] A few minor pharmacogenomic discoveries have been made, for instance the higher incidence of rash due to carbamazepine in persons with certain HLA (human leukocyte antigen) types. The effect is slight, and the relevance of even this effect depends on the population studied. In a few rare forms of epilepsy, some treatment specificity has been demonstrated, but to date pharmacogenomics has had no major impact in the field of epilepsy.

greater emphasis on such aspects as lifestyle, psychical aspects, diet and occupation than now, and by 2020 a commonly voiced accusation was that epilepsy medicine was too focused on the study of the disease and not the individual, treating the patient more as a physiological study than as someone in distress. Whilst no sensible person would exchange the therapy of 1860 or of 1950 for that of 2020, it remains a concern that many patients in 2020 find pharmacological medicine impersonal and inflexible and yearn for more holistic and personalised measures. Novels, memoirs and movies in recent times have repeatedly highlighted the imperfections of technological medicine, and have been critical of its attitudes and concepts, and of some of its practitioners. The writer Kurt Eichenwald considered that the quality most needed in a physician was humility and the good grace to say 'I don't know', but humility too has been seldom forthcoming.[32]

Surgical Treatment of Epilepsy

In the 1860s, whilst brain areas were being mapped by amongst others his colleague David Ferrier, Hughlings Jackson formulated his famous postulation that epileptic seizures were the result of an excessive discharge of brain cells in a localised area of the cerebral cortex – the epileptic 'focus' ('bastard cells', as he colourfully named them). He pointed out that the symptoms of the seizure indicated the part of the brain in which the focus was located.[33] This was indeed one of the greatest paradigm shifts in epilepsy theory (perhaps the greatest) in the whole long twentieth century, and it led directly to epilepsy surgery. In 1886, the first cutting out ('resection') of brain tissue to remove the area of the brain containing the 'discharging lesion' was undertaken, based on clinical localisation, and was a success. After this, similar attempts at epilepsy surgery were carried out in a variety of centres. But, by 1900 enthusiasm had diminished as the risks of surgery and its only modest long-term effects on epilepsy became apparent.

In the interwar years, influenced by military necessity, emphasis switched to surgery for post-traumatic epilepsy. Then after 1960, civilian resective surgical treatment was revitalised by the introduction first of EEG and later by MRI. Both provided additional ways of predicting the location of the discharging lesion. Linked to this, and to advances in surgical technique and equipment (for instance, the operating microscope) and more effective antibiotics and anaesthesia, the potential for epilepsy surgery was again re-examined. A small coterie of surgeons, often trained in one of a handful of bigger centres, introduced epilepsy surgery to many countries in the world, but the numbers of operated cases remained quite small. In 1986, a landmark conference was

---

[32] Eichenwald, 'A mind unraveled.'   [33] Jackson, 'A suggestion for the treatment of epilepsy'.

held in Palm Desert, California. It was estimated there that, up until then, around 3,000 surgeries had been carried out in 47 centres worldwide. A plea was made for more activity and the second conference reported that in the intervening 5 years, more than 8,000 surgeries had been performed in 113 centres. The ILAE heavily promoted epilepsy surgery, and it became a fashionable and much vaunted topic.

By 2020, interest had also grown in non-resective methods interfering with the physiology of epileptic seizures. The most common non-resective surgical procedure was not 'brain surgery' at all, but vagal nerve stimulation, which by 2020 had been performed in more than 125,000 persons. Although a simple and safe operation, its effects proved modest. Whether this was more effective than cervical sympathectomy and other non-cerebral operations performed in the past is unknown, and in the author's view it was probably not, but its success was no doubt aided by the skilfull promotion of the manufacturers of the stimulator device. Other forms of brain stimulation were being developed by 2020, involving implanted electrodes in a range of targets including the cerebellum, caudate nucleus, centromedian nucleus of the thalamus, anterior thalamus, subthalamic nuclei and hippocampus, and also 'responsive' stimulation into neocortical seizure foci (i.e. stimulation that was triggered by a developing seizure recorded by implanted electrodes). Of these, only anterior thalamic and responsive stimulation were robustly shown to have positive effects on seizures, and even then benefit was often uncertain.

By 2020, epilepsy surgery was still offered to relatively few persons, and despite encouragement from many epilepsy specialists, there remained a general reluctance amongst a sizeable number of neurologists to recommend surgery even to patients whose epilepsy remained wholly uncontrolled on drug therapy. This was probably because the long-term results were often disappointing (even in the most favourable cases of temporal lobe epilepsy, only around 60% of patients achieve long-term seizure freedom after temporal lobectomy), the side effects of brain resection were potentially severe and because of a well-founded suspicion of over-promotion.

There remain four other more general reservations. First, is the objection that in many patients with focal epilepsy, the idea that there is a well-localised 'seizure focus' may be an illusion. As experimental results since at least the 1970s had shown, so-called focal epileptic seizures often depend on large, widely distributed systems, rendering the idea of a discrete, small focus of limited validity.[34] This was true both for neocortical seizures, especially from the frontal lobe, and also for limbic seizures, and may be why surgery fails to

---

[34] Indeed, Gastaut in the 1906s realised this and named such seizures as 'partial' not 'focal' seizures.

control seizures in many patients. Even where surgery is effective, this could be because, rather than removing a discrete focus, the operation degrades, desynchronises or disconnects the epileptic network. If this is the case, then the increasingly complex and elaborate methods to refine localisation are hardly logical, and Rasmussen's view that the bigger the resection, the better is the outcome, makes more therapeutic sense.

A second and related criticism is that the assessment of patients for surgery is, to a significant degree, based on empiricism dressed up as technology. The idea has arisen that outcome is best when there is concordance of findings from diverse tests – having 'all the ducks lined up', as it is often put. Epilepsy, though, is not a shooting gallery and this is an intellectually lazy concept. Despite this, in the last decades of the twentieth century ever more complex and lucrative methods of assessment were being implemented – for instance, with chronic invasive EEG and computerised correlation of EEG and imaging data – resulting in an increasingly phrenological approach to epilepsy which is surely wrong. The question of whether such high-technology assessment has added value or cost effectiveness over less complex methods of assessment, in terms of the surgical outcome, has remained an unanswered question, as no proper independent health technology assessment has ever been made. This is a grievous omission.

Thirdly, is the reservation that the potentially negative effects of removing brain tissue have been only very poorly evaluated. The major side effects – death, hemiplegia, severe memory disturbance – are well studied, but a host of more subtle effects on personality and behaviour are far less understood. A standard temporal lobectomy, for instance, removes about 15% of an individual's cortical brain tissue and it is clear that this can have subtle (and sometimes less subtle) effects. Furthermore, the risk of late effects, such as intellectual deterioration due to the reduction in cerebral reserve caused by large resections, is also completely unknown. There have been numerous case reports of psychological and behavioural deficits following epilepsy surgery which have not been systematically studied. Proponents of epilepsy surgery have always been keen to avoid its designation as psychosurgery, but there is no doubt that psychological deficits can be a consequence (as in many types of neurosurgery). Despite the long history of surgery, these aspects remain largely under-studied and unresolved.

Finally, when it comes to epilepsy surgery, there is another elephant in the capitalistic room: the potential for income and profit to interfere with medical judgment. In the free-market system, the financial underpinning of epilepsy surgery has come to have a significant influence in its medical promotion. Expensive epilepsy surgical units had been established in many hospitals world-wide and are a large investment with potentially large financial returns to hospitals and surgeons. The claims made for resective surgery have been propagandist in tone, and a strangely macho culture has arisen amongst some surgical centres, which vie each with the other to claim they have 'operated on more patients'. The extent to which the marketing effort has influenced the processes involved in presurgical assessment and obscured some of its problems is not clear; but it has certainly prevented a truly objective evaluation.

Despite all, it should also be emphasised epilepsy surgery can be strikingly effective – and for some individuals can provide the only path out of intractable epilepsy and all the baggage carried with it. There are many patients who are forever indebted to the skill of the surgeon and investigatory teams, and in many cases the benefits have greatly outweighed any side-effects. As has been the case with psychosurgery, separating the wheat and the chaff, the benefits and the drawbacks for any individual patient is difficult. Like all treatment, the skill of the physician and surgeon is in drawing a balance between benefit and risk, but the risks and side effects of surgery are irreversible (unlike those of drug therapy) and so the balance is even more difficult to adjudicate upon; underlying all is the nagging thought that there must be a better way of controlling epilepsy than by cutting out or damaging bits of the human brain.

The Harm Caused by Medicine

This brings us to the question of harm. The Hippocratic oath dictates that above all, doctors should 'first, do no harm' (primum non nocere) but it is clear that, throughout the long twentieth century, many patients have been harmed irrevocably by the medical interventions they were subjected to. Examples are numerous and include eugenic actions; institutionalisation; involuntary sterilisation; surgical procedures to control autointoxication; actions taken on other misguided theories of cause, including psychoanalysis and reflex theories; brain operations based on false ideas of localisation which failed or damaged memory or personality; and drug side effects (see Appendices 1 and 2).

Harm has been inflicted by physicians, surgeons, psychiatrists and psychologists, and other practitioners, and a whole variety of so-called medical advances have injured individuals, sometimes gravely. In the early years of the modern era of epilepsy, there was little regulation of medical action and how many suffered as a result cannot be known, but I suspect that some ill effects were experienced by the great majority. Whether the benefits of medicine in those days outweighed the negative effects for the generality of patients is uncertain. But if there were overall benefits, they must on balance have been rather slight. Furthermore, few if any mechanisms existed for patients to complain, seek recourse or even express their views.

In the post-war years the issue of benefit versus risk rose rapidly up the public agenda. Although the manifest advances of medicine were widely and rightly praised, a sense of suspicion and unease developed. Society responded by becoming increasingly directive from the 1960s onwards. In the pharmaceutical arena as described earlier, the regulatory environment became much more restrictive, and this may well have prevented unforeseen dangers, although it also rendered the cost of drug development much higher and the drug approval process much longer.

Perhaps more important has been a change in attitude to litigation which reflects a growing mistrust of medicine. Litigation gives patients (in most Western countries at least) more opportunity to obtain financial damages for medical harm than was common in the past, and has moved the cost of mismanagement from patient to provider, which in countries with public health services means the taxpayer. There has been a dramatic increase in litigation in the last few decades, and whether the huge cost has been beneficial to the generality of the population is arguable – the only invariable beneficiaries of these bitter actions have been the swelling wallets of lawyers.

In most cases, the harm inflicted by medicine was not intentional. Doctors had usually acted in accord with current thinking and because the nature and extent of damage becomes clarified usually only through the lens of history. For the same reason, it is highly unlikely that some of today's practices will be judged unblemished in future generations. This is the warning of history. Candidates for future censure could be the extrapolation of genetic findings, of drug side effects, of invasive investigations (notably stereo EEG), of ill-advised surgery and, perhaps overriding all, the focus on medicalisation of a condition in which the societal impact is as important as the medical.

THE PERSON WITH EPILEPSY: THE INSIDER'S VIEW

Accruing knowledge of epilepsy has not always been a cause for celebration 'for in much wisdom is grief: and he that increaseth knowledge increaseth sorrow' (Ecclesiastes 1:18). There has indeed been wisdom, sorrow and grief, and this brings us to what is surely the most important perspective on epilepsy: that of the insider, the person with epilepsy. Of course, there is no single or uniform emotional response to the experience of epilepsy, and, in the final analysis, no universally valid explanatory model can describe what is essentially personal, entangled and chimerical.[35]

Furthermore, few first-person accounts of what it felt like to have epilepsy exist before the later decades of the century, and so in this book much reliance has

---

[35] There is an inherent impossibility of knowing another's experience, as famously explored, for instance, by Nagel, 'What is it like to be a bat?'. But as Sherlock Holmes also noted: 'While the individual man is an insoluble puzzle, in the aggregate he becomes a mathematical certainty' (Doyle, *Sign of the Four*, p. 196).

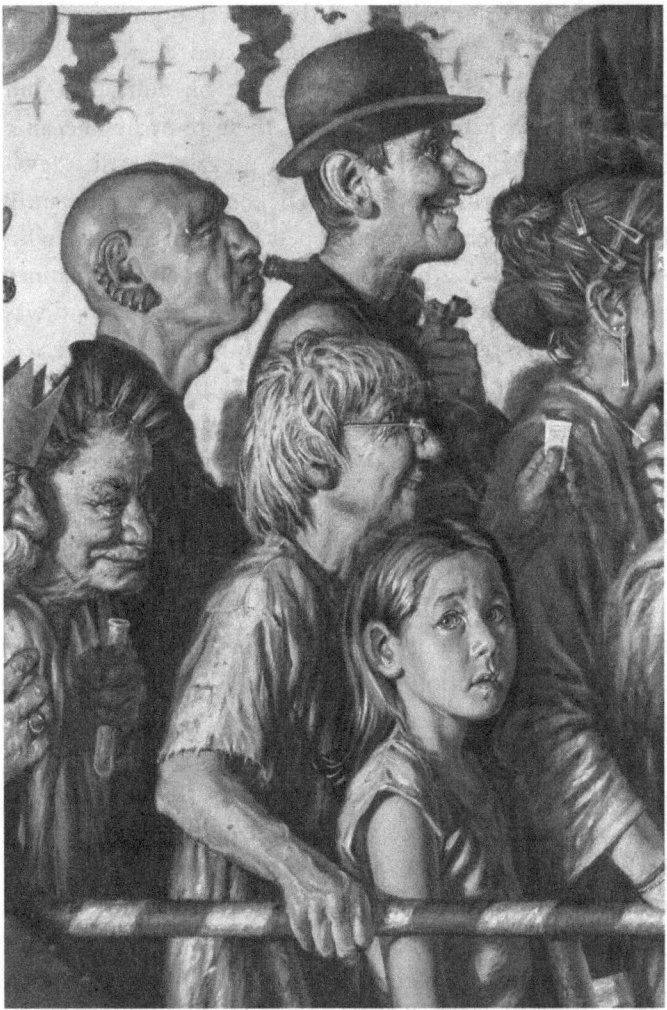

45. 'Bandwagon to Oblivion'. A detail of a painting by David Cobley when he was artist in residence at the Chalfont Centre for Epilepsy in 1992. It represents the uncertainty of life.

had to be placed not only on memoirs but also medical texts, creative literature and film. These can act only as surrogates for exploring the changing epilepsy experience, but do help flesh out its reality and its symbolism. A kaleidoscopic picture is painted, but certain common themes emerge. Only generalisations can be made but what is abundantly clear is that striking changes did occur as the century progressed.

The Doctor–Patient Relationship

One aspect of this experience is encapsulated in the doctor–patient relationship. In the late nineteenth century, the status of doctors rose rapidly, in part due to the regulation of medicine and medical training, which cemented the differentiation of doctors from quacks and charlatans, and the industrialisation of society, which put a premium on education and science. The power of doctors also increased as their remedies became more efficacious, and the ridicule which had been prevalent earlier (evidenced, for instance, in the works of Charles Dickens) was significantly reduced. This rubbed off on specialists and especially neurologists, who increasingly in those years adopted a patrician and condescending manner and a patronising stance. Doctors gave instructions and the patient was expected to follow these without query or explanation. This was a period when medicine was doctor- and disease-centred, and the stereotype of a neurologist, in particular, was of a man (there were no female neurologists then) intellectually superior but cold and arrogant. These postures reflected the gap in knowledge between the doctor, who tended to obscure facts in technical jargon, and the patient, to whom disease was mysterious and whose knowledge of physiology and pathology was generally negligible. There was thus an intensely unequal power relationship which encouraged a style of behaviour among doctors that today would be considered abusive and intimidating.

In the post-war years, these attitudes began to change. This was partly because science had become a fundamental feature of the school curriculum and the population as a whole had become much better informed about medicine. The process accelerated at the end of the century, and by 2020 the gap in knowledge between physician and patient, at least in the advanced economies, had narrowed considerably. Furthermore, in the commercialised culture of the late twentieth century, the power of the consumer (the patient) rose and the patient perceived there to be 'rights' where previously there were just privileges. The demeanour of epilepsy doctors had changed palpably, as reflected in their writings on epilepsy, which showed more respect, less prejudice and more compassion. Empathy and communication skills even entered into the curriculum at medical school and indeed were given much more teaching time than was epilepsy itself. Nevertheless, as Schneider and Conrad's interviewees demonstrated in 1983, attitudes to doctors were still at the time 'on balance ambivalent'.[36]

By 2020, in most Western countries the relationship between doctor and patient had evolved to be seen as a partnership in which the doctor advised on options for treatment and the patient made the choice. The primary responsibility of the doctor was to provide information and to

[36] Schneider and Conrad, *Having Epilepsy*, p. 211.

seek informed consent – changes that became enshrined in law. The prior idea that physicians could withhold information if they believed it was not material or not in the patient's 'best interest' was replaced by the legally enforceable requirement to give all accurate and relevant information. Thus, the societal pressure for a patient-centric consultation became cemented in legislation.[37] This was a trend in medicine in general, and epilepsy was in the vanguard in view of its chronic and multifaceted nature.

'Being Epileptic' – What it Feels Like to Have Epilepsy

Most patients are less concerned with epilepsy as a biological phenomenon of disease – the preoccupation of medicine, industry and science – than with epilepsy as an illness – in other words, how the experience of epilepsy is 'felt'. To many, it is the fact of *being epileptic* (having the illness) which matters far more than just having seizures. A seizure is usually short lived, often infrequent and the non-convulsive variants are sometimes (but obviously not always) slight in their manifestations. Yet being epileptic has a continuous impact on, for instance, social interactions, social relationships, marriage, domestic life, driving, education and employment; seizures may be brief and transient, but the impact of *being epileptic* is long-lasting and continuous. The consequences depend not only on the external attitudes of others, but also on internal factors such as personality, life experience, identity, self-esteem, self-confidence, affect and over-dependency. This is a complex brew. To the person with epilepsy, the medical and scientific aspects may simply be irrelevant; to the doctor, the experiential aspects are hardly comprehended.

At the centre of the patient experience has been the issue of stigma. This was probably always the case throughout this period of history, but the impact of the label 'epileptic' has greatly varied. In the nineteenth century, epilepsy

---

[37] In British common law (and in many countries in the common-law jurisdiction) this change was enshrined in litigation law. From 1957, a doctor was said to have acted appropriately if the information he provided was deemed acceptable and sufficient by other competent doctors (the so-called Bolam test, a case in which the complaint had been made that the side effects of electroconvulsive therapy had not been explained). There was no obligation to provide patients with unsolicited information about risks if the doctor believed that such information could have a detrimental effect on the patients or have deterred them from undergoing the treatment that the doctor believed was in their best interest. This changed in 2014 when consent to treatment was said to be sufficient only if the patient has enough information to make a well-thought-out decision (including the benefits and risks, even if the risk itself is very small, and the risks and benefits of not having the treatment – the so-called Montgomery test (based on Montgomery v. the Lanarkshire Health Board in the UK, and Rogers v. Whitaker in Australia ('Rogers v. Whitaker').

was considered a mental disorder, associated with cerebral degeneration, madness and dementia. Seizures were seen as a sign of this degeneration (as Edward Sieveking had written: 'We should regard the fit as the flower of a noxious weed'[38]). Epilepsy was associated with violence, criminality, amorality and perversity, and its sufferers were shunned and held in contempt. It was furthermore considered to be largely inherited and the reproduction of people with epilepsy was thought potentially to weaken the genetic health of a population. These concepts were slow to die, and persisted in some form or other well into the twentieth century. By then, a more materialistic and agnostic attitude seemed to prevail, and eugenic solutions were increasingly proposed and enacted. Hostility was commonplace, and from the extreme perspective of racial hygiene those with epilepsy were even considered subhuman. Not surprisingly, the almost universal reaction of individuals with epilepsy, and their families, was to deny or conceal the condition. Epilepsy in those days lurked in the shadows and was seldom voluntarily disclosed. This damaged the sense of existential being, self-confidence and self-esteem, and increased feelings of rejection and isolation. As a sign of this, there were almost no published first-person writings or memoirs concerning the experience of epilepsy.

The experience of the Second World War changed social perceptions, and also the experience of those with epilepsy. In the new social and political environment, stigma progressively lessened, and by 2020, although still present, was certainly much less intense, at least in Western countries. By then, laws had been put in place to prevent discrimination, and expressing stigmatising attitudes or behaviour became frankly illegal. Similarly, lobbying by patient organisations such as the IBE, and open discussion of the issues, not least by those suffering from epilepsy, led to significant shifts in self-esteem and feelings of self-worth. Surveys showed a progressively more tolerant attitude amongst the public. Slowly the condition was emerging from the shadows. This is not to say that stigma had disappeared entirely by 2020, and sadly many people with epilepsy still laboured under the burden of the disease. Although enacted stigma was certainly less evident, the felt stigma and the self-stigma of epilepsy proved harder nuts to crack.

The experience of having epilepsy, and of its stigma, became the subject of academic sociological study in the 1970s and 1980s, focusing on public education and legislation and changing the public discourse about epilepsy, and a better understanding of these issues developed. It also became clear that in some countries of the world, where political regimes have been more authoritarian, less progress had been made.

---

[38] Sieveking, *On epilepsy*, p. 10 (2nd ed, p. 12).

Stigma of course is a societal creation, the parameters of which are set mostly by mutable social and political norms, and should not be considered inevitable. But the extent of felt stigma due to epilepsy has also depended on internal factors. Because of epilepsy, a person had always needed greater strength of character and greater fortitude to enter social space. Not all had managed this, but many did. And by 2020, for a large number of people with epilepsy, self-respect and dignity had been restored, and a quality of life equal to that of non-epileptic peers had become possible.

Reflecting the more open and accepting public mood, one of the most striking features of epilepsy in the last decades of this history has been the willingness of people to declare and discuss their epilepsy in a manner which could not have occurred in earlier years. For the first time, memoirs had been written detailing personal experiences of epilepsy, and films and books produced with epilepsy as a central theme. These provide a richer, more detailed and more nuanced picture of epilepsy than ever before, and the thoughts and experiences of those with epilepsy were explored in more depth and with more subtlety. The advent of social media also, in the last decade, provided an easy and accessible method of expression. The true emotional and personal impact of epilepsy had in the last decades of the twentieth and early decades of the twenty-first centuries been exposed to an unprecedented degree, as individuals openly explored their personal experiences, and the wider effects and symbolism of epilepsy.

I would argue that the reduction in prejudice and stigma achieved at the end of the long twentieth century, the new openness about epilepsy, the more accepting public attitudes and the alleviation of many of the discriminatory features of being epileptic have been the *most significant and beneficial developments in the lives of people with epilepsy* and in many ways of *greater importance than any scientific or medical advances*. This is an achievement to be celebrated, but is a transformation not yet by any means complete. Altering deep-rooted social and personal attitude is a long-drawn-out process.

THE END OF EPILEPSY?

In 1945 (and in the 1971 second edition), Owsei Temkin entitled the final section of his history of epilepsy, which reached up to the time of Hughlings Jackson, 'The end of the falling sickness?'[39] It is an intriguing and enigmatic thought, and I would like to conclude this book by addressing his question – and by considering whether we are, or could or should be, witnessing the end of epilepsy.

---

[39] Dieter Schmidt and I published a short book using Temkin's title, musing on the evolution of modern epilepsy (Schimdt and Shorvon, *End of Epilepsy*).

The prologue of this book is a brief discourse on the changing meaning of the disease 'epilepsy' as the twentieth century evolved, and ends with the suggestion that now perhaps epilepsy should not be considered to be a disease at all. This is not simply a dance on the pin-head of semantics; it is an issue which has been in the past of great significance and still matters greatly.

Let us start with definitions. First, consider epilepsy as a disease from the medical perspective. According to the medical model, as outlined in the prologue, a disease is an entity defined by three typical features: (a) a unique grouping of symptoms, signs and clinical contexts; (b) a reasonably well-defined pathogenesis; and (c) a reasonably well-defined aetiology. This medical conceptualisation of 'what a disease is' is now the dominant orthodoxy, in medical and scientific circles at least. Within this model, the emphasis has veered over time from the symptom (the seizure), to the physiology (especially EEG) to the cause; illustrating the difficulty of fitting 'epilepsy' into this medical concept of disease.

Starting first with the 'symptom'. It has often been said the *epileptic seizure* is the symptom and *epilepsy* the disease. This was not the case in the pre-modern period, when no distinction was made and the terms *epileptic seizure* (the 'fit') and *epilepsy* were effectively synonymous; then the symptom was the disease. Around the beginning of our historical period, in 1873, Jackson proposed his famous definition of an epileptic seizure, and stated that a seizure was the manifestation of a sudden discharge of neurons caused by disordered cellular biochemistry (he called this disturbed 'nutrition') and this opened the modern era of epilepsy, He moved the idea of epilepsy away from mere clinical symptoms towards the mechanism of the seizure (or the 'pathophysiology'). Then, with the rise of theories of heredity, in the late nineteenth century, the entity known as *idiopathic epilepsy* came to be known as *genuine* epilepsy, and was considered to be a specific disease-entity because it had a unitary cause and pathophysiology (inherited cerebral degeneration). It thus met all the criteria of a *disease*. Seizures in other conditions, such as brain tumours, were 'symptomatic seizures' and were not part of the disease epilepsy but simply symptoms of other diseases (for instance an underlying tumour). However, as knowledge advanced, and particularly as more causes were uncovered with seizure types and clinical features identical to those of idiopathic epilepsy, and with identical treatment, the illogicality of limiting the term 'epilepsy' to the idiopathic condition became increasingly clear. In parallel, the view grew up that idiopathic epilepsy had an underlying cause but one which had *not yet* been identified, and thus was not in categorical terms any different from any other condition with seizures. As a result, by mid-century, leading figures such as Kinnier Wilson and Cobb were suggesting that the word 'epilepsy' should be replaced by the term *the epilepsies* or discarded altogether. But then came EEG, and this changed the equation again. The disease of epilepsy came to be defined much more by the pathophysiology of seizures. Epilepsy evolved again to be seen as a physiological concept, a *cerebral dysrhythmia*, and included cases whatever their cause. In fact, this emphasis on physiology blurred the distinction between seizures and epilepsy, and that there was some confusion between these concepts can be perhaps inferred from the fact that the ILAE classifications of the epilepsies (in 1981) had the same major subdivisions (partial/generalised and symptomatic/idiopathic) as the 1969 ILAE classifications of seizure type (i.e. of seizures).

After the 1980s, the concept of epilepsy again began to change. The focus turned back to underlying causes, as the application of new technologies of neuroimaging and then later of molecular genetics revealed many hundreds of new pathologies that 'caused' seizures, and at the same time molecular studies demonstrated a huge range of different pathogenic mechanisms – rendering the idea of a unitary condition inadmissible. What made more sense was the concept of the *epileptic syndrome* (introduced in the 1980s) which was defined as specific constellation of symptoms, signs and EEG features, but without a fixed aetiology, and this in effect filled the void between the idea of epilepsy as a symptom (the epileptic seizure) and a disease'.

In the post-war period, the formal definitions of epilepsy[40] have, perhaps in recognition of the inherent ambiguities in the medical conception of epilepsy, avoided any consideration of cause or mechanism and returning to what was in essence the pre-modern conception, defined *'epilepsy'* as an entity characterised by the occurrence of seizures or the 'propensity to have seizures'. This has a circularity of which Escher would have been proud, but is not satisfactory.[41] A lexical confusion has been ignored by successive epilepsy nosologists. It would not matter were it not for the fact that persisting to conceptualise epilepsy in this way sets an illogical framework for scientific discovery and research – the equivalent of framing research on pneumonia by studying the cough.

By 2020, in my view, the many advances in science have stretched the idea that there is a single disease called epilepsy beyond its logical limits. An analogy would be to define headache or cough or anaemia as *a disease* and this of course makes little medical sense. From the medical and scientific perspective, the case

---

[40] For instance in 1973: Gastaut, *WHO Dictionary of Epilepsy*; 2001: Blume et al., 'Glossary of descriptive terminology'; 2005: Fisher et al., *Definitions*.

[41] See Béjoint, *Lexicography of English*, pp. 325–6. This book started with a citation from Pascal, and to end it here is another. Pascal thought circular definitions were "ridiculous: "There are some who go "as far as this absurdity of explaining a word by the word itself. I know some who have defined light in this way: "Light is a luminous movement of luminous bodies"; as if we could hear the words luminary and luminous without that of light'; translated from Pascal, *De l'Esprit géométrique, 1657*, p. 11). I suspect Pascal would have as much fun with 'Epilepsy is the propensity to have epileptic seizures'.

for dropping the term *epilepsy* as a disease seems overwhelming; and, at the same time, recognises that the *epileptic seizure* is a clinical manifestation (i.e. symptom) of a large number of conditions and diseases, with a wide range of pathophysiological mechanisms, a large number of highly diverse clinical features (symptom/sign constellations) and contexts, and a large number of causes (even if in many cases, the cause is not known).

If the medical and scientific advances of the twentieth century have challenged the concept of epilepsy, why has it persisted? The reason is of course neither medical nor scientific but the fact that epilepsy is also an idea laden with social and personal signification, and, from these other perspectives, epilepsy is indeed a disease entity and a valid concept. As Walther Riese described,[42] throughout history there have been many concepts of disease that have little similarity to the medical model. These have included what he called anthropological, stoic, cosmological, historical, Galenic, moral, social, psychologic, biographic and metaphysic conceptions of disease – all of which have been prevalent at one time or another, all of which have some validity, and all have an internal logic.[43] He had a further point –that, in his view, nosography in Western medicine – the process in which the 'nosographer outlines a scheme of classification of diseases' and thus no longer has to deal with the sick individual (p. 87) – was a most precarious step. He considered this to decompose individual life histories into anonymous entities, and he detected, at the time of his writing (1945), a backlash, 'a steadily threatening revival of ontologic views of disease' in which the focus was increasingly turning on to 'diseased individuals calling for help' rather than 'on the disturbed mechanics and dynamics of life-processes' (p. 96). Rivers, whose views were coloured by his experiences in treating shell shock in the Great War, makes a similar point, emphasising the importance of mind and unconscious psychological mechanisms in the production of disease. These elements are currently completely ignored in scientific medicine.[44]

Another aspect of the use of the word epilepsy is its utility as a *shorthand for combining the fact of having epileptic seizures with the consequences of these seizures.* Indeed, the use of the term throughout this book is an example of this. From the societal perspective, cause and pathogenesis are less important than the consequences of the condition and its wider implications. It is a word thus used, for instance, to set standards for employment and driving, or makes its appearance in legal or legislative proceedings, and to determine resource allocation

---

[42] Riese, *Conception of Disease*.

[43] Rivers explored ethnological concepts of disease in his landmark book *Medicine, Magic and Religion* (based in part on his earlier Fitzpatrick lectures of 1915 and 1916). From his work amongst the Melanesian people he showed that the ascribing of causation of disease by science, religion and magic, and the approaches to treatment, share surprising parallels.

[44] Rivers, *Medicine, Magic and Religion*, chp 5 (based on a lecture given in April 1919).

and stimulate political debate.[45] If this were the whole story, then it would seem sensible to retain the term and to recognise that this is simply a 'societal' label. However, it is this very label of epilepsy that has caused stigma and social exclusion and, at times, loss of liberty, involuntary sterilisation and euthanasia – and whilst useful as a shorthand for medical and societal purposes, the linguistic sleight of hand, by which epileptic seizures are turned into the *disease* called epilepsy, has had dire consequences for the sufferer in the scientific age.[46] Many people with epilepsy continue to sag under the weight of this cultural baggage, which has been at times hostile and prejudicial and has led to bitter philippic and extreme action. As a result, for many sufferers (but not all) the consequences of having the disease (*'being epileptic'*) have been far worse than the occurrence of seizures.

Temkin wrote in the Epilogue of his book that 'The ideal history of a disease is a blend of its natural history, as far as it has revealed itself in the past, and its human history, if this term may be used to designate what man knew, thought and did about it' (p. 383, ed. 2). This is of course true, but the incorporation of 'human history', with its complex and sometimes unsavoury nature, has led to the persistence of a term, and an idea, now outmoded from a scientific or medical perspective. Temkin, by entitling his final chapter 'The end of epilepsy', probably recognised this. My interpretation of his meaning is that he was not conveying the idea that epileptic seizures would disappear, since they have existed since the beginning of recorded history, and, like height and weight, are surely very much part of mammalian physiology. Even today, let alone in Temkin's time, with the rapid advances of science, no one seriously considers that seizures can be abolished; this is far too optimistic a hope to be realised in any foreseeable future. It seems more likely that Temkin had believed that, through modernity and societal improvement, the social concept of epilepsy might disappear, and thus cease to be the 'paradigm of the suffering of both body and soul'.[47] And that the cultural ideas inherent in the concept of 'being *epileptic'* might be vanquished. This is a hope that I also feel is feasible and capable of realisation.

Perhaps one step towards achieving this would be for medicine to abolish the term *epilepsy* altogether. Clinicians and scientists could (and should) refer to epileptic seizures, and see these as symptoms of many underlying conditions and physiologies. At the same time, we could and should desist from using the word 'epilepsy' – for if there is no longer a disease called epilepsy, from the medical perspective, why retain the name? The abolition of the term epilepsy from medical discourse would be a first step towards rendering redundant its usage in societal settings. Abolishing the concept of a disease called epilepsy

[45] The change in the ILAE definition of epilepsy in 2005 was in recognition of this.
[46] And this was at the heart of my Indian interlocutor's anger (p.18).
[47] Temkin, *Falling Sickness*, p. 388.

thus might prevent the prejudicial social and personal consequences that *being epileptic* can entail. In my view, it should be possible to look forward to a day when a seizure is treated in the same way as a headache or a cough, and not taken to signify a disease, with its negative archetypes and ancient historical echoes. Although the abolition or reduction of epileptic seizures is of course the ultimate goal of science, the greatest *interim benefit* to a person suffering from seizures would be the abolition of the negative and stigmatising social attitudes that *having epilepsy* or *being epileptic* can still sometimes bring about. This in my view might make a more fundamental difference than anything that medical technologies, markets, industry or finance can currently deliver.

Since the 1970s, campaigns have been launched to avoid the labelling of a person as 'epileptic' but, unfortunately, in my view, this was achieved by substituting the term 'a person with epilepsy' (a 'PWE'). The emphasis on the individual and not the condition (an example of Riese's ontology) is of course absolutely to be celebrated, but the unintended consequence of relabelling a person as a PWE confirms the existence of the disease which is almost as prejudicial. In Eastern cultures, in recent years, the word for epilepsy has attracted much attention because of its linguistic association with madness and disturbed personality states. In Korea, for instance, in 2007 the Korean Epilepsy Association organised an 'Epilepsy Renaming Task-force' which came up with the recommendation of changing the Korean name for epilepsy, *gan-jil* (간질, 癎疾: a crazy, convulsive disease), to a neutral and scientifically explainable name: *noi-jeon-jeung* (뇌전증; 腦電症; cerebroelectric disorder).[48] In Japan, too, it has been pointed out that the word used for epilepsy – *tenkan* – carries connotations of 'to become mad' and to have 'a violent temperament'; moves to rename the condition have been made there, and similarly in Hong Kong, China and Malaysia.[49] In each country, efforts have been made to replace epilepsy by a more neutral and scientific term. This is progressive and enlightened, but I wonder whether reform should be more far-reaching – not just renaming but abandoning the term, and hence the idea the term implies, altogether.

The consequences of abolishing the use of the term epilepsy, and thus of 'having epilepsy' might improve self-esteem and reduce stigma in employment, education and social and personal relationships. It would also directly benefit medicine. The framework of research could more profitably focus on seizures and individuals, which would have the added advantage of making redundant the frequent and largely pointless changes to the 'classification of epilepsy' – perhaps too the International League Against Epilepsy should be renamed.

---

[48] Kim et al., 'Changing name of epilepsy in Korea'.

[49] See Lim et al., 'Name of epilepsy, does it matter?' This article also lists the meaning of the word for epilepsy in various Eastern languages.

Of course, the counter-argument is that there needs to be a term that does indicate that a person is liable to have seizures, and this has utility in many societal settings and legislation, etc. This is a valid justification. Finding an alternative expression that is usable might be difficult, and furthermore some would say it is dishonest to avoid difficult terms. There is force in this argument, but accuracy in the use of words also matters, and is such a term now *really needed?* Many stigmatising phrases have been removed from usage and are now outlawed. And, generally, their removal has improved the lives of those so labelled. I hesitate even to put these words in print, but in the field of learning disability, for instance, the outlawing of the terms 'mental defective', 'mentally handicapped', 'moron', 'spastic', 'idiot', etc., or in psychiatry 'lunatic', 'madman' and so on, has had a manifestly beneficial effect.

Given that it does not exist as a disease, that it carries with it dark and deeply engrained archetypal memories of heredity, mental disease and impairment, and that it confers prejudice and social exclusion, I think the removal of the term 'epilepsy' from public discourse is at least worthy of debate.[50] My personal opinion is that the gain might well outweigh the drawbacks. Much as Temkin had hoped, perhaps at this juncture, the end of epilepsy is possible to envisage. This would indeed be a goal worth achieving.

[50] The introduction of this book closed with a quotation from Robert Burton, and so lets also finish this epilogue with another of his many elegant statements: 'It is an old saying, "A blow with a word strikes deeper than a blow with a sword"; and many men are as much galled with a calumny, a scurrilous [scurrile] and bitter jest, a libel, a pasquil, satire, apologue, epigram, stage-play, or the like, as with any misfortune whatsoever"' (*Anatomy of Melancholy*, part 1, section 2, mem. 4, subsection 4),

APPENDIX 1

'THE EPILEPSY BALANCE SHEET'

APPENDIX 1: *The epilepsy balance sheet*

Some theories and practices that have improved epilepsy in the long twentieth century	Some theories and practices that have harmed epilepsy in the long twentieth century
SCIENCE AND MEDICINE	**SCIENCE AND MEDICINE**
• The adoption of science as the principal explanatory model of epilepsy	• Erroneous scientific theories of pathogenesis
• The elucidation of the physiochemical mechanisms of seizure production	• Erroneous hereditarian theories of degeneration and the neurological diathesis
• The development of diagnostic technologies such as EEG, CT and MRI, and biochemical and genetic technologies	• Eugenics
• Targeted processes of pharmaceutical discovery	• Erroneous psychiatric theories including that of the 'epileptic' personality, the association of epilepsy with criminality, violence, inherent mental handicap, insanity
• The advances in all the basic biomedical fields (pathology, histology, immunology, etc.)	• Psychoanalytical explanations of the nature of epilepsy
• Specialisation in medicine	• Scientifically flawed surgical and medical treatments
• Discovery of many diverse aetiologies	• False belief in objectivity of science
• Improvement in diagnosis	• Wasteful redundancy and poor science
• Effective new drugs	• Fraud
• Improvements in monitoring of therapy	• Hyperbole
• Improvement in surgical techniques	• Medicine as a 'doctor-inspired conspiracy'
• Improvement of the clinical assessment of medical therapies	• Unethical experimentation
• Increased pharmaceutical regulation	• Irrelevance of medicine and science to health
• Identification of syndromes	• Poor assessment of medical and surgical therapies in epilepsy
	• Side-effects of medical and surgical treatment
	• Changing schemes of classification and terminology

(continued)

APPENDIX 1: *(continued)*

Some theories and practices that have improved epilepsy in the long twentieth century	Some theories and practices that have harmed epilepsy in the long twentieth century
	• Surgical assessment based on resecting the epileptic 'focus' in widely distributed epilepsies • Poor understanding of the true impact of treatment advances on epilepsy. • Lack of regulation of surgery and invasive devices
SOCIETY AND THE PERSON WITH EPILEPSY • Liberal democratic policies in health care • Improving societal attitudes • Reduction in stigma • Legislation to protect rights and remove discrimination • Better access to care and treatment • Foundation of professional and lay associations (e.g. ILAE and IBE) • Increased openness/visibility • Increased self-respect/self-esteem • Louder patient voice • Improved communication technologies and access to information • More balanced doctor–patient relationship	**SOCIETY AND THE PERSON WITH EPILEPSY** • Fake news and propaganda • Disproportionate influence of the pharmaceutical industry • Unethical and illegal pharmaceutical marketing practices • Inequalities of care • Treatment gap • The label 'genetic' • Failure to end stigma • Persisting prejudice and inequalities • Abusive use of social media

APPENDIX 2

OBSOLETE OR FAILED THEORIES AND TREATMENTS

Throughout history, theories and therapies have come and gone; some of these are listed here. These are the 'non-enduring' elements of the history of epilepsy (the 'leaves' not the 'trunk'). Some were universally accepted or practised in their time, and there can be no doubt that a similar fate awaits theories and therapies of today.

TABLE A2.1 *Some of the theories of pathogenesis and aetiology of epilepsy, previously widely held but now largely disregarded or dismissed*

- Aberrant sexual practices as a cause of epilepsy
- Acid-base defects as a cause of epilepsy
- Autotoxins and autocytotoxins as a cause of epilepsy
- Bacillus epilepticus and infective theories of causation of epilepsy
- Chemical theories of causation of epilepsy
- Centroencephalic mechanisms of seizures
- Concept of a highly localised epileptic focus
- Consumptive hypoxia as a cause of epilepsy
- Defects in acetylcholine metabolism as a cause of epilepsy
- Defective dentition and dental caries as a cause of epilepsy
- Epilepsy due to cardiac disease
- Epilepsy due to endocrine disease (pituitary, thyroid, parathyroid, adrenals, thymus, generative organs)
- Eugenic theories of propagation and control
- Eyestrain and disorders of extraocular muscles as a cause of epilepsy
- Gastrointestinal disorders (constipation, worms) as a cause of epilepsy
- Histopathological changes in idiopathic epilepsy
- Hormonal theories of causation of epilepsy
- Inherited degeneration as an inherent feature of epilepsy
- Larval epilepsy resulting in behavioural change
- Link of epilepsy with criminality and moral defect
- Link of epilepsy with physical stigmata (including abnormalities of ears, nose, throat, face, digits, bones, etc.)
- Lymphoid, hyperplasia (adenoids, thymus) as a cause of epilepsy
- Masturbation (and sexual excess/perversion/deviance) as a cause of epilepsy
- Menstrual disorders and menstruation as a cause of epilepsy

(continued)

TABLE A2.1 *(continued)*

- Mental deterioration, dementia and amentia in epilepsy
- Neurological diathesis (neurological trait/taint)
- Nutritional theories as a cause of epilepsy
- Peripheral nerve injury as a cause of epilepsy
- Psychoanalytical theories of seizures and the epileptic personality
- Psychosis or insanity as an inherent feature of epilepsy
- Reflex theories as a cause of epilepsy
- Rickets as a cause of epilepsy
- Seizure equivalents as explanation of behavioural changes
- Sensory-limbic hyperconnection theories of personality
- Systemic infection as a cause of epilepsy
- Toxins (including alcohol, lead) as a cause of epilepsy
- Vasoconstriction and other vascular abnormalities as a cause of seizures
- Various genetic theories of causation of epilepsy (including neurological trait, defective germ plasm)

TABLE A2.2 *Drugs used in clinical practice in the long twentieth century but now largely discarded*

Drugs introduced prior to 1914 (a selection only of the more commonly used or recommended)	<ul><li>Animal derivatives such as: cantharides, chloralamide, crotalin, mole, musk.</li><li>Herbals and alkaloids, including: aconite, adonis vernalis, asafoetida, belladonna, bryonia, camphor, cannabis, castor, cimicifuga, cinnamon, conium, cotyledon umbilicus, curare, decandra, digitalis, ergot, *Gelsemium sempervirens*, hydrastin, hyoscyamus (and other solanaceae), indigo, mistletoe, opioids, peppermint, pilocarpine, phytolacca, picrotoxin, santonin, selinum palustre, physostigmine, rue, simulo, strychnine, turpentine, valerian, veratrum viride.</li><li>Metals, metal salts and minerals: bismuth, borax, bromide (many salts), calcium, iron, lithium, mercury iodide, mercury chloride (calomel), sodium bicarbonate, sodium phosphate, zinc and zinc salts.</li><li>Synthetic chemicals: acetanilide, acetophenetidin (phenacetin), ammonia, amylene hydrate, amyl nitrite, antipyrine, beta-naphthol, chloretone, chloral, chloroform glycothymidine, hydrocyanic acid, nitroglycerine, osmic acid, paraldehyde, pepto-mangan, quinoline (chinolin), resorcin, sodium eosinate sodium salicylate, sulphonal, trional, urethane.</li><li>Others: anti-malarials, anti-rheumatics, anti-syphilitics, bowel antiseptics, evacuants, glandular extracts, serum and antiserum.</li></ul>

(continued)

TABLE A2.2 *(continued)*

Drugs introduced 1914–60	• Barbiturates: phenylethyl barbituric acid, phenylethyl malonylurea, methylphenyl barbituric acid, metharbital, methylphenylethyl barbituric acid, methyldiethyl barbituric acid. • Hydantoins: dimethyldithio hydantoin, ethylphenylhydantoin, methyldiphenyl hydantoin (mephenytoin), methyldibromophenylethyl hydantoin, methylphenyl hydantoin, methylphenylethyl hydantoin, sodium phenylthienyl hydantoin. • Oxazolidinediones: allylmethyl oxazolidine dione, dimethylethyl oxazolidine dione, diphenyl oxazolidine dione, ethotoin, trimethyl oxazolidine dione. • Succinimides: methsuximide, methylalphaphenyl succinimide, phensuximide. • Vital dyes: brilliant vital red, methyl blue. • Others: alkaline borotartrates, allylparacetaminophenol, anti-rabies vaccine, beclamide, chlormethiazole, glutamic acid, N-benzyl-β-chloropropionamide, neoprontosil, paraldehyde, phenthenylate, phenylacetylurea (phenacemide).
Drugs introduced 1960–2020	• Albutoin • Deltoin • Eterobarbitone • Felbamate • Progabide • Retigabine • Tiagabine

TABLE A2.3 *Some non-resective surgical operations and procedures used to relieve epilepsy in the long twentieth century but now discarded*

Cranial operations	• Craniotomy alone • Drainage of cerebral cysts • Dural splitting and 'valve' formation • Multiple subpial transection • Stimulation of subcortical targets (fields of Forel, cingulum, thalamic nuclei, subthalamic nuclei, mammillary bodies, etc.) • Subtemporal decompression • Trepanation/trephination
Operations to affect vascular supply	• Arterialisation of the internal jugular vein • Carotid artery occlusion/ligation • Carotid body removal • Carotid sinus denervation • Cervical sympathectomy/cervicothoracic sympathetic ganglionectomy • Vertebral artery occlusion/ligation

(continued)

TABLE A2.3 *(continued)*

Systemic operations and procedures★	• Adenoidectomy • Adrenalectomy • Circumcision, removal of tight prepuce • Clitoridectomy • Colectomy and other bowel resections • Correction of urethral strictures • Hysterectomy • Ocular tenotomise and operations to relieve eye strain and astigmatism • Ovarectomy • Peripheral nerve section • Removal of teeth and treatment of caries • Section of peripheral nerves • Testectomy • Tonsillectomy • Tracheostomy

★ On the basis of such theories as: removing peripheral irritations, disrupting reflex arcs, stopping masturbation and other sexual practices, removing sources of autointoxication

TABLE A2.4 *Some other physical treatments used in the long twentieth century but now largely disregarded or dismissed*

• Blood letting
• Cauterisation
• Cupping
• Drainage of cerebrospinal fluid
• Endocrine therapy
• Enemas
• Fasting
• Galvanism and other electrical treatments
• Hydrotherapy
• Induction of fever or infection
• Leeches
• Organotherapy
• Serotherapy
• Setons/ligatures and other counter-irritation procedures

THE INTERNATIONAL LEAGUE AGAINST EPILEPSY

The International League Against Epilepsy has been the most important professional organisation in the field of epilepsy; here are details of its international and regional congresses, its journal *Epilepsia* and its executive committee membership.

TABLE A3.1 *International and regional Congresses of the International League Against Epilepsy*

Year	Title of the meeting	Location	Country
1909	ILAE Meeting	Budapest	Hungary
1910	ILAE Meeting	Berlin	Germany
1912	ILAE Meeting	Zurich	Switzerland
1913	ILAE Meeting	London	Great Britain
1935	ILAE Meeting	Lingfield	Great Britain
1939	ILAE Meeting	Copenhagen	Denmark
1946	ILAE Meeting	New York	USA
1949	ILAE Meeting	Paris	France
1953	ILAE Meeting	Lisbon	Portugal
1957	ILAE Meeting	Brussels	Belgium
1961	ILAE Meeting	Rome	Italy
1965	ILAE/IBE Meeting	Vienna	Austria
1969	11th ILAE/IBE Congress	New York	USA
1973	12th ILAE/IBE Congress	Barcelona	Spain
1977	13th ILAE Congress/9th IBE Symposium	Amsterdam	Netherlands
1978	10th Epilepsy International Symposium	Vancouver	Canada
1979	11th Epilepsy International Symposium	Florence	Italy
1980	12th Epilepsy International Symposium	Copenhagen	Denmark
1981	13th Epilepsy International Symposium	Kyoto	Japan
1982	14th Epilepsy International Symposium	London	Great Britain
1983	15th Epilepsy International Symposium	Washington	USA
1985	16th Epilepsy International Symposium	Hamburg	Germany
1987	17th Epilepsy International Epilepsy Congress	Jerusalem	Israel
1989	18th Epilepsy International Epilepsy Congress	New Delhi	India
1991	19th Epilepsy International Epilepsy Congress	Rio de Janeiro	Brazil
1993	20th Epilepsy International Epilepsy Congress	Oslo	Norway
1994	1st European Congress on Epileptology	Oporto	Portugal
1995	21st Epilepsy International Epilepsy Congress	Sydney	Australia
1996	2nd European Congress on Epileptology	The Hague	Netherlands
	1st Asian and Oceanian Epilepsy Congress	Seoul	South Korea

(continued)

TABLE A3.1 *(continued)*

Year	Title of the meeting	Location	Country
1997	22nd Epilepsy International Epilepsy Congress	Dublin	Ireland
1998	3rd European Congress on Epileptology	Warsaw	Poland
	2nd Asian and Oceanian Epilepsy Congress	Taipei	Taiwan
1999	23rd Epilepsy International Epilepsy Congress	Prague	Czechoslovakia
2000	4th European Congress on Epileptology	Florence	Italy
	3rd Asian and Oceanian Epilepsy Congress	New Delhi	India
	1st Latin American Epilepsy Congress	Santiago	Chile
2001	24th International Epilepsy Congress	Buenos Aires	Argentina
2002	5th European Congress on Epileptology	Madrid	Spain
	4th Asian and Oceanian Epilepsy Congress	Nagano	Japan
	2nd Latin American Epilepsy Congress	Fos do Iguaçu	Brazil
2003	25th International Epilepsy Congress	Lisbon	Portugal
2004	6th European Congress on Epileptology	Vienna	Austria
	5th Asian and Oceanian Epilepsy Congress	Bangkok	Thailand
	3rd Latin American Epilepsy Congress	Mexico City	Mexico
2005	26th International Epilepsy Congress	Paris	France
2006	7th European Congress on Epileptology	Helsinki	Finland
	6th Asian and Oceanian Epilepsy Congress	Kuala Lumpur	Malaysia
	4th Latin American Epilepsy Congress	Guatemala	Guatemala
	1st North American Epilepsy Congress	San Diego	USA
2007	27th International Epilepsy Congress	Singapore	Singapore
2008	8th European Congress on Epileptology	Berlin	Germany
	7th Asian and Oceanian Epilepsy Congress	Xiamen	China
	5th Latin American Epilepsy Congress	Montevideo	Uruguay
	2nd North American Epilepsy Congress	Seattle	USA
	1st East Mediterranean Epilepsy Congress	Luxor	Egypt
2009	28th International Epilepsy Congress	Budapest	Hungary
2010	9th European Congress on Epileptology	Rhodes	Greece
	8th Asian and Oceanian Epilepsy Congress	Melbourne	Australia
	6th Latin American Epilepsy Congress	Cartegena	Colombia
	3rd North American Congress	San Antonio	USA
	2nd East Mediterranean Epilepsy Congress	Dubai	UAE
2011	29th International Epilepsy Congress	Rome	Italy
2012	10th European Congress of Epileptology	London	Great Britain
	9th Asian and Oceanian Epilepsy Congress	Manila	Philippines
	4th North American Epilepsy Congress	San Diego	USA
	1st African Epilepsy Congress	Nairobi	Kenya
2013	30th International Epilepsy Congress	Montreal	Canada
2014	11th European Congress of Epileptology	Stockholm	Sweden
	10th Asian and Oceanian Epilepsy Congress	Singapore	Singapore
	7th Latin American Epilepsy Congress	Quito	Ecuador
	5th North American Epilepsy Congress	Philadelphia	USA
	3rd East Mediterranean Epilepsy Congress	Dubai	UAE
	2nd African Epilepsy Congress	Cape Town	South Africa
2015	31st International Epilepsy Congress	Istanbul	Turkey

(continued)

TABLE A3.1 *(continued)*

Year	Title of the meeting	Location	Country
2016	12th European Congress of Epileptology	Prague	Czech Republic
	11th Asian and Oceanian Epilepsy Congress	Hong Kong	China
	8th Latin American Epilepsy Congress	Buenos Aires	Brazil
	6th North American Epilepsy Congress	Houston	USA
2017	32nd International Epilepsy Congress	Barcelona	Spain
	4th East Mediterranean Epilepsy Congress	Luxor	Egypt
	3rd African Epilepsy Congress	Dakar	Senegal
2018	13th European Congress of Epileptology	Vienna	Austria
	12th Asian and Oceanian Epilepsy Congress	Bali	Indonesia
	9th Latin American Epilepsy Congress	Cancun	Mexico
	7th North American Epilepsy Congress	New Orleans	USA
2019	33rd International Epilepsy Congress	Bangkok	Thailand
	5th East Mediterranean Epilepsy Congress	Marrakech	Morocco
	4th African Epilepsy Congress	Entebbe	Uganda

Note: The international meetings were in the earlier years were held initially as part of, and then in conjunction with, meetings of other organisations: International Medical Congress (1909 and 1913, International Congress for the Care of the Insane (1910), International Congress for Psychology and Psychotherapy (1912), International Congress of Neurology (1939, 1949, 1953, 1957, 1961,1965, 1973, 1967, 1977), Association for Research in Nervous and Mental Disease (1946), International Congress of Neurology (1949, 1953), the International Congress of Electroencephalography and Clinical Neurophysiology 1949, 1957, 1961,1965, 1967, 1981), the International Congress of Neuropathology (1957), Symposium Neuroradiologicum (1957), World Congress of Neurological Sciences (1969), World Congress of Neurology (1981, 1985). From 1978 the international meetings have been held jointly with the IBE, and between 1978 and 1983 under the auspices of Epilepsy International.

The regional meetings of the Asian and Oceanian, Latin American, Eastern Mediterranean and African regions are held in conjunction with IBE. The European meetings are stand-alone meetings, and the North American meetings are held as part of the meeting of the American Epilepsy Society. In 2020, the congresses were either cancelled or held virtually due to the Covid-19 pandemic.

TABLE A3.2 *The four series of Epilepsia*

Series I	
Volume 1	4 instalments: 1909–10
Volume 2e	4 instalments: 1910–11
Volume 3e	4 instalment issues and Ergänzungsheft (supplement): 1911–12
Volume 4e	4 instalments: 1912–13
Volume 5e	6 instalments: 1914–15
Series II	
Volume I	4 issues: 1937, 1938, 1939, 1940
Volume II	4 issues: 1941, 1942, 1943, 1944
Volume III	4 issues: 1945, 1946, 1947, 1948
Volume IV	2 issues: 1949, 1950

(continued)

TABLE A3.2 *(continued)*

Series I	
Series III	
Volume 1	1952
Volume 2	1953
Volume 3	1954
Volume 4	1955
Series IV	
Volume 1	5 issues: 1959–60
Volume 2–18	4 issues a year: 1961–77 (except for the printing of extra issues in 1972 (6 issues) and 1975 (5 issues))
Volume 19–35	6 issues a year: 1978–94
Volume 36–61	12 issues a year: 1995–2020

Note: *Epilepsia* has had a complicated system of numbering issues and volumes, due to the interruption of publication on three occasions (creating 4 'series') and changes in editorial policy. This has caused considerable confusion, not only to readers but also to libraries and archives.

1st series: The original concept was of a single volume annually, each comprising four quarterly issues. Actually, in six years of its existence, only five volumes were produced. The first issue was undated but was almost certainly published in March 1909, covering the first three months of that year.

2nd series: It was planned to have one volume covering a four-year period, with one issue a year. This scheme was followed between 1937 and 1948, but the last volume (IV) comprised only two issues before publication again ceased.

3rd series: It was intended to publish one volume in a single issue each year. This plan was followed for four years and again publication ceased.

The 4th series: The initial plan was for one volume a year comprising initially four issues each year. The first volume actually occupied two years and contained five issues. In 1978, the journal expanded to six issues a year, and in 1995 there was a further major increase in size with twelve issues a year. The term 'series IV' was dropped in 1974, although the volume numbering (i.e. 1974 = volume 15) was continued (i.e. 2020 = volume 62).

In the late 2010s, the numbering system of the previous series was changed again (for reasons which are obscure). The term 'series' was dropped and the names of the volumes and issues changed retrospectively. Series I was renamed A and the volumes 1–5 were renamed as A1–A5. Similarly, the volumes of series II were renamed B1–B4 and the volumes of series III were renamed volumes C1–4. The volumes of series IV were renamed simply Volume 1–61.

TABLE A3.3 *Members of the ILAE Executive Committee*

1909–1914
Initiators: J. Van Deventer (Amsterdam, Holland); Auguste Marie (Villejuif, France); Gyula Donáth (Budapest, Austrian-Hungarian Empire); Louis Muskens (Amsterdam, Holland)

Provisional Members of the Board 1909
(*German version*) Gyula Donáth, William Graves, Boris Greidenberg, Otto Hebold, Auguste Marie, Ernō Moravcsik, Juliano Moreira, Louis Muskens, Heinrich Obersteiner, Augusto Tamburini

(*French version*) Otto Hebold, Auguste Marie, Louis Muskens, Heinrich Obersteiner, Bernard Sachs, Robert Sommer, Jacob Van Deventer

(continued)

TABLE A3.3 *(continued)*

Augusto Tamburini is apparently chosen chairman/president. In 1912, he is replaced by David Weeks (USA).

Comité de patronage
Otto Hebold, Adolf Friedländer, Vladimir Beckterev, Antoine Rémond, Louis Landouzy, Robert Sommer, Wilhelm Weygandt, Augusto Tamburini
Bureau permanent: Gyula Donáth
Secrétaire général: Louis Muskens

1935–1939
William Lennox, USA, President
Louis Muskens, Holland, Vice-President
Hans Jacob Schou, Denmark, Secretary/Editor *Epilepsia*
Joseph Tylor Fox, England, Treasurer

1939–1946
William Lennox, USA, President
Karl-Heinz Stauder, Germany, Vice-President
Hans Schou, Denmark, Secretary/Editor *Epilepsia*
Joseph Tylor Fox, England, Treasurer

1946–1949
William Lennox, USA President/Editor *Epilepsia*
Bernard Ledeboer, Heemstede, Holland, Vice-President
Hans Schou, Dianalund, Denmark, Secretary
Denis Williams, London, England, Treasurer

1949–1953
Macdonald Critchley, England, President
Hans Stubbe Teglbjaerg, Dianalund, Denmark, Vice-President
Frederic Gibbs, USA, Vice-President
Bernard Ledeboer, Heemstede, Holland, Secretary-General
Antoine Rémond, France, Recording Secretary
Denis Williams, England, Treasurer
William Lennox, USA, Editor *Epilepsia*/Hon. Pres.
Jerome Merlis, USA, Assistant Editor

1953–1957
A. Earl Walker, Albuquerque, New Mexico, USA, President
Henri Gastaut, Marseilles, France, President-Elect
Denis Williams, London, England, Vice-President
Paulo Niemeyer, Brazil, Vice-President
Bernard Ledeboer, Heemstede, Holland, Secretary-General
Hans Stubbe Teglbjaerg, Dianalund, Denmark, Treasurer
Jerome Merlis, Framingham, USA, Editor *Epilepsia*

1957–1961
A. Earl Walker, Albuquerque, New Mexico, USA, President
Henri Gastaut, Marseilles, France, Secretary-General
Jerome Merlis, Framingham, USA, Treasurer
Francis Walshe, UK, Editor-in-Chief *Epilepsia*

(continued)

TABLE A3.3 *(continued)*

1961–1965
Francis McNaughton, Canada, President
Bartolomé Fuster, Uruguay, Vice-President
Albert Lorentz de Haas, Netherlands, Vice-President/Editor *Epilepsia*
Henri Gastaut, Marseilles, France, Secretary-General/Editor *Epilepsia*
Jerome Merlis, USA, Treasurer

1965–1969
Albert Lorentz de Haas, Netherlands (died 1967), President/Editor *Epilepsia*
Jerome Merlis, Framingham, USA, President
Heinrich Landolt, Switzerland, Vice-President
Francis McNaughton, Canada, Past President
Henri Gastaut, France, Secretary-General/Editor *Epilepsia*
David Daly, Arizona, USA, Treasurer

1969–1973
Henri Gastaut, France, President
Jerome Merlis, USA, Past President
Karl-Axel Melin, Sweden, Vice-President
Luis Oller-Daurella, Spain, Vice-President
Otto Magnus, Netherlands, Secretary-General
David Daly, Arizona, USA, Treasurer
Margaret Lennox-Buchthal, Denmark, Editor-in-Chief *Epilepsia*

1973–1977
David Daly, USA, President
Henri Gastaut, France, Past President
Dieter Janz, Germany, Vice-President
Francisco Rubio Donnadieu, Mexico, Vice-President
J. Kiffin Penry, USA, Secretary-General
Karl-Axel Melin, Sweden, Treasurer
Ellen Grass, USA, Ex Officio IBE
George Burden, UK, Ex Officio IBE
Arthur Ward, Jr., USA, Editor-in-Chief *Epilepsia*

1977–1981
J. Kiffin Penry, USA, President
David Daly, USA, Past President
Dieter Janz, Germany, Vice-President
Toyoji Wada, Japan, Vice-President
Francisco Rubio Donnadieu, Mexico, Secretary-General
Karl-Axel Melin, Sweden, Treasurer
Harry Meinardi, Netherlands, Ex Officio IBE
Richard Grant, UK, Ex Officio IBE
Arthur Ward, Jr., USA, Editor-in-Chief *Epilepsia*

1981–1985
Mogens Dam, Denmark, President
J. Kiffin Penry, USA, Past President
Carlo Alberto Tassinari, Italy, Vice-President
Masakazu Seino, Japan, Vice-President

(continued)

TABLE A3.3 *(continued)*

Fred Dreifuss, USA, Secretary-General
Francisco Rubio Donnadieu, Mexico, Treasurer
Francesco Castellano, Italy, Ex Officio IBE
Richard Grant, Ex Officio IBE
Arthur Ward, Jr., USA, Editor-in-Chief *Epilepsia*

1985–1989
Fred Dreifuss, USA, President
Mogens Dam, Denmark, Past President
Masakazu Seino, Japan, Vice-President
Pierre Loiseau, France, Vice-President
Harry Meinardi, Netherlands, Secretary-General
Francisco Rubio Donnadieu, Mexico, Treasurer
Joop Loeber, Netherlands, Ex Officio IBE
Richard Masland, USA, Ex Officio IBE
Arthur Ward, Jr., USA, until 1986 Editor-in-Chief *Epilepsia*
James Cereghino, USA, from 1986 Editor-in-Chief *Epilepsia*

1989–1993
Harry Meinardi, Netherlands, President
Fred Dreifuss, USA, Past President
Paulo de Bittencourt, Brazil Vice-President
Edward Reynolds, UK, Vice-President
Roger Porter, USA, Secretary-General
Masakazu Seino, Japan, Treasurer
William McLin, USA, Ex Officio IBE
Hanneke M. de Boer, Netherlands, Ex Officio IBE
James Cereghino, USA, Editor-in-Chief *Epilepsia*

1993–1997
Edward Reynolds, UK, President
Harry Meinardi, Netherlands, Past President
Giuliano Avanzini, Italy, Vice-President
Simon Shorvon, UK, Vice-President
Peter Wolf, Germany, Secretary-General
Jerome Engel, Jr., USA, Treasurer
Hanneke M. de Boer, Netherlands, Ex Officio IBE
Michael Hills, New Zealand, Ex Officio IBE
Timothy Pedley, USA, Editor-in-Chief *Epilepsia*

1997–2001
Jerome Engel, Jr., USA, President
Edward Reynolds, UK, Past President
Yoshiaki Mayanagi, Japan, Vice-President
Natalio Fejerman, Argentina, Vice-President
Peter Wolf, Germany, Secretary-General
Giuliano Avanzini, Italy, Treasurer
Richard Holmes, Ireland, Ex Officio IBE
Michael Hills, New Zealand, Ex Officio IBE
Timothy Pedley, USA, Editor-in-Chief *Epilepsia*
Simon Shorvon, UK, Editor-in-Chief *Epigraph*

(continued)

TABLE A3.3 *(continued)*

2001–2005
Giuliano Avanzini, Italy, President
Jerome Engel, USA, Past President
Fred Andermann, Canada, 1st Vice-President
Martin Brodie, Scotland, UK, 2nd Vice-President
Natalio Fejerman, Argentina, Secretary-General
Josimir Sander, UK, Treasurer
Robert Fisher, USA, Editor-in-Chief *Epilepsia*
Simon Shorvon, UK, Information Officer
Philip Lee, UK, President IBE, Ex Officio
Esper Cavalheiro, Brazil, Secretary-General IBE, Ex Officio
Johan Falk Pederson, Norway, Treasurer IBE, Ex Officio

2005–2009
Peter Wolf, Germany, President
Solomon Moshe, USA, Secretary-General
Martin Brodie, Scotland, UK, Treasurer
Giuliano Avanzini, Italy, Past President
Emilio Perucca, Italy, Vice-President
Chong Tin Tan, Singapore, 1st Vice-President
Fred Andermann, Canada, 2nd Vice-President
Simon Shorvon, UK, Editor-in-Chief *Epilepsia*
Philip Schwartzkroin, USA, Editor-in-Chief *Epilepsia*
Edward Bertram, USA, Information Officer
Susanne Lund, Sweden, President IBE
Eric Hargis, USA, Secretary-General IBE
Mike Glynn, Ireland, Treasurer IBE

2009–2013
Solomon Moshé, USA, President
Samuel Wiebe, Canada, Secretary-General
Emilio Perucca, Italy, Treasurer
Peter Wolf, Germany, Past President
Tatsuya Tanaka, Japan, First Vice President
Michel Baulac, France, Second Vice Presdient
Marco Medina, Honduras, Third Vice President
Philip Schwartzkroin, USA, Editor-in-Chief Epilepsia
Simon Shorvon, UK, Editor-in-Chief Epilepsia
Edward Bertram, USA, Information Officer
Mike Glynn, Ireland, IBE President
Carlos Acevedo, Chile, IBE Secretary-General
Grace Tan, Singapore, IBE Treasurer

2013–2017
Emilio Perucca, Italy, President
Helen Cross, UK, Secretary-General
Samuel Wiebe, Canada, Treasurer
Tatuya Tanaka, Japan, Vice-President
Solomon Moshé, USA, Past President
Amadou Gallo Diop, Senegal, Commission on African Affairs

(continued)

TABLE A3.3 *(continued)*

Byung-In Lee, Korea, Commission on Asian and Oceanic Affairs
Hassan Hosny, Egypt, Commisson on Eastern Mediterranean Affairs
Meir Bialer, Israel, Commission on European Affairs
Marco Medina, Honduras, Commission on Latin American Affairs
Sheryl Haut, USA, Commission on North American Affairs
Gary Mathern, USA, Epilepsia Co-Editor-in-Chief
Astrid Nehig, France, Epilepsia Co-Editor-in-Chief
Mike Sperling, USA, Epilepsia Co-Editor-in-Chief
Thanos Covanis, Greece, IBE President
Sari Tervonen, Finland, IBE Secretary-General
Robert Cole, Australia, IBE Treasurer

Invitees
Alexis Arzimanoglou, France, *Epileptic Disorders* Editor-in-Chief
Edward Bertram, USA, Information Officer
Jaime Carrizosa, Chair Education Comission
Jean Gotman, Canada, Director of Interactive Media
Torbjörn Tomson, Sweden, Strategic Planning
Gary Mathern, USA, *Epilepsia Open* Co-Editor-in-Chief
Aristea Galanopoulou, USA, *Epilepsia Open* Co-editor-in-Chief
Dieter Schmidt, Germany, *Epilepsia Open* Co-editor-in-Chief
Xufeng Wang, China, *Epilepsia Open* Co-editor-in-Chief

2017–2021
Samual Wiebe, Canada, President
Edward Bertram, USA, Secretary General
J. Helen Cross, UK, Treasurer
Alla Guekht, Russia, Vice President
Emilio Perucca, Italy, Past President
Mike Sperling, USA, *Epilepsia* co-Editor-in-Chief
Astrid Nehlig, France, *Epilepsia* co-Editor-in-Chief
Angelina Kakooza-Mwesige, Uganda, Chair ILAE-Africa
Akio Ikeda, Japan, Chair ILAE-Asia Oceania
Eugen Trinka, Austria, Chair ILAE-Europe
Roberto Caraballo, Argentina, Chair ILAE-Latin America
Nathalie Jette, USA, Chair ILAE-North America
Chahnex Triki, Tunisia, Chair ILAE-Eastern Mediterranean
Martin Brodie, UK, IBE President
Mary Secco, Canada, IBE Secretary-General
Anthony Zimba, Zambia, IBE Treasurer

Invitees
Jean Gotman, Canada, Strategic advisor
Alexis Arzimanaglou, France, *Epileptic Disorders* Editor-in-Chief
Aristea Galanopoulou, USA, *Epilepsia Open* Co-editor-in-Chief
Dieter Schmidt, Germany, *Epilepsia Open* Co-editor-in-Chief
Xufeng Wang, China, *Epilepsia Open* Co-editor-in-Chief
Shichuo Li, China, Advisor on Public Health
Ingmar Blücke, Germany, Chair Education Council
Gunter Krämer, Switzerland, *Wikipedia* Editor-in-Chief
Nicola Maggio, Israel, *Wikipedia* Editor-in-Chief

GLOSSARY

Medicine and medical science are littered with technical terms (so much so that it has been said that medical students double the number of words in their vocabulary during their training). This glossary is constructed to assist the non-medical reader by explaining in lay terms a small selection of the terms used in this book, the meaning of which may not be immediately obvious. The terms are here only briefly and informally defined. For fuller and more technical descriptions, the reader is referred to Gastaut 'Dictionary of Epilepsy' (1973), Blume 'Descriptive terminology' (2001) and standard medical and scientific text books.

ABSENCE (syn: absence seizure) A type of epileptic seizure in which there is a very brief clouding of consciousness manifested as a 'blankness'. Originally describing any such seizure but, following the introduction of EEG, the term has become restricted to a seizure with generalised spike–wave patterns on the EEG. There are two types: typical absence seizures, in which the EEG shows rhythmic 3/second spike and wave discharge; and atypical absence seizures, in which the spike and wave discharge rate is slower (2–2.5/second).

ACETYLCHOLINE A neurotransmitter in the brain and other sites in the nervous system. At one time it was thought to be a key neurotransmitter in epilepsy, but now this is known not to be the case.

ACETYLCHOLINESTERASE The enzyme in the body that metabolises acetylcholine.

ACIDOSIS Increased acidity of the blood or other body fluid. This is a common transient finding during and after convulsive seizures.

ACTION POTENTIAL (in neurophysiology) The sudden change in electrical potential, created by the movement of ions across a neuronal membrane. The action potential underpins the passage of a nerve impulse down the neuron and is the basis of all neuronal activity.

ACTIVITY, EEG EEG patterns of cerebral origin.

AFTER-DISCHARGE EEG discharges which continue to occur in the brief period after the cessation of electrical stimulation.

AGNOSIA, VISUAL The inability to perceive or recognise an object (or person) despite the preservation of the ability to see. Klüver and Bucy named this 'psychic blindness'.

AGONIST (of receptors) A chemical substance that binds to a receptor on a cell membrane, and in doing so activates the receptor.

ALPHA RHYTHM (of EEG) EEG activity taking the form of waves occurring at a frequency of 8–13 Hz.

ALIENIST A psychiatrist working in an asylum.

ALKALOID Nitrogen-containing organic compounds which have physiological actions. Most are derived from plants.

ALKALOSIS Increased alkalinity (i.e. base content) of blood or other body fluid.

AMAUROTIC IDIOCY (syn: Tay-Sachs disease) An inherited disease due to a mutation in the HEXA gene, which results in a deficiency of the enzyme beta-hexaminidase A.

AMENTIA A term which was used, in the early twentieth century, synonymously with mental deficiency

AMMON'S HORN (CORNU AMMONIS) An anatomical structure that is part of the hippocampus. The term arises from its resemblance to the ram shaped horns on the head of the Egyptian God Ammon-Ra. It is often the site of damage in temporal lobe epilepsy.

AMNESIA Absence of memory. Amnesia for the events during a seizure, and briefly in its aftermath, is a feature of many epileptic seizures, as well as a variety of other neurological and psychiatric conditions. The anatomical or physiological basis of amnesia is largely unknown.

AMPA α-amino-3-hydroxy-5-methyl-4-isoxazolepropionic acid. An agonist of the AMPA receptor, mimicking the action of glutamate.

AMPA RECEPTOR A subtype of glutamate receptor that is activated by AMPA.

AMYGDALA A structure of the brain in the mesial temporal region lying in front of the hippocampus. It is one part of the limbic system.

ANAEMIA, HYPOPLASTIC A potentially serious abnormality in the red cells of the blood. This can be a side effect of some antiepileptic drugs.

ANATOMY, FUNCTIONAL The study of the function of anatomical structures. In epilepsy, the functional anatomy of the cerebral cortex has been an area of particular study, via stimulation and ablation experiments. The reason for the special interest is the concept that the symptoms of the epileptic seizure reflect activation of the anatomical structure in which it originates. So, knowledge of the functional anatomy of the brain will help identify (localise) the anatomical origin of the epileptic discharge.

ANATOMY, MORBID The study of anatomical abnormalities caused by disease.

ANERGIA, MORAL Loss or lack of mental or physical energy.

ANGIOGRAPHY (cerebral) A radiological technique for rendering visible on X-ray the position and anatomy of blood vessels of the brain. It was originally performed by taking an X-ray after the injection of a radiopaque contrast medium into the blood stream. MRI and CT angiography are similar techniques for visualising blood vessels using MRI and CT scanning.

ANOMALY, ANATOMICAL A structure the anatomy of which deviates from normal. In epilepsy structural anomalies are found especially in congenital diseases.

ANOXAEMIA Absence of oxygen in the blood.

ANTAGONIST (of receptors) A chemical substance which binds to a receptor on a cell membrane, and in doing so blocks the activation of a receptor.

ANTIEPILEPTIC DRUG A drug used to prevent epileptic seizures. A preferred term now is antiseizure drug.

AURA A term introduced by Galen to describe the sensation of a breeze or puff of air (from the Latin aura). Now used to describe the initial symptoms of a focal seizure prior to the loss of consciousness (and sometimes occurring without subsequent loss of consciousness). It is sometimes perceived as the 'warning' of a seizure. An aura can take many forms – motor, sensory, autonomic or psychic. Common auras include a sensation of déjà vu, a cephalic sensation and epigastric sensation.

AUTOINTOXICATION, THEORY OF A theory, now dismissed, in which the cause of epilepsy was thought to be circulating toxins created internally, for instance by gut bacteria. One variant of this theory was that of an autocytotoxin, a toxin latent in the blood cells which is released during a convulsion.

AUTOMATISM An involuntary motor activity occurring during a state of clouding or loss of consciousness/awareness during or immediately after an epileptic seizure. The sufferer has no control over the movements and no memory of them. The automatism can take many forms, can appear purposive, and is often a continuation of an activity that was going on when the seizure occurred.

AUTONOMIC (in neurophysiology) Functions of the body which occur without conscious effort, such as control of heart beat, blood pressure, breathing and sweating. These functions are often transiently affected in epileptic seizures.

AUTOSOMAL DOMINANT FRONTAL LOBE EPILEPSY (ADFLE) An epilepsy syndrome due to a mutation in genes coding for the nicotinic acid acetylcholine receptor.

AXON The long cable-like process of a nerve cell along which nerve impulses are conducted.

AYURVEDIC A traditional Indian system of medicine in which health is maintained by keeping mind, body and spirit in balance. Treatment is usually with herbs and other natural substances.

BACKGROUND ACTIVITY (of EEG in epilepsy) The underlying EEG rhythm upon which epileptic transients are superimposed. Background slowing is a background rhythm which is slower than normal for age and state of consciousness and is a common finding in epilepsy.

BINDING, BINDING SITES (of antiepileptic drugs) Antiepileptic drugs act by binding to receptors in the brain – either activating or inhibiting the receptor function, and in this way effecting a physiological change. Drugs also bind to plasma proteins in the blood and this may affect the concentration of drug which is available to exert an effect (the 'free drug concentration').

BRAIN SLICE An experimental model in which a portion (a thin slice) of brain tissue is kept 'alive' by immersion in an nutrient-filled and oxygenated fluid in the laboratory. Brain slices have been frequently used in physiological and chemical studies in epilepsy.

BURSTING/BURST FIRING A property of neurons in epilepsy in which a train of rapid repetitive discharges is triggered by an action potential. It is a hallmark of epilepsy.

CA1, CA2, CA3 Anatomical regions of the hippocampus. CA1 is sometimes referred to as Sommer's Sector, and CA2 as the resistant sector.

CAROTID ARTERY An artery in the neck supplying the brain with blood.

CAVERNOMA (cerebral) (syn: cavernous angioma, cavernous haemangioma) A structural abnormality in the brain comprising a cluster of abnormal blood vessels. Epilepsy is a common symptom of a cavernoma situated in grey matter.

CENTRAL NERVOUS SYSTEM The brain and the spinal cord.

CENTRENCEPHALIC SYSTEM An ill-defined neural network involving brain stem areas and the cerebral cortex. The existence of this network (or system) was proposed by Wilder Penfield, who suggested its function was to 'integrate' cortical activity. Whether the network exists as a valid anatomical or physiological concept remains contentious.

CEREBRAL LOCALISATION A theory in which it is postulated that different locations in the cerebral cortex are responsible for different bodily functions: for instance, that the precentral gyrus is responsible for movement, the occipital lobe for vision and Broca's area in the left frontal lobe for speech. The functions of different parts of the cortex can be 'mapped' experimentally by direct electrical stimulation and by resection. The theory was fundamental to the beginning of epilepsy surgery.

CEREBROSPINAL FLUID A liquid substance occupying ventricular and subdural spaces of the brain and spinal cord.

CHANNEL, ION (in the brain) Transmembrane protein structures situated in the neuron and along the length of its axons. They form a pore through which charged ions can pass between the extracellular fluid and the interior of the neuron. This passage of charged ions maintains the voltage difference (a 'gradient') across the membrane, necessary for the conduction of nerve impulses. Ion channel mutations can result in abnormal voltage gradients causing electrical hyperexcitability and epileptic seizures.

CHANNELOPATHY A disease caused by mutations in ion channels.

CHOLINERGIC Enhancing acetylcholine functions. Cholinergic substances can bind to cholingergic receptors and mimic the action of acetylcholine at cholinergic synapses (synapses where acetylcholine is the neurotransmitter).

CHOREA A disorder of the brain in which there are involuntary, irregular and unpredictable movements. There are many different causes, but in the nineteenth century chorea and epilepsy were considered to be inherited as part of the neuropathic trait.

CHROMATOGRAPHY A scientific technique for separating out chemicals in a mixture. It is used in clinical epilepsy to measure the concentrations of antiepileptic drugs in blood. In experimental epilepsy it is used to measure the concentration of various biochemicals.

CHYMUS The semi-fluid substance comprising partly digested food that moves from the stomach to the duodenum during the process of digestion.

CLONIC Jerks or jerky movements occurring in an epileptic seizure.

COLECTOMY A surgical operation in which all or part of the colon (the lower bowel) is removed.

COLONY, EPILEPSY A residential home for people with epilepsy. Usually located in the country with opportunities for simple employment and sometimes also medical attention. The 'colony movement', a medical fashion promoting the establishment of colonies, had its apogee in the early twentieth century.

COMA, INSULIN / BARBITURATE Coma induced by the administration of insulin or barbiturate, as a treatment for psychiatric disorders. In epilepsy barbiturate coma is sometimes induced in the treatment of status epilepticus.

COMPUTERISED AXIAL TOMOGRAPHIC IMAGING (CT) A form of brain scanning involving multiple images taken by a rotating X-ray tube, processed by computer and reconstructed to produced tomographic (cross sectional) images in the form of 'slices'.

CONGENITAL Present at birth.

CONTRAST MEDIUM A substance used in radiology to increase the visibility of tissues; for instance, in brain to help differentiate brain tissue from blood vessels and cerebrospinal fluid.

CONVULSANT A chemical or other material which induces epileptic seizures.

CONVULSION, FEBRILE Convulsions precipitated by fever. These are most commonly encountered in children between the ages of six months and three years. In that situation, they are usually benign. Prolonged febrile convulsions and or those with focal features may damage temporal lobe structures, leading to later temporal lobe epilepsy.

CONVULSION, JACKSONIAN A form of focal motor seizure restricted to one side of the body or one limb. It is often the clinical manifestation of seizure discharges in the contralateral motor cortex. It can take the form of a 'Jacksonian March' in which the seizure spreads progressively along a limb or one side of the body.

CORPUS CALLOSECTOMY / CALLOSOTOMY A form of brain operation, carried out to control epilepsy, in which the corpus callosum is cut, thus partly disconnecting the two cerebral hemispheres from each other.

CORPUS CALLOSUM A structure in the brain comprising a bundle of nerve fibres which connect the two cerebral hemispheres.

CORTEX, CEREBRAL The most superficial layer of the brain, which contains the cell bodies of neurons. It mostly comprises six layers and has a convoluted folded form with ridges (gyri) and grooves (sulci). It comprises the cell bodies of neurons (hence its colour). Seizure discharges originate in cerebral cortical cells. It occupies 40% of brain tissue and contains 14–16 billion neurons. It is divided into four 'lobes': frontal, temporal, parietal and occipital. The term 'motor cortex' is used to describe the most posterior part of the frontal lobe and sensory cortex the most anterior part of the parietal lobe.

CRETINISM A disease caused by congenital thyroid hormone deficiency.

DELTA RHYTHM (of EEG) EEG activity taking the form of waves occurring at a frequency of 0.25–2 per second.

DEGENERATION (DÉGÉNÉRESCENCE) THEORY OF A theory of brain disease, now dismissed but widely held in the late nineteenth century, in which it was postulated that epilepsy and other physical, mental or social disorders are inherited diseases which tended to worsen over generations.

DEMENTIA, EPILEPTIC A term used in the early twentieth century to refer to the occurrence of dementia during the course of epilepsy. At that time, it was (incorrectly) believed that epilepsy often resulted in mental deterioration and dementia.

DENDRITE Short tree-like branched structures of a nerve cell along which nerve impulses are conducted.

DEOXYRIBONUCLEIC ACID (DNA) A complex molecule composed of two chains that coil around each other to form a double helical structure. DNA provides the substrate for the coding and transfer of genetic information.

DETERMINISM, BIOLOGICAL The belief that a person's behaviour is dictated by their physiological make-up (and usually their genetic make-up) and less by the environment, experience or external factors. In epilepsy this term was usually employed in relation to abnormal or violent behaviour.

DIENCEPHALON The most caudal part of the forebrain that lies in front of the midbrain and consists of the thalamic nuclei, part of the hypothalamus, other nuclei around the thalamus and the subthalamus.

DISCHARGE, EPILEPTIC The sudden and excessive neuronal activity in the cerebral cortex that is characteristic of epilepsy. The ictal discharge is that which occurs during an epileptic seizure. The inter-ictal discharge is that which occurs at other times. A subclinical discharge is that which occurs without any obvious clinical sign or symptom.

DNA, RECOMBINANT A piece of DNA that has been created by combining fragments of DNA from different sources. It is one form of gene editing.

DURA MATER (syn: Dura) The tough outermost membrane covering the brain and spinal cord.

DYSCRASIA Abnormality or disordered function. (A drug-induced blood dyscrasia is a term used to describe a severe reduction in the number of blood cells often as an allergic reaction to a drug).

DYSPLASIA, CORTICAL (dysplasia, cerebral) An area of abnormal development of the cerebral cortex. Many are caused by genetic mutations. Epilepsy is a common symptom of cortical dysplasia. There are a range of different types.

ECLAMPSIA A rare but serious condition in which high blood pressure and epileptic seizures occur in late pregnancy.

EEG ACTIVITY, FOCAL EEG activity arising from a localised area of the brain.

EEG ACTIVITY, GENERALISED EEG discharges appearing approximately symmetrically and synchronously over widespread regions of both hemispheres. It is the EEG signature of generalised seizures.

EEG ACTIVITY, ICTAL The pattern of EEG discharges during a seizure.

EEG ACTIVITY INTER-ICTAL The pattern of EEG discharges seen in epilepsy at times when there is no seizure occurring.

ELECTRICAL STATUS EPILEPTICUS DURING SLOW-WAVE SLEEP (ESES) (syn: Continuous spike and wave during slow-wave sleep; CSWS). An EEG pattern seen in some severe epilepsies.

ELECTROCONVULSIVE THERAPY (ECT) A form of physical psychiatric therapy in which an electric current is passed through the brain to induce an epileptic seizure.

ELECTROCORTICOGRAPHY (syn: Corticography) The recording of EEG directly from the surface of the brain (in contrast to routine EEGs which are recorded from the scalp). The recording is called an electrocorticogram.

ELECTRODE, EEG The conducting device which is applied to the patient to record an EEG. There are various types of electrode and various positions of placement. A scalp electrode is one placed on the scalp during a routine EEG; a depth electrode is one placed within the substance of the brain with the insertion often performed stereotactically to improve precision and to avoid causing haemorrhage by perforation of a major cerebral vessel; a subdural electrode is one placed underneath the dura; an epidural electrode is one placed on the dura; a sphenoidal electrode is one placed into the sphenoid bone.

ELECTROENCEPHALOGRAPHER A person who records and/or analyses the EEG record.

ELECTROENCEPHALOGRAM (EEG) A tracing (a record) of the voltage fluctuations over time recorded by electrodes placed over the head. It is an amplified recording of the fluctuating potentials from neurons in the vicinity of the electrodes. In a routine (scalp) EEG, the electrodes are placed on top of the scalp according to an internationally agreed convention – the '10-20' system. Initially, the fluctuating voltages were visualised by transferring the recording onto paper moving at a constant speed via an ink and pen writer. More recently, the EEGs are recorded digitally and displayed electronically.

ELECTROENCEPHALOGRAPH A machine to record EEG; an EEG record.

ELECTROENCEPHALOGRAPHY (EEG) The study of EEG; the practice of recording EEG.

ELECTROENCEPHALOGRAPHY, DEPTH EEG recorded from within the brain substance, obtained by recording electrodes inserted into the brain.

EPILEPSIA PARTIALIS CONTINUA A rare form of epilepsy with focal seizures persisting for long periods of time.

EPILEPSY Defined currently as a chronic brain disorder, regardless of aetiology or mechanism, characterised by recurrent seizures. In the early twentieth century, it was a term often restricted to idiopathic epilepsy. Whether the term has any useful function is discussed in the Epilogue.

EPILEPSY, ACQUIRED A form of symptomatic epilepsy due to non-inherited factors.

EPILEPSY, BENIGN WITH CENTROTEMPORAL SPIKES A common epileptic syndrome of childhood.

EPILEPSY, CATAMENNIAL A form of epilepsy in which the seizures occur in a fixed temporal relationship to menstruation (usually during or just before or just after menstruation).

EPILEPSY, FRONTAL LOBE An epilepsy in which the focal seizures arise from the frontal lobe.

EPILEPSY, GENERALISED An epilepsy in which there are exclusively generalised seizures.

EPILEPSY, IDIOPATHIC (syn: essential epilepsy, primary epilepsy) Epilepsy in which the cause is not known but is presumed to be geneticor developmental in origin. *Idiopathic Generalised Epilepsy* is a common epilepsy syndrome in which there are characteristic clinical and EEG features.

EPILEPSY, POST-TRAUMATIC Epilepsy caused by head trauma.

EPILEPSY, LARVAL (syn: epileptic equivalent) An obsolete term that refers to mental manifestations thought to be due to epileptic activity but in the absence of an overt seizure. It was used to describe paroxysmal mental abnormalities thought to be due to epilepsy.

EPILEPSY, PROGRESSIVE MYOCLONIC A form of epilepsy in which the main seizure type is myoclonus and is associated with additional neurological features and a progressive course resulting in death. There were a variety of different genetic causes, including forms of Ceroid lipofuscinosis, Unverricht–Lundborg Disease (Lafora body disease), some forms of mitochondrial disease and Baltic myoclonus.

EPILEPSY, REFLEX A form of epilepsy in which seizures are provoked by sensory stimuli. One example is musicogenic epilepsy, in which seizures are provoked by music. There are many other types, although reflex epilepsies are rare.

EPILEPSY, SECONDARY GENERALISED A form of epilepsy in which a focal seizure evolves into a generalised seizure.

EPILEPSY, SYMPTOMATIC Epilepsy arising from a pathological condition.

EPILEPSY, TEMPORAL LOBE An epilepsy in which the focal seizures arise from the temporal lobe.

EPILEPTIC (of a person) A person who has epilepsy. The use of this term is now strongly discouraged as prejudicial. PWE (A person with epilepsy) is often suggested as an alternative (but see objections to this term in the Epilogue of this book).

EPILEPTIC, INSANE/SANE These terms, now obsolete, were used in the nineteenth century to refer to people with epilepsy who had/did not have psychiatric disturbance or learning disability.

EPILEPTIC SEIZURE, AUDIOGENIC A form of reflex seizure precipitated by sounds.

EPILEPTIC SEIZURE, GENERALISED Epileptic seizure in which the epileptic discharges arise in wide areas of the brain in both cerebral hemispheres. Secondary generalised seizures are those which are initially focal and then spread to become generalised discharges.

EPILEPTIC SEIZURE, PARTIAL (syn: focal epileptic seizure) Epileptic seizure which arise from and are confined to a restricted area of the brain (the focus).

EPILEPTIC SEIZURE, TONIC–CLONIC (syn: grand mal seizure, convulsive seizure). A severe type of seizure, in which there is convulsive motor activity, usually involving all four limbs, and the jaw and facial muscles, and often associated with autonomic features, tongue biting and urinary incontinence.

EPILEPTOGENESIS The process of the development of epilepsy; the abnormal brain mechanisms which result in epilepsy.

EPILEPTOLOGY/EPILEPTOLOGIST The study or medical specialism of epilepsy; a doctor specialising in epilepsy.

ENCEPHALOPATHY, EPILEPTIC An altered mental state, often with other clinical features, that occurs in the context of frequent electrographic epileptic discharges.

EPHAPTIC TRANSMISSION The direct passage of nerve impulses from one cell to another without chemical transmission

EPILOIA (syn: Tuberose Sclerosis) A genetic disorder in which epileptic seizures are a common feature.

EPSP (excitatory post synaptic potential). An electrical phenomenon which may trigger an electrical impulse in the post-synaptic neuron.

EQUIPOTENTIALITY (in neurophysiology) A theory which considers that all (or many) parts of the cerebral cortex are involved for all functions (in opposition to the theory of cerebral localisation).

EUGENICS The study (science or social policy) of human reproduction with the purpose of increasing the proportion of characteristics regarded as desirable or reducing the proportion regarded as undesirable within a population or species.

EXOGENOUS A cause or origin from outside the body (or outside the brain).

EXPERIENTIAL (in epilepsy) The sensation of past memories or experiences. This is a not uncommon aura of an epileptic seizure. Experiential responses can be produced by stimulating areas of the temporal lobe.

EXON The portion of a gene that codes for an amino acid. Exons lie between introns.

FEEBLE-MINDED An obsolete term meaning 'lacking normal mental powers'. In the late nineteenth and early twentieth centuries, most (or all) people with epilepsy were assumed to be feeble-minded. Later, Godard divided feeble-mindedness into three categories, based on the newly introduced IQ measures: idiots, imbeciles and morons.

DOPAMINE A neurotransmitter, not considered to be of great importance in epilepsy or its treatment.

FIXATION (in histology) A chemical process which prevents biological material or histological staining from deteriorating.

GABA RECEPTOR A receptor activated by GABA. The GABA A and GABA B receptors are both important in epilepsy. Activation of these receptors exerts an inhibitory action on the spread of epileptic discharges.

GALACTOSAEMIA A rare genetic disorder in which there is a deficiency in enzymes which metabolise galactose.

GALVANOMETER An apparatus for detecting the existence and determining the direction and intensity of an electrical current.

GENOME The complete set of genetic material in an individual, stored in DNA.

GENOME WIDE ASSOCIATION STUDY (GWAS) A method of genetic investigation in which markers across the complete genome are scanned to identify genetic variants (mutations and others).

GERM PLASM An obsolete term which was used to refer to material which transmits heritable information, and which is contained in germ cells (cells involved in reproduction).

GLIOSIS (GLIA, NEUROGLIA) A pathological finding characterised by hypertrophy of glial cells. It is a response to damage and a frequent finding in epilepsy.

GLUTAMATE The principal excitatory neurotransmitter in the brain. Of great importance in epilepsy and its treatment (adjectival form: glutaminergic).

GLUTAMATE RECEPTOR Synaptic and non-synaptic receptors in neurons and glial cells to which glutamate binds. Activation of the synaptic glutamate receptor underpins the transmission of an action potential from the presynaptic to the post-synaptic cell. It has a central role of the generation and spread of epileptic discharges. There are several subtypes: ionotropic and metabotropic. Ionotropic receptors are subdivided into NMDA, AMPA and Kainate subtypes. Metabotropic receptors are subdivided into eight subtypes (mGluR1-8).

GLYCOLYTIC PATHWAY A process of steps involved in the metabolism of glucose in the body. Each step is controlled by one enzyme.

GRAND MAL SEIZURE An obsolete term for a generalised convulsion.

GREY MATTER/GRAY MATTER The brain substance containing cell bodies.

GYRUS A ridge-like fold of cerebral cortex (bordered by 'sulci').

HHE SYNDROME A syndrome comprising hemiconvulsions, hemiplegia and epilepsy, resulting from brain damage caused by a prolonged febrile convulsion.

HEMIMEGALENCEPHALY A form of cortical dysplasia in which one hemisphere of the brain is abnormally large. It is a developmental disorder, of unknown cause, in which epilepsy is a common symptom.

HEMISPHERECTOMY A form of surgical operation in which large areas of one hemisphere of the brain are resected (anatomical hemispherectomy) or disconnected (functional hemispherectomy).

HERBAL (In pharmacology) A drug produced from plants.

HETEROTOPIA, SUBEPENDYMAL A form of congenital dysplasia in which foci of grey matter cells are located deep in the brain, in the subependymal region. These maldeveloped cells often cause epileptic seizures.

HIPPOCAMPUS A curved anatomical structure, of infolded cerebral cortex, located in the floor of the inferior (temporal) horn of the lateral ventricle. It is often involved in epilepsy.

HIPPOCAMPAL SCLEROSIS (syn: incisural sclerosis, mesial temporal sclerosis, Ammon's Horn sclerosis) A pathological state in which the hippocampus is damaged. It is hardened (gliotic) and histological examination reveals cell loss, dispersion of cells and gliosis. It is a common lesion in epilepsy. It is a form of damage commonly considered to be caused by a prolonged febrile seizure.

HISTOPATHOLOGY The study of the microscopic appearance of disease in tissues.

HOMUNCULUS (in epilepsy) A diagram in which a small human-like form is used to represent the functions of the sensory-motor cortex.

HOSPITAL, VOLUNTARY A term used in the nineteenth century to refer to a hospital funded by voluntary, often philanthropic, gifts of money (in contrast to state or regionally funded or private hospitals).

HUNTINGTON CHOREA A genetic disorder, caused by abnormal trinucleotide repeats in the Huntington gene. It is inherited in an autosomal dominant fashion.

HYPEREXCITABLE (of neurons) Neurons which generate or transmit discharges more readily than normal. Such cells are a feature of epileptic brain tissue.

HYPERPLASIA The pathological finding of hypertrophy with excessive cellular formation.

HYGIENE, MEDICAL A form of medical treatment aimed at the maintenance of health by diet and healthy lifestyle.

HYPOGLYCAEMIA Abnormally low concentration of sugar in the blood.

HYPOTHALAMUS A small structure in the base of the brain which is involved in autonomic control and hormone release. A hamartoma situated within the hypothalamus is a rare cause of epilepsy.

HYSTERIA A condition considered to have a psychological cause. Seizure-like episodes can occur as one manifestation of hysteria.

IBE International Bureau for Epilepsy. An association of lay persons involved in the field of epilepsy.

ICTAL Events or EEG appearances that occur during an epileptic seizure.

IFSECN International Federation of Societies for Electroencephalography and Clinical Neurophysiology. A professional association of medical persons in the field of EEG and clinical neurophysiology.

ILAE International League Against Epilepsy. An association of medical and other professionals involved in the field of epilepsy.

INBORN ERRORS OF

METABOLISM Inherited genetic defects (usually single gene defects) which result in specific clinical diseases.

INHERITANCE, COMPLEX Inheritance with does not follow a simple Mendelian pattern. This is due to the interaction between genes (epistasis) and/or the interaction of genes and environmental factors (epigenetics).

INHERITANCE, MENDELIAN An inheritance pattern which follows simple Mendelian principles – i.e. autosomal dominant autosomal recessive or X-linked inheritance.

INHERITANCE, MITOCHONDRIAL Inheritance of a trait encoded by mitochondrial DNA (in contrast to DNA in cell nuclei). Inheritance is through the maternal line (i.e. transmitted by the mother, not the father). Epilepsy can be caused by a range of mitochondrially inherited genetic defects.

IONOTROPIC RECEPTORS Receptors to which binding of neurotransmitters results directly in the opening of ion channels.

INSANITY A term which in the past was used loosely to refer to a wide range of mental illnesses and also to mental handicap.

INTRAPERITONEAL Contained within the peritoneum, the membrane-lined abdominal cavity containing the abdominal organs.

INTER-ICTAL Events or EEG appearances that occur in between epileptic seizures in a person with epilepsy.

INTERNEURON A neuron which transmits impulses between other neurons. These can be excitatory or inhibitory, and abnormal interneuronal activity is important in the generation of epilepsy in the hippocampus.

INTRON The portion of DNA that does not code for an amino acid. Introns lie in between exons.

KETOGENIC DIET A low carbohydrate and high fat diet that induces ketosis and is used as a treatment for epilepsy. Ketosis is a metabolic process that converts fat into energy during which ketone is produced. It is a source of energy utilised by the body when carbohydrate sources are insufficient.

KINDLING (in neurophysiology) The process by which repeated sub-threshold electrical stimuli result eventually in the occurrence of spontaneous epileptic seizures.

KREBS CYCLE A series of chemical steps that release energy from glucose. Each step is mediated by one enzyme.

LEUCOTOMY (syn: lobotomy). A form of brain operation in which white matter tracts are cut ('disconnected'), in contrast to operations which involve resection of brain tissue. This is an operation usually performed in the frontal lobe to relieve severe psychiatric symptoms.

LESION A localised area of abnormal tissue.

LESIONECTOMY A form of brain operation in which a lesion is removed (resected). This operation is often performed for epilepsy.

LESIONING The act of creating an area of damage. In brain lesioning, the damage can be created by surgical means, focused radiation or ultrasound, or via an implanted electrode by heat or electrical current.

LIMBIC SYSTEM (syn: Papez circuit) A network of anatomical structures in the brain which are thought to be involved with emotions and drives. It is commonly involved in epileptic seizures.

LUMBAR PUNCTURE A medical investigation in which a sample of cerebrospinal fluid is taken via a needle inserted in the lower back (lumbar) region.

MAGNETIC RESONANCE IMAGING (MRI) A form of radiological investigation in which images are obtained by measuring changes in directions of the rotational axis of protons in bodily structures placed in a strong magnetic field and subjected to pulsed beams of high-frequency radio waves. The images produced by an MRI scanner provide a very high level of anatomical detail.

MAGNETOENCEPHALOGRAPHY (MEG) A technique of recording the magnetic fields generated by cortical neurons (in contrast to electroencephalography, which records the electrical currents generated by cortical neurons).

MAPS, CORTICAL Diagrams of brain structure often indicating the functions of localised areas.

MEDICAL TREATMENT Non-surgical methods of treatment.

MEDULLA The most caudal part of the brain, at the junction with the spinal cord.

MENDELIAN CONDITION A condition in which the inheritance is via a single gene, and follows the basic laws propounded by Gregor Mendal of dominant or recessive genetics (i.e. classical or simple inheritance, in contrast to complex inheritance).

MENTAL DEFICIENCY A condition in which measures of cognition and/or behaviour are below normal (usually defined as less than 2 standard deviations from the mean).

META-ANALYSIS A statistical technique in which results from different clinical studies (for instance, randomised clinical trials) are amalgamated.

METABOTROPIC RECEPTOR A form of receptor in which the binding of a neurotransmitter exerts its effects by a series of metabolic steps. It can be indirectly linked to ion channel function by activating a metabolic step which in turn activates an ion channel.

MICROCEPHALY This term refers to a small head size, and can be caused of a range of different pathologies, both inherited and acquired.

MIRROR FOCUS (in neurophysiology). A term used to describe the induction of epileptic discharges in brain structures of one cerebral hemisphere by similar discharges in homologous structures in the other hemisphere. The mechanism of this effect is not known.

MITOCHONDRION A structure found in cells. It is involved in the production of chemical energy for use in the cell's biochemical reactions.

MONGOLISM (syn: trisomy 21) An obsolete tern for Down syndrome, a condition caused by an extra copy of chromosome 21.

MORAL DEFICIENCY Defined in the British Parliamentary Mental Deficiency Act in 1927 as 'mental defectiveness coupled with strongly vicious or criminal propensities'.

MORPHOLOGY The structure of an organism – its size, shape and constitution.

MOSAICISM (of genetics) A term referring to the condition in which there are two different genetic cell lines in a single individual. It is caused when a mutation occurs early in the development of the foetus but after other cell lines have already begun to be formed. This mutation is then carried only in structures derived from the affected cell line.

MOSSY FIBRES This term refers to the histological appearance of axons of cells in the hippocampus. Mossy fibre sprouting is the excessive abnormal development of mossy fibres within their own dendritic field, thus creating recurrent circuits. This might be an explanation of increased hippocampal excitability in epilepsy.

MTOR Mammalian target of rapamycin. An enzyme (a kinase) which is at the centre of biochemical pathways that play a major regulatory role in the brain.

MYOCLONUS A shock-like muscle jerk, often multiple or repeated. It can sometimes be a form of epileptic seizure.

NEUROCYSTICERCOSIS A condition in which calcified larva of the tapeworm are located in the brain. Epileptic seizures are a common symptom.

NEUROFIBROMATOSIS A genetic disorder due to mutations in either the NF1 or NF2 gene. The mutations cause a variety of abnormalities. Epileptic seizures can occur in both types.

NEUROLOGY The branch of medicine and science that deals with organic diseases and disorders of the nervous system. Behavioural neurology is a synonym of neuropsychiatry.

NEURON Nerve cell.

NEUROPATHIC TRAIT, THEORY OF (Syn: Neuropathic diathesis; neuropathic taint; neurological trait) The theory that epilepsy is inherited together with other conditions, some neurological, some social and some psychological. The theory was almost universally held in the late nineteenth and early twentieth centuries but is now discarded.

NEUROPHYSIOLOGY, CLINICAL The medical specialty concerned with the use of physiological techniques (such as EEG) to investigate neurological disease.

NEUROPHYSIOLOGY The study of the physiology of the nervous system.

NEUROPSYCHIATRY The branch/school of psychiatry that emphasises the organic and biological mechanisms of psychiatric disease. Also, the specialty that is concerned with the psychiatric aspects of neurological disease.

NEUROSIS The term is used today to refer to a range of relatively mild mental disorders (including depression, anxiety and OCD). In the past, it was used more widely to describe any mental disorder (especially those without any overt cause).

NEUROTRANSMITTER A chemical substance that is released at the presynaptic nerve ending in response to the arrival of a nerve impulse and which then crosses the synapse to excite or inhibit the post-synaptic cell membrane. It thus effects the transfer of the nerve impulse from one cell to the next. This is the principal mechanism by which brain cells 'communicate' with each other.

NMDA N-Methyl-D-aspartic acid or N-Methyl-D-aspartate. An agonist of NMDA receptors, mimicking the action of glutamate.

NMDA RECEPTOR A subtype of glutamate receptor that is activated by NMDA. It is an excitatory receptor of great importance in epilepsy.

NON-CONVULSIVE A form of epileptic seizure in which there are no motor symptoms. There are various types, including generalised absence and atonic seizures, and some forms of focal seizure including temporal lobe seizures.

NORMALISATION, FORCED (of EEG) A phenomenon in epilepsy in which psychiatric symptoms coincide with the reduction or disappearance of EEG abnormalities.

NOSOLOGY A systematic classification and division of disease; also the study of classification of disease.

ONTOGENY The study of the development of an organism from conception to maturity (ontogenesis).

ONTOGENETIC A term used to describe the appearance of an organism during its development.

OSCILLOSCOPE (syn Oscillograph obs.) In electrophysiology, an apparatus for graphically displaying a varying voltage.

PARACLISIS Differential sensitivity (for instance, of a tissue to damage).

PAROXYSM (of EEG) Sudden onset transient EEG activity, either in an epileptic seizure or as an inter-ictal feature.

PAROXYSMAL DEPOLARISATION SHIFT (PDS) A neurophysiological phenomenon referring to the abnormal change in the neuronal membrane voltage that follows an action potential. It is a hallmark of epilepsy.

PAROXYSMAL DISORDERS Disorders/diseases in which the symptoms are intermittent. Epilepsy is a common example.

PATHOGENESIS The process/mechanism by which a disease develops; the events occurring during this process.

PATHOLOGY The study of the causes and effects of disease, especially related to the examination of anatomy and body tissues.

PEDIGREE CHART Inherited traits displayed in family tree diagram, used in genetic studies.

PERSONALITY, EPILEPTIC Behavioural characteristics that were said to be inherent in, and typically exhibited by, persons with epilepsy. In the late nineteenth and early twentieth centuries, many features were included in this category, but the existence of specific personality traits in epilepsy has been repeatedly dismissed in more recent times.

PES HIPPOCAMPI An anatomical structure at the lower end of the hippocampus.

PETIT MAL SEIZURE A traditional term for a generalised absence seizure. It is now not used in official classifications, but often still widely used by patients and doctors (and the author) as it is linguistically more elegant than 'generalised absence seizure'.

PHARMACOKINETICS The study of drug absorption, distribution, protein binding, metabolism, excretion and of drug interactions.

PHENYLKETONURIA A congenital disease caused by a genetic defect resulting in the deficiency of the enzyme phenylalanine hydroxylase.

PHOTIC STIMULATION (of EEG) The delivery of intermittent flashes of light at different frequencies (usually 1–60 Hz) during an EEG. It is a technique for inducing EEG abnormalities (an EEG activation procedure) in epilepsy, to assist in the diagnosis of epilepsy.

PHOTOPAROXYSMAL RESPONSE (PPR) (of EEG). Abnormal pattern which develops during photic stimulation. It is characterised by spike-and-slow wave or polyspike-and-slow-wave complexes. It is strongly suggestive of the presence of epilepsy.

PHYLOGENY The history of development of a species during its evolution (also phylogenetics: the branch of genetics that is the study of phylogeny).

PHYSIOGNOMY The study of the features of the face, or general form of the body, which is supposed to provide a clue to aetiology and to character traits in those with epilepsy. Most physiognomic theories have been thoroughly discredited.

PLACEBO A substance that has no pharmacological activity. It is often used as a 'control' substance in clinical trials. Although having no pharmacological action, a placebo can have a beneficial effect (the placebo effect) for psychological or other reasons. There is a strong placebo effect in trials of antiepileptic drugs, for reasons which are unclear.

PLASTICITY (of neurons or networks) The ability of a neuron or network to change its structure or function.

PNEUMOENCEPHALOGRAPHY (syn: air encephalography) A radiological investigation in which the cerebral ventricular system is visualised by using air as a contrast medium, usually introduced by lumbar puncture.

POLYMERASE CHAIN REACTION (PCR) A method of making numerous copies of pieces of DNA, thus amplifying a small sample of DNA into one large enough for detailed study.

POLYMICROGYRIA A congenital disorder of brain structure in which gyral patterns are disrupted. It is a condition in which epilepsy is a prominent symptom.

POLYP Abnormal tissue growths, either on a stalk or flat base.

POLYVALENT (in psychoanalysis) Having several different types or forms.

PRIMATE The order in the animal kingdom that includes monkeys, lemurs, apes and humans. Some primates have naturally occurring epilepsies, and epilepsy can be induced experimentally in many primate species.

PSYCHIATRY The branch of medicine concerned with mental illness. For many years, psychiatrists (doctors specialising in psychiatry) were the specialists principally responsible for managing epilepsy; this role was then largely surpassed by neurologists.

PSYCHOANALYSIS A psychological treatment based on theories of mind developed by Sigmund Freud.

PSYCHOMETRY The measurement of psychological traits by means of quantifiable tests (psychometric tests; an example is the IQ test).

PSYCHOPATHY When coined in the 1890s, this term referred to a wider range of mental and behavioural conditions than it does today.

Currently, it is confined to conditions in which the individual engages in antisocial and/or amoral behaviour and who has specific personality features (lack of remorse, failure to establish loving relationships, etc.).

PSYCHOSIS Psychosis is a severe disorder in which mental processes become deranged. It can occur in epilepsy, and can be subdivided into cases in which transient psychosis occurs prior to seizures (pre-ictal psychosis), during seizures (ictal psychosis) or just after seizures (post-ictal psychosis) or in which there is no clear temporal relationship to the occurrence of seizures (inter-ictal psychosis). Psychosis can also be produced as a side-effect of some drug treatment (drug-induced psychosis). Other subdivisions are described in the text.

REFLEX SEIZURES Epileptic seizures which are reliably triggered by a specific precipitant (e.g. photic stimulation, music, etc.)

REFLEX THEORY OF EPILEPSY A now discredited theory that seizures are a form of reflex with an input (afferent) and output (efferent) arm.

RESECTION, SURGICAL The act of excising bodily tissue in a surgical operation. In resective epilepsy surgery, parts of the brain are removed in the hope that the resected parts contain the 'epileptic focus' and that resecting these will prevent the occurrence of further epileptic seizures.

RNA Ribonucleic acid. A single-stranded molecule which carries genetic information from DNA to the cell microsome where proteins are formed.

SCHIZOPHRENIA A form of psychosis. Schizophreniform is a term used in epilepsy practice to refer to the symptoms of an epileptic psychosis which resemble those in schizophrenia.

SCLEROSIS A hardening of bodily tissue, often colloquially referred to as scarring. Hippocampal sclerosis is a common finding in epilepsy and a cause of temporal lobe epilepsy.

SEQUENCING, GENETIC A technique for identifying the sequence of nucleic acids in DNA (or RNA).

SHARP WAVE An EEG pattern, similar to a spike in amplitude, but less pointed and of a duration of 70–200 milliseconds. It suggests the presence of epilepsy but is less specific than a spike.

SOMATOSENSORY A physiological term referring to the ability to detect such sensations as touch, pressure, pain, warmth and vibration.

SPECTROPHOTOMETER An instrument for measuring the intensity of radiation at different wavelengths. It is used in epilepsy mainly in the measure of drug levels in blood and other bodily fluids.

SPECTROSCOPY The study or measurement of the absorption and emission of radiation. In epilepsy practice, it is used to measure drug or biochemical concentrations in bodily fluids. Magnetic resonance spectroscopy is a form of spectroscopy using magnetic resonance scanning.

SPHENOID BONE The ridged bone of the skull lying underneath the temporal lobe.

SPIKE An EEG pattern of duration 20–70 milliseconds with high amplitude giving it a sharp and pointed appearance. It can occur ictally or inter-ictally and is strongly suggestive of the presence of epilepsy.

SPIKE AND WAVE (syn: Spike–wave) An EEG pattern comprising a spike followed by a slow wave. It is a waveform that is highly predictive of the presence of epilepsy. It can occur ictally or inter-ictally. Generalised 3/second spike–wave is a typical finding in Idiopathic Generalised Epilepsy.

STATUS EPILEPTICUS A condition in which epileptic seizures are prolonged, or repeated without recovery in between attacks.

STEREOTACTIC ELECTRO-ENCEPHALOGRAPHY (SEEG) Technique of recording EEG using intracerebral electrodes implanted stereotactically.

STEREOTAXIS A method of surgery in which the surgical target is defined in 3D space by calculation from spatially defined coordinates (fiducials).

STIGMA The negative and hostile attitudes of the public to individuals with epilepsy are sometimes referred to as the stigma associated with epilepsy. It has been divided into enacted and felt forms of stigma. Enacted stigma refers to attitudes which result in overt actions and felt stigma is an internal perception of stigma. Self-stigma is another term used to refer to the negative attitudes held by a person to his/her condition.

STIGMATA Distinguishing marks or characteristics of a specific disorder, such as epilepsy. These can be physical or mental marks. In the late nineteenth and early twentieth centuries it was widely held that epilepsy had specific stigmata, indicating the presence of degenerative germ plasm, a theory now discredited.

STIMULATION, CORTICAL The application of small electrical currents directly to the cerebral cortex. This is used for such purposes as mapping the cortex, detecting hyperexcitable regions and triggering epileptic seizures.

SUDDEN UNEXPECTED DEATH IN EPILEPSY (SUDEP) An occurrence in which a person with epilepsy dies suddenly without any obvious additional cause, usually in the aftermath of a seizure.

SULCUS The grooves (depressions) in the cerebral cortex seen on the surface of the brain.

SUSCEPTIBILITY GENES Genes in which variants contribute to the occurrence of a trait, such as epilepsy, but only to a relatively small degree. Such genetic variants contribute 'a susceptibility' to epilepsy but are not in themselves sufficient on their own to be a predominant cause.

SYMPTOMATIC SEIZURES/EPILEPSY Seizures/epilepsy occurring as a result of an identified pathological condition.

SYNDROME, EPILEPTIC This was defined in 1989 by the ILAE as '[a]n epileptic disorder characterised by a cluster of signs and symptoms customarily occurring together; these include such items as type of seizure, etiology, anatomy, precipitating factors, age of onset, severity, chronicity, diurnal and circadian cycling, and sometimes prognosis. However, in contradistinction to a disease, a syndrome does not necessarily have a common etiology and prognosis.' This definition still applies today (the syndromes identified by the ILAE in 1989 are show in Table 4.1.

SYNDROME, DOUBLE CORTEX A congenital anomaly of the cerebral cortex in which grey matter cells are embedded in white matter. It is due to a failure of the process of neuronal migration. Epilepsy is a common symptom.

SYNDROME, KLÜVER–BUCY A syndrome caused by bilateral medial temporal lobe ablation or lesioning.

SYNAPSE The microscopic structure which takes the form of a fluid filled gap, 20–40 nanometres wide, between two nerve cells. Transmission of nerve impulses across synapses is mediated by chemical neurotransmitters, released from the presynaptic neuron by an action potential, diffusing across the synapse and then binding to receptors on the surface of the post-synaptic neuron.

SYNCOPE The medical term for fainting. This occurs when the blood supply to the brain is critically decreased. It therefore has a different mechanism entirely from an epileptic seizure, which is due to excessive excitation in the brain and in which blood supply is actually increased. However, there are superficial clinical similarities and the diagnosis of the two conditions can be confused. Convulsive syndrome is a term used when convulsive movements are one of the symptoms of the syncope.

TELEMETRY, VIDEO-EEG A clinical investigation in which EEG and video are recorded simultaneously for long periods of time (sometimes days) in order to record epileptic discharges on the EEG and to correlate these with clinical symptoms.

TEMPORAL LOBECTOMY An operation in which a large portion of the temporal lobe is resected. An 'en bloc' temporal lobectomy is one in which the lobe is resected in one piece, allowing a detailed post-operative pathological analysis of its structure.

TENTORIUM A large dural fold which divides the brain and the cranial cavity into superior and inferior sections.

TERATOGENICITY (of antiepileptic drugs) The occurrence of congenital defects in the growing foetus caused by the ingestion of the drug by the mother when pregnant.

THALAMUS A grey matter structure deep in the cerebral hemispheres.

THALAMOCORTICAL CIRCUIT A neuronal network of thalamic and cortical neurones. Abnormalities of this network are thought to underpin the occurrence of absence seizures.

THERAPEUTIC DRUG MONITORING (TDM) An investigation in which the concentration of a drug in blood, or another body fluid/tissue, is measured as a way of monitoring drug effectiveness or side effects.

THERAPEUTIC RANGE (of antiepileptic drugs) The range of drug concentrations in the blood in which effectiveness is maximised and side effects minimised.

TOXAEMIA Poisoning in the blood by toxins or infection.

TRANSECTION, MULTIPLE SUBPIAL A form of epilepsy operation in which multiple superficial cuts are made through the cerebral cortex but no brain tissue is resected.

TREPANATION (Syn: trepanning) A form of operation in which a hole is cut through the bones of the skull. It has been a procedure used to treat epilepsy (by 'letting out the evil spirits') since the earliest recorded history and continued to be used until the early twentieth century (verb form: to trepan or trephine).

TRIAL, RANDOMISED CONTROLLED (RCT) A technique by which a drug effectiveness is assessed. It is a type of clinical trial in which bias is minimised and is considered the gold standard of clinical trials. This now usually has a 'parallel group' design in which patients are randomised to either placebo or the trial drug, and the effects of the drug are then observed over time in both arms. Previously a 'cross-over' design was preferred, in which the subject takes both the placebo and the trial drug in a randomised sequence.

UNCUS OR UNCINATE GYRUS An anatomical structure in the anterior hippocampus, commonly involved in epilepsy. Uncinate seizures were first described and localised by Hughlings Jackson in the celebrated case of Dr Z.

URIC ACID A chemical, the breakdown product (waste product) of proteins, found in blood. Most uric acid passes into the urine and is excreted from the body.

VACUOLATION The formation of 'vacuoles' (space, vesicles, bubbles). Vacuolation of brain tissue occurs in some brain diseases and also is produced as a side effect of the antiepileptic drug vigabatrin.

VENTRICULOGRAPHY A radiological technique in which the cerebrospinal fluid of the ventricles is replaced by air or some other substance (a contrast medium) to allow the ventricules to be visualised in a plain X-ray.

VERTEBRAL ARTERY An artery in the neck supplying the brain with blood.

WEST SYNDROME One form of infantile epileptic encephalopathy. It has characteristic symptoms and EEG findings, but many different causes.

WFN World Federation of Neurology, a professional association of neurologists and other medical personnel in the field of neurology.

X-RAY, PLAIN An X-ray taken with no computerised enhancements. The image is made up by a beam of X-rays directed at a bodily structure (such as the head) and recording the degree to which X-rays are able to pass through the tissues in their path.

BIBLIOGRAPHY

BOOKS, CHAPTERS, REPORTS AND MISCELLANEOUS MEDIA

Abstracts Read at the First International Eugenics Congress, University of London, July 1912 (London: Charles Knight and Co. Ltd., 1912).

Adie, W. J. and W. W. Wagstaffe, *A Note on a Series of 656 Cases of Gunshot Wound of the Head, with a Statistical Consideration of the Results Obtained*. Medical Research Committee Statistical Reports 1 (London: HMSO, 1918).

Adrian, E. D., *The Mechanism of Nervous Action: Electrical Studies of the Neurone* (Philadelphia: University of Pennsylvania Press, 1932).

Aicardi, J., *Diseases of the Nervous System in Childhood* (London: Mac Keith Press, 1992, 1998, 2009).

Aicardi, J., *Epilepsy in Children* (New York: Raven Press, 1986, 1994).

Aicardi, J., *Movement Disorders in Children*, with E. Fernandez Alvarez (Mac Keith Press, 2001).

Album du XVIe Congrès International de Médicine (Budapest: n.p., 1909), p. 123.

Alexander, W., *The Treatment of Epilepsy* (Edinburgh: Young J. Pentland, 1889).

Alvarez, L. W., 'Alfred Lee Loomis', in *Biographical Memoirs*, vol. 51 (Washington, DC: National Academies Press, 1980), pp. 308–41.

Aminoff, M. J., *Brown-Séquard: An Improbable Genius Who Transformed Medicine* (Oxford: Oxford University Press, 2011).

Andermann, F. (ed.), *Chronic Encephalitis and Epilepsy: Rasmussen's Syndrome* (Boston: Butterworth-Heinemann, 1991).

Anderson, T., *Mot Kveld* (Oslo: Aschehoug, 2003 [1900]).

Antony and the Johnsons, 'Epilepsy is dancing', available at www.youtube.com/watch?v=h32WC1aUQsc.

Armstrong, D., *Political Anatomy of the Body: Medical Knowledge in the Twentieth Century* (Cambridge: Cambridge University Press, 1983).

Armstrong, K., *Beginning the World* (London: MacMillan, 1983).

Arzimanaglou, A., A. Guerrini and J. Aicardi, *Aicardi's Epilepsy in Children* (Philadelphia: Lippencott, Williams and Wilkins, 2004).

Atlas: Epilepsy Care in the World (Geneva: World Health Organization, 2005).

Avanzini, G. and S. Franceschetti, 'Mechanisms of epileptogenesis', in S. Shorvon, E. Perucca and J. Engel (eds.), *The Treatment of Epilepsy*, 4th ed. (Oxford: Wiley-Blackwell, 2016), pp. 38–59.

B, David., *L'Ascension du Haut Mal* (Brussels: L'Association, 1996–2004).

B, David., *Epileptic*, trans. K. Thompson (London: Jonathan Cape, 2006).

Bagley, C., *The Social Psychology of the Child with Epilepsy* (London: Routledge and Kegan Paul, 1971).

Bailllarger, J., 'Théorie de l'automatisme', in *Recherches sur les maladies mentales*, vol. 1 (Paris: Impr. municipale, 1890), pp. 494–500.

Baldini, E., *Come il lupo* (Torino: Einaudi, 2006).

Baldwin, M. and Bailey, P. (eds.), *Temporal Lobe Epilepsy* (Springfield: Charles C. Thomas, 1958).

Bancaud, K., Talairach, J, Bonis, A., Szikla, G., Morel, P. and M. Bordas-Ferrer, *La stéréo-électro-encéphalographie dans l'épilepsie* (Paris: Masson, 1965).

Barclay, J. A., *A Caring Community: A Centenary History of the National Society for Epilepsy and the Chalfont Centre, 1892–1992* (London: National Society for Epilepsy, 1992).

Barker, P., *Regeneration* (London: Viking Press, 1991).

Barr, M. W., *The King of Thomond: A Story of Yesterday* (Boston: H. B. Turner, 1907).

Barr, M. W., *Mental Defectives: Their History, Treatment and Training* (Philadelphia: P. Blakiston's Son, 1904).

Barrow, R. L. and H. Fabing, *Epilepsy and the Law* (New York: Hoeber-Harper, 1956).

Barton, R., *Institutional Neurosis* (Bristol: John Wright, 1959).

Bateson, W. *Materials for the Study of Variation Treated with Especial Regard to Discontinuity in the Origin of Species* (London: Macmillan and Co., 1894).

Beers, C. W., *A Mind That Found Itself: An Autobiography* (New York: Longmans, Green, 1908).

Béjont, H., *The Lexicography of English: From Origins to Present* (Oxford: Oxford University Press, 2010).

Berger, J. A., *Fortunate Man: The Story of a Country Doctor* (London: Allan Lane, Penguin Press, 1967).

'Bernarr Macfadden', in *Encyclopedia Britannica* online (www.britannica.com/biography/ Bernarr-Macfadden, accessed 5 December 2019).

Berridge, V., *Health and Society in Britain since 1939* (Cambridge: Cambridge University Press, 1999).

Bevis, M. and J. Williams, *Edward Lear and the Play of Poetry* (Oxford: Oxford University Press, 2016).

Binet, A., *The Intelligence of the Feeble-Minded* (Baltimore: Williams & Wilkins, 1916).

Binet, A. and T. Simon, *Mentally Defective Children*, trans. W. B. Drummond (London: Edward Arnold, 1914).

Binswanger, O., *Die Epilepsie* (Vienna: Alfred Holder, 1899).

Bladin, P. F., *A Century of Prejudice and Progress: A Paradigm of Epilepsy in a Developing Society: Medical and Social Aspects: Victoria, Australia 1835–1950* (Melbourne: Epilepsy Society of Australia, 2001).

Blatty, W. P., *The Exorcist* (New York: Harper & Row, 1971).

Bloch, S. and P. Reddaway, *Russia's Political Hospitals: The Abuse of Psychiatry in the Soviet Union* (London: Victor Gollancz, 1977).

Bogen, J. E., 'Some historical aspects of callosotomy for epilepsy', in A. G. Reeves and D. W. Roberts (eds.), *Epilepsy and the Corpus Callosum 2* (New York: Plenum, 1985), pp. 107–21.

Bourke, J., 'Wartime', in R. Cooter and J. Pickstone (eds.), *Medicine in the Twentieth Century* (New York: Harwood, 2000), pp. 589–601.

Bourneville, D.-M., 'L'état de mal épileptique', in D.-M. Bourneville (ed.), *Recherches cliniques et thérapeutiques sur l'épilepsie & l'hystérie: Compte-rendu des observations recueillies à la Salpêtrière de 1872 à 1875* (Paris: Delahaye, 1876), pp. 1–24.

Bourneville, D.-M. and P. Regnard, *Iconographie photographique de la Salpêtrière, Service de M. Charcot*, 3 vols. (Paris: Delahaye, 1877–80).

Brand, R. and P. Kumar, 'Detailing gets personal: Integrated segmentation may be Pharma's key to "repersonalizing the selling process"', *PharmExec.com*, 1 August 2003 (www .pharmexec.com/view/detailing-gets-personal, accessed 31 October 2020).

Brandt, A. M. and M. Gardner, 'The golden age of medicine?', in R. Cooter and J. Pickstone (eds.), *Companion to Medicine in the Twentieth Century* (Amsterdam: Harwood, 2003), pp. 21–37.

Bratty v. *Attorney General for Northern Ireland* [1963] AC 386; House of Lords archive HL/ PO/JU/4/3/1079.

Bravais, L. F., *Recherches sur les symptômes et le traitement de l'épilepsie hémiplégique* (Paris: Didot le jeune, 1827).

Brazier, M. A. B. (ed.), *Epilepsy: Its Phenomena in Man* (New York: Academic Press, 1973).

Brazier, M. A. B., 'Historical introduction: The role of electricity in the exploration and elucidation of the epileptic seizure', in M. A. B. Brazier (ed.), *Epilepsy: Its Phenomena in Man* (New York: Academic Press, 1973), pp. 1–9.

Brazier, M. A. B., *A History of the Electrical Activity of the Brain: The First Half-Century* (London: Pitman Medical Publishing, 1961).

Broad, W. J. and N. Wade, *Betrayers of the Truth: Feud and Deceit in the Halls of Science* (New York: Simon and Schuster, 1982).

Brown-Séquard, E., *Researches on Epilepsy: Its Artificial Production in Animals and Its Etiology, Nature and Treatment in Man* (Boston: David Clapp, 1857).

Bruns, L., A. Cramer and T. Ziehen, *Handbuch der Nervenkrankheiten im Kindesalter* (Berlin: Karger, 1912).

Buck v. Bell, 274 U.S. 200 (1927).

Bucknill, J. and D. Tuke, *A Manual of Psychological Medicine* (London: J. Churchill, 1862).

Burleigh, M., *Ethics and Extermination: Reflections on Nazi Genocide* (Cambridge: Cambridge University Press, 1997).

Bumke, O., *Richtlinien für Schwangerschaftsunterbrechung und Unfruchtbarmachung aus gesundheitlichen Gründen* (Munich: Lehmann, 1936).

Burton, R., *The Anatomy of Melancholy, What It Is, with all the Kinds, Causes, Symptoms, Prognostics, and Several Cures of it. In Three Partitions. With their Several Sections, Members, and Subsections, Philosophically, Medically, Historically, Opened and Cut Up. By Democritus Junior. With a Satirical Preface, Conducing to the Following Discourse.* (1st edition. Oxford: printed for Henry Cripps, 1621). (n.b: The page numbers in text refer to the new edition published by Claxton [Philadelphia] in 1883).

Bucy, P. C., *Percival Bailey 1892–1973* (Washington, DC: National Academy of Sciences 1989).

Bush, V., *Science: The Endless Frontier. A Report to the President* (Washington, DC: United States Government Printing Office, 1945).

Calmeil, L. F., *De l'épilepsie, étudiée sous le rapport de son siège et de son influence sur la production de l'aliénation mentale* (Paris: Thése de Université de Paris, 1824).

Care of Epileptics: The Reid Report, Hansard, HL, vol. 327, cols. 474–87, 27 January 1972.

Carlyle, T., *On Heroes, Hero-Worship and the Heroic in History* (London: James Fraser, 1840).

Carpenter, W. B., *Principles of Human Physiology, with Their Chief Applications to Psychology, Pathology, Therapeutics, Hygiène, and Forensic Medicine* (Philadelphia: Blanchard and Lea, 1858).

Cartright, L., *Screening the Body: Tracing Medicine's Visual Culture* (Minneapolis: University of Minnesota Press, 1995).

Census of England and Wales for the Year 1861. Population Tables. Vol II. Ages, Civil Condition, Occupations, and Birth-Places of the People: With the Ages and Occupations of the Blind, of the Deaf-and-Dumb, and of the Inmates of Certain Public Institutions (London: HMSO, 1863).

Central Health Services Council, Ministry of Health, *Medical Care of Epileptics: Report of the Sub-Committee of the Central Health Services Council* (London: HMSO, 1956).

Chandler, R., *The Big Sleep* (New York: Knopf, 1939).

Charity Organisation Society, *The Epileptic and Crippled Child and Adult: A Report on the Present Condition of These Classes of Afflicted Persons, with Suggestions for their better Education and Employment* (London: Swan Sonnenschein, 1893).

Chat, L., *Electro Girl: Living a Symbiotic Existence with Epilepsy* (Raw Encounters Media, 2017).

Chauvel, P., 'Contribution of Jean Talairach and Jean Bancaud to epilepsy surgery', in H. O. Lüders and Y. G. Comair (eds.), *Epilepsy Surgery*, 2nd ed. (Philadelphia: Lippincott Williams and Wilkins, 2001), pp. 35–41.

The Chinese Classics, vol. 1, Confucian Analects, the Great Learning, and the Doctrine of the Mean, trans. J. Legge (Oxford: Clarendon, 1893).

Choyce, G. L., *The Potter's Wheel: How Epilepsy Changed My Life* (Atlanta: BDI Publishers, 2017).

Christie, A., *The ABC Murders* (London: Collins, 1936).

Christie, A., *Murder on the Links* (London: John Lane, 1923).

Christie, A., *Nemesis* (London: Collins, 1971).

Christie, D. A. and E. M. Tansey, 'Making the human body transparent: The impact of nuclear magnetic resonance and magnetic resonance imaging. The transcript of a Witness Seminar held at the Wellcome Institute for the History of Medicine, London, on 2 July 1996', in E. M. Tansey, D. A. Christie and L. A. Reynolds (eds.), *Wellcome Witnesses to Twentieth Century*

Medicine, 2 vols. (London: Wellcome Trust, 1998), pp. 1–74.

Clark, L. P., *Clinical Studies in Epilepsy* (New York: Utica NY State Hospitals Press, 1917).

Clark, L. P., 'Status epilepticus', ch. 12, in W. Spratling, *Epilepsy and Its Treatment* (Philadelphia: Saunders, 1904), pp. 195–220.

Clark, L. P. *Napoleon, Self-Destroyed* (New York: Jonathan Cape and Harrison Smith, 1929).

Clinical Standards Advisory Group (CSAG). *Services for Patients with Epilepsy* (London: The Department of Health, 2000).

Coatsworth, J. J., *Studies on the Clinical Efficacy of Marketed Antiepileptic Drugs*, NINDS Monograph No. 12, DHEW Publication No. (NIH) 73–51 (Washington, DC: US Government Printing Office, 1971).

Cobb, S., A. M. Frantz, W. Penfield and H. A. Riley (eds.), *The Circulation of the Brain and Spinal Cord: A Symposium on Blood Supply* (Baltimore: Williams & Wilkins, 1938).

Cochrane, A. L., *Effectiveness and Efficiency: Random Reflections on Health Services* (London: Nuffield Provincial Hospitals Trust, 1972).

Cockerell, O. and S. Shorvon, 'The economic cost of epilepsy', in S. Shorvon, D. Fish, D. Thomas (eds). *The Treatment of Epilepsy* (Oxford: Blackwell Science, 1996), pp. 114–19.

Coles, A., 'Temporal lobe epilepsy, Dostoyevsky and irrational significance', in A. Coles and J. Collicut (eds.), *Neurology and Religion* (Cambridge: Cambridge University Press, 2020), pp. 89–100.

Collier, C. K., 'Social implications and management', in P. H. Hoch and R. P. Knight (eds.), *Epilepsy: Psychiatric Aspects of Convulsive Disorders* (New York: Grune & Stratton, 1947), pp. 58–68.

Collins, W., *Poor Miss Finch* (New York: Harper, 1872).

Comfort, N., *The Science of Human Perfection* (New Haven: Yale University Press, 2012).

Committee for Proprietary Medicinal Products, *Opinion following an Article 12 referral for Vigabatrin: Background Information*, CPMP/1357/99 (Amsterdam: European Medicines Agency, 1999).

Committee on the Public Health Dimensions of the Epilepsies of the Institute of Medicine of the National Academies. *Epilepsy across the Spectrum, promoting health and understanding* (Washington, DC: National Academies Press, 2012).

Cook-Deegan, R., *The Gene Wars: Science, Politics and the Human Genome* (New York: Norton, 1994).

Cope, V. Z., *The Medical Balance-Sheet of War*. In *Some Famous General Practitioners and Other Medical Historical Essays* (London: Pitman Medical Publishing, 1961), pp. 169–83.

Cotton, H., *The Defective, Delinquent and Insane: The Relation of Focal Infections to Their Causation, Treatment and Prevention* (Princeton: Princeton University Press, 1921).

The Craig Colony for Epileptics at Sonyea in Livingston County, New York. Thirteenth Annual Report to the State Board of Charities, 1906 (https://ia803100.us.archive.org/1/items/b31687210/b31687210.pdf, accessed 27 July 2020).

Crichton, M. *The Andromeda Strain* (New York: Alfred A. Knopf, 1969).

Crichton, M., *The Terminal Man* (New York: Alfred A. Knopf, 1972).

Crichton, M., *Jurassic Park* (New York: Alfred A. Knopf, 1990).

Crichton, M., *Timeline* (New York: Alfred A. Knopf, 1999).

Crick, F., *What Mad Pursuit: A Personal View of Scientific Discovery* (New York: Basic Books, 1988).

Critchley, M., *Sir William Gowers, 1845–1915: A Biographical Appreciation* (London: Heinemann, 1949).

Critchley, M. and E. A. Critchley, *John Hughlings Jackson: Father of English Neurology* (Oxford: Oxford University Press, 1998).

Critser, G., *Generation RX: How Prescription Drugs Are Altering American Lives, Minds, and Bodies* (New York: Houghton Mifflin, 2005).

Currell, S. and C. Cogdell, *Popular Eugenics: National Efficiency and American Mass Culture in the 1930s* (Athens: Ohio University Press, 2006).

Cushing, H., *The Life of Sir Willliam Osler* (Oxford: The Clarendon Press, 1925).

Dam, M. and L. Gram, *Comprehensive Epileptology* (New York: Raven Press, 1991).

D'Amico, A., *Short Circuit: An Epileptic Journey* (Manchester Center: Shires Press, 2017).

Dana, F., *Text-book of Nervous Diseases for the Use of Students and Practitioners of Medicine* (New York: Willam Wood and Co., 1st ed., 1892).

Dandy, W. E., *Benign, Encapsulated Tumors in the Lateral Ventricles of the Brain: Diagnosis and Treatment* (Baltimore: Williams & Wilkins, 1934).

Dandy, W. E., 'The brain', in D. Lewis (ed.), *The Practice of Surgery: Clinical, Diagnostic Operative, Post-operative*, in association with J. Shelton Horsley, E. Starr Judd, G. P. Muller, T. S. Cullen and H. L. Kretschemer, vol. 12 (Hagerston: W. F. Prior Company, 1932), pp. 556–605.

Darwin, C., *On the Origin of Species by Means of Natural Selection, or Preservation of Favoured Races in the Struggle for Life* (London: John Murray, 1959).

De Haas, A. M. L. (ed.), *Lectures on Epilepsy* (Amsterdam: Elsevier, 1958).

Dejerine, J. J., *L'hérédité dans les maladies du système nerveux* (Paris: Asselin et Houzeau, 1886).

Delasiauve, L. I. F., *Traité de l'épilepsie: histoire, traitement, medicine légale* (Paris: Masson, 1854).

Delgado, J. M. R., *Physical Control of the Mind: Toward a Psychocivilized Society* (New York: Harper and Row, 1989).

De Swaan, A., *In Care of the State: Health Care, Education and Welfare in Europe and the USA in the Modern Era* (New York: Oxford University Press, 1988).

Deutsch, A., *The Shame of the States* (New York: Harcourt, Brace, 1948).

Devinsky, O. and M. D'Esposito (eds.), *Neurology of Cognitive and Behavioral Disorders* (Oxford: Oxford University Press, 2004).

Diätophilus, *Physische und psychologische Geschichte einer siebenjährigen Epilepsie. Nebst angehaengten Beitraegen zur körperlichen und Seelendiaetetik für Nervenschwache. Erste Haelfte. Reine Geschichte in chronologischer Ordnung. Zweite Haelfte. Beurtheilende Zergliederung und*

Ergaenzung der Thatsachen (Zurich: Orell, Füssli, 1798–9).

Dickens, C., *Bleak House* (London: Bradbury & Evans, 1853).

Dickens, C., *Oliver Twist*, 3 vols. (London: Richard Bentley, 1838).

Dickens, C., *Our Mutual Friend*, 2 vols. (London: Chapman and Hall, 1864–5).

Dicks, H., *Clinical Studies in Psychopathology* (London: Edward Arnold, 1939).

Dittrick, L., *Patient H. M.: A Story of Memory, Madness and Family Secrets* (New York: Random House, 2016).

Dollery, C., *The End of an Age of Optimism: Medical Science in Retrospect and Prospect* (London: Nuffield Provincial Hospitals Trust, 1978).

Dostoevsky, F, *Brothers Karamazov* ([English edition, trans. C. Garnett]. London: William Heinemann Ltd., 1912).

Dostoevsky, F. *The Idiot* ([English edition, trans. C. Garnett]. London: William Heinemann Ltd., 1913).

Dostoevsky, F. *The Possessed* ([English edition, trans. C. Garnett]. London: William Heinemann Ltd., 1914).

Dowbiggin, I., *Keeping America Sane* (Ithaca: Cornell University Press, 1997).

Doyle, A. C., *The Sign of the Four* (London: Spencer Blackett, 1890).

Doyle, A. C., *The Adventures of Sherlock Holmes* (London: George Newnes, 1892).

Dreifuss, F., 'Development of a comprehensive epilepsy program', in P. Robb (ed.), *Epilepsy Updated: Causes and Treatment* (Chicago: Year Book Medical Publishers, 1981), pp. 303–12.

Duckworth Williams, S. W., *On the Efficacy of the Bromide of Potassium in Epilepsy and Certain Psychical Affections* (London: John Churchill and Sons, 1860).

Duroselle, J. B., *Clemenceau* (Paris: Fayard, 1988).

Eadie, M. J., *The Flowering of a Waratah* (Sydney: John Libbey, 2000).

Echeverria, M. C., *De la trépanation dans l'épilepsie par traumatismes du crane* (Paris: Asseli, 1878).

Echeverria, M. C., *On Epilepsy: Anatomo-pathological and Clinical Notes* (New York: William Wood, 1870).

Eichenwald, K., *A Mind Unraveled* (New York: Ballantine Books, 2018).

Eiselsberg, A. von, *Lebensweg eines Chirurgen* (Innsbruck: Deutscher Alpenverlag, 1939).

Eiselsberg, A. von, 'Report on gunshot injuries of the brain', in Office of the Surgeon General, *War Surgery of the Nervous System: A Digest of the Important Medical Journals and Books Published during the European War* (Washington, DC: Government Printing Office, 1917), pp. 187–98.

Eissler, K. R., *Freud as an Expert Witness: The Discussion of War Neurosis between Freud and Wagner-Jauregg* (New York: International Universities Press, 1986).

Ellison, R. H., M. Placencia, A. Guvenor, et al., 'A programme of transcultural studies of epilepsy: Outline of objectives and study design', in J. Manelis, E. Bental, J. N. Loeper et al. (eds.), *Advances in Epileptology: The XVIIth Epilepsy International Congress* (New York: Raven Press, 1989), pp. 435–40.

Engel, J. Jr, 'Overview of surgical treatment of epilepsy', in S. Shorvon, E. Perucca and J. Engel (eds.), *The Treatment of Epilepsy*, 3rd edn (Oxford: Wiley-Blackwell, 2009), pp. 743–56.

Engel, J. Jr, *Seizures and Epilepsy*, 2nd ed. (Oxford: Oxford University Press, 2013).

Engel, J. Jr (ed.), *The Surgical Treatment of the Epilepsies* (New York: Raven Press, 1987).

Engel, J. Jr and D. A. Shewmon, 'Who should be considered as a surgical candidate?', in J. Engel Jr (ed.), *The Surgical Treatment of the Epilepsies*, 2nd ed. (New York: Raven Press, 1993), pp. 23–34.

Epilepsy Management at Primary Health Level in Rural China (Geneva: World Health Organization, 2009).

Ernst, R., *Weakness Is a Crime: The Life of Bernarr Macfadden* (New York: Syracuse University Press, 1991).

Esquirol, J.-É., *Des maladies mentales considerées sous les rapports médical, hygiénique et médico-légal* (Paris: J. B. Ballière, 1838).

Estabrook, A. H. and C. B. Davenport, *The Nam Family: A Study in Cacogenics*, Memoir No. 2 (Cold Spring Harbour: Eugenics Record Office, 1912).

Ettinger, A. B. and A. M. Kanner, *Psychiatric Issues in Epilepsy* (Philadelphia: Wolters Kluwer, 2001).

Evans, M., *The Nightingale Silenced and Other Late Unpublished Writings* (Dinas Powys: Honno, 2020).

Evans M., *A Ray of Darkness* (London: Arthur Barkar Ltd, 1952)

Ey, H., *Études psychiatriques* (Paris: Desclée de Brower, 1954).

Fadiman, A., *The Spirit Catches You and You Fall Down: A Hmong Child, Her American Doctors, and the Collision of Two Cultures* (New York: Farrar, Straus and Giroux, 1997).

Falret, J. P., *Maladies mentales et des asiles d'aliénés* (Paris: Ballière 1864).

Farmer, P., *Snakes and Ladders* (London: Little Brown and Co., 1993).

Farmer, P., *Snakes and Ladders* (London: Abacus, 1994).

Farreras, I. G., 'Establishment of the National Institute of Neurological Diseases and Blindness', in I. G. Farreras, C. Hannaway and V. A. Harden (eds.), *Mind, Brain, Body and Behavior* (Amsterdam: IOS Press, 2004), pp. 19–32.

Farreras, I. G., C. Hannaway and V. A. Harden (eds.), *Mind, Brain, Body and Behavior* (Amsterdam: IOS Press, 2004).

Feeble-Minded Persons (Control) Bill, Hansard, HC, vol. 38, col. 1474, 17 May 1912.

Feindel, W. and R. Leblanc, *The Wounded Brain Healed: The Golden Age of the Montreal Neurological Institute, 1934–1984* (Montreal: McGill-Queen's University Press, 2016).

Feinstein, A. R., *Clinical Judgment* (Baltimore: Williams & Wilkins, 1967).

Féré, C., *Épilepsie* (Paris: Gautier-Villars et fils, 1892).

Féré, C., *La famille névropathique. Théorie tératologique de l'hérédité et de la prédisposition morbides et de la dégénérescence* (Paris:Felix Alcan, 1894).

Féré, C., *Les épilepsies et les épileptiques* (Paris: Baillière, 1890).

Ferenczi, S., 'On epileptic fits, observations and reflections', in M. Balint (ed.), *Final Contributions to the Problems and Methods of*

Psycho-analysis (London: Howarth Press and the Institute of Psycho-analysis, 1955), pp. 197–204.

Ferenczi, S., 'The unwelcome child and his death instinct', in M. Balint (ed.), *Final Contributions to the Problems and Methods of Psycho-analysis* (London: Howarth Press and the Institute of Psycho-analysis, 1955), pp. 102–3.

Ferrier, D., *The Croonian Lectures on Cerebral Localisation Delivered before the Royal College of Physicians, June 1890* (London: Smith Elder, 1890).

Ferrier, D., *Functions of the Brain* (London: Smith Elder, 1876).

Ferrier, D., *Localisation of Cerebral Disease* (London: Smith, Elder, 1878).

Feyerabend, P., *Against Method* (London: Verso, 1975).

Feyerabend, P., *The Tyranny of Science*, ed. Eric Oberheim (London: Polity, 2011).

'Fifty-third day: Thursday, 7 February 1946, morning session', in *Nuremberg Trial Proceedings*, vol. 7 (New Haven: Lillian Goldman Law Library, 2008) (https://avalon.law.yale.edu/imt/02-07-46.asp, accessed 11 April 2021).

Flemming, F. *Pathologie und Therapie der Psychosen. Nebst Anhang: Über das gerichtsärztliche Verfahren bei Erforschung krankhafter Seelenzustände* (Berlin: Hirschwald, 1859).

Flexner, A., *Medical Education in the United States and Canada* (Washington, DC: Science and Health Publications, 1910).

Flood, E., 'What has been gained for the epileptics?', in *Transactions of the National Association for the Study of Epilepsy and the Care and Treatment of Epileptics*, vol. 4 (New York: Owen, 1906), pp. 120–30.

Foster, M., *A Text Book of Physiology*, assisted by C. S. Sherrington, 7th ed. (London: Macmillan, 1897).

Foucault, M. *Folie et Déraison: histoire de la folie à l'âge classique* (Paris: Plon, 1961). [English translation: *Madness and Civilisation* (London: Tavistock, 1964)].

Frank, L., *The Pleasure Shock: The Rise of Deep Brain Stimulation and Its Forgotten Inventor* (New York: Dutton, 2018).

Freud, S., 'Dostoevsky and parricide', in J. Strachey (ed. and trans.), *The Standard Edition of the Complete Psychological Works of Sigmund Freud*, vol. 21 (London: Hogarth, 1961), pp. 173–96.

Freud, S., *The Interpretation of Dreams*, trans. J. Strachey (New York: Basic Books, 1955).

Friedlander, W. J., *History of Modern Epilepsy: The Beginning, 1865–1914* (Westport: Greenwood Press, 2001).

Fukuyama, F., *The End of History and the Last Man* (New York: Free Press, 1992).

Fukuyama, Y., *Epilepsy Bibliography* (Tokyo: Child Neurology Institute, 2004).

Fulton, J. F., *Harvey Cushing: A Biography* (Springfield: Charles C. Thomas, 1946).

Gallo Diop, A. and I. Ndiae, 'Senegal', in J. Engel Jr and T. Pedley, *Epilepsy: A Comprehensive Textbook*, 2nd ed. (Philadelphia: Lippincott William & Wiilllkins, 2008), pp. 2909–18.

Garrod, A. E, *Inborn Errors of Metabolism* (London: Henry Frowde and Hodder & Stoughton, 1909).

Gastaut, H., *Dictionary of Epilepsy: Part 1: Definitions* (Geneva: World Health Organization, 1973).

Gastaut, H. and J.-L. Gastaut, 'Computerized axial tomography in epilepsy', in J. K. Penry (ed.), *Epilepsy: The Eighth International Symposium* (New York: Raven Press, 1977), pp. 5–15.

Gastaut, H., J. Roger and H. Lob (eds.), *Les états de mal épileptique* (Paris: Masson, 1967).

Geschwind, N., 'Pathogenesis of behavioural change in temporal lobe epilepsy', in A. A. Ward, J. K. Penry and D. Purpura, *Epilepsy*, vol. 61 (New York: Raven Press, 1983), pp. 355–70.

Gibbs, F. and E. Gibbs, *Atlas of Electroencephalography* (Cambridge, MA: Addison-Wesley, 1941).

Gibson, W. C., 'Sir Charles Sherrington O.M. P.R.S. (1847–1952)', in F. C. Rose (ed.), *Twentieth Century Neurology: The British Contribution* (London: Imperial College Press, 2001), pp. 1–7.

Glaser, G. H., J. K. Penry and D. M. Woodbury, *Antiepileptic Drugs: Mechanisms of Action* (New York: Raven Press, 1980).

Glasner, P., *Splicing Life: The New Genetics and Society* (London: Ashgate, 2004).

'Global actions on epilepsy and other neurological disorders', draft resolution, in *Seventy-third World Health Assembly*, A73/A/CONF./2, 9 November 2020 (Geneva: World Health Organization, 2020).

Global Burden of Epilepsy and the Need for Coordinated Action at the Country Level to Address Its Health, Social and Public Knowledge Implications, EB136/CONF./4 Rev.1 (Geneva: World Health Organization, 2015).

Gloor, P., *The Temporal Lobe and Limbic System* (Oxford: Oxford University Press, 1997).

Goddard, H. H., *Feeble-Mindedness, Its Causes and Consequences* (New York: Macmillan, 1914).

Goddard H. H., *The Criminal Imbecile* (New York: Macmillan, 1915).

Goddard, H. H., *The Kallikat Family: A Study in the Heredity of Feeble-Mindedness* (New York: Macmillan, 1916).

Goddard, H. H., *Psychology of the Normal and Subnormal* (New York: Dodd, Mead, 1919).

Goffman, E., *Asylums: Essays on the Condition of the Social Situation of Mental Patients and Other Inmates* (New York: Anchor Books, 1961).

Goffman, E., *Stigma: Notes on the Management of Spoiled Identity* (Englewood Cliffs: Prentice Hall, 1963).

Goldstein, J., *Console and Classify: The French Psychiatric Profession in the Nineteenth Century* (Cambridge: Cambridge University Press, 1987).

Goldstein, K., *Aftereffects of Brain Injuries in War, Their Evaluation and Treatment: The Application of Psychologic Methods in the Clinic* (London: William Heinemann, 1942).

Goncharov, I. A., *Oblomov*, trans. C. H. Hogarth (New York: Macmillan, 1915).

Goodman, J., 'Pharmaceutical industry', in R. Cooter and J. Pickstone (eds.), *Medicine in the Twentieth Century* (New York: Harwood, 2000), pp. 141–55.

Gotman, J., J. R. Ives and P. Gloor (eds.), *Long-Term Monitoring in Epilepsy* (Amsterdam: Elsevier, 1985).

Gould, S. J., *The Mismeasure of Man* (New York: Norton, 1981).

Gowers, W. *A Manual of Diseases of the Nervous System* (2 vols. London: J. & A. Churchill, 1886–8).

Gowers, W. R., *The Border-Land of Epilepsy: Faints, Vagal Attacks, Vertigo, Migraine, Sleep Symptoms, and Their Treatment* (London: J. & A. Churchill, 1907).

Gowers, W. R., *Epilepsy and Other Chronic Convulsive Disorders: Their Causes, Symptoms, & Treatment* (London: J. & A. Churchill, 1881).

Gowers, W. R., *Epilepsy and Other Chronic Convulsive Diseases: Their Causes, Symptoms, and Treatment*, 2nd ed. (London: Old Hickory Bookshop, 1901).

Grant, M. *The Passing of the Great Race* (New York: Charles Schribner's Sons, 1916).

Greyling, A. C., *Towards the Light: The Story of the Struggles for Liberty and Rights That Made the Modern West* (London: Bloomsbury, 2007).

Griesinger, W., *Mental Pathology and Therapeutics*, trans. C. L. Roberson and J. Rutherford (New York: New Sydenham Society, 1867).

Grinspoon, L. and P. Hedblom, *The Speed Culture: Amphetamine Use and Abuse in America* (Boston: Harvard University, 1975).

Groper, J., She Must Be Brought to Reason Somehow: Depictions of Epilepsy in Charles Dickens, George Eliot and Wilkie Collins, PhD Dissertation, Claremont Graduate University, 2011.

Grove, V. *Laurie Lee. The Well-Loved Stranger* (London: Viking, 1999).

Guelaen, P., E. Van Der Kleijn and U. Woudstra, 'Statistical analysis of pharmacokinetic parameters in epileptic patients chronically treated with anti-epileptic drugs', in H. Schneider, D. Janz, C. Gardner-Thorpe, H. Meinardi and A. Sherwin, A. (eds.) *Clinical Pharmacology of Anti-Epileptic Drugs* (Berlin: Springer-Verlag, 1975), pp. 2–10.

Guerreiro, C., 'Brazil', in J. Engel Jr and T. Pedley, *Epilepsy: A Comprehensive Textbook*, 2nd ed. (Philadelphia: Lippincott William & Wilkins, 2008), pp. 2849–57.

Hall, M., *On the Threatenings of Apoplexy and Paralysis; Inorganic Epilepsy; Spinal Syncope; Hidden Seizures; the Resultant Mania; etc.* (London: Longman, Brown, Breeen, and Longman, 1851).

Halstead, W. C., *Brain and Intelligence: A Quantitative Study of the Frontal Lobes* (Chicago: University of Chicago Press, 1947).

Hammond, W. A., *A Treatise on the Diseases of the Nervous System* (New York: D. Appleton, 1871).

Hardy, T., *The Mayor of Casterbridge: The Life and Death of a Man of Character*, 2 vols. (London: Smith, Elder, 1886).

Harvald, B., *Heredity in Epilepsy: An Electroencephalographic Study of Relatives of Epileptics* (Copenhagen: Ejnar Munksgaard, 1954).

Haward, F., *Report of the Medical Officer*, National Society of Epilepsy (1929).

Hearings before the subcommittee on children and youth of the Committee on Labor and Public Welfare United States Senate (93rd congress), parts 1–4. Washington, DC: US Government Printing Office, 1974.

Healy, D. *Pharmageddon* (Berkeley: University of California Press, 2012).

Heath, R. G., *Studies in Schizophrenia: A Multidisciplinary Approach to Mind–Brain Relationships* (Cambridge: Harvard University Press, 1954).

Heron, D., *Mendelism and the Problem of Mental Defect. 1. A Criticism of Recent American Work* (London: Delau, 1913).

Herpin, T., *Des accès incomplets d'épilepsie* (Paris: J.-B. Ballière, 1867).

Herpin, T., *Du prognostic et du traitement curatif de l'épilepsie* (Paris: J.-B. Ballière, 1852).

Hill, A. B., *Principles of Medical Statistics* (London: Lancet, 1937).

Hill, D., and G. Parr (eds.), *Electroencephalography: A Symposium on Its Various Aspects* (London: Macdonald, 1950).

Hill, D., and G. Parr (eds.), *Electroencephalography: A Symposium on Its Various Aspects* (2nd ed.) (London: Macdonald, 1963).

Hill, S. R. *Hannah Arendt* (London: Reaktion Books, 2021).

Himwich, H. E., *Brain Metabolism and Cerebral Disorders* (London: Bailière, Tindall & Cox, 1951).

History of the Epilepsy Movement in the United States (Washington, DC: Epilepsy Foundation of America).

Hobsbawm, E., *The Age of Extremes: The Short Twentieth Century History 1914–1991* (London: Abacus, 1995).

Hoch, P. H. and R. P. Knight (eds.), *Epilepsy: Psychiatric Aspects of Convulsive Disorders* (New York: Grune & Stratton, 1947).

Hoche, A. and R. Binding, *Die Freigabe der Vernichtung Lebensunwerten Lebens* (Meiner: Leipzig, 1920).

Hodgson, H. and S. Shorvon, *Physicians and War* (London: Royal College of Physicians, 2016).

Hollingsworth, J. R., *A Political Economy of Medicine: Great Britain and the United States* (Baltimore: Johns Hopkins University Press, 1986).

Hopkins, A. *Epilepsy.* (London: Chapman and Hall, 1987).

Hopkins, A., S. Shorvon, G. Cascino (eds.), *Epilepsy.* 2nd ed. (London: Chapman and Hall, 1995).

Höring, C. F. F., Über Epilepsie, inaugural dissertation (Tübingen, 1859).

Howard, T. and J. Rifkin, *Who Shall Play God?* (New York: Dell, 1977).

Hughes, J. R., *EEG in Clinical Practice* (Boston: Butterworths, 1982).

Hume, D., *A Treatise of Human Nature*, reprinted from the Original Edition in three volumes and edited, with an analytical index, by L. A. Selby-Bigge (Oxford: Clarendon Press, 1896).

Hunter, R. and I. Macalpine, *Psychiatry for the Poor: 1851 Colney Hatch Asylum – Friern Hospital 1973. A Medical and Social History* (London: Wm Dawson & Sons, 1974).

ILAE, British Branch, *Bylaws* (London: Privately published, 1984).

Illich, I., *Limits to Medicine. Medical Nemesis: The Expropriation of Health* (London: Pelican Books, 1977).

Jackson, H. A., 'A suggestion for the treatment of epilepsy', unpublished manuscript labelled

'For private circulation', December 1899, Queen Square Archive, QSA/837, London.

Jackson, J. H., 'On classification and on methods of investigation', in J. Taylor (ed.), *Selected Writings of John Hughlings Jackson, vol. 1, On Epilepsy and Epileptiform Convulsions* (London: Hodder and Stoughton, 1931), pp. 191–2.

Jaffe, R., *After the Reunion* (New York: Delacorte Press, 1985).

Janz, D., *Die Epilepsien, Spezielle Pathologie und Therapie* (Stuttgart: Georg Thieme, 1969).

Janz, D., M. Dam, A, Richens, L. Bossi, H. Helge and D. Schmidt, *Epilepsy, Pregnancy, and the Child* (Proceedings of a Conference held 14–16 Sept., 1980, West Berlin, Germany) (New York: Raven Press, 1982).

Jasper, H., 'Electroencephalography', in W. Penfield and T. C. Erickson, *Epilepsy and Cerebral Localization* (Springfield: Charles C. Thomas, 1941), pp. 380–454.

Jasper, H. H., A. A. Ward Jr and A. Pope, *Basic Mechanisms of the Epilepsies* (Boston: Little, Brown, 1969).

Jelliffe, S. E., 'Fifty years of American neurology', in *Semi-centennial Anniversary Volume of the American Neurological Association (1875–1044)* (Albany: Boyd, 1924), pp. 386–438.

Jennett, B., *Epilepsy after Blunt Head Injuries* (London: William Heinemann Medical Books, 1962).

Jennett, B., *Epilepsy after Non-missile Head Injuries* (London: William Heinemann Medical Books, 1975).

Jilek-Aall, L., *Call Mama Doctor: African Notes of a Young Woman Doctor* (Saanichton: Hancock House, 1979).

Jones, K., *Asylums and After: A Revised History of the Mental Health Services: From the Early 18th Century to the 1990s* (London: Athlone Press, 1993).

Judt, T., *Postwar: The History of Europe since 1945* (London: William Heinemann, 2005).

Kapur, J. and R. L. Macdonald, 'Status epilepticus: A proposed pathophysiology', in S. D. Shorvon, F. Dreifuss, D. R. Fish, et al., *The Treatment of Epilepsy* (Oxford: Blackwell Science, 1996), pp. 258–68.

Kater, M. H., *Doctors under Hitler* (Chapel Hill: University of North Carolina Press, 1989).

Kerr, A. and T. Shakespeare, *Genetic Politics: From Eugenics to Genome* (Cheltenham: New Clarion Press, 2002).

Kesey, K., *One Flew over the Cuckoo's Nest* (New York: Viking, 1962).

Kevles, B. H., *Naked to the Bone: Medical Imaging in the Twentieth Century* (New Brunswick: Rutgers University Press, 1997).

Kevles, D. J., *In the Name of Eugenics: Genetics and the Uses of Human Heredity* (Cambridge, MA: Harvard University Press, 1985).

Kleinman, A., *The Illness Narratives: Suffering, Healing and the Human Condition* (New York: Basic Books, 1988).

Koch, J. L. A., *Die psychopathischen Minderwertigkeiten* (Ravensburg: Otto Maier, 1891–93).

Kopeloff, N., L. M. Kopeloff and B. L. Pacella, 'The experimental production of epilepsy in animals', in P. H. Hoch and R. P. Knight (eds.), *Epilepsy: Psychiatric Aspects of Convulsive Disorders* (London: Heineman, 1948), pp. 163–80.

Kraepelin, E., *Psychiatrie: ein kurzes Lehrbuch für Studierende und Ärzte*, 2nd ed. (Leipzig: Verlag von Ambr. Abel, 1887).

Kraepelin, E., *Ein Lehrbuch der Psychiatrie* (Leipzig: Barth, 1903–4).

Krause, F., *Surgery of the Brain and Spinal Cord: Based on Personal Experiences*, vols. 2 and 3, trans. M. Thorek (New York: Rebman, 1912).

Krause, F. and H. Schum, 'Die spezielle Chirurgie der Gihirnkrankheiten', in *Die epileptischen Erkrankungen*, vol. 2 (Stuttgart: Enke, 1932).

Kubin, A., *The Other Side: A Fantastic Novel*, trans. D. Lindley (New York: Crown, 1967).

Kuhn, T. S., *The Structure of Scientific Revolutions* (Chicago: University of Chicago Press, 1962).

Lader, M., *Psychiatry on Trial* (Harmondsworth: Penguin, 1977).

Laidlaw, J. and M. Laidlaw, 'People with epilepsy – living with epilepsy', in J. Laidlaw and A. Richens (eds.), *A Textbook of Epilepsy* (Edinburgh: Churchill Livingstone, 1976), pp. 355–85.

Laidlaw, J. and A. Richens (eds.), *A Textbook of Epilepsy* (Edinburgh: Churchill Livingstone, 1976).

Laing, R. D., *The Divided Self: An Existential Study in Sanity and Madness* (London: Harmondsworth, 1960).

Laing, R. D., *The Self and Others* (London: Tavistock Publications, 1961).

Landolt, H., 'Serial EEG investigations during psychotic episodes in epileptic patients and during schizophrenic attacks', in A. M. L. De Haas (ed.), *Lectures on Epilepsy* (Amsterdam: Elsevier, 1958), pp. 91–133.

Thomson, L. A., *Half a Century of Medical Research*, 3 vols. (London: HMSO, 1973–5).

Lawrence, C., 'Continuity in crisis: medicine 1914–1945', ch. 3 in W. F. Bynum, A. Hardy, S. Jacyna et al., *The Western Medical Tradition 1800–2000* (Cambridge: Cambridge University Press, 2006), pp. 247–390.

Lawrence, C., *Medicine in the Making of Modern Britain 1700–1920* (London: Routledge, 1994).

Lear, E., *Edward Lear Diaries*, 5 January 1858, Houghton Library, Harvard University, MS Eng. 797.3 (https://iiif.lib.harvard.edu/manifests/view/drs:44446328$5i, accessed 26 July 2020).

Le Fanu, J., *The Rise and Fall of Modern Medicine* (London: Little, Brown, 1999).

Lekka, V., *The Neurological Emergence of Epilepsy: The National Hospital for the Paralysed and Epileptic (1870–1895)* (Heidelberg: Springer, 2015).

Lennox, M. A., 'Professor Gastaut's contribution to the International League Against Epilepsy', in R. J. Broughton (ed.), 'Henri Gastaut and the Marseilles school's contribution to the neurosciences', *Electroencephalogr. Clin. Neurophysiol. Suppl.*, 35 (1982), 9–12.

Lennox, W. G., *Epilepsy and Related Disorders*, with the collaboration of Margaret A. Lennox, 2 vols. (Boston: Little, Brown, 1960).

Lennox, W. G., *The Health and Turnover of Missionaries* (New York: Advisory Committee, 1933).

Lennox, W. G. and S. Cobb, *Epilepsy, from the Standpoint of Physiology and Treatment* (Baltimore: Williams & Wilkins, 1928).

Lennox, W. G., H. H. Merritt and T. E. Bamford, *Epilepsy* (Baltimore: Williams & Wilkins, 1947).

Letchworth, W. P., *Care and Treatment of Epileptics* (New York, G. P. Putnam's Sons, 1900).

Letchworth, W. P., *The Insane in Foreign Countries* (New York: G. P. Putnam's Sons, 1889).

Lévi-Strauss, C., *Wild Thought*, trans. J. Mehlman and J. Leavitt (Chicago: University of Chicago Press, 2021 [1962]).

Lévi-Strauss, C. and D. Eribon, *Conversations with Claude Lévi-Strauss*, trans. P. Wissig (Chicago: Chicago University Press, 1988).

Lewis, D. (ed.), *Practice of Surgery: Clinical, Diagnostic Operative, Post-operative*, in association with J. Shelton Horsley, E. Starr Judd, G. P. Muller et al., 12 vols. (Hagerstown, MD, 1927–33).

Lewis, W. B (Bevan Lewis), *A Text-Book of Mental Diseases* (London: Charles Griffin, 1889).

Lifton, R. J., *The Nazi Doctors: Medical Killing and the Psychology of Genocide* (New York: Basic, 1986).

Lives of the Fellows of the Royal College of Physicians (Munk's Roll), vol. 6 (http://munksroll.rcplondon.ac.uk/Biography/Details/1801, accessed 1 December 2019).

Lombardo, P. A., *Three Generations, No Imbeciles: Eugenics, the Supreme Court, and Buck v. Bell* (Baltimore: Johns Hopkins University Press, 2008).

Lombroso, C., *Criminal Man*, trans. M. Gibson and N. H. Rafter (Durham: Duke University Press, 2006). [This contains an English language translation of all the Italian editions of Lombroso's book: 1st, 1876; 2nd, 1878; 3rd, 1884; 4th, 1889 and 5th, 1896–7].

Lombroso, C., *The Man of Genius* (London: W. Scott, 1896).

London, J., *Told in the Drooling Ward* (New York: Macmillan, 1910).

Lorenz, F., 'Über den Status epilepticus', unpublished medical dissertation, University of Kiel (1890).

Love, A. G. and C. B. Davenport, *Defects in Drafted Men* (Washington, DC: Government Printing Office, 1920).

Lucas, R. C., *Bradshaw Lecture on Some Points in Heredity* (London: Adlard, 1912).

Lüders, H. O., 'History of invasive EEG', in S. D. Lhatoo, P. Kahane and H. O. Lüders (eds.), *Invasive Studies of the Human Epileptic Brain* (Oxford: Oxford University Press, 2019), pp. 3–18.

Lüders, H. O., *Textbook of Epilepsy Surgery* (London: Informa, 2008).

Lüders, H. O. and Y. G. Comair (eds.), *Epilepsy Surgery*, 2nd ed. (Philadelphia: Lippincott Williams and Wilkins, 2001).

Lundborg, H. B. *Die progressive Myoklonus-Epilepsie (Unverricht's Myoklonie)* (Uppsala: Almqvist and Wiksell, 1903).

Mad Doctors, by One of Them. Being a Defence of Asylum Physicians Against Recent Aspersions Cast on Them, and An Examination into the Functions of the Lunacy Commission, Together with a Scheme of Lunacy Reform (London: Swan Sonnenschein & Co, 1890).

Maddox, B., *Freud's Wizard: The Enigma of Ernest Jones* (London: John Murray, 2006).

Maeder, A., *Die Sexualität der Epileptiker* (Leipzig: Franz Deuticke, 1909).

Magoni, L. B., *All Eyes on Me: Epilepsy 'You Are Not Alone'* (self-published, 2019).

Malzberg, B., 'The incidence and prevalence of intramural epilepsy', in P. H. Hoch and R. P. Knight (eds.), *Epilepsy: Psychiatric Aspects of Convulsive Disorders* (New York: Grune & Stratton, 1947).

Mann, T., *Buddenbrooks: The Decline of a Family*, trans. H. T. Lowe-Porter (London: Martin Secker, 1952 [1901]).

Mann, T., *Confessions of Felix Krull, Confidence Man*, trans. D. Lindley (London: Secker & Warburg, 1955 [1922]).

Mann, T., 'Dostoyevsky – within limits', in J. W. Angell (ed.), *The Thomas Mann Reader* (New York: Knopf, 1930), pp. 434–49.

Mann, T., *The Magic Mountain*, trans. H. T. Lowe-Porter (London: Vintage, 1999 [1924]).

Mark, V. H. and F. R. Ervin, *Violence and the Brain* (New York: Harper and Row, 1970).

Mason, D., *The Secret Vice: Masturbation in Victorian Fiction and Medical Culture* (Manchester: Manchester University Press, 2008).

Maudsley, H., *Body and Mind* (London: D. Appleton, 1871).

Maudsley, H., *The Physiology of Mind*, 3rd ed., rev. and enlarged (London: Macmillan, 1878).

Maudsley, H., *Responsibility in Mental Disease* (New York: H. S. King, 1874).

McKeown, T., *The Role of Medicine: Dream, Mirage or Nemesis?* (London: Nuffield Provincial Hospitals Trust, 1976).

McKim, W. D., *Heredity and Human Progress* (New York: G. P. Putnam's, 1900).

McLuhan, M. and B. R. Powers, *The Global Village: Transformations in World Life and Media in the 21st Century* (Oxford: Oxford University Press, 1992).

McMillan, T., *Disappearing Acts* (New York: Viking Penguin, 1989).

Medical Research Committee, *4th Annual Report* (London: HMSO, 1918).

Menninger, K., *The Vital Balance: The Life Process in Mental Health and Illness* (New York: Viking Penguin, 1963).

The Mental Deficiency Act (London: HMSO, 1913).

Meyrink, G., *The Golem*, trans. M. Pemberton (London: Victor Gollancz, 1928).

Millichap, J. G., *Febrile Convulsions* (New York: Macmillan, 1968).

Millichap, J. G., 'William Lennox', in S. Ashwal (ed.), *The Founders of Child Neurology* (San Francisco: Norman, 1990), pp. 758–63.

Ministry of Health, *National Assistance Act. 1948. Welfare of Handicapped Persons: The Special Welfare Needs of Epileptics and Spastics* (London: HMSO, 1953).

Mitchell, W. P., *Recent Social Trends in the United States: Report of the President's Research Committee on Social Trends*, 2 vols. (New York: McGraw-Hill, 1933).

Mittelmann, B., 'Psychopathology of epilepsy', in P. H. Hoch and R. P. Knight (eds.), *Epilepsy: Psychiatric Aspects of Convulsive Disorders* (New York: Grune & Hatton, 1947), pp. 136–48.

Moll, A. and F. Balke, *Die Fürsorge für die Epileptischen. Zwei Vorträge, gehalten auf der zweiten südwestdeutschen Conferenz für innere*

Mission in Bruchsal am 11. Oktober 1865 (Stuttgart: J. F. Steinkopf, 1866).

Moniz, A. E., Diagnostic des tumeurs cérébrales et épreuve de l'encéphalographie artérielle (Paris: Masson & Cie).

Morante, E., History: A Novel, trans. W. Weaver (New York: Alfred Knopf, 1977).

Moreau, L. L., La psychologie morbide dans ses rapports avec la philosophie de l'histoire (Paris: Masson, 1859).

Morel, B. A., Études cliniques sur les maladies mentales considérés dans leur nature, leur traitement, et dans leur rapport avec la médecine légale des aliénés, 2 vols. (Nancy: Grimblot et Veuve Raybois, 1852–3).

Morel, B. A., Traité des dégénérescences physiques, intellectuelles et morales de l'espèce humaine et des causes qui produisent ces variétés maladives (Paris: J. B. Baillière, 1857).

Morel, B. A., Traité des maladies mentales (Paris: Masson, 1860).

Müller, J., Über den feineren Bau und die Formen der krankhaften Geschwülste (Berlin: G Reimer, 1838).

Murphy, E., After the Asylums: Community Care for People with Mental Illness (London: Faber and Faber, 1991).

Muskens, L. J. J., Epilepsy: Comparative Pathogenesis, Symptoms, Treatment, foreword by C. S. Sherrington (London: Baillière, Tindall and Cox, 1928). (The Dutch language edition was published in 1924).

Myerson, A., The Inheritance of Mental Diseases (Baltimore: Wiliiams & Wilkins, 1925).

Myerson, A., J. B. Ayer, T. J. Putnam et al., Eugenical Sterilization: A Reorientation of the Problem (New York: Macmillan, 1936).

National Epilepsy Act. Hearing before the subcommittee on health of the committee on labor and public welfare, United States senate, eighty-first congress. First session on S.659, May 4 1949. (Washington, DC: United States Government Printing Office, 1949)

Nevins, M., A Tale of Two 'Villages': Vineland and Skillman, NJ (Bloomington: Universe, 2009).

Newmark, M. E. and J. Kiffin Penry, The Genetics of Epilepsy: A Review (New York: Raven Press, 1980).

Niedermeyer, E. and F. Lopes Da Silva. Electroencephalography: Basic Principles, Clinical

Applications and Related Fields (Philadelphia: Lippincott Williams & Wilkin 5 editions, 1983, 1987, 1993, 1999, 2005, 2011). [6th and 7th editions renamed: Schomer, D. L. and F. Lopes da Silva (eds.) Niedermeyer's Electroencephalography: Basic Principles, Clinical Applications and Related Fields (6th ed. Philadelphia: Lippincott Williams & Wilkins, 2011; 7th ed. Oxford: Oxford University Press, 2017)].

Niedermeyer, E., 'Depth electroencephalography', in E. Niedermeyer and F. Lopes da Silva (eds.), Electroencephalography: Basic Principles, Clinical Applications and Related Fields, 5th edn (Philadelphia: Lippincott Williams & Wilkins, 2005), pp. 733–48.

Nordau, M., Degeneration, translated from the second edition of the German work (London: William Heinemann, 1895).

Norman, M. Night Mother (London: Josef Weinberger Ltd, 1982).

Nothnagel, H., 'Epilepsy and eclampsia', trans. J. H. Emerson, in H. von Ziemssen (ed.), Cyclopaedia of the Practice of Medicine, vol. 14 (New York: William Wood, 1877), pp. 182–314.

O'Connor, N. and J. Tizard, The Social Problem of Mental Deficiency (London: Pergamon, 1956).

O'Donohoe, N. V, Epilepsies of Childhood (London: Butterworths, 1979).

OECD Health Data 2000 (Paris: CREDDOC/ OECD, 2000).

Oppenheim, H. Lehrbuch der nervenkrankheiten (Berlin: S. Karger, 1894).

Ormerod, J. On Heredity in Relation to Disease (London: Adlard and Son, 1908).

Orwell, G., 'Looking back at the Spanish war', in A Collection of Essays 1903–1950 (San Diego: Harcourt, 1953).

Osler, W. The Principles and Practice of Medicine: Designed for the Use of Practitioners and Students of Medicine (New York: D. Appleton and Company, 1892).

Otolano, G., The Two Cultures Controversy: Science, Literature and Cultural Politics in Postwar Britain (Cambridge: Cambridge University Press, 2009).

Ounsted, C., J. Lindsay and R. Normal, Biological Factors in Temporal Lobe Epilepsy, Clinics in

Developmental Medicine 22 (London: Spastics Society Education and Information Unit and William Heinemann Medical Books, 1966).

Overy, R., *The Morbid Age: Britain between the Wars* (London: Allen Lane, 2009).

Page, I. H., *Chemistry of the Brain* (London: Baillière, Tindall & Cox, 1937).

Pagel, J., *Biographisches Lexikon hervorragender Ärzte des neunzehnten Jahrhunderts* (Berlin: Urban und Schwarzenberg, 1901).

Pollak, R., *The Episode* (New York: New American Library, 1986)

Panayiotopoulos, T., *The Epilepsies: Seizures, Syndromes and Management* (Chipping Norton: Bladon, 2005).

Pappworth, M. H., *Human Guinea Pigs: Experimentation on Man* (London: Routledge and Kegan Paul, 1967).

Parsons, T. *The Structure of Social Action*. (New York: Free Press, 1937).

Pascal, B., *De l'Esprit géométrique et de l'Art de persuader*. In Pascal, B. *Œuvres complètes*, vol. 3 (Paris: Hachette, 1871), pp. 163–82.

Pascal, B., *Pensées*, ed. and trans. R. Ariew (Indianapolis: Hackett, 2005).

Pellock, J. M., D. R. Nordli Jr, R. Sankar et al., *Pediatric Epilepsy: Diagnosis and Therapy* (New York: Demos Medidical, 2016).

Penfield, W., 'The anatomy of temporal lobe seizures', in L. van Bogaert and J. Radermecker (eds.), *First International Congress of Neurological Sciences*, vol. 3 (London: Pergamon Press, 1949), pp. 514–27.

Penfield, W. G. (ed.), *Cytology and Cellular Pathology of the Nervous System*, 3 vols. (New York: Paul B. Hoeber, 1932).

Penfield, W. G., *The Difficult Art of Giving: The Epic of Alan Gregg* (Boston: Little, Brown, 1967).

Penfield, W. G., *No Man Alone* (Boston: Little, Brown, 1977).

Penfield, W. and T. C. Erickson, *Epilepsy and Cerebral Localization* (Springfield: Charles C. Thomas, 1941).

Penfield, W. and H. Jasper, *Epilepsy and the Functional Anatomy of the Human Brain* (Boston: Little, Brown, 1954).

Penfield, W. and K. Kristiansen, *Epileptic Seizure Patterns* (Springfield: Charles C. Thomas, 1950).

Penfield, W. and T. Rasmussen, *The Cerebral Cortex of Man: A Clinical Study of Localisation of Function* (New York: Macmillan, 1950).

Pennybacker, J., Unpublished memoirs (The Royal College of Surgeons of England, 1961).

Penry, J. K., R. G. Porter, A. A. Wolf et al., *The Absence Seizure* [film] (Washington, DC: National Audiovisual Archive, 1972).

Penrose, L. S., *The Biology of Mental Defect*, with a preface by J. B. S. Haldane, rev. ed. (London: Sidgwick and Jackson, 1959).

Penrose, L. S., *A Clinical and Genetic Study of 1280 Cases of Mental Defect (the 'Colchester Survey')* (London: Her Majesty's Stationery Office, 1938).

Penrose, L. S., *Mental Defect* (London: Sidgwick & Jackson, 1933).

Penrose, L. S., *The Social Problem of Mental Deficiency* (London: Pergamon Press, 1956).

People with Epilepsy: Report of a Joint Sub-Committee of the Standing Medical Advisory Committee and the Advisory Committee on the Health and Welfare of Handicapped Persons (Chairman: J. J. A. Reid) (London: Department of Health and Social Security, 1969).

Pernick, M. S., *The Black Stork: Eugenics and the Death of 'Defective' Babies in American Medicine and Motion Pictures since 1915* (Oxford: Oxford University Press, 1996).

Piotrowski, Z. A., 'The personality of the epileptic', in P. H. Hoch and R. P. Knight (eds.), *Epilepsy: Psychiatric Aspects of Convulsive Disorders* (New York: Grune & Hatton, 1947), pp. 89–108.

Pippenger, C. E., J. K. Penry and H. Kutt, *Antiepileptic Drugs: Quantitative Analysis and Interpretation* (New York: Raven Press, 1978).

Polanyi, K., *Origins of Our Time: The Great Transformation* (New York: Farrar & Rinehart, 1944).

Polanyi, M. *Science, Faith and Society* (Oxford: Oxford University Press, 1946).

Poliakoff, S., *The Lost Prince* (London: Methuen, 2003).

Policy Implications of the Computed Tomography (CT) Scanner: An Update (Washington, DC: US Government Printing Office, 1981).

Pope, A., A. A. Morris, H. Jasper et al., 'Histochemical and action potential studies on epileptogenic areas of cerebral cortex in man and the monkey', ch. 15 in W. G. Lennox, H. H. Merritt and T. E. Bamford (eds.), *Epilepsy: Proceedings of the Association Held Jointly with the International League Against Epilepsy, December 13 and 14, 1946* (Baltimore: Williams & Wilkins, 1947), pp. 218–33.

Portal, Le Baron, *Observations sur la nature et le traitement de l'épilepsie* (Paris: J.-B. Baillière, 1827).

Porter, R., *The Greatest Benefit to Mankind: A Medical History of Humanity from Antiquity to the Present* (London: Harper Collins, 1997).

Powell, E., *Address to the National Association of Mental Health Annual Conference, 9 March 1961*, Nuffield Trust (www.nuffieldtrust.org .uk/public/health-and-social-care-explained/ the-history-of-the-nhs/enoch-powell-address-to-the-national-association-of-mental-health-annual-conference-9-march-1961/#address-to-the-national-association-of-mental-health-annual-conference-9-march-1961, accessed 15 August 2020).

Powys, J. C., *The Art of Growing Old* (London: Jonathan Cape, 1944).

Powys, J. C., *Auto Biography* (London: John Lane, 1934).

Powys, J. C., *Dostoievsky* (London: John Lane, 1946).

Powys, J. C., *Ducdame* (Garden City: Doubleday, Page, 1925).

Powys, J. C., *A Glastonbury Romance* (London: John Lane, 1933).

Powys, J. C., *Owen Glendower: An Historical Novel* (New York: Simon and Schuster, 1941).

Powys, J. C., *Visions and Revisions: A Book of Literary Devotions* (New York: G. Arnold Shaw, 1915).

Powys, J. C., *Wolf Solent* (New York: Simon and Schuster, 1929).

Preston, J., 'Paul Feyerabend', in *Stanford Encyclopedia of Philosophy*, Stanford University,

1997. Article published 26 August 1997; last modified 24 August 2020 (https://plato.stanford .edu/entries/feyerabend/, accessed 22 December 2020).

Preston, R., *Epilepsy: A Review of Basic and Clinical Research*, PHS Publication No. 1357, NINDS Monograph No. 1 (Washington, DC: US Department of Health, Education, and Welfare, 1965).

Price, J. C., K. L. Kogan and L. R. Tompkins, 'The prevalence and incidence of extramural epilepsy', in P. H. Hoch and R. P. Knight, *Epilepsy: Psychiatric Aspects of Convulsive Disorders* (New York: Grune & Stratton, 1947), pp. 48–57.

Pritchard, J. C., *A Treatise on Diseases of the Nervous System: Part the First, Comprising Convulsive and Maniacal Affections* (London: Thomas and George Underwood, 1822).

Procter, R. N., *Racial Hygiene: Medicine under the Nazis* (Cambridge, MA: Harvard University Press, 1988).

Prout, T. P. and L. P. Clark, 'Pathology of epilepsy', in W. Spratling, *Epilepsy and Its Treatment* (Philadelphia: Saunders, 1904), pp. 309–35.

Public Health Service Advisory Committee on the Epilepsies, *Minutes of Meeting, 9 February 1967* (Bethesda MD: National Institutes of Health, 1967).

Purkinje, J. E. and G. Valentin, *De phaenomeno Generali et Fundamentali motus Vibratorii Continui in Membranis tum Externis tum Internus Animalium Plurimorum et Superiorum et Inferiorum Ordinuum Obvii. Commentatio Physiologica*, vol. 1 (Breslau: Aug. Schultz, 1835).

Purpura, D. P., J. K. Penry, D. B. Tower et al. (eds.), *Experimental Models of Epilepsy: A Manual for the Laboratory Worker* (New York: Raven Press, 1972).

Putnam, J. J. *Addresses on Psycho-Analysis*. With a preface by Sigmund Freud. (Vienna: The International Psycho Analytic Press, 1921; published posthumously)

Putnam, T. J., 'The demonstration of the specific anti convulsant action of diphenylhydantoin and related compounds', in F. J. Ayd and B. Blackwell (eds.), *Discoveries in Biological Psychiatry* (Philadelphia: Lippincott, 1970), pp. 85–90.

Putney, M. J., *Dearly Beloved* (London: Penguin Publishing Group, 1990)

Quadfasel, F. A. and A. E. Walker, 'Problems of posttraumatic epilepsy in an army general hospital', in W. G. Lennox, H. H. Merritt and T. E. Bamford (eds.), *Epilepsy: Proceedings of the Association held jointly with the International League Against Epilepsy, December 13 and 14, 1946* (New York: Williams and Wilkins, 1947), pp. 461–75.

Qvarnström, G., *Från Öbacka till Urbs. Ludvig Nordströms Småstad och Världsstadsdröm* (Stockholm: Albert Bonniers Förlag, 1954).

Quinn, N. A., 'A year at the Salpêtrière', unpublished, Queen Square Archives (2020).

Rabot, L. *De la myoclonie épileptique* (Paris: Georges Carré et C. Naud, 1899).

Rasmussen, T., 'The role of surgery in the treatment of focal epilepsy', in P. Carmel (ed.), *Clinical Neurosurgery. Proceedings of the Congress of Neurological Surgeons in Toronto, Ontario, Canada* (Baltimore: Williams and Wilkins, 1969), pp. 288–314.

Rechtin, E., *Systems Architecting of Organizations: Why Eagles Can't Swim* (Boca Raton: CRC Press, 2000).

Recore, K., *Brain Storm: An Electrifying Journey* (Bandon: Robert D. Reed, 2019).

Reeves, A. G. and D. W. Roberts (eds.), *Epilepsy and the Corpus Callosum 2* (New York: Plenum, 1985).

Report of the Global Campaign Against Epilepsy Demonstration Project: Epilepsy Management at Primary Health Level in Rural China (Geneva: World Health Organization, 2009).

Report of the Mental Deficiency Committee (London: HMSO, 1929).

Report of the Royal Commission on the Care and Control of the Feeble-Minded (London, 1908).

Report of the Royal Commission on University Education in London (Haldane) (London: HMSO, 1913).

Report of the War Office Committee of Inquiry into 'shell-shock' (London: HMSO, 1922).

Report of the Working Group on Services for People with Epilepsy: A Report to the Department of Health and Social Security, The Department of Education and Science and The Welsh Office (Winterton Report) (London: HMSO, 1986).

Reynolds, J. R., *Epilepsy: Its Symptoms, Treatment, and Relation to Other Chronic Convulsive Diseases* (London: John Churchill, 1861).

Reynolds, J. R., *A System of Medicine* (3 vols.) (London: John Macmillan, 1866–79).

Richens, A., 'Clinical pharmacology and medical treatment', in J. Laidlaw and A. Richens (eds.), *A Textbook of Epilepsy* (Edinburgh: Churchill Livingstone, 1976), pp. 185–247.

Richens, A., 'The St Bartholomew's Hospital quality control scheme for antiepileptic drugs', in H. Meinardi and A. J. Rowan, *Advances in Epileptology 1977 (Proceedings of the 13th Congress of the International League Against Epilepsy and 9th Symposium of the International Bureau for Epilepsy)* (Amsterdam: Swets and Zeitlingere, 1978), pp. 239–42.

Riese, W., *The Conception of Disease: Its History, Its Versions and Its Nature* (New York: Philosophical Library, 1945).

Rinck, P. A., *Magnetic Resonance in Medicine: The Basic Textbook of the European Magnetic Resonance Forum*, 11th edn (BoD, 2017) (www.magnetic-resonance.org, accessed 15 August 2020).

Rivers, W. H. R., *Medicine Magic and Religion* (London: Keegan Paul, 1917).

Rivett, G., *The Development of the London Hospital System, 1823–1982* (London: King Edward's Hospital Fund for London, 1986).

Rivett, G., *National Health Service History, Nuffield Trust, London, UK* (www.nuffieldtrust.org.uk/files/2019-11/nhs-history-book/58-67/powell-s-water-tower-speech.html, accessed 15 August 2020).

Robb, B., *Sans Everything* (London: Nelson, 1967).

Roberts, F., *Seizure Mama and Rose: An Epilepsy Memoir* (self-published, 2020).

Robinson, R., *Electricity* (London: Picador, 2007).

Rodin, E., *The Prognosis of Patients with Epilepsy* (Springfield: Thomas, 1968).

Roger, J., C. Dravet, M. Bureau et al. (eds.), *Epileptic Syndromes in Infancy, Childhood and Adolescence* (London: J. Libbey Eurotext, 1985).

Rogers v. *Whitaker* [1992] HCA 58; (1992) 175 CLR 479 F.C. 92/045.

Romberg, M. H., *A Manual of the Nervous Diseases of Man*, vol. 1 and vol 2, trans. and ed. E. H. Sieveking (London: Sydenham Society, 1853).

Rose, F. C., *History of British Neurology* (London: Imperial College Press, 2012).

Roth, J., *Job: The Story of a Simple Man*, trans. D. Thompson (New York: Viking, 1931).

Rowland, L. P., *NINDS at 50: An Incomplete History Celebrating the Fiftieth Anniversary of the National Institute of Neurological Disorders and Stroke*, NINDS Publication 01-4161 (Washington, DC: National Institutes of Health, 2001).

Rushdie, S. *Midnight's Children* (London: Jonathan Cape, 1981).

Rushdie, S. *Satanic Verses* (London: Jonathan Cape, 1986).

Salzman, M., *Lying Awake* (New York: Knopf, 2000).

Sale of Food and Drug Act 1875, Chapter 63. (www.legislation.gov.uk/ukpga/1875/63/ enacted, accessed 24 May 2022).

Scambler, G., *Epilepsy: The Experience of Illness* (London: Tavistock/Routledge, 1989).

Schmidt, D. and S. Shorvon, *The End of Epilepsy* (Oxford: Oxford University Press, 2016).

Schneider, J. F., *Burnet – Ferguson – Schneider: A Family History* (Lulu, 2013).

Schneider J. F. and P. Conrad, *Having Epilepsy: The Experience and Control of Illness* (Philadelphia: Temple University Press, 1983)

Scholz, W., *Die Krampfschädigungen des Gehirns* (Berlin: Springer, 1951).

Schroeder van der Kolk, J., *On the Minute Structure and Functions of the Medulla Oblongata and the Proximate Causes and Rational Treatment of Epilepsy.* (Translated from the original) (London: Sydenham Society, 1859).

Schweitzer, A. *Decay and the Restoration of Civilization The Philosophy of Civilization* (London: A&C Black Ltd, 1923).

Séguin, É., *Traitement moral, hygiène et éducation des idiots et des autres enfants arriérés ou retardés dans leur développement, agités de mouvements involontaires, débiles, muets non-sourds, bègues, etc.* (Paris: Baillière, 1846).

Shakespeare, W., *Othello* (Oxford: Clarendon Press, 1622).

Shelley, M., *Frankenstein; or, The Modern Prometheus*, 3 vols. (London: Lackington, Hughes, Harding, Mavor, & Jones, 1818).

Shephard, B., *Headhunters: The Search for the Science of the Mind* (London: Bodley Head, 2014).

Sherrington, C. S., *The Integrative Action of the Nervous System* (London: Archibald Constable, 1906).

Shorvon, S. D., 'The concept of causation in epilepsy', in S. D. Shorvon, R. Guerrini, S. Schachter et al. (eds), *Causes of Epilepsy*, 2nd ed. (Cambridge: Cambridge University Press, 2019), pp. 1–7.

Shorvon, S. D., 'Definition (terminology) and classification in epilepsy: A historical survey and current formulation, with special reference to the ILAE', in S. D. Shorvon, E. Perucca and J. Engel Jr (eds.), *Treatment of Epilepsy*, 4th ed. (Oxford: Wiley-Blackwell, 2016), pp. 1–23.

Shorvon, S. D., 'The enigmatic figure of Leon Pierce Clark and his contribution to epilepsy', *Epilepsia Open,* 5 Mar (2022). doi: 10.1002/epi4.12589.

Shorvon, S. D., *Status Epilepticus: Its Clinical Features and Treatment in Children and Adults* (Cambridge: Cambridge University Press, 1994).

Shorvon, S. D, The Drug Treatment of Epilepsy: Towards More Effective Anticonvulsant Assessment and Therapeutics, MD thesis, University of Cambridge, 1982.

Shorvon, S. D., F. Andermann, G. Bydder et al. (eds.), *Magnetic Resonance Scanning and Epilepsy* (London: Plenum Press, 1994).

Shorvon, S. D., F. Andermann and R. Guerrini, *The Causes of Epilepsy: Common and Uncommon*

Causes in Adults and Children (Cambridge University Press: Cambridge, 2011).

Shorvon, S. and A. Compston, *Queen Square: A History of the National Hospital and Its Institute of Neurology* (Cambridge: Cambridge University Press, 2019).

Shorvon, S. D. and P. J. Farmer, 'Epilepsy in developing countries: A review of epidemiological, sociocultural and treatment aspects', in M. R. Trimble (ed.), *Chronic Epilepsy, Its Prognosis and Management* (Chichester: Wiley & Sons, 1989).

Shorvon, S. D., R. Guerrini, S. Schachter et al. (eds), *Causes of Epilepsy: Common and Uncommon Causes in Adults and Children*, 2nd ed. (Cambridge: Cambridge University Press, 2019).

Shorvon, S. D., Y. M. Hart, J. W. A. S. Sander et al., *The Management of Epilepsy in Developing Countries: An 'ICEBERG' Manual* (London: Royal Academy of Medical Services, 1991).

Shorvon, S. and G. Weiss, 'The International League Against Epilepsy – the first period: 1909–1952', in S. Shorvon, G. Weiss, G. Avanzini, et al. (eds.), *The International League Against Epilepsy 1909–2009: A Centenary History* (Oxford: Wiley-Blackwell, 2009), pp. 1–44.

Shorvon, S., G. Weiss, G. Avanzini et al., *The International League Against Epilepsy 1909–2009: A Centenary History* (Chichester: Wiley-Blackwell, 2009).

Shorvon, S. D., F. Dreifuss, D. Fish and D. Thomas (eds), *The Treatment of Epilepsy* (Oxford: Blackwell Science, 1996).

Shorvon, S. D., E. Dodson, D. R. Fish and E. Perucca (eds), *The Treatment of Epilepsy*, 2nd ed. (Oxford: Blackwell Science, 2004).

Shorvon, S. D., E. Perucca and J. Engel (eds), *Treatment of Epilepsy*, 3rd ed. (Oxford: Wiley-Blackwell, 2009).

Shorvon, S. D., E. Perucca and J. Engel (eds), *Treatment of Epilepsy*, 4th ed. (Oxford: Wiley, 2016).

Shryock, R. H., *American Medical Research: Past and Present* (New York: The Commonwealth Fund, 1947).

Sieveking, E. H., *On Epilepsy and Epileptiform Seizures, Their Causes, Pathology, and Treatment* (London: John Churchill, 1859; 2nd ed., rev. and enlarged: London: John Churchill, 1861).

Silverman, M., P. R. Lee and M. Lydecker, *Prescriptions for Death: The Drugging of the Third World* (Berkelely: University of California Press, 1982).

Singer, P. *Animal Liberation* (New York: Random House, 1975).

Skidelsky, R., *Keynes: The Return of the Master* (London: Allen Lane, 2009).

Slater, L. J., *Lying: A Metaphorical Memoir* (New York: Random House, 2000).

Snow, C. P., *The Two Cultures and the Scientific Revolution* (Cambridge: Cambridge University Press, 1959).

Spark, M., *The Bachelors* (New York: Avon Books, 1960).

Spielmeyer, W., 'Zur Pathogenese örtlich elektiver Gehirnveränderungen', *in Arbeiten aus der Deutschen Forschungsanstalt für Psychiatrie in München (Kaiser-Wilhelm-Institut)* (Berlin: Springer, 1926), pp. 313–36.

Spratling, W., *Epilepsy and Its Treatment* (Philadelphia: Saunders, 1904).

Srinivas, H. V., *A Saga of Indian Epilepsy Association: 40 Years of Journey* (Bangalore: Indian Epilepsy Association, 2013).

Starr, P., *The Social Transformation of American Medicine: The Rise of a Sovereign Profession and the Making of a Vast Industry* (New York: Basic Books, 1982).

Stern, K., *The Pillar of Fire* (New York: Harcourt, Brace, 1951).

Sternbach, L. H., 'The benzodiazepine story', in E. Jucker (eds.), *Progress in Drug Research*, vol. 22 (Basel: Birkhäuser, 1978), pp. 230–64.

Sternbach, L., 'The story of the benzodiazepines', in R. G. Priest, U. Vianna Filho, R. Amrein et al. (eds.), *Benzodiazepines Today and Tomorrow. Proceedings of the 1st International Symposium on Benzodiazepines in Rio de Janeiro, 28–30 September 1979* (Lancaster: MTP Press, 1980), pp. 5–18.

Stevenson, R. L., *Strange Case of Dr Jekyll and Mr Hyde* (London: Longmans, Green and Co., 1886).

Stirling, J., *Representing Epilepsy: Myth and Matter* (Liverpool: Liverpool University Press, 2010).

Stoker, B., *Dracula* (London: Archibald Constable, 1897).

Sussman, R. W., *The Myth of Race: The Troubling Persistence of an Unscientific Idea* (Cambridge, MA: Harvard University Press, 2014).

Szasz, T., *The Myth of Mental Illness: Foundations of a Theory of Personal Conduct* (New York: Hoeber-Harper, 1961).

Talairach, J., M. David, P. Tournoux et al., *Atlas d'anatomie stéréotaxique: repérage radiologique indirect des noyaux gris centraux des régions mésencéphalo-sous-optique et hypothalamique de l'homme* (Paris: Masson, 1957).

Talairach, J., and G. Szikla, *Atlas of Stereotaxic Anatomy of the Telencephalon* (Paris: Masson, 1967).

Talbot, F., *The Treatment of Epilepsy* (London: Cassell, 1930).

Tallis, R., *Aping Mankind: Neuromania, Darwinitis and the Misrepresentation of Humanity* (Durham: Acumen, 2011).

Taylor, B., *The Last Asylum: A Memoir of Madness in our Times* (London: Hamish Hamilton, 2014).

Taylor, J. (ed.), *Selected Writings of John Hughlings Jackson, vol. 1, On Epilepsy and Epileptiform Convulsions* (London: Hodder and Stoughton, 1931).

Temkin, O., *The Falling Sickness: A History of Epilepsy from the Greeks to the Beginnings of Modern Neurology*, 2nd ed. (Baltimore: Johns Hopkins University Press, 1971).

Thomas, R., *The Modern Practice of Physic* (London: Longman, 1813).

Thomson, M., *The Problem of Mental Deficiency: Eugenics, Democracy and Social Policy in Britain c. 1870–1959* (Oxford: Clarendon Press, 1998).

Thompson, J. W., *A History of Historical Writing, vol. 2, The Eighteenth and Nineteenth Centuries* (New York: Macmillan, 1942).

Timmermann, C. 'Clinical research in postwar Britain: The role of the Medical Research Council', in C. Hannaway (ed.), *Biomedicine in the Twentieth Century* (Amsterdam: IOS Press, 2008), pp. 231–54.

Tissot, S. *Onanism: or, a Treatise upon the Disorders Produced by Masturbation; or, the Dangerous Effects of Secret and Excessive Venery* (trans. A. Hume). (London: printed for the translator, 1776) [The Frenchlanguage edition was: L'Onanisme. Dissertation sur les maladies produites par la Masturbation. Lausanne, Chapuis, 1773].

Tissot, S. *Traité de l'épilepsie* (Paris: Didot de jeune, 1770).

Toman, J. and L. S. Goodman, 'Conditions modifying convulsions in animals', ch. 10 in W. G. Lennox, H. H. Merritt and T. E. Bamford (eds.), *Epilepsy: Proceedings of the Association, Held Jointly with the International League Against Epilepsy, December 13 and 14, 1946* (Baltimore: Williams & Wilkins, 1947), pp. 141–63.

Tonnini, S., *Le epilessie in rapporto alla degenerazione* (Torino: Bocca, 1891).

Tower, D. G., 'The evidence for a neurochemical basis of seizures', in M. Baldwin and P. Bailey (eds.), *Temporal Lobe Epilepsy* (Springfield: Charles C. Thomas, 1958), pp. 301–48.

Tredgold, A. F., *Mental Deficiency (Amentia)* (London: Ballière, Tindall and Cox, 1908).

Tredgold, A. F., *A Text-Book of Mental Deficiency*, 6th ed. (Baltimore: W. Wood, 1937).

Trimble, M. R. (ed.), *The Psychopharmacology of Epilepsy* (Wiley: Chichester, 1985).

Trimble, M. R. and B. Schmitz, *Forced Normalisation and Alternative Psychoses of Epilepsy* (Peterfield: Wrightson Biomedical, 1998).

Trostle, J. 'Social aspects: Stigma, beliefs and measurement', in J. Engel Jr and T. Pedley, *Epilepsy: A Comprehensive Textbook*, vol. 2. (Philadelphia: Lippincott William & Wilkins, 1997), pp. 2183–9.

Tucker, W. H., *The Science and Politics of Racial Research* (Urbana: University of Illinois Press, 1994).

Turda, M., *The History of East-Central European Eugenics, 1900–1945: Sources and Commentaries* (London: Bloomsbury, 2015).

Turner, W. A., *Epilepsy: A Study of the Idiopathic Disease* (London: Macmillan, 1907).

US Commission for the Control of Epilepsy and Its Consequences, *Plan for Nationwide Action on Epilepsy*, 4 vols. (Bethesda: National Institutes of Health, 1977).

Vaizey, J., *National Health* (Oxford: Martin Robertson, 1984).

Valentin, A. and G. Alarcon, *Introduction to Epilepsy* (Cambridge, Cambridge University Press, 2012).

Van Bogaert, L. and J. Radermecker (eds.), *First International Congress of Neurological Sciences, Brussels, July 21 –28, 1957*, 5 vols. (London: Pergamon Press, 1959).

Van Emde Boas, W. and P. Boon. 'The development of epilepsy surgery in the Netherlands and Belgium', ch 10, in H. Luders (ed.), *Textbook of Epilepsy Surgery* (London: Informa, 2008), 84–96

Veith, G. and R. Wicke, *Cerebrale Differenzierungsstörungen bei Epilepsie. Jahrbuch 1968* (Köln-Opladen: Westdeutscher Verlag, 1968).

Vincent, J., *Inside the Asylum* (London: George Allen & Unwin, 1948).

Virchow, R., *Die Cellularpathologie in ihrer Begründung auf physiologische und pathologische Gewebelehre* (Berlin: Verlag von August Hirschwald, 1858).

Vogt, H., *Die Epilepsie des Kindesalters* (Berlin: Karger, 1910).

Voisin, J., *L'épilepsie* (Paris: Félix Alcan, 1897).

Von Eiselsberg, A., 'Report on gunshot injuries of the brain', in Office of the Surgeon General, *War Surgery of the Nervous System: A Digest of the Important Medical Journals and Books Published during the European War* (Washington, DC: Government Printing Office, 1917).

Von Krafft-Ebing, R., *Psychopathia Sexualis*, trans. F. J. Redman (New York: Rebman, 1900).

Wada, J. and J. K. Penry, *Advances in Epileptology: the Xth Epilepsy International Symposium* (New York: Raven Press, 1980).

Walker, A. E., *Posttraumatic Epilepsy* (Oxford: Blackwell Scientific, 1949).

Walker, A. E., C. Marshall and E. N. Beresford, 'Electrocorticographic characteristics of the cerebrum in posttraumatic epilepsy', in W. G. Lennox, H. H. Merritt and T. E. Bamford (eds.), *Epilepsy: Proceedings of the Association Held Jointly with the International League Against Epilepsy, December 13 and 14, 1946* (New York: Williams & Wilkins, 1947), pp. 502–15.

Wallace, F. A., *Pushing for Cushing in War and Peace* (Framingham: Damianos Publishing, 2015).

Wallace, S. J., *The Child with Febrile Seizures* (London: Wright, 1988).

Wallace D. J. and K. Farrell. *Epilepsy in Children*. (London: Arnold, 2004).

Wallin, J. *Children with Mental and Physical Handicaps* (New York: Prentice Hall, 1949).

Walker, A. S. *Clinical Problems of War* (Canberra: Australian War Memorial, 1956).

Walshe, F. M. R., *Diseases of the Nervous System*, 5th ed. (Baltimore: Williams and Wilkins, 1947).

Walter, W. G., *The Living Brain* (London: Duckworth, 1952).

Ward, A. A., 'Perspectives for surgical therapy of epilepsy', in A. A. Ward, J. K. Penry and D. Purpura (eds.), *Epilepsy (Research Publications: Association for Research in Nervous and Mental Disease Publications, Vol. 61)* (New York: Raven Press, 1983), pp. 371–90.

Ware, M. and M. Mabe, *The STM Report: An Overview of Scientific and Scholarly Journal Publishing*, 4th ed. (Lincoln: STM, 2015).

Watson, P., *The German Genius: Europe's Third Renaissance, the Second Scientific Revolution and the Twentieth Century* (London: Simon & Schuster, 2010).

Watson, P., *A Terrible Beauty: The People and Ideas That Shaped the Modern Mind – A History* (London: Weidenfeld & Nicolson, 2000).

Watson, W., 'The incidence of epilepsy following cranio-cerebral injury', in W. G. Lennox, H. H. Merritt and T. E. Bamford (eds.), *Epilepsy: Proceedings of the Association, Held*

Jointly with the International League Against Epilepsy December 13 and 14, 1946 (New York. Baltimore: Williams & Wilkins, 1947), pp. 216–28.

Webster, C., 'Medicine and the welfare state 1930–1970', in R. Cooter and J. Pickstone (eds.), *Medicine in the Twentieth Century* (Amsterdam: Harwood, 2000), pp. 121–42.

Weindling, P., *Health, Race and German Politics between National Unification and Nazism 1870–1945* (Cambridge: Cambridge University Press, 1989).

Weiss, G. and S. D. Shorvon, 'International League Against Epilepsy – the second period: 1953–1992', in S. Shorvon, G. Weiss, G. Avanzini et al., *The International League Against Epilepsy 1909–2009: A Centenary History* (Chichester: Wiley-Blackwell, 2009), pp. 45–96.

Weisz, G., *Divide and Conquer: A Comparative History of Medical Specialization* (Oxford: Oxford University Press, 2006).

Wellcome Trust Genetic Timeline (originally available at: https://wellcomelibrary.org/collections/digital-collections/makers-of-modern-genetics/genetics-timeline [URL defunct at time of publication]).

Wells, H. G., *Kipps: The Story of a Simple Soul* (London: Macmillan, 1905).

Wernicke, C., *Der Aphasische Symptomencomplex: eine psychologische Studie auf anatomischer Basis* (Breslau: Max Cohn & Weigert, 1874).

West, J. B., *High Life: A History of High-Altitude Physiology and Medicine* (New York: Oxford University Press, 1989).

Whiteley, W. W., 'Department of Neurosurgery', ch. 40 in F. B. Wagner Jr. (ed.), *Thomas Jefferson University – Tradition and Heritage* (Philadelphia Thomas Jefferson University, 1989), pp. 639–40 (http://jdc.jefferson.edu/wagner2/34, accessed 2 August 2020).

Whitman, W., 'One's-self I sing', in F. Murphy (ed.), *Walt Whitman: The Complete Poems* (London: Penguin, 2004), p. 37.

Willis, T., *Pathologiae cerebri et nervosi generis specimen. In quo agitur de morbis convulsivis et de scorbuto* (Amsterdam: Danielem Elzevirium, 1668).

Wilson, C., *The Anatomy of Courage* (London: Constable, 1945).

Wilson, S. A. K., 'The epilepsies', in O. Bumke and O. Foerster (eds.), *Handbuch der Neurologie*, vol. 17 (Berlin: Springer, 1935), pp. 1–87.

Wilson, S. A. K. (finshed posthumously by Bruce, A. N.), *Neurology*, 2 vols. (Baltimore: Williams & Wilkins, 1940).

Wittkower, E. and J. P. Spillane, 'Survey of the literature of neurosis in war', in E. Miller (ed.), *The Neuroses in War* (London: Macmillan, 1940), pp. 1–32.

Wolf, P. (ed.), *Epileptic Seizures and Symptoms* (London: J. Libbey, 1994).

Wood, J. C., *Clinical Gynecology* (Philadelphia: Boericke and Tafel, 1917).

Woodbury, D. M., J. K. Penry and R. P. Schmidt *Antiepiletic Drugs* (New York: Raven Press, 1972).

Wyllie, E., *Treatment of Epilepsy* (Philadelphia: Lippincott Williams & Wilkins; 4 editions: 1992, 1997, 2001, 2005).

Wyllie, E., G. Cascino, B. Gidal and H. Goodkin, *Wyllie's Treatment of Epilepsy* (Philadelphia: Lippincott Williams & Wilkins, 2010).

Wyllie, E., G. Cascino, B. Gidal and H. Goodkin, *Wyllie's Treatment of Epilepsy* (Philadelphia: Wolters Kluwer, 2015).

Wyllie, E., B. Gidal, H. Goodkin and T. Loddenkemper, J. Sirven, *Wyllie's Treatment of Epilepsy* (Philadelphia: Wolters Kluwer, 2021).

York, G. K. and D. A. Steinberg, *An Introduction to the Life and Work of John Hughlings Jackson with a Catalogue Raisonné of His Writings* (London: Wellcome Trust, 2006).

Yealland, L. R., *Hysterical Disorders of Warfare* (London: Macmillan, 1918).

Zeepvat, C., *Prince Leopold: The Untold Story of Queen Victoria's Youngest Son* (London: Sutton, 1998).

Zielinski, J. J., 'Epidemiology', in J. Laidlaw and A. Richens (eds.), *A Textbook of Epilepsy* (Edinburgh: Churchill Livingstone, 1976).

Zola, É., *Le Bête Humaine*, trans. R. Pearson (Oxford: Oxford University Press, 1996).

JOURNALS AND WEBSITES

Abbott Labs to pay $1.5 billion to resolve criminal & civil investigations of off-label promotion of Depakote', *Justice News* (www.justice.gov/opa/pr/abbott-labs-pay-15-billion-resolve-criminal-civil-investigations-label-promotion-depakote, accessed 15 December 2020).

Adrian, E. D. and B. H. C. Matthews, 'The Berger rhythm: Potential changes from the occipital lobes in man', *Brain*, 57 (1934), 355–85.

Adrian, E. D. and B. H. C. Matthews, 'The interpretation of potential waves in the cortex', *J. Physiol.*, 81 (1934), 440–71.

Adrian, E. D. and G. Moruzzi, 'Impulses in the pyramidal tract', *J. Physiol.*, 97 (1939), 153.

Aicardi, J. 'Jean Aicardi: My circuitous path to becoming a French child neurologist and epileptologist', *J. Child. Neurol.* 28 (2013), 409–15.

Aicardi, J. and J. J. Chevrie, 'Consequences of status epilepticus in infants and children', *Adv. Neurol.*, 34 (1983), 115–25.

Aicardi, J. and J. J. Chevrie, 'Convulsive status epilepticus in infants and children: a study of 239 cases', *Epilepsia*, 11 (1970), 187–97.

Aird, R. B., 'Mode of action of brilliant vital red in epilepsy', *Arch. Neurol. Psychiatry*, 42 (1939), 700–23.

Akelaitis, A. J., 'Studies on the corpus callosum. II. The higher visual functions in each homonymous field following complete section of the corpus callosum', *Arch. Neurol. Psychiatry*, 45 (1941), 788–96.

Akelaitis, A. J., 'Studies on the corpus callosum. VII. Study of language functions (tactile and visual lexia and graphia) unilaterally following section of the corpus callosum', *J. Neuropath. Exp. Neurol.*, 2 (1943), 226–62.

Akelaitis, A. J., 'A study of gnosis, praxis, and language following section of the corpus callosum and anterior commissure', *J. Neurosurg.*, 1 (1944), 94–102.

Alkhamees, H. A., C. E. Selai and S. D. Shorvon, 'The beliefs among patients with epilepsy in Saudi Arabia about the causes and treatment of epilepsy and other aspects', *Epilepsy Behav.*, 53 (2015), 135–9.

Alonso-Deflorida, F. and J. M. Delgado, 'Lasting behavioral and EEG changes in cats induced by prolonged stimulation of amygdala', *Am. J. Physiol.*, 193 (1958), 223–9.

Alström, C. H., 'A study of epilepsy in its clinical, social and genetic aspects', *Acta Psychiatr. Neurol. Suppl.*, 63 (1950), 1–284.

Álvaro, L. C., 'Dr Jekyll and Mr Hyde: A case of epilepsy in the late nineteenth century', *Neurosci. Hist.*, 1 (2013), 21–7.

'Amateur medical statisticians', *Lancet*, 1 (1943), 19.

Andermann F. 'In memoriam - Herbert Henri Jasper 1906–1999'. *Epilepsia*, 41 (2000), 113–120.

'An epitome of current medical literature', *BMJ* 2 (8 Sept.) (1906), 35–6.

Annegers, J. F., W. A. Hauser and L. R. Elveback, 'Remission of seizures and relapse in patients with epilepsy', *Epilepsia*, 20 (1979), 729–37.

Ascroft, P. B., 'Traumatic epilepsy after gunshot wounds of the head', *BMJ*, 1 (1941), 739–44.

Austin, J. K., P. O. Shafer and J. B. Deering, 'Epilepsy familiarity, knowledge, and perceptions of stigma: Report from a survey of adolescents in the general population', *Epilepsy Behav.* 3 (2002), 368–75.

Avanzini, G., P. Manganotti, S. Meletti et al., 'The system epilepsies: A pathophysiological hypothesis', *Epilepsia*, 53 (2012), 771–8.

Axtell, W., 'Acute angulation and flexure of the sigmoid: a causative factor in epilepsy. Preliminary report of thirty-one cases', *Am. J. Surg.*, 24 (1910), 385–7.

Bagley, C., 'Social prejudice and the adjustment of people with epilepsy', *Epilepsia*, 13 (1972), 33–45.

Bailey, P., 'The past, present and future of neurology in the United States', *Neurology*, 1 (1951), 1–9.

Bailey, P., 'Surgical treatment of psychomotor epilepsy: five year follow-up', *South. Med. J.*, 54 (1961), 299–301.

Baird J. B. 'Mindbending controversy', *Harvard Crimson*, Jan 16 1974.

Ballentine, C., 'Taste of raspberries, taste of death: the 1937 Elixir Sulfanilamide incident', *FDA Consumer Mag.*, June 1981 (www.fda.gov/files/about%20fda/published/The-Sulfanilamide-Disaster.pdf, accessed 20 May 2020).

Baulac, M., H. de Boer, C. Elger et al., 'Epilepsy priorities in Europe: A report of the ILAE-IBE Epilepsy Advocacy Europe Task Force', *Epilepsia*, 56 (2015), 1687–95.

Baxendale, S., 'Epilepsy at the movies: Possession to presidential assassination', *Lancet Neurol.*, 3 (2003), 764–70.

Baxendale, S., 'The representation of epilepsy in popular music', *Epilepsy Behav.*, 12 (2008), 165–9.

Bear, D. M., 'Temporal lobe epilepsy – a syndrome of sensory-limbic hyperconnection', *Cortex*, 15 (1979), 357–84.

Bear, D. M. and P. Fedio, 'Quantitative analysis of interictal behavior in temporal lobe epilepsy', *Arch. Neurol.*, 34 (1977), 454–67.

Baird, J. 'Mindbending controversy', *The Harvard Crimson*, 16 Jan. 1974.

Beevor, C. E. and V. Horsley, 'A Record of the Results Obtained by Electrical Excitation of the So-Called Motor Cortex and Internal Capsule in an Orang-Outang (Simia satyrus)'. *Philos Trans R Soc Lond B Biol Sci.*, vol. 181 (1890), 129–58.

Ben-Ari, Y., 'Limbic seizure and brain damage produced by kainic acid: mechanisms and relevance to human temporal lobe epilepsy', *Neuroscience*, 14 (1985), 375–403.

Berg, A. T., S. F. Berkovic, M. J. Brodie et al., 'Revised terminology and concepts for organization of seizures and epilepsies: report of the ILAE Commission on Classification and Terminology, 2005–2009', *Epilepsia*, 51 (2010), 676–85.

Berger, H., 'Über das Elektrenkephalogramm des Menschen. III', *Arch. Psychiatr. Nervenkr.*, 94 (1931), 16–60.

Berger, H., 'Über das Elektrenkephalogramm des Menschen. IV', *Arch. Psychiatr. Nervenkr.*, 97 (1932), 6–26.

Berger, H., 'Über das Elektrenkephalogramm des Menschen. V', *Arch. Psychiatr. Nervenkr.*, 98 (1932), 231–54.

Berger, H., 'Über das Elektrenkephalogramm des Menschen. VII', *Arch. Psychiatr. Nervenkr.*, 100 (1933), 301–20.

Berger, H., 'Über das Elektrenkephalogramm des Menschen. XIV', *Arch. Psychiatr. Nervenkr.*, 108 (1938), 407–31.

Berkeley-Hill, O., 'A short analysis of eighty-nine cases of epilepsy in the Punjab Lunatic Asylum', *Ind. Med. Gaz.*, 49 (1914), 136–7.

Berrios, G. E., 'Epilepsy and insanity during the early 19th century. A conceptual history', *Arch. Neurol.*, 41 (1984), 978–81.

Betts, T. and H. Betts, 'A note on a phrase in Shakespeare's play *King Lear.* "A plague upon your epileptic visage"', *Seizure*, 7 (1998), 407–9.

Bharucha, E. P., S. M. Katrak and B. S. Singham, 'In memoriam: Noshir H Wadia', *World Neurol.*, 31 (2016), 5.

Bialer, M., S. I. Johannessen, H. J. Kupferberg et al., 'Progress report on new antiepileptic drugs: A summary of the Eighth Eilat Conference (EILAT VIII)', *Epilepsy Res.*, 73 (2007), 1–52.

Biervert, C. and O. K. Steinlein, 'Structural and mutational analysis of KCNQ2, the major gene locus for benign familial neonatal convulsions', *Hum. Genet.*, 104 (1999), 234–40.

Bird, C. A. K., B. P. Griffen, J. Miklazewska et al., 'Tegretol (carbamazepine): A controlled trial of a new anticonvulsant', *Br. J. Psychiatry*, 112 (1966), 737–42.

Bishop, M. P., S. T. Elder and R. G. Heath, 'Intracranial self-stimulation in man', *Science*, 140 (1963), 394–6.

Bjerkedal, T., A. Czeizel, J. Goujard et al., 'Valproic acid and spina bifida', *Lancet*, 2 (1982), 1096.

Bladin, P. F., 'A century of prejudice and progress: Paradigm of epilepsy in a developing society – medical and social aspects', *Epilepsy Australia*, 3 (2001), 234.

Bladin, P. F., 'John William Springthorpe, 1855–1933: Early Australian epileptologist and keeper of the flame for neurosciences', *J. Clin. Neurosci.*, 11 (2004), 6–15.

Bladin, P. F., 'Reflections on a life in epilepsy: Evolution of epileptology in Australia: early days', *Epilepsy Behav.*, 71 (2017), 108–55.

Blume, W. T., H. O. Lüders, E. Mizrahi et al., 'ILAE Commission Report: glossary of descriptive terminology for ictal semiology: report of the ILAE Task Force on Classification and Terminology', *Epilepsia*, 42 (2001), 1212–18.

Blumgart, H. L., 'Care for the patient', *N. Engl. J. Med.*, 270 (1964), 449–56.

Boodman S. and G. Frankel, 'Over 7,500 sterilized by Virginia', *Washington Post*, 23 February 1980.

Bouchet, C. and G. Cazauvieihl, 'De l'épilepsie considérée dans ses rapports avec l'alienation mentale: recherches sur la nature et le siege de ces deux maladies', *Arch. Gen. Med.*, 9 (1825), 510–42; 10 (1826), 5–50.

Bourke, J., 'Enjoying the high life: Drugs in history and culture', *Lancet*, 376 (2010), 1817.

Brain, W. R., 'The inheritance of epilepsy', *Quart. J. Med.*, 19 (1926), 299–310, 1925–6.

Brain, W. R., 'Neurology: Past, present, and future', *BMJ*, 1 (1958), 355–60.

Brand, R. and P. Kumar, 'Detailing gets personal: Integrated segmentation may be Pharma's key to "Repersonalizing the selling process"', *PharmExec.com*, 1 August 2003 (www.pharmexec.com/detailing-gets-personal, accessed 31 October 2020).

Braslow, J. T., 'In the name of therapeutics: the practice of sterilization in a California state hospital', *J. Hist. Med. Allied Sci.*, 51 (1996), 29–51.

'British Medical Association, proceedings of sections at the annual meeting, Bradford, 1924', *BMJ*, 2 (1924), 1043–56.

Brown, R. R., 'A study of the mental and physical traits of the relatives of epileptics', *J. Appl. Psychol.*, 14 (1930), 620–36.

Brown, S. and E. A. Schäfer, 'An investigation into the functions of the occipital land temporal lobes of the monkey's brain', *Phil. Trans. Roy. Soc. Lond.*, 179B (1888), 303–27.

Bull, J. W. D., 'The history of neuroradiology', *Proc. R. Soc. Med.*, 63 (1970), 637–43.

Burkholder, D. B., 'Pearce Bailey: The "Fifth Horseman" and the National Institute for Neurological Diseases and Blindness', *J. Hist. Neurosciences*, 27 (2018), 303–9

Burnside, J., 'Voyage around my brother', *Guardian*, 4 April 2009 (www.theguardian .com/books/2009/apr/04/the-music-room-william-fiennes, accessed 5 April 2020).

Bury, J. S., 'The treatment of epilepsy by biborate of soda', *Lancet*, 135 (1890), 1206.

Bydder, G. M., R. E. Steiner, I. R. Young et al., 'Clinical NMR imaging of the brain: 140 cases', *Am. J. Roentgenol.*, 139 (1982), 215–36.

Camerman, A. and N. Camerman, 'Diphenylhydantoin and diazepam: molecular structure similarities and steric basis of anticonvulsant activity', *Science*, 168 (1980), 1457–8.

Capeda C, Tanaka T, Stutzmann J-M, Korn H. 'Robert Naquet (1923-2005): The Scientific Odyssey of a French Gentleman', *Epilepsy and Seizure* 2 (2009), 1–16

Carey, M. J., 'Cushing and the treatment of brain wounds during World War 1', *J. Neurosurg.*, 114 (2011), 1495–1501.

Caton, R., 'The electric currents of the brain', *BMJ*, 2 (1875), 278.

Caveness, W., 'A survey of public attitudes toward epilepsy', *Epilepsia*, 4 (1949), 19–26 and 3 (1954), 99–102.

Caveness, W. and G. H. Gallup Jr, 'A survey of public attitudes toward epilepsy in 1979 with an indication of trends over the past thirty years', *Epilepsia*, 21 (1980), 509–18.

Caveness, W., H. H. Merritt, G. H. Gallup et al., 'A survey of public attitudes toward epilepsy in 1964', *Epilepsia*, 6 (1965), 75–86.

Caveness, W. F., H. H. Merritt and G. H. Gallup, 'A survey of public attitudes toward epilepsy in 1969 with an indication of trends over the past twenty years', *Epilepsia*, 10 (1969), 429–40.

Cecil, R. L., 'Henry Rawle Geyelin', *Trans. Am. Clin. Climatolog. Assoc.*, 58 (1946), xciii–xcv.

Cereghino, J. J., 'The major advances in epilepsy in the 20th century and what we can expect (hope for) in the future', *Epilepsia*, 50 (2009), 351–7.

Chabris, C. F., J. J. Lee, D. Cesarini et al., 'The fourth law of behavior genetics', *Curr. Dir. Psychol. Sci.*, 24 (2015), 304–12.

Chagnac-Amitai, Y. and B. W. Connors, 'Synchronized excitation and inhibition driven by intrinsically bursting neurons in neocortex', *J. Neurophysiol.*, 62 (1989), 1149–62.

Chan, C. K. 'Eugenics on the rise: a report from Singapore' *International Journal of Health Services*, 15 (1985), 707–12.

'Charge against a vivisectionist', *London Daily News*, 4 November 1881.

Claes, L., J. Del-Favero, B. Ceulemans et al., 'De novo mutations in the sodium-channel gene SCN1A cause severe myoclonic epilepsy of infancy', *Am. J. Hum. Genet.*, 68 (2001), 1327–32.

Clark, L. P., 'A digest of recent work on epilepsy', *J. Nerv. Ment. Dis.*, 27 (1900), 387–404.

Clark, L. P., 'The nature and pathogenesis of epilepsy', *N. Y. Med. J.*, 101 (1915), 385–92, 442–8, 515–22, 623–8.

Clark, L. P., 'A psychological interpretation of essential epilepsy', *Brain*, 43 (1920), 38–49.

Clark, L. P., and A. Busby, 'Value of roentgen analysis of gastro-intestinal tract in some types of so-called functional nervous disorders. A preliminary report', *Trans. Am. Neurol. Assoc.*, 39 (1913), 125–41.

Clark, L. P. and T. P. Prout, 'Status epilepticus: A clinical and pathological study in epilepsy' [article in three parts], *Am. J. Insanity*, 60 (1903–4), 291–306 and 645–75, and 61 (1903–4), 81–108.

Clark, R. A. and J. M. Lesko, 'Psychoses associated with epilepsy', *Am. J. Psychiatry*, 40 (1939–40), 595.

Clifford, A. 'Science and fiction: The world turned upside down', *New Scientist*, 20 March 1993.

Clow, H. and I. R. Young, 'Britain's brains produce first NMR scan', *New Sci.*, 80 (1978), 588.

Cobb, S., M. E. Cohen and J. Ney, 'Anticonvulsive action of vital dyes', *Arch. Neurol. Psychiatry*, 40 (1938), 1156–77.

Cobb, S., M. E. Cohen and J. Ney, 'Brilliant Vital Red as an anticonvulsant', *Arch. Neurol. Psychiatry*, 37 (1938), 463–5.

Cochrane, A., 'The randomised controlled trial', *Lancet*, 1 (1972), 985.

Coenen, A. and O. Zayachkivska, 'Adolf Beck: A pioneer in electroencephalography between Richard Caton and Hans Berger', *Adv. Cogn. Psychol.*, 9 (2013), 216–21.

Coenen, A., E. Fine and O. Zayachkivska, 'Adolf Beck: A forgotten pioneer in electroencephalography', *J. Hist. Neurosci.*, 23 (2014), 276–86.

Cohen, B., N. Showstack and A. Myerson, 'The synergism of phenobarbital, Dilantin sodium and other drugs in the treatment of institutional epilepsy', *JAMA*, 114 (1940), 480–4.

Cohen, M. M. 'In memoriam, *Frank Morrell'*, *Neurology* 49 (1997), 905–6.

Collier, J., 'Discussion on the nature and treatment of epilepsy', *BMJ*, 2 (1924), 1045–54.

Collura, T. F., 'History and evolution of electro-encephalographic instruments and techniques', *J. Clin. Neurophysiol.*, 10 (1993), 476–504.

Commission on Classification and Terminology of the International League Against Epilepsy, 'Proposal for revised classification of epilepsies and epileptic syndromes', *Epilepsia*, 30 (1989), 389–99.

'Compounds of boron and potassium in epilepsy', *Lancet*, 199 (1922), 446.

Compton, K., 'Big pharma and medical device manufacturers', *Drug Watch*, n.d., www.drugwatch.com/manufacturers/, accessed 23 October 2020.

Conrad, K., 'Erbanlage und Epilepsie. Untersuchungen an einer Serie von 253 Zwillingspaaren', *Zschr. Neurol.*, 135 (1935), 271–326.

Cook, M. J. 'Advancing seizure forecasting from cyclical activity data', *Lancet Neurology*, 20 (2021), 86–7.

Cook, M. J., D. R. Fish, S. D. Shorvon et al., 'Hippocampal volumetric and morphometric studies in frontal and temporal lobe epilepsy', *Brain*, 115 (1992), 1001–15.

Credner, L., 'Klinische und sociale Auswirkungen von Hirnshädigungen', *Z. Gesamte Neurol. Psychiatr.*, 126 (1930), 721–57.

Crichton-Browne, J., 'The actions of the bromide of potassium upon the nervous system', *J. Ment. Sci.*, 11 (1866), 598–602.

Crichton-Browne, J., 'On the actions of picrotoxine, and the antagonisms between picrotoxine and chloral hydrate', *BMJ*, 1 (1875), 409–11, 442–4, 476–8, 506–7, 540–2.

Crichton-Browne, J., 'William Bevan-Lewis', *BMJ*, 2 (1929), 833–5.

Critchley, M., 'Musicogenic epilepsy', *Brain*, 60 (1937), 13–27.

Critchley, M., 'Remembering Kinnier Wilson', *Mov. Disord.*, 3 (1988), 2–6.

Crombie, D. L., K. W. Cross, J. Fry et al., 'A survey of the epilepsies in general practice: A report by the Research Committee of the College of General Practitioners', *BMJ*, 2 (1960), 416–22.

Cromie, R., 'Is Crichton bestseller unjust to epileptics?' *Chicago Tribune*, 6 August 1972.

Currie, S., W. Heathfield, R. Hensona et al., 'Clinical course and prognosis of temporal lobe epilepsy: a survey of 666 patients', *Brain*, 94 (1971), 173–90.

Curtis, D. R., A. W. Duggan, D. Felix et al., 'GABA, bicuculline and central inhibition', *Nature*, 226 (1970), 1222–4.

Cushing, H., 'A study of a series of wounds involving the brain and its enveloping structures', *Br. J. Surg.*, 5 (1918), 558–684.

Daly, D., 'In memoriam A. B. Baker', *Epilepsia*, 31 (1990), 116–17.

Dam, M., 'Message from the President of the International League Against Epilepsy', *Epilepsia*, 23 (1982), 239–41.

Dam, M., R. Ekberg, Y. Løyning et al., 'A double-blind study comparing oxcarbazepine and carbamazepine in patients with newly diagnosed, previously untreated epilepsy', *J. Neurol. Neurosurg. Psychiatry*, 52 (1989), 472–6.

Dana, C., 'The future of neurology', *J. Nerv. Ment. Dis.*, 40 (1913), 753.

Daroff, R. B., 'NINDS at 50: An incomplete history celebrating the fiftieth anniversary of the National Institute of Neurological Disorders and Stroke', *J. Neurol. Neurosurg. Psychiatry*, 75 (2004), 348.

Davenport, C. B., 'The Nams: feeble-minded as country dwellers', *The Survey*, 27 (1912), 1844–5.

Davenport, C. and D. Weeks, 'A first study of inheritance of epilepsy', *J. Nerv. Ment. Dis.*, 38 (1911), 641–70.

Davidson, W., 'Book excerpt: The letters of Joseph Roth', *New Yorker*, 6 January 2012 (www.new yorker.com/culture/culture-desk/book-excerpt-the-letters-of-joseph-roth, accessed 26 July 2020).

De Kovel, C. G. F., H. Trucks, I. Helbig et al., 'Recurrent microdeletions at 15q11.2 and 16p13.11 predispose to idiopathic generalized epilepsies', *Brain*, 133 (2010) (Pt 1), 23–32.

Delgado, J. M., H. Hamlin and W. P. Chapman, 'Technique of intracranial electrode implacement for recording and stimulation and its possible therapeutic value in psychotic patients', *Confin. Neurol.*, 12 (1952), 315–9.

Delgado Escueta, A. V., R. H. Mattson, D. B. Smith et al., 'Principles in designing clinical ltrials for antiepileptic drugs', *Neurology*, 33 (1983) (3 Suppl 1), 8–13.

Demonic possession or just epilepsy? by Dr Jack', *Sort Your Brain Out* (blog), 8 December 2011 (www.drjack.co.uk/epileptic-seizures-mis taken-for-demonic-possession-by-our-ances tors-by-dr-jack-lewis/, accessed 15 December 2020).

Denny-Brown, D., 'The clinical aspects of traumatic epilepsy', *Am. J. Psychiatry*, 100 (1944), 585–91.

'Discussion', *Epilepsia*, 2 (1953), 76–96.

Dobbs, D., 'What is your DNA worth?', *BuzzFeed News*, (www.buzzfeed.com/david dobbs/weighing-the-promises-of-big-genomics, accessed 17 July 2021).

Dodrill, C. B., 'A neuropsychological battery for epilepsy', *Epilepsia*, 19 (1978), 611–23.

Dollery, C. T., 'Clinical pharmacology – the first 75 years and a view of the future', *Br. J. Clin. Pharmacol.*, 61 (2006), 650–5.

Dravet, C. and J. Roger, 'In memoriam, Henri Gastaut, 1915–1995', *Epilepsia* 37 (1996), 410–5.

Dreifuss, F., J. K. Penry, S. W. Rose, et al. 'Serum clonazepam concentrations in children with absence seizures', *Neurology* 25 (1975), 255–8.

Duffy, T. P., 'The Flexner Report – 100 years later', *Yale J. Biol. Med.*, 84 (2011), 269–76.

Eadie, M., 'Louis François Bravais and Jacksonian epilepsy', *Epilepsia*, 51 (2010), 1–6.

Earle, K. M., M. Baldwin and W. Penfield, 'Incisural sclerosis and temporal lobe seizures produced by hippocampal herniation at birth', *Arch. Neurol. Psychiatry*, 69 (1953), 27–42.

Eccles, J. and W. Feindel, 'Wilder Graves Penfield', *Biograph. Mem. Roy. Soc.*, 24 (1978), 472–513.

Echeverria, M. G., 'On epileptic insanity', *Am. J. Insanity*, 30 (1873), 1–51.

Edson, L. 'For the mentally ill, a court of last resort', *New York Times*, 30 Sept., 1973

Ehrlich, P., 'On immunity with special reference to cell life', *Proc. R. Soc. London*, 66 (1900), 424–33.

Eichenwald, K., *A Mind Unraveled* (New York: Ballantine Books, 2018).

Eichenwald, K., 'A mind unraveled', interview by K. Cervantes, 9 October 2019 (rebroadcast), in *Seizing Life*, podcast, 10: 50 (www.cureepilepsy.org/seizing-life/a-mind-unraveled-a-memoir-by-kurt-eichenwald/, accessed 21 December 2020).

Eke, T., J. Talbot and M. Lawden, 'Severe persistent visual field constriction associated with vigabatrin', *Br. Med. J.*, 314 (1997), 180–1.

Elian, M., 'Youngsters with epilepsy within the framework of the social institutions of Israel, with special reference to the Armed Services', *Epilepsia*, 13 (1972), 51–6.

Eling, P. and A. Keyser, 'Louis Muskens: A leading figure in the history of Dutch and world epileptology', *J. Hist. Neurosci.*, 12 (2003), 276–85.

Elliott, B., E. Joyce and S. Shorvon, 'Delusions, illusions and hallucinations in epilepsy: 1. Elementary phenomena', *Epilepsy Res.*, 85 (2009), 162–71.

Elliott, B., E. Joyce and S. Shorvon, 'Delusions, illusions and hallucinations in epilepsy: 2. Complex phenomena and psychosis', *Epilepsy Res.*, 85 (2009), 172–86.

Engel, J. R. Jr, 'The legacy of Frank Morrell', *Int. Rev. Neurogiol.*, 45 (2001), 571–84.

Engel, J. Jr, 'More on the history of temporal lobe surgery', *Epilepsia*, 49 (2008), 1481–2.

Engel, J. Jr, 'A proposed diagnostic scheme for people with epileptic seizures and with epilepsy: Report of the ILAE Task Force on Classification and Terminology', *Epilepsia*, 42 (2001), 796–803.

Engel, J. Jr, 'Report of the ILAE Classification Core Group', *Epilepsia*, 47 (2006), 1558–68.

Engel, J., 'Update on surgical treatment of the epilepsies: A summary of the second international Palm Desert conference on the surgical treatment of the epilepsies (1992)', *Neurology*, 43 (1993), 1612–7.

Engel, J., S. Wiebe, J. French et al., 'Practice parameter: Temporal lobe and localized neocortical resections for epilepsy: Report of the Quality Standards Subcommittee of the American Academy of Neurology, in association with the American Epilepsy Society and the American Association of Neurological Surgeons', *Neurology*, 25 (2003), 538–47.

'Epilepsy in movies and television', on *Your Life Protected* website (www.yourlifeprotected.co.uk/news/epilepsy-in-movies-and-television/, accessed 15 December 2020).

Erickson, T. C., 'Spread of epileptic discharges', *Arch. Neurol. Psychiatry*, 43 (1940), 449–52.

Escayg, A. P., B. T. MacDonald, M. H. Meisler et al., 'Mutations of SCN1A, encoding a neuronal sodium channel, in two families with GEFS$^+$ 2', *Nat. Genet.*, 24 (2000), 343–5.

Falconer, M. A., 'Reversibility by temporal-lobe resection of the behavioural abnormalities of temporal-lobe epilepsy', *New Engl. J. Med.*, 289 (1973), 451–5.

Falret, J., 'De l'état mental des épileptiques', *Arch. gén. med.*, 16 (1860), 661–79.

'Fasting as epilepsy cure', *New York Times*, 6 July 1922, p. 25.

Fay, T., 'The therapeutic dehydration of epileptic patients', *Arch. Neurol. Psychiatry*, 33 (1930), 920–45.

Feindel, W., 'Osler and the "medico-chirurgical neurologists: Horsley, Cushing and Penfield"', *J. Neurosurg.*, 99 (2003), 188–99.

Féré, C., 'La famille névropathique', *Arch. Neurol.*, 9 (1884), 9–25.

Ferenczi, S., 'Stages in the development of the sense of reality' (E. Jones (trans.), *First Contributions to Psycho-Analysis*, 45 (1952), 213–39.

Ferlisi, M. and S. Shorvon, 'The outcome of therapies in refractory and super-refractory convulsive status epilepticus and recommendations for therapy', *Brain*, 135 (2012) (Pt 8), 2314–28.

Ferrier, D., 'Cerebral localization in its practical relations', *Brain*, 12 (1889), 36–58.

Ferrier, D., 'Experimental researches in cerebral physiology and pathology', *West Riding Lunatic Asylum Med. Rep.*, 3 (1873), 30–96.

F. G. C., 'Epilepsy and genius', *BMJ*, 1 (1902), 301.

Feindel, W., R. Leblanc, and A. N. De Almeida, 'Epilepsy surgery: Historical highlights 1909–2009'. *Epilepsia*, 50 (2009), 131–51

Fiennes, W., *The Music Room* (London: Picador, 2009).

Fiest, K. M., K. M. Sauro, S. Wiebe, et al. 'Prevalence and incidence of epilepsy: A systematic review and meta-analysis of international studies', *Neurology*, 88 (2017), 296–303.

Fine, E. J., D. L. Fine and L. Sentz, 'The importance of Spratling', *Arch. Neurol.*, 151 (1994), 82–8.

Fischer, M. H. and H. Löwenbach, 'Aktionsströme des Zentralnervensystems unter der Einwirkung von Krampfgiften. I. Mitteilung: Strychnin und Pickrotoxin', *Arch. Exp. Pathol. Pharmakol.*, 174 (1934), 357–82.

Fischer, M. H. and H. Löwenbach, 'Aktionsströme des Zentralnervensystems unter der Einwirkung von Krampfgiften. II. Mitteilung: Cardiazol, Coffein und andere', *Arch. Exp. Pathol. Pharmakol.*, 174 (1934), 502–16.

Fisher, D., 'The Rockefeller Foundation and the development of scientific medicine in Great Britain', *Minerva*, 16 (1978), 20–41.

Fischer, H., 'What made Hanno Buddenbrook sick?', *N. Engl. J. Med.*, 350 (2004), 419–20.

Fisher, R. S., C. Acevedo, A. Arzimanoglou et al., 'ILAE official report: A practical clinical definition of epilepsy', *Epilepsia*, 55 (2014), 475–82.

Fisher, R. S., W. van Emde Boas, W. Blume et al., 'Epileptic seizures and epilepsy: Definitions proposed by the International League Against Epilepsy (ILAE) and the International Bureau for Epilepsy (IBE)', *Epilepsia*, 46 (2005), 470–2.

Foerster, O., 'Zur operativen Behandlung der Epilepsie', *Dtsch. Z. Nervenheilkd.*, 89 (1926), 137–47.

Foerster, O. and H. Altenburger, 'Elektro biologische Vorgänge an der menschlichen Hirnrinde', *Dtsch. Z. Nervenheilkd.*, 135 (1935), 277–88.

Foerster, O. and W. Penfield, 'The structural basis of traumatic epilepsy and results of radical operation', *Brain*, 53 (1930), 99–120.

Fölling, A., 'Über Ausscheidung von Phenylbrenztraubensäure in den Harn als Stoffwechselanomalie in Verbindung mit Imbezillität', *Hoppe Seylers Z. Physiol. Chem.*, 227 (1934), 169–81.

Fox, T., 'Accommodation for epileptic patients in Great Britain', *Epilepsia*, 1 (1937), 45–9.

Freud, S., 'L'Hérédité et l'étiologie des névroses', *Rev. Neurol.*, 4 (1896), 161–9.

Friedlander, W. J., 'Putnam, Merritt, and the discovery of Dilantin', *Epilepsia*, 27 (Suppl 3) (1986), S1–S21.

Friedlander, W. J., 'Who was "the father of bromide treatment of epilepsy"?', *Arch. Neurol.*, 43 (1986), 505–7.

Fritsch, G. and Hitzig, E., 'Über die elektrische Erregbarkeit des Grosshirns', *Arch. Anat. Physiol.*, 37 (1870), 300–32.

Fuchs, W., 'Epilepsie und Luminal', *Munch. Med. Wochenschr.*, 61 (1914), 873–5.

Gaitatzis, A., A. L. Johnson, D. W. Chadwick et al., 'Life expectancy in people with newly diagnosed epilepsy', *Brain*, 127 (2004), 2427–32.

Gallagher, C. E., 'The return of lobotomy and psychosurgery', *Cong. Rec.*, vol. 118, part 5, 24 February 1972, 5575.

Galton, F., 'The history of twins as a criterion of the relative powers of nature and nurture', *Fraser's Magazine*, 12 (1875), 566–76.

Gandhoke, G. S., E. Belykh, X. Zhao et al., 'Edwin Boldrey and Wilder Penfield's homunculus: A life given by Mrs. Cantlie (in and out of realism)', *World Neurosurg.*, 132 (2019), 377–88.

Garceau, E. L. and H. Davis, 'An amplifier, recording system and stimulation devices for the study of cerebral action currents', *Am. J. Physiol.*, 107 (1934), 305–10.

Garceau, E. L. and H. Davis, 'An ink-writing electroencephalograph', *Arch. Neurol. Psych.*, 34 (1935), 1292–4.

Garrod, A. E., 'The Croonian Lectures on inborn errors of metabolism', *Lancet*, 4 July (1908), 1–7.

Gastaut, H., 'Classification of the epilepsies: proposal for an international classification', *Epilepsia*, 10 (Suppl.) (1969), 14–21.

Gastaut, H., 'Classification of status epilepticus', *Adv. Neurol.*, 34 (1983), 15–35.

Gastaut, H., 'Clinical and electroencephalographical classification of epileptic seizures', *Epilepsia*, 10 (Suppl.) (1969), 2–13.

Gastaut, H., 'Clinical and electroencephalographical classification of epileptic seizures', *Epilepsia*, 11 (1970), 102–13.

Gastaut, H., 'Conclusions: Computerized transverse axial tomography in epilepsy', *Epilepsia*, 17 (1976), 337–8.

Gastaut, H., 'The effect of benzodiazepines on chronic epilepsy in man', in R. J. Broughton (ed.), 'Henri Gastaut and the Marseilles school's contribution to the neurosciences', *Electroencephalogr. Clin. Neurophysiol. Suppl.*, 35 (1982), 239–50.

Gastaut, H., 'So-called "psychomotor" and "temporal" epilepsy', *Epilepsia*, 2 (1953), 59–76.

Gastaut, H., W. F. Caveness and H. Landolt et al., 'A proposed international classification of epileptic seizures', *Epilepsia*, 5 (1964), 297–306.

Gastaut, H., J. Courjon, R. Poiré et al., 'Treatment of status epilepticus with a new benzodiazepine more active than diazepam', *Epilepsia*, 12 (1971), 197–214.

Gastaut, H., Gastaut, Y. and Broughton, R., 'Gustave Flaubert's illness: A case report in evidence against the erroneous notion of psychogenic epilepsy', *Epilepsia*, 25, (1984), 622–37.

Gastaut, H., G. Morin and N. Lesevre, 'Étude du comportement des épileptiques psychomoteurs dans l'intervalle de leurs crises: les troubles de l'activité gobale et de la sociabilité', *Ann. Med. Psychol.*, 113 (1955), 1–29.

Gastaut, H., R. Naquet, R. Poiré et al., 'Treatment of status epilepticus with diazepam (Valium)', *Epilepsia*, 6 (1965), 167–82.

Gastaut, H. and A. Rémond, 'Études électroencéphalographiques des myoclonies', *Rev. Neurol.*, 86 (1952), 596–609.

Gastaut, H., J. Roger, R. Soulayrol et al., 'Childhood epileptic encephalopathy with diffuse spike-waves (otherwise known as "petit mal variant") or Lennox syndrome', *Epilepsia*, 7 (1966), 139–79.

GBD 2016 Neurology Collaborators. 'Global, regional, and national burden of neurological disorders, 1990–2016: A systematic analysis for the Global Burden of Disease Study 2016', *Lancet Neurol.*, 18 (2019), 357–75.

Geschwind, N., 'Behavioural changes in temporal lobe epilepsy', *Psycholog. Med.*, 9 (1979), 217–19.

Gibbs, F. A., 'William Gordon Lennox 1884–1960', *Epilepsia*, 2 (1961), 1–8.

Gibbs, F. A. and H. Davis, 'Changes in the human electroencephalogram associated with loss of consciousness', *Am. J. Physiol.*, 113 (1935), 49–50.

Gibbs, F. A., H. Davis and W. G. Lennox, 'The electroencephalogram in epilepsy and in conditions of impaired consciousness', *Arch. Neurol. Psychiatry*, 34 (1935), 1133–48.

Gibbs, E., F. Gibbs and B. Fuster, 'Psychomotor epilepsy', *Arch. Neurol. Psychiatry*, 60 (1948), 331–9.

Gibbs, F. A., E. L. Gibbs and W. G. Lennox, 'Cerebral dysrhythmias of epilepsy: measures for their control', *Arch. Neur. Psych.*, 39 (1938), 298–314.

Gibbs, F. A., E. L. Gibbs and W. G. Lennox, 'Epilepsy: A paroxysmal cerebral dysrhythmia', *Brain*, 60 (1937), 377–88.

Gibbs, F. A., W. G. Lennox and E. Gibbs, 'The electro-encephalogram in diagnosis and in localization of epileptic seizures', *Arch. Neurol. Psychiatry*, 36 (1936), 1225–35

Gilliatt, P, The Dashing Novellas of Muriel Spark. *Grand Street*, 8 (1989), 139–46

'GlaxoSmithKline to plead guilty and pay $3 billion to resolve fraud allegations and failure to report safety data', *Justice News* (www.justice.gov/opa/pr/glaxosmithkline-plead-guilty-and-pay-3-billion-resolve-fraud-allegations-and-failure-report, accessed 15 December 2020).

Glazko, A. J., 'Discovery of phenytoin', *Ther. Drug Monit.*, 8 (1986), 490–7.

Gloor, P., 'Hans Berger on the electroencephalogram of man: The fourteen original reports on the human electroencephalogram', *Electro encephalogr. Clin. Neurophysiol.*, 28 (1969), 1–350.

Godber, G., 'Measurement and mechanisation in medicine', *Lancet*, 2 (1964), 1194.

Goddard, G. V., 'Development of epileptic seizures through brain stimulation at low intensity', *Nature*, 214 (1967), 1020–1.

Golla, F., 'Luminal contrasted with bromide in epilepsy', *BMJ*, 2 (1921), 320–1.

Goodkin, H. P., J. L. Yeh and J. Kapur, 'Status epilepticus increases the intracellular accumulation of GABAA receptors', *J. Neurosci.*, 25 (2005), 5511–20.

Goodridge, D. M. and S. D. Shorvon, 'Epileptic seizures in a population of 6000. II: Treatment and prognosis', *BMJ*, 287 (1983), 645–7.

Gorman, C., 'Taming the brain storms', *Time Magazine*, 16 Aug. 1993, 42.

Gowers, W. R., 'The new neurology', *Lancet*, 153 (1899), 71–3.

Gowers, W. R., 'The Gulstonian Lectures on epilepsy. Lecture III', *BMJ*, 1 (1880), 547–9.

Gram, L., B. B. Lyon and M. Dam, 'Gamma-vinyl-GABA: A single-blind trial in patients with epilepsy', *Acta Neurol. Scand.*, 68 (1983), 34–9.

Grass, A. M., 'The electroencephalographic heritage', *Am. J. EEG Tech.*, 24 (1984), 133–73.

Graves, W. C., 'The Baltimore-Meeting May 25th 1914 of the American Association for the Study of Epilepsy and the Care of and Treatment of Epileptics. A. President's address', *Epilepsia*, 5 (1915), 248–53.

Green, J. R., R. E. H. Duisberg and W. B. McGrath, 'Focal epilepsy of psychomotor type', *J. Neurosurg.*, 8 (1951), 157–72.

Gregoris, N. and S. Shorvon, 'What is the enduring value of research publications in clinical epilepsy? An assessment of papers published in 1981, 1991, and 2001', *Epilepsy Behav.*, 28 (2013), 522–9.

Grinkler, J., 'Further experiences with phenobarbital (Luminal) in epilepsy', *JAMA*, 79 (192), 788–93.

Gruhle, H. W., 'Über den Wahn bei Epilepsie', *Zeitschr. ges. Neur. Psychiatrie*, 154 (1935), 395–9.

Grzywo-Dybrowski, W., 'Die Wirkung des Luminals bei epileptischer Demenz', *Monatsschr. Psychiatr. Neurol.*, 36 (1914), 248–54.

Gunn, J. and J. Bonn, 'Criminality and violence in epileptic prisoners', *Br. J. Psychiatry*, 118 (1971), 337–43.

Gunn, J. and G. Fenton, 'Epilepsy, automatism, and crime', *Lancet*, 297 (1971), 1173–6.

Haas, L. F., 'Hans Berger (1873–1941), Richard Caton (1842–1926) and electroencephalography', *J. Neurol. Neurosurg. Psychiatry*, 74 (2003), 9.

Haefely, W., A. Kulcsár, H. Möhler et al., 'Possible involvement of GABA in the central actions of benzodiazepines', *Adv. Biochem. Psychopharmacol.*, 14 (1975), 131–51.

Handley, R. and A. S. R. Stewart, 'Mysoline: A new drug in the treatment of epilepsy', *Lancet*, 259 (1952), 742–4.

Harary, M. and G. Rees Cosgrove, 'Talairach: A cerebral cartographer', *Neurosug. Focus*, 47 (2019), 1–7.

Harding, J. R., 'Epilepsy as seen in the laboratory of penal institution', *J. Am. Inst. Crim. Law Criminol.*, 9 (1918), 260–6.

Hauptmann, A., 'Erfahrungen aus der Behandlung der Epilepsie mit Luminal', *Munch. med. Wochenschr.*, 46 (1919), 1319–21.

Hauptmann, A., 'Luminal bei Epilepsie', *Munch. med. Wochenschr.*, 59 (1912), 1907–12.

Hauser, W. A. and L. T. Kurland, 'The epidemiology of epilepsy in Rochester, Minnesota, 1935 through 1967', *Epilepsia*, 16 (1975), 1–66.

Hayne, R., I. Belinson and F. Gibbs, 'Electrical activity of subcortical areas in epilepsy', *Electroencephalogr. Clin. Neurophysiol.*, 1 (1949), 437–45.

H. B. D., 'Popular Freudism', *BMJ*, 2 (1914), 1048.

Heath, R. G., 'Correlation of electrical recordings from cortical and subcortical regions of the brain with abnormal behavior in human subjects', *Confin. Neurol.*, 18 (1958), 305–15.

Heath, R. G., 'Psychosis and epilepsy: Similarities and differences in the anatomic-physiologic substrate', *Advances in Biological Psychiatry*, 8 (1982), 106–16.

Heck, C. N., D. King-Stephens, A. D. Massey, et al. 'Two-year seizure reduction in adults with medically intractable partial onset epilepsy treated with responsive neurostimulation: Final results of the RNS System Pivotal trial', *Epilepsia* 55 (2014), 432–41.

Henderson, C., 'Rise of the German Inner Mission', *Am. J. Sociol.*, 1 (1896), 583–95.

Heptinstall, C., 'Psichiatria democratica: Italy's revolution in caring for the mentally ill', *Commun. Care*, 3 (1984), 17–19.

Herberg, L. J. and P. J. Watkins, 'Epileptiform seizures induced by hypothalalmic stimulation in the rat: Resistance to fits following fits', *Nature*, 209 (1966), 515–16.

Hermann, B., '100 years of *Epilepsia*: Landmark papers and their influence in neuropsychology and neuropsychiatry', *Epilepsia*, 51 (2010), 1107–19.

Hermann, B. P. and J. L. Stone, 'A historical review of the epilepsy surgery program at the University of Illinois Medical Center: The contributions of Bailey, Gibbs, and collaborators to the refinement of anterior temporal lobectomy', *J. Epilepsy*, 2 (1989), 155–63.

Hill, D., 'Discussion on the surgery of temporal lobe epilepsy: The clinical study and selection of patients', *Proc. Roy. Soc. Med.*, 46 (1953), 965–71.

Hill, D., D. A. Pond, W. Mitchell et al., 'Personality changes following temporal lobectomy for epilepsy', *J. Ment. Sci.*, 103 (1957), 18–27.

Hirsch, C. S. and D. L. Martin, 'Unexpected death in young epileptics', *Neurology*, 21 (1971), 682–90.

Hodgkin, A., 'Edgar Douglas Adrian, Baron Adrian of Cambridge, 30 November 1889–4 August 1977', *Biogr. Mem. Fellows R. Soc.*, 25 (1979), 1–73.

Hodgkin, A. L. and A. F. Huxley, 'A quantitative description of membrane current and its application to conduction and excitation in nerve', *J. Physiol.*, 117 (1952), 500–44.

Hoefle, M. L., 'The early history of Parke-Davis and Company', *Bull. Hist. Chem.*, 25 (2000), 28–34.

Holland, O., 'Exploration and high adventure: The legacy of Grey Walter', *Phil. Trans. Roy. Soc. Lond. A*, 361 (1811), 2085–2121.

Horsley, V., 'Advances in the surgery of the central nervous system', *Lancet*, 2 (1886), 346–7.

Horsely, V., 'Brain-surgery', *BMJ*, 2 (1886), 670–5.

Horsley, V., 'British Medical Association', *BMJ*, 2 (1886), 670–677.

Horsley, V., 'Remarks on ten consecutive cases of operations upon the brain and cranial cavity to illustrate the details and safety of the method employed', *BMJ*, 1 (1887), 853–65.

Horwitz, N. H., 'Fedor Krause (1857–1937)', *Neurosurgery*, 38 (1996), 844–8.

Hounsfield, G. N., 'Computer medical imaging', Nobel lecture, 8 December 1979, *The Nobel Prize* (www.nobelprize.org/prizes/medicine/1979/hounsfield/lecture/, accessed 4 April 2020).

Hughes, C. H., 'The quarter and semi-decade treatment and curability of epilepsia', *Alien. Neurol.*, 25 (1904), 326–34.

Hunter, J. and H. H. Jasper, 'A method of analysis of seizure pattern and electroencephalogram: A cinematographic technique', *Electroencephalogr. Clin. Neurophysiol.*, 1 (1949), 113.

Huxley, J., 'Eugenics and society', *Eugenics Rev.*, 728 (1938), 11–31.

Huxley, T. H., 'The connexion of the biological sciences with medicine', *Lancet*, 2 (1881), 272–6.

'Institutional care of epileptics in the United States', *Epilepsia*, 1 (1937), 35–9.

'Institutions for the care and treatment of epilepsy in different countries of the world', *Epilepsia*, 2 (1938), 105–13.

'International list of anti-epilepsy drugs', *Epilepsia*, 4 (1955), 121–2.

'International Neurological Congress in London', *BMJ*, 2 (1935), 223–5, 269–72.

'International Neurological Congress: the first day's proceedings', *Lancet*, 226 (1935), 268–9, 332–6.

'Interview with Tony Coelho', podcast, A11y Rules, episodes 92 and 93 (https://a11yrules.com/podcast/e092-interview-with-tony-coelho-part-1/ and https://a11yrules.com/ podcast/e093-interview-with-tony-coelho-part-2/, accessed 17 July 2021).

Ioannidis, J. P. A., 'The mass production of redundant, misleading and conflicted systemic reviews and meta-analyses', *Milbank Q*, 94 (2016), 485–514.

Ioannidis, J. P. A., 'Spin, bias, and clinical utility in systematic reviews of diagnostic studies', *Clin. Chem.*, 66 (2020), 863–5.

Ioannidis, J. P. A., 'Why most clinical research is not useful', *PLoS Med.*, 13 (2016), e1002049.

Ioannidis, J. P. A., 'Why most published research findings are false', *PloS Med.*, 2 (2005), e124.

Ioannidis, J. P. A., R. Klavans and K. W. Boyack, 'Thousands of scientists publish a paper every five days', *Nature*, 561 (2018), 167–9.

Jack, C. R. Jr, F. W. Sharbrough, C. K. Twomey et al., 'Temporal lobe seizures: Lateralization with MR volume measurements of the hippocampal formation', *Radiology*, 175 (1990), 423–9.

Jackson, G. D., A. Connelly, J. S. Duncan et al., 'Detection of hippocampal pathology in tractable partial epilepsy: Increased sensitivity with quantitative magnetic resonance T2 relaxometry', *Neurology*, 43 (1992), 1793–9.

Jackson, J. H., 'The Lumleian Lectures on convulsive seizures', *Lancet*, 135 (1890), 735–8.

Jackson, J. H., 'Notes on the physiology and pathology of the nervous system', *Med. Times Gaz.*, 2 (1868), 177–9.

Jackson, J. H., 'On the anatomical, physiological, and pathological investigation of epilepsies', *West Riding Lunatic Asylum Med. Rep.*, 3 (1873), 315–49.

Jackson, J. H., 'On a particular variety of epilepsy ("Intellectual Aura"), one case with symptoms of organic brain disease', *Brain*, 11 (1888), 179–207.

Jackson, J. H., 'On the scientific and empirical investigation of epilepsies', *Med. Press Circular*, 21 (1875), 312, 351, 487.

Jackson, J. H., 'Remarks on the diagnosis and treatment of diseases of the brain', *BMJ*, 2 (1888), 111–17.

Jackson, J. H., 'A study of convulsions', *Trans. St. Andrews Med. Graduates' Assoc.*, 3 (1869), 162–204.

Jackson, J. H., 'A suggestion for the treatment of epilepsy', unpublished manuscript labeled 'For private circulation', December 1899, Queen Square Archive, QSA/837, London.

Jackson, J. H. and W. S. Colman, 'Case of epilepsy with tasting movements and "dreamy state" – very small patch of softening in the left uncinate gyrus', *Brain*, 21 (1898), 580–90.

Jackson, J. H. and P. Stewart, 'Epileptic attacks with a warning of a crude sensation of smell and with the intellectual aura (dreamy state) in a patient who had symptoms pointing to gross organic disease of the right temporo-sphenoidal lobe', *Brain*, 22 (1899), 534–9.

Jacoby, A., 'Felt versus enacted stigma: A concept revisited', *Epilepsia*, 28 (1994), 269–74.

Jacoby, A., J. Gorry, C. Gamble et al., 'Public knowledge, private grief: A study of public attitudes to epilepsy in the United Kingdom and implications for stigma', *Epilepsia*, 45 (2004), 1405–15.

Jacoby, A., D. Snape and G. A. Baker, 'Epilepsy and social identity: The stigma of a chronic neurological disorder', *Lancet Neurol.*, 4 (2005), 171–8.

Jasper, H., 'The centrencephalic system', *Can. Med. J.*, 16 (1977), 1371–2.

Jasper, H. 'Preface', *Electroencephalogr Clin Neurophysiol.* 28 (suppl), (1969), v–vii.

Jasper, H. and J. Kershman, 'Electroencephalographic classification of the epilepsies', *Arch. Neurol. Psychiatry*, 45 (1941), 903–43.

Jennett, B., 'Epilepsy and acute traumatic intracranial haematoma', *J. Neurol. Neurosurg. Psychiatry*, 38 (1975), 378–81.

Jennett, B., J. D. Miller and R. Braakman, 'Epilepsy after nonmissile depressed skull fracture', *J. Neurosurg.*, 41 (1974), 208–16.

Jensen, J. P. A., 'The rise and fall of borax as an antiepileptic drug', *Arch. Neurol.*, 63 (2006), 621–2.

Jones, E., 'Mental characteristics of epileptics', *Maryland Med. J.*, 53 (1910), 223–9.

Jones, E., 'Obituary', *J. Psychoanal.*, 25 (1944), 177.

Kaelber, L., 'Eugenics: Compulsory sterilization in 50 American states. Massachusetts', presentation at the Social Science History Association (2012) (www.uvm.edu/~lkaelber/eugenics/MA/MA .html, accessed 8 April 2021).

Kapur, J. and R. L. Macdonald, 'Rapid seizure-induced reduction of benzodiazepine and $Zn2^+$ sensitivity of hippocampal dentate granule cell GABAA receptors', *J. Neurosci.*, 17 (1997), 7532–40.

Kendrick, J. F. and F. A. Gibbs, 'Origin, spread and neurosurgical treatment of the psychomotor type of seizure dischárge', *J Neurosurg.* 14 (1957), 270–84.

Kennard, M. A., J. F. Fulton and C. G. de Gutierrez-Mahoney, 'Otfrid Foerster 1873–1941: An appreciation', *J. Neurophysiol.*, 5 (1942), 1–17.

Kerr, M., A. Sen and J. Hanna, 'Prevent 21: SUDEP Summit – time to listen', *Epilepsy Behav.*, special issue, 103 (2020) (Part B).

Kerson, T. S. and L. A. Kerson, 'Implacable images: Why epileptiform events continue to be featured in film and television', *Epileptic Disord.*, 8 (2006), 103–13.

Kerson, T. S. and L. A. Kerson, 'Truly enthralling: Epileptiform events in film and on television – why they persist and what we can do about them', *Soc. Work Health Care*, 47 (2008): 320–37.

Kesselring, J., 'Early globalization of neurology – the first International Congress of Neurology 1931 Bern, Switzerland', *Clin. Translat. Neurosci.*, 4 (2020), 1–5.

Kim, H. D., H. C. Kang, S. A. Lee, K. Huh and B. I. Lee, 'Changing name of epilepsy in Korea; Cerebroelectric disorder (noi-jeon-jeung, 뇌전증,): My epilepsy story', *Epilepsia*, 55 (2014), 384–6.

Kimball, O. P., 'The treatment of epilepsy with sodium diphenyl hydantoinate', *JAMA*, 112 (1939), 1244–5.

Kinnier Wilson, J. V. and E. H. Reynolds, 'Translation and analysis of a cuneiform text forming part of a Babylonian treatise on epilepsy', *Med. Hist.*, 34 (2012), 185–98.

Kissiov, D., T. Dewall and B. Hermann, 'The Ohio Hospital for Epileptics – the first 'epilepsy colony' in America', *Epilepsia*, 54 (2013), 1524–34.

Kleinman, A., W. Wang, S. Li et al., 'The social course of epilepsy: Chronic illness as social experience in interior China', *Soc. Sci. Med.*, 40 (1995), 1319–30.

Kligman, D. and D. A. Goldberg, 'Temporal lobe epilepsy and aggression', *J. Nerv. Ment. Dis.*, 160 (1975), 324–41.

Klüver, H. and P. C. Bucy, 'Preliminary analysis of functions of the tempora lobes in monkeys', *Arch. Neurol. Psychiatry*, 42 (1939), 979–1000.

Klüver, H. and P. C. Bucy, 'Psychic blindness and other symptoms following bilateral temporal lobectomy', *Am. J. Physiol.*, 119 (1937), 254–84.

Knott, J. R., 'Educational efforts in EEG technology – a view through the retrospectroscope', *Am. J. Electroneurodiagnostic Technol.*, 49 (2009), 154–61.

Krauss, G. L., S. Gondek, A. Krumholz, S. Paul, and F. Shen, '"The scarlet E": The presentation of epilepsy in the English language print media'. *Neurology* 54 (2000), 1894–8.

Krnjević, K. and S. Schwartz, 'The action of g-aminobutyric acid on cortical neurones', *Exp. Brain Res.*, 3 (1967), 320–36.

Kubista, H., S. Boehm and M. Hotka, 'The paroxysmal depolarization shift: Reconsidering its role in epilepsy, epileptogenesis and beyond', *Int. J. Mol. Sci.*, 20 (2019), 577.

Kumbier, E. and K. Haack, 'Pioneers in neurology: Alfred Hauptmann (1881–1948)', *J. Neurol.*, 251 (2004), 1288–9.

Kuramochi, I., N. Horikawa, S. Shimotsu et al., 'The self-stigma of patients with epilepsy in Japan: A qualitative approach', *Epilepsy Behav.*, 109 (2020), 106994.

Kurland, L. T., 'The incidence and prevalence of convulsive disorders in a small urban community', *Epilepsia*, 1 (1959), 143–61.

Kutt, H. and F. McDowell, 'Management of epilepsy with diphenylhydantoin sodium: Dosage regulation for problem patients', *JAMA*, 203 (1968), 969–72.

Kutt, H., W. Winters, R. Kokenge et al., 'Diphenylhydantoin metabolism: Blood levels and toxicity', *Arch. Neurol.*, 11 (1964), 642–8.

Kutzinski, A., 'Luminalbehandlung bei Epilepsie', *Monatsschr. Psychiatr. Neurol.*, 36 (1914), 174–180.

Lamb, R. J., M. J. Leach, A. A. Miller et al., 'Anticonvulsant profile in mice of lamotrigine, a novel anticonvulsant', *Br. J. Pharmacol.*, 85 (1985), 235.

Lau, K. K., P. W. Ng, C. W. Chan et al., 'Announcement of a new Chinese name for epilepsy', *Epilepsia*, 52 (2011), 420–1.

'The League and *Epilepsia*', *Epilepsia*, 3 (1945), 7–8.

Leão, A. P. P., 'Spreading depression of activity in the cerebral cortex', *J. Neurophysiol.*, 7 (1944), 359–90.

Ledeboer, B. C., 'Care for epileptics in Holland', *Epilepsia*, 1 (1940), 268–70.

Lees, A. J., 'The strange case of Dr. William Gowers and Mr. Sherlock Holmes', *Brain*, 138 (2015), 2103–8.

Leestma, J. E., M. B. Kalelkar, S. S. Teas et al., 'Sudden unexpected death associated with seizures: Analysis of 66 cases', *Epilepsia*, 25 (Feb. 1984), 84–8.

Leestma, J. E., T. Walczak, J. R. Hughes et al., 'A prospective study on sudden unexpected death in epilepsy', *Ann. Neurol.*, 26 (1989), 195–203.

Lenz, F., 'Eugenics in Germany', *J. Heredity*, 15 (1924), 223–31.

Lennox, W. G., 'Epilepsy', *Hygeia* (October 1931), 904–6.

Lennox, W. G., 'The problem of epilepsy', *Epilepsia*, second series, vol 1, iss. 1 (1937), 22–30

Lennox, W. G., 'Contributions to epilepsy in 1939', *Epilepsia*, 2 (1941), 12–13.

Lennox, W. G., 'Contributions to epilepsy in 1940', *Epilepsia*, 2 (1942), 96–7.

Lennox, W. G., 'The future of the International League Against Epilepsy', *Epilepsia*, 1 (1939), 174–6.

Lennox, W. G., 'The International League', *Epilepsia*, 3 (1947), 175.

Lennox, W. G., 'Marriage and children for epileptics', *Hum. Fertil.*, 10 (1945), 97–106.

Lennox, W. G., 'Message from the president', *Epilepsia*, 1 (1952), 7–8.

Lennox, W. G., 'The moral issue', *N. Engl. J. Med.*, 241 (1941), 321.

Lennox, W. G., 'Phenomena and correlates of the psychomoter triad', *Neurology*, 1 (1951), 35–71.

Lennox, W. G., 'Should they live? Certain economic aspects of medicine', *Am. Scholar*, 7 (1938), 454–366.

Lennox, W. G., 'Study of Epilepsy in America in 1938', *Epilepsia*, 1 (1940), 279–91.

Lennox, W. G. and S. Cobb, 'Studies in epilepsy. VIII. The clinical effect of fasting', *Arch. Neurol. Psychiatry*, 20 (1928), 771–9.

Lennox, W. G., E. L. Gibbs and F. A. Gibbs, 'The brain-wave pattern, an hereditary trait; evidence from 74 "normal" pairs of twins', *J. Hered.*, 36 (1945), 233–43.

Lennox, W. G., E. L. Gibbs and F. A. Gibbs, 'Inheritance of cerebral dysrhythmia and epilepsy', *Arch. Neurol. Psychiatry*, 44 (1940), 1155–83.

Lennox, W. G., F. A. Gibbs and E. I. Gibbs, 'The relationship in man of cerebral activity to blood flow and to blood constituents', *J. Neurol. Psychiatry*, 1 (1938), 211–25.

Lennox, W. G., M. McBride and G. Potter, 'The higher education of epileptics', *Epilepsia*, 3 (1947), 182–98.

Lerche, H., K. Jurkat-Rott and F. Lehmann-Horn, 'Ion channels and epilepsy', *Am. J. Med. Genet. (Semin. Med. Genet.)*, 106 (2001), 146–59.

Levin, S., 'Epileptic clouded states', *J. Nerv. Ment. Dis.*, 116 (1952), 215–25.

Lewis, J., 'Demonic possession or just epilepsy? by Dr Jack', *Sort Your Brain Out* (blog), 8 December 2011 (www.drjack.co.uk/epileptic-seizures-mistaken-for-demonic-possession-by-our-ancestors-by-dr-jack-lewis/, accessed 15 December 2020).

Lichterman, B. L., 'The Moscow Colloquium on Electroencephalography of Higher Nervous Activity and its impact on international brain research', *J. Hist. Neurosci.*, 10 (2010), 313–32.

Liddle, D. W. 'Discussion on the surgery of temporal lobe epilepsy', *Proc. Roy. Soc. Med.*, 46 (1953), 976.

Lim, K. S., S. C. Li, J. Casanova-Gutierrez, C. T. Tan, 'Name of epilepsy, does it matter?' *Neurology Asia* 17(2) (2012), 87–91.

Linden, S. C., V. Hess and E. Jones, 'The neurological manifestations of trauma: Lessons from World War I', *Eur. Arch. Psychiatry Clin. Neurosci.*, 262 (2012), 253–64.

Linden, S. C. and E. Jones, 'German battle casualties: The treatment of functional somatic disorders during World War I', *J. Hist. Med. Allied Sci.*, 63 (2013), 627–58.

Linden, S. C. and E. Jones, '"Shell shock" revisited: An examination of the case records of the National Hospital in London', *Med. Hist.*, 58 (2014), 519–45.

Lipicky, R. J., D. L. Gilbert and I. M. Stillman, 'Diphenylhydantoin inhibition of sodium conductance in squid giant axon', *Proc. Natl. Acad. Sci. USA*, 69 (1972), 1758–60.

Lishman, A., 'What is neuropsychiatry?', *J. Neurol. Neurosurg. Psychiatry*, 55 (1992), 983–5.

Liu, J., Z. Liu, Z. Zhang et al., 'Internet usage for health information by patients with epilepsy in China', *Seizure*, 22 (2013), 787–90.

Löwenstein, O., 'Über klinisch-kinematographische Epilepsiebeobachtung und die Prinzipien einer experimentellen "Anfalls"-Analyse', *Schweiz. Arch. Neurol. Psychiatrie*, 32 (1933), 44–73.

Lund, M., R. S. Jörgensen and V. Kühl, 'Serum diphenylhydantoin (phenytoin) in ambulant patients with epilepsy', *Epilepsia*, 5 (1964), 51–8.

MacLean, P. D., 'Psychosomatic disease and the visceral brain: Recent developments bearing on the Papez theory of emotion', *Psychosom. Med.* 11 (1949), 338–53.

Malerba, F. and L. Orsenigo, 'The evolution of the pharmaceutical industry', *Bus. Hist.*, 57 (2015), 664–87.

'The march of specialism', *Lancet*, 1 (1863), 183.

Marie, A., 'Ligue international contre l'épilepsie', *Epilepsia*, 1 (3), (1909), 2–3 (published in French, The English translation is by Giselle Weiss).

Marshall, L. H., W. A. Rosenblith, P. Gloor et al., 'Early history of IBRO: The birth of organized neuroscience', *Neuroscience*, 72 (1996), 283–306.

Martinson, B., M. Anderson and R. De Vries, 'Scientists behaving badly', *Nature*, 435 (2005), 737–8.

Masland, R. L., 'Classification of the epilepsies', *Epilepsia*, 1 (1959–60), 512–20.

Masland, R. L., 'Comments on the classification of epilepsy', *Epilepsia*, 10 (Suppl.) (1969), 22–7.

Mathews, M. S., M. E. Linskey and D. K. Binder, 'William P. van Wagenen and the first corpus callosotomies for epilepsy', *J. Neurosurg.*, 108 (2008), 608–13.

Matsumoto H, and C. Ajmone-Marsan, 'Cortical cellular phenomena in experimental epilepsy: Interictal manifestations', *Exp. Nerurol.*, 9 (1964), 286.

Mattson, R. H., J. A. Cramer, J. F. Collins et al., 'Comparison of carbamazepine, phenobarbital, phenytoin, and primidone in partial and secondarily generalized tonic–clonic seizures', *N. Engl. J. Med.*, 313 (1985), 145–51.

Mattson, R. H., J. A. Cramer, A. V. Delgado Escueta et al., 'A design for the prospective evaluation of the efficacy and toxicity of anti-epileptic drugs in adults', *Neurology*, 33 (1983) (3 Suppl. 1), 14–25.

McCarthy, J., 'Big pharma sinks to the bottom of U.S. industry rankings', *Gallop*, 3 September 2019 (https://news.gallup.com/poll/266060/big-pharma-sinks-bottom-industry-rankings.aspx, accessed 23 October 2020).

McCartney, J., 'Further notes on treatment of epilepsy', *BMJ*, 1 (1923), 16–17.

McDougall, A., 'The David Lewis Manchester Epileptic colony', *Epilepsia*, 1 (1909), 132.

McNaughton, F. L., 'The classification of the epilepsies', *Epilepsia*, 3 (1952), 7–16.

McNeil, K., P. Brna and K. Gordon, 'Epilepsy in the Twitter era: a need to re-tweet the way we think about seizures', *Epilepsy Behav.*, 23 (2012), 127–30.

Meadow, S. R. 'Anticonvulsant drugs and congenital abnormalities'. *Lancet*, 2 (1968), 1296

Meinardi, H., 'A tribute to K. S. Mani, 1928–2001', *Epilepsia*, 44 (2003) (Suppl. 1), 2–4.

Meldrum, B. S., 'Cell damage in epilepsy and the role of calcium in cytotoxicity', *Adv. Neurol.*, 44 (1986), 849–55.

Meldrum, B. S. and J. B. Brierley, 'Prolonged epileptic seizures in primates: Ischemic cell change and its relation to ictal physiological events', *Arch. Neurol.*, 28 (1973), 10–17.

Meldrum, B. and R. Horton, 'Blockade of epileptic responses in the photosensitive baboon, *Papio papio*, by two irreversible inhibitors of GABA-transaminase, gamma-acetylenic GABA 4-amino-hex-5-ynoic acid) and gamma-vinyl GABA (4-amino-hex-5-enoic acid)', *Psycho pharmacology*, 59 (1978), 47–50.

Meldrum, B. S. and R. W. Horton, 'Physiology of status epilepticus in primates', *Arch. Neurol.*, 28 (1973), 1–9.

Meldrum, B. S., R. A. Vigouroux and J. B. Brierley, 'Systemic factors and epileptic brain damage: Prolonged seizures in paralyzed, artificially ventilated baboons', *Arch. Neurol.*, 29 (1973), 82–7.

Meng, Y., L. Elkaim, J. Wang et al., 'Social media in epilepsy: a quantitative and qualitative analysis', *Epilepsy Behav.*, 71 (2017), 79–84.

'Mental disorder in relation to eugenics', *BMJ*, 1 (1927), 886.

Merlis, J. K., 'Proposal for an international classification of the epilepsies', *Epilepsia*, 11 (1970), 114–19.

Merritt, H. H. and T. J. Putnam, 'Experimental determination of anticonvulsive activity of chemical compounds', *Epilepsia*, 5 (1945), 51–75.

Merritt, H. H. and T. J. Putnam, 'Further experiences with the use of sodium diphenyl hydantoinate in the treatment of convulsive disorders', *Am. J. Psychiatry*, 96 (1940), 1023–7.

Merritt, H. H., T. J. Putnam and W. G. Bywater, 'Anticonvulsant activity of sulfoxides and sulfones', *Arch. Neurol. Psychiatry*, 54 (1945), 319–22.

Metrakos, K. and J. Metrakos, 'Genetics of convulsive disorders', *Neurology*, 10 (1960), 228–40.

Metrakos, K. and J. Metrakos, 'Genetics of convulsive disorders', *Neurology*, 11 (1961), 474–83.

Meyer, A., M. A. Falconer and F. Beck, 'Pathological findings in temporal lobe epilepsy', *J. Neurol. Neurosurg. Psychiatry*, 17 (1954), 276–85.

Meyers, R. and R. Hayne, 'Electrical potentials of the corpus striatum and cortex in parkinsonism and hemiballismus', *Trans. Am. Neurol. Assoc.*, 73 (1948), 10–14.

Millett, D., 'Hans Berger: From psychic energy to the EEG', *Perspect. Biol. Med.*, 44 (2001), 522–42.

Milner, B., Intellectual Effects of Temporal Lobe Damage (Thesis, McGill University, 1952).

Mizrahi, E. M., T. A. Pedley and S. H. Apple, 'In memoriam Peter Kellaway', *Neurology*, 82 (2004), 361–2.

'The moral treatment, hygiene, and education of idiots, and of other children backward or retarded in their development, agitated with involuntary movements, weak, dumb, but not deaf, stammering, &c. by Edward Séguin', *Br. Foreign Med. Rev.*, 24 (1847), 1–22.

Moran, N., 'A more balanced and inclusive view of the history of temporal lobectomy', *Epilepsia*, 49 (2008), 543–4.

Morel, B. A., 'D'une forme de délire, suite d'une surexitation nerveuse se rattachant à une variété non encore décrite d'épilepsie', *Gaz. Hebd. Méd. Chir.*, 7 (1860), 773–5, 819–21, 836–41.

Morrell, F., 'Secondary epileptogenic lesions', *Epilepsia*, 1 (1960), 538–60.

Morell F. 'Graham Goddard: an appreciation', *Epilepsia* 28 (1987), 717–20.

Morrell, F., W. W. Walter and T. P. Bleck, 'Multiple subpial transection: A new approach to the surgical treatment of focal epilepsy', *J. Neurosurg.*, 70 (1989), 231–9.

Morris, A. A., 'The surgical treatment of psychomotor epilepsy', *Med. Ann. Dist. Columbia*, 19 (1950), 121–31.

Morris, A. A., 'Temporal lobectomy with removal of uncus, hippocampus and amygdala: Results for psychomotor epilepsy three to nine years after operation', *Arch. Neurol. Psychiatry*, 76 (1956), 479–96.

'The motor cortex in man', *BMJ*, 2 (1935), 260.

Moynihan, R. and D. Henry, 'The fight against disease mongering: generating knowledge for action', *PLoS Med*, 3(2006), e191.

Muskens, L. J. J., 'The International League Against Epilepsy in war and post-war', *Epilepsia*, 1 (1937), 14–22.

Myers, C. S., 'A contribution to the study of "Shell-Shock"', *Lancet*, 1 (1914), 316–18.

Myerson, A., 'Certain medical and legal phases in eugenic sterilization', *Yale Law J.*, 52 (1943), 618–33.

Nagel, T., 'What is it like to be a bat?', *Philosoph. Rev.*, 83 (1974), 435–50.

Narabayashi, H., T. Nagao, Y. Saito et al., 'Stereotaxic amygdalotomy for behavior disorders', *Arch. Neurol.*, 9 (1963), 1–16.

Nashef, L., 'Sudden unexpected death in epilepsy: Terminology and definitions', *Epilepsia*, 38 (1997) (Suppl. 11), S6–8.

Naquet, R., 'In memoriam, Henri Gastaut', *Electroencephalography and Clinical Neurophysiology* 98 (1996), 231–5.

Naylor, D. E., H. Liu and C. G. Wasterlain, 'Trafficking of GABA(A) receptors, loss of inhibition, and a mechanism for pharmacoresistance in status epilepticus', *J. Neurosci.*, 25 (2005), 7724–33.

Neher, E., B. Sakmann and J. H. Steinbach, 'The extracellular patch clamp: A method for resolving currents through individual open channels in biological membranes', *Pflugers Arch.*, 375 (1978), 219–28.

'Notice and review of Alexander, L. *Neuropathology and Neurophysiology, Including Electroencephalography in Wartime Germany*. Report No. 359, Office of Pub. Board, Dept. of Commerce, Washington, D. C.', *Epilepsia*, B3 (1948), 309.

'Nouvelles', *Epilepsia*, 5 (1915), 282.

Nuwer, M. R. and C. H. Lücking, 'Wave length and action potentials: History of the IFCN', *Clin. Neurophysiol.*, 51 (Suppl.) (2010), 3–10.

Kreft, G., G. G. Kovacs, T. Voigtländer, et al., '125th anniversary of the Institute of Neurology (Obersteiner Institute) in Vienna.

"Germ cell" of interdisciplinary neuroscience', *Clin. Neuropathol.*, 27 (2008), 439–43.

'Obituary', *New Engl. J. Med.*, 244 (1951), 774.

Obrador, S., 'Personal recollections of the development of human stereotactic neurosurgery', *Confin. Neurol.*, 37 (1975), 378–83.

Offen, M. L., 'Dealing with "defectives", Foster Kennedy and William Lennox on eugenics', *Neurology*, 61 (2003), 668–3.

'Ohio's many imbeciles', *New York Times*, 25 September 1912, p. 24.

Okamoto, S., 'Epileptogenic action of glutamate directly applied into the brains of animals and inhibitory effects of protein and tissue emulsions on its action', *J. Physiol. Soc. Jpn.*, 13 (1951), 555–62.

Olle-Daurella, L. and L. Oller Ferrer-Vidal, 'Considerations on the International Classification of Epileptic Seizures, compiled in Marseilles in 1964', in R. J. Broughton (ed.), 'Henri Gastaut and the Marseilles school's contribution to the neurosciences', *Electroencephalogr. Clin. Neurophysiol. Suppl.*, 35 (1982), 197–209.

Osborne, J., 'A comparative view of the effects of some remedies used in epilepsy', *Dublin Quart. J. Med. Sci.*, 22 (1856), 337–50.

Olsen, R. W. and A. J. Tobin, 'Molecular biology of GABAA receptors', *FASEB J.*, 4 (1990), 1469–80.

O'Neil, C. M., C. M. Baker, C. Glenn et al., 'Dr. Robert G. Heath: A controversial figure in the history of deep brain stimulation', *Neurosurg. Focus*, 43 (2017), E12.

Osler, W., 'An address to the medical clinic: A retrospect and a forecast', *BMJ*, 1 (1914), 10–16.

Osler, W., 'Sir Victor Horsley, a study of his life and work', *Oxford Mag.*, 38 (1920), 175.

Ozer, L. J., 'Images of epilepsy in literature', *Epilepsia* 32 (1991): 798–809.

Pain, S., 'High times: the Victorian doctor who promoted medical marijuana', *New Sci.*, 2 May 2018.

Papez, J. W., 'A proposed mechanism of emotion', *Arch. Neurol. Psychiatry*, 38 (1937), 725–43.

Parker, C. S. and C. Breakell, 'The radio-electrophysiologogram: radio transmission of electrophysiological data from the ambulant and active patient', *Lancet* (1953), 1285–8.

Pecheux, A. and L. Lotte, '"Le Luminal" comme anti-épileptique', *Echo Med: Nord Lille*, 17 (1913), 353–7.

Penfield, W., 'The cerebral cortex in man. I. The cerebral cortex and consciousness', *Arch. Neurol. Psychiatry*, 40 (1938), 417–42.

Penfield, W., 'Epilepsy and surgical therapy', *Arch. Neurol. Psychiatry*, 3 (1936), 449–84.

Penfield, W., 'Epileptic automatism and centrencephalic integrating system', *Res. Publ. Assoc. Nerv. Ment. Dis.*, 30 (1952), 513–28.

Penfield, W., 'Mechanisms of voluntary movement', *Brain* 77 (1954), 1–17.

Penfield, W. and M. Baldwin, 'Temporal lobe seizures and the technic of subtotal temporal lobectomy', *Ann. Surg.*, 136 (1952), 625–34.

Penfield, W. and E. G. Boldrey, 'Somatic motor and sensory representation in the cerebral cortex of man as studied by electrical stimulation', *Brain*, 60 (1937), 389–43.

Penfield, W., T. C. Erickson and L. Tarlov, 'Relation of intracranial tumors and symptomatic epilepsy', *Arch. Neurol. Psychiatry*, 44 (1940), 300–15.

Penfield, W. and H. Flanigin, 'Surgical therapy of temporal lobe seizures', *Arch. Neurol. Psychiatry*, 64 (1950), 491–500.

Perucca, E. and E. H. Reynolds, 'In memoriam: Harry Meinardi (February 20, 1932–December 20, 2013)', *Epilepsia*, 55 (2014), 621.

Perucca, P. and M, Mula, 'Antiepileptic drug effects on mood and behavior: Molecular targets'. *Epilepsy & Behavior*, 26 (2013), 440–9.

Peterman, M. G., 'Idiopathic epilepsy in childhood', *Nerv. Child*, 6 (1947), 49–51.

'Philadelphia Neurological Society, November 24, 1903', *J. Nerv. Ment. Dis.*, 31 (1904), 104–12.

Platt, L., 'Medical science: master or servant?', *BMJ*, 4 (1967), 439–44.

Poiré, R., R. Royer, M. Degraeve et al., 'Traitement des états de mal épileptiques par le "CTZ" base', *Rév. Neurolog.*, 108 (1963), 112–26.

Pols, H. and S. Oak, 'War and military mental health: the US psychiatric response in the 20th century', *Am. J. Public Health*, 97 (2007), 2132–42.

Pond, D. A., 'Psychiatric aspects of epilepsy', *J. Ind. Med. Prof.*, 3 (1957), 1141.

Pond, D. A., 'The psychological disorders of epileptic patients', *Psychiatr. Neurol. Neurochir.*, 74 (1971), 159–62.

Porter, R. J., 'In memoriam: Fritz E. Dreifuss, 1926–1997', *Epilepsia*, 39 (1998), 556–9.

Porter, R. J. and H. J. Kupferberg, 'The anticonvulsant screening program of the National Institute of Neurological Disorders and Stroke, NIH: History and contributions to clinical care in the twentieth century and beyond', *Neurochem*, 42 (2017), 1889–93.

Preul, M. and W. Feindel, 'The art is long and the life is short: The letters of Wilder Penfield and Harvey Cushing', *J. Neurosurg.*, 95 (2001), 148–61.

Preul, M. and W. Feindel, 'The origins of Penfield's surgical technique', *J. Neurosurg.*, 75 (1991), 812–20.

Prince, D. A., 'The depolarization shift in "epileptic" neurons', *Exp. Neurol.*, 21 (1968), 467–85.

Prince, M., 'American neurology of the past – neurology of the future', *J. Nerv. Ment. Dis.*, 42 (1915), 445.

'Princeton State Village for Epileptics', *Wikipedia* (www.asylumprojects.org/index.php/Princeton_State_Village_for_Epileptics, accessed 30 March 2021).

Putnam, T. J. and H. H. Merritt, 'Experimental determination of the anticonvulsant properties of some phenyl derivatives', *Science*, 85 (1937), 525–6.

Putnam, T. J. and H. H. Merritt, 'Chemistry of anticonvulsant drugs', *Arch. Neurol. Psychiatry*, 45 (1941), 505–16.

Ramón y Cajal, S., 'Estructura de los centros nerviosos de las aves', *Rev. Trim. Histol. Norm. Patol.*, 1 (1888), 1–10.

Rasmussen, T., 'Surgical treatment of complex partial seizures: results, lessons, and problems', *Epilepsia*, 24 (Suppl. 1) (1983), 65–76.

Reed, C. A. L., 'The bacillus epilepticus: Third report', *JAMA*, 66 (1916), 1607–11.

'Report of the Committee on Methods of Clinical Examination in Electroencephallography: 1957', *Electroencephalogr. Clin. Neurophysiol.*, 10 (1958), 370–5.

Reynolds, E. H., 'Chronic antiepileptic toxicity', *Epilepsia*, 16 (1975), 319–62.

Reynolds, E. H. (ed.), 'Epilepsy in the world: Launch of the second phase of the ILAE/IBE/WHO Global Campaign Against Epilepsy', *Epilepsia*, 43 (2002) (Suppl. 6), 9–11.

Reynolds, E. H., 'The ILAE/IBE/WHO Global Campaign "Out of the Shadows": Bringing epilepsy "out of the shadows"', *Epilepsy Behav.*, 1 (2000), S3–8.

Reynolds, E. H., 'ILAE/IBE/WHO Global Campaign "Out of the Shadows": Global and regional developments', *Epilepsia*, 42 (2001), 1094–100.

Reynolds, E. H., S. D. Shorvon, A. W. Galbraith et al., 'Phenytoin monotherapy for epilepsy: A long-term prospective study, assisted by serum level monitoring in previously untreated patients', *Epilepsia*, 22 (1981), 475–88.

Richens, A., 'Drug level monitoring – quantity and quality', *Br. J. Clin. Pharmacol.*, 5 (1978), 285–8.

Richens, A. and S. Ahmad, 'Controlled trial of sodium valproate in severe epilepsy', *BMJ*, 4 (1975), 255–6.

Riechert, T., 'Development of human stereotactic surgery', *Confin. Neurol.*, 37 (1975), 399–409.

Rinaldi, C. and M. J. A. Wood, 'Antisense oligonucleotides: the next frontier for treatment of neurological disorders', *Nat. Rev. Neurol.*, 14 (2018), 9–21.

Risien Russell, J. S. and J. Taylor, 'The treatment of epilepsy by biborate of soda', *Lancet*, 135 (1890), 1061–3.

Robertson, E. G. R., 'Epilepsy as a symptom of organic lesions of the brain', *Med. J. Australia*, 2 (1937), 831–40.

Roeber, H., 'Physiological action of picrotoxin', *Glasgow Med. J.*, 1 (1869), 361–8.

Ross, E. M., C. Peckham and N. R. Butler, 'Epilepsy in childhood: Findings from National Child Development Study', *BMJ*, 1 (1980), 207–11.

Ryan, R., 'The stigma of epilepsy as a self-concept', *Epilepsia*, 21 (1980), 433–44.

Rzany, B., O. Correia, J. P. Kelly et al., 'Risk of Stevens-Johnson syndrome and toxic epidermal necrolysis during first weeks of antiepileptic therapy: A case-control study. Study Group of the International Case Control Study on Severe Cutaneous Adverse Reactions', *Lancet*, 354 (1999), 1033–4.

Salanova, V., T. Witt and R. Worth et al. 'Long-term efficacy and safety of thalamic stimulation for drug-resistant partial epilepsy', *Neurology* (2015), 1017–25.

Salomone, G. and R. Arnone, 'The care of epileptics: From the madhouse to the League against Epilepsy', *Ital. J. Neurol. Sci.*, 14 (1993), 181–3.

Samt, P., 'Epileptische Irreseinsformen', *Arch. Psychiatr. Nervenkr.*, 5 (1875), 393–444; 6 (1876), 110–216.

Sander, J. W., J. Barclay and S. D. Shorvon, 'The neurological founding fathers of the National Society for Epilepsy and of the Chalfont Centre for Epilepsy', *J. Neurol. Neurosurg. Psychiatry*, 56 (1993), 599–604.

Sargent, P., 'Some observations on epilepsy', *Brain*, 44 (1921), 312–28.

Sargent, P., 'Some observations on epilepsy. President's address, the Section of Neurology', *Proc. Roy. Soc. Med.*, 15 (1922), 1–12.

Saunie, R. and C. Vaille, 'Pharmaceutical preparations in the treatment of epilepsy', *Epilepsia*, 4 (1955), 116–23.

Scambler, G. and A. Hopkins, 'Being epileptic: Coming to terms with stigma', *Soc. Health Illness*, 8 (1986), 26–43.

Scambler, G. and A. Hopkins, 'Generating a model of epileptic stigma: The role of qualitative analysis', *Soc. Sci. Med*, 30 (1990), 1187–94.

Scambler, G. and A. Hopkins, 'Social class, epileptic activity and disadvantage at work', *J. Epidemiol. Comm. Health*, 34 (1980), 129–33.

Scheffer, I. E., K. P. Bhatia, I. Lopes-Cendes et al., 'Autosomal dominant nocturnal frontal lobe epilepsy: A distinct clinical disorder', *Brain*, 118 (1995), 61–73.

Schiff, T. H., 'Tryggve Andersen's novel Mot "Kvaeld" and its motto', *Scand. Studies*, 48 (1976), 146–55.

Schijns O. E., G. Hoogland, P. L. Kubben and P. J. Koehler, 'The start and development of epilepsy surgery in Europe: A historical review', *Neurosurg Rev*, 38 (2015), 447–61.

Schirmann, F., 'The wondrous eyes of a new technology – a history of the early electroencephalography (EEG) of psychopathy, delinquency, and immorality', *Front. Hum. Neurosci.*, 8 (2014), 232.

Schofield, P. R., M. G. Darlison, N. Fujita et al., 'Sequence and expression of the $GABA_A$ receptor shows a ligand-gated receptor super-family', *Nature*, 328 (1987), 221–7.

Schou, H. I., 'The care of epileptics in Scandinavia', *Epilepsia*, 2 (1937), 53–5.

Schou, H. I., 'Subjects for discussion at the meeting of the League in Copenhagen and Dianalund', *Epilepsia*, 1 (1939), 176–9.

Schou, M., 'Reorganisation of the International League Against Epilepsy', *Epilepsia*, 1 (1937), 12.

Schou, M., 'Report of the Scandinavian Branch of the League', *Epilepsia*, 1 (1937), 51–3.

Schou, H. J., 'Institutional care of epileptics in different countries of the world and how to improve it', *Epilepsia* 1(4) (1940), 252–60.

Schurr, P. H. and W. R. Merrington, 'The Horsley-Clarke stereotaxic apparatus', *Br. J. Surgery*, 65 (1978), 33–6.

Schwab, R. S., M. W. Schwab, D. Withee et al., 'Synchronized moving pictures of patient and EEG', *Electroencephalogr. Clin. Neurophysiol.*, 6 (1954), 684–6.

Schwartz, J. G., 'Heredity as a factor in epilepsy', *Ohio State Inst. J.*, 2 (1920), 53–4.

Sen, A., S. Mahone and T. Kadzviti et al. 'A neurological letter from Zimbabwe', *Practical Neurology*, 18, 3 (2018), 255.

Serafetinides, E. A., 'Aggressiveness in temporal lobe epileptics and its relation to cerebral dysfunction and environmental factors', *Epilepsia*, 6 (1965), 33–42.

Serafetinides, E. A., and M. A. Falconer, 'The effects of temporal lobectomy in epileptic patients with psychosis', *J. Ment. Dis.*, 108 (1962), 584–93.

Shah, P. and S. Seshia, 'Dr. Eddie Phiiroz Bharucha (December 28, 1916–December 14, 2017)', *Ann. Ind. Acad. Neurol.*, 21 (2018), 91–2.

Shanahan, W. T., 'Therapeutics: Epilepsy', *JAMA*, 52 (1909), 1667.

Shannon, J. A., 'The advancement of medical research: A twenty-year view of the role of the National Institutes of Health', *J. Med. Edu.*, 42 (1967), 97–108.

Shepherd, M., 'Neurolepsis and the psychopharmacological revolution: Myth and reality', *Hist. Psychiatry*, 5 (1994), 89–96.

'Shorter Notices', *Brain*, 83 (1960), 191–4.

Shorvon, S. D., 'Drug treatment of epilepsy in the century of the ILAE: The second 50 years, 1959–2009', *Epilepsia*, 50 (Suppl. 3) (2009), 93–130.

Shorvon, S. D., 'An episode in the history of temporal lobe epilepsy: The quadrennial meeting of the ILAE in 1953', *Epilepsia*, 47 (2006), 1288–91.

Shorvon, S. D., 'The first 100 years of the ILAE (1909–2009): its landmarks, achievements, and challenges', *Epilepsia Open*, 4 (2019), 237–46.

Shorvon, S. D., 'A history of neuroimaging in epilepsy 1909–2009', *Epilepsia*, 50 (2009) (Suppl. 1), 39–49.

Shorvon, S. D., 'The outcome of therapies in refractory and super-refractory convulsive status epilepticus and recommendations for therapy', *Brain*, 135 (2012) (Pt 8), 2314–28.

Shorvon, S. D., 'Specialized services for the non-institutionalized patient with epilepsy: Developments in the US and the UK', *Health Trends*, 15 (1983), 40–5.

Shorvon, S. D., 'We live in the age of the clinical guideline', *Epilepsia*, 47 (2006), 1091–3.

Shorvon, S. D. and P. J. Farmer, 'Epilepsy in developing countries: A review of epidemiological, sociocultural, and treatment aspects', *Epilepsia*, 29 (1988) (Suppl. 1), S36–S54.

Shorvon, S. and M. Ferlisi, 'The treatment of super-refractory status epilepticus: A critical review of available therapies and a clinical treatment protocol', *Brain*, 134 (2011) (Pt 10), 2802–18.

Shorvon, S. D., and D. M. Goodridge, 'Longitudinal cohort studies of the prognosis of epilepsy: Contribution of the National General Practice Study of Epilepsy and other studies', *Brain*, 136 (2013), 3497–510.

Shorvon, S. D. and E. H. Reynolds, 'Reduction of polypharmacy for epilepsy', *Br. Med. J.*, 1 (1979), 1023–5.

Shorvon, S. D. and E. H. Reynolds, 'Unnecessary polypharmacy in the treatment of epilepsy', *Br. Med. J.*, 1 (1977), 1635–7.

Shorvon, S., E. Trinka and M. Walker, 'The seventh London-Innsbruck Colloquium on Status Epilepticus and Acute Seizures', *Epilepsy Behav.*, 101 (2019) (Pt B), 106532.

Shorvon S. D., G. Weiss and H. P. Goodkin, 'Notes on the origins of *Epilepsia* and the International League Against Epilepsy', *Epilepsia*, 50 (2009), 368–76.

Sicard, J. and J. Forestier, 'Méthode radiographique d'exploration de la cavité épidurale par la lipoidol', *Rev. neurol.*, 28 (1921), 1264–6.

Sieveking, E. H., 'Medical societies, Royal Medical & Chirurgical Society, Tuesday, May 11th 1857: Sir C. Locock, President, in the Chair. Analysis of fifty-two cases of epilepsy observed by the author', *Lancet*, 70 (1857), 527–9.

Silverman, D., 'Clinical and electroencephalographic studies on criminal psychopaths', *Arch. Neurol. Psychiatry*, 50 (1945), 18–33.

Simon, D. and J. K. Penry, 'Sodium di-N-propylacetate (DPA) in the treatment of epilepsy: A review', *Epilepsia*, 16 (1975), 549–73.

Siontis, C. K. and J. P. A. Ioannidis, 'Replication, duplication, and waste in a quarter million systematic reviews and meta-analyses', *Circ. Cardiovasc. Qual. Outcomes*, 11 (2018), e005212.

Siró, B. Jr., 'Eugenics in neurology and psychiatry in Hungary between the two World Wars' [article in Hungarian], *Orvosi Hetilap*, 144 (2003), 1737–42.

'The Sixteenth International Congress of Medicine', *BMJ*, 2 (1909), 706–9, 797–801, 887–90.

'The Sixteenth International Medical Congress', *Lancet*, 174 (1909), 482–3, 691–766, 907–76.

Slater, E. and A. W. Beard, 'The schizophrenia-like psychosis of epilepsy', *Br. J. Psychiatry*, 109 (1963), 95–150.

Slinn, J., 'Patents and the UK pharmaceutical industry between 1945 and 1970', *Hist. Technol.*, 24 (2008), 191–206.

Sommer, W., 'Erkrankung des Ammons horns als ätiologisches Moment der Epilepsie', *Arch. Psychiatr. Nervenkr.*, 10 (1880), 631–75.

Sorel, L. and A. M. Dusaucy-Bauloye, 'A propos de 21 cas d'hypsarrhythmia of Gibbs. Son traitement spectaculaire par l'ACTH', *Acta Neurol. Psychiat. Belg.*, 48 (1958), 130–41.

Southard, E., 'On the mechanism of gliosis in acquired epilepsy', *Am. J. Insanity*, 64 (1907–8), 607–41.

Sperling, M. R., G. Wilson, J. Engel Jr et al., 'Magnetic resonance imaging in intractable partial epilepsy: Correlative studies', *Ann. Neurol.* 20 (1986), 57–62.

Spiegel, E. and H. Wycis, 'Thalamic recordings in man with special reference to seizure discharges', *Electroencephalogr. Clin. Neurophysiol.*, 2 (1950), 23–9.

Spiegel, E., H. Wycis, M. Marks and A. Lee, 'Stereotactic apparatus for operations on the human brain', *Science*, 106 (1947), 349–50.

Spiegel, E. A., H. T. Wycis and V. Reyes, 'Diencephalic mechanisms in petit mal epilepsy', *Electroencephalogr. Clin. Neurophysiol.*, 3 (1951), 473–5.

Spillane, J. 'A memorable decade in the history of neurology 1874–1884', *BMJ* 4 (1974), 701–6, 757–9.

Spratling, W. 'An ideal colony for epileptics and the necessity for the broader treatment of epilepsy'. Transactions of the National Association for the Study of Epilepsy and the Care and Treatment of Epileptics at the first annual meeting held in Washington, D.C., 14th and 15th May, 1901. (Ed: W. P. Letchworth). Buffalo: Brinkworth, 1901, pp. 25–40.

Squires, P. C., 'Charles Dickens as criminologist', *J. Crim. Law Criminol.*, 29 (1938), 170–201.

Starr, M. A., 'Is epilepsy a functional disease?', *J. Nerv. Ment. Dis.*, 31 (1904), 145–56.

'Statement of C. E. Gallagher', 118 Cong. Rec., vol. 118, part 5, 24 February 1972, pp. 5567–77.

'State take over doctors, hospitials and dentists', Evening Standard, 21 March 1948, p. 1.

Stauder, K. H., 'Epilepsie und schläfenlappen', Arch. Psychiatr., 104 (1935), 181–212.

Stein, C., 'Hereditary factors in epilepsy', Am. J. Psychiatry, 12 (1933), 989–1027.

Stein, C., 'Studies in endocrine therapy in epilepsy', Am. J. Psychiatry, 90 (1934), 739–60.

Steinhoff, B., M. Chatrou and H. Hjalfrim (eds.), 'The European Association of Epilepsy Centres (EAEC) – a unique cooperation of traditional institutions devoted to epilepsy care of today and tomorrow', Epilepsy Behav., 76 (2017) (Suppl.), S1–54.

Steinman, M. A., L. A. Bero, M. M. Chren et al., 'Promotion of gabapentin: An analysis of internal industry documents', Ann. Intern. Med., 145 (2006), 284–93.

Stempel, J., 'Pfizer pay $325 million in Neurontin settlement', Reuters, 2 June 2014.

Sterling, F., dir., Dirty Work in a Laundry (1915) (www.historicfilms.com/tapes/6157_457.73_2249.73, accessed February 2020).

Sternbach, L. H., 'The benzodiazepine story', J. Med. Chem., 22 (1979), 1–7.

Stevens, J. R. and B. P. Hermann, 'Temporal lobe epilepsy, psychopathology, and violence: The state of the evidence', Neurology, 31 (1981), 1127–32.

Stone, J. L. and J. R. Hughes, 'Early history of electroencephalography and establishment of the American Clinical Neurophysiology Society', J. Clin. Neurophysiol., 30 (2013), 28–44.

'Streptomycin in pulmonary tuberculosis', Lancet, 2 (1948), 733.

Stubbe Teglbjaerg, H. P., 'Lines to be followed by modern hospitals for epileptics', Epilepsia, 2 (1939), 180–91.

Swann, J. P., 'Evolution of the American pharmaceutical industry', Pharm. Hist., 37 (1995), 79–82.

Swartz, B. E. and E. S. Goldensohn, 'Timeline of the history of EEG and associated fields', Electroencephalogr. Clin. Neurophysiol., 106 (1988), 173–6.

Symonds, C.P, 'Classification of the epilepsies', BMJ, 1 (1955), 1235–8.

Symonds, C. P., 'Traumatic epilepsy', Lancet, 2 (1935), 1217–20.

'Symposium on laboratory evaluation of antiepileptic drugs', Epilepsia, 10 (1969), 101–336.

Talairach, J., 'Mes travaux' (1965) (https://histoire.inserm.fr/les-femmes-et-les-hommes/jean-talairach/(page)/3, accessed 3 May 2021).

Takeuchi Y., P. M. Harangozó, T. Földi, G. Kozák, Q. Li and A. Berényi, 'Closed-loop stimulation of the medial septum terminates epileptic seizures', Brain, 144 (2021), 885–908,

Taylor, J., 'Epilepsy considered as a symptom not as a disease', BMJ, 1 (1921), 4–6.

Taylor, D. and S. Marsh, 'Hughlings Jackson's Dr Z: The paradigm of temporal lobe epilepsy revealed', J. Neurol. Neurosurg. Psychiatry, 43 (1980), 758–67.

Teasdale, G. and B. Jennett, 'Assessment of coma and impaired consciousness: a practical scale', Lancet, 2 (1974), 81–4.

Temin, P., 'Technology, regulation, and market structure in the modern pharmaceutical industry', Bell J. Econ., 10 (1979), 429–46.

'The charge against Professor Ferrier under the vivisection act: Dismissal of the summons.' BMJ, 2 (1881), 836–42.

'The treatment of the epileptic status', JAMA, 44 (1905), 1686–7.

'Therapeutics. Epilepsy', JAMA, 52 (1909), 1667.

Thom, D. A., 'Epilepsy and its rational extra-institutional treatment', Am. J. Psychiatry, 87 (1931), 623–35.

Thurman, D. J., G. Logroscino, E. Beghi, et al., and Epidemiology Commission of the International League Against Epilepsy. 'The burden of premature mortality of epilepsy in high-income countries: A systematic review from the Mortality Task Force of the International League Against Epilepsy', Epilepsia, 58 (2017), 17–26.

Toman, J. E., 'The neuropharmacology of antiepileptics', Electroencephalogr. Clin. Neurophysiol., 1 (1949), 33–44.

Tredgold, A. F. 'Mental disease in relation to eugenics: the Galton Lecture', Eugen. Rev., (1927), 1–11.

Trimble, M. R., 'Anticonvulsant drugs and cognitive function: A review of the literature', *Epilepsia*, 28 (1987) (Suppl. 3), S37–45.

Turner, E., 'A new approach to unilateral and bilateral lobotomies for psychomoter epilepsy', *J. Neurol. Neurosurg. Psychiatry*, 26 (1963), 285–99.

Turner, J., R. Hayword, K. Angel, et al., 'The history of mental health services in modern England: Practitioner memories and the direction of future research', *Med. Hist.*, 59 (2015), 599–624.

Turner, W. A., 'The Morison Lectures on Epilepsy. Lecture I. – The problem of epilepsy', *BMJ*, 1 (1910), 737–7.

Turner, W. A., 'Reviews. (1) *Care and Treatment of Epileptics*. By William Pryor Letchworth, LL.D. New York, 1900 ... (2) *Transactions of the National Association for the Study of Epilepsy and the Care and Treatment of Epileptics*, vol. i. Buffalo, 1901', *Brain*, 25 (1902), 387–9.

Turner, W. A., 'Statistics from England relative to epilepsy', *Epilepsia*, 4 (1913), 369–74.

Twitchell, E. W., 'Recent work in epilepsy', *Cal. State J. Med.*, 14 (1916), 483–6.

Umbach, W., 'Long-term results of fornicotomy for temporal epilepsy', *Confin. Neurol.*, 27 (1966), 121–3.

van Dijk, J. C., B. C. Ledeboer and H. W. Duyvendak, Het verzet van de inrichtingen Meer en Bosch en Bethesda – Sarepta te Heemstede en Haarlem gedurende de bezettingsjaren. Brochure, uitgegeven door de Christelijke Vereeniging voor de Verpleging van Lijders aan Vallende Ziekte, Heemstede, 1946.

Van Gieson, I., 'A contribution to the pathology of traumatic epilepsy', *Medical Record*, 43 (1893), 513–21.

Vannemreddy, P. S. S. V. and J. L. Stone, 'Sanger Brown and Edward Schäfer before Heinrich Klüver and Paul Bucy: Their observations on bilateral temporal lobe ablations', *Neursurg. Focus*, 43 (2017), E2.

Van Wagenen W. P. and R. Y. Herren, 'Surgical division of the commissural pathways in the corpus callosum: Relation to spread of an epileptic attack', *Arch. Neurol. Psychiatry*, 44 (1940), 740–59.

Vedula, S. S., P. S. Goldman, I. J. Rona et al., 'Implementation of a publication strategy in the context of reporting biases: A case study based on new documents from Neurontin litigation', *Trials*, 13 (2012), 136.

Veeramah, K. R., J. E. O'Brien, M. H. Meisler et al., 'De novo pathogenic SCN8A mutation identified by whole-genome sequencing of a family quartet affected by infantile epileptic encephalopathy and SUDEP', *Am. J. Hum. Genet.*, 9 (2012), 502–10.

Verbeek, E., 'John Cowper Powys: Tempting the gods', *Powis Rev.*, 26 (1991), 40–8.

Vogt C. and O. Vogt, 'Allgemeine Ergebnisse unserer Hirnforschung'. *J. Psychol. Neurol* 25 (1919), 273–462.

Vogt, O., 'Der Begriff der Pathoklise', *J. Psychol. Neurol.*, 31 (1925), 245–55.

Vogt C. and O. Vogt, 'Allgemeine Ergebnisse unserer Hirnforschung'. *J. Psychol. Neurol.*, 25 (Suppl. 1) (1919), 273–462.

Walker, A. E., 'The president's report', *Epilepsia*, 4 (1955), 109.

Wallin, J. E., 'Eight months of psycho-clinical research at the New Jersey State Village for Epileptics, with some results from the Binet-Simon testing', *Epilepsia*, 3 (1912), 366–80.

Walshe, F. M. R., 'The brain-stem conceived as the "highest level" of function in the nervous system; with particular reference to the "automatic apparatus" of carpenter (1850) and to the "centrencephalic integrating system" of Penfield', *Brain*, 80 (1957), 510–39.

Walshe, F. M. R., 'Editorial note', *Epilepsia*, 1 (1959), 1.

Walshe, F. M. R., 'Mind and brain', *Blackfriars*, 41 (1960), 246–56.

Walshe, F. M. R., 'The present and future of neurology', *A. M. A. Arch. Neurol.*, 2 (1960), 93–8.

Walter, W. G., 'Electro-encephalography in the study of epilepsy', *J. Ment. Sci.*, 85 (1939), 932–94.

Walusinski, O., 'Louis Delasiauve (1804–1893), an alienist at the dawn of epileptology and pediatric psychiatry', *Rev. Neurolog.*, 74 (2018), 106–14.

Wang, J., Z. J. Lin, L. Liu et al., 'Epilepsy-associated genes', *Seizure*, 44 (2017), 11–20.

Wang, W. Z., J. Z. Wu, D. S. Wang et al., 'The prevalence and treatment gap in epilepsy in China: An ILAE/IBE/WHO study', *Neurology*, 60 (2003), 1544–5.

Watkins, J. C. and D. A. Jane, 'The glutamate story', *Br. J. Pharmacol.*, 147 (2006), S100–8.

Waxman, S. G. and N. Geschwind, 'The interictal behavior syndrome of temporal lobe epilepsy', *Arch. Gen. Psychiatry*, 32 (1975), 1580–6.

Weatherall, D., 'The centenary of Garrod's Croonian lectures', *Clin. Med.*, 8 (2008), 309–11.

Weber, M. M., 'Ernst Rüdin, 1874–1952: A German psychiatrist and geneticist', *Am. J. Med. Gen.*, 67 (1996), 323–31.

'The Wellcome Trust', *BMJ*, (1937), 224.

Westphal, A., 'Myoklonusepilepsie und Rechklinghausesche Krankeheit (mit Vorführung kinematographischer Bilder)', *Zentralb. Neurol. Psychiatrie*, (1929), 51–123.

Wiebe, S., W. T. Blume, J. P. Girvin et al., 'Effectiveness and efficiency of surgery for temporal lobe epilepsy study group: A randomized, controlled trial of surgery for temporal-lobe epilepsy', *N. Engl. J. Med.*, 345 (2001), 311–8.

Welzel, J. J., 'Ernst Rüdin: Hitler's racial hygiene mastermind', *J. Hist. Biol.*, 46 (2014), 1–30.

West, W. J., 'On a peculiar form of infantile convulsions', *Lancet*, 1 (1841), 724.

Westphal, K., 'Körperbau und Charakter der Epileptiker', *Nervenarzt*, 4 (1931), 96–9.

Wheless, J. W., 'History of the ketogenic diet', *Epilepsia*, 49 (Suppl. 8) (2008), 3–5.

Wieser, H. G., 'Depth recorded limbic seizures and psychopathology', *Neurosci. Biobehav. Rev.*, 7 (1983), 427–40.

Wieser, H. G., 'Temporal lobe or psychomotor status epilepticus: A case report', *Electroen cephalogr. Clin. Neurophysiol.*, 48 (1980), 558–72.

Wilder, R. M., 'The effect on ketonemia on the course of epilepsy', *Mayo Clin. Bull.*, 2 (1921), 307.

Wilder, R. M. and M. D. Winter, 'The threshold of ketogenesis', *J. Biol. Chem.*, 52 (1922), 393–401.

Wilkinson, M, W. Jacobson and D. A. Wilkinson, 'Brain slices in radioligand binding assays: Quantification of opiate, benzodiazepines and beta-adrenergic ([3 H] CGP-12177) receptors', *Prog. Neuropsychopharmacol. Biol. Psychiatry*, 8 (1984) 621–6.

'William Lennox, physician, 76, dies', *New York Times*, 23 July 1960, p. 19.

William, P., 'Surgery of the last resort', *BBC*, 11 March 1981.

Williams, D., 'The effect of cholin-like substances on the cerebral electrical discharges in epilepsy', *J Neurol. Psychiatry*, 4 (1941), 32–47.

Wilson, G., 'The Brown Animal Sanatory Institution', *J. Hyg.*, 82 (1979), 155–76, 337–52, 501–21; 83 (1979), 171–97.

Wilson, S., P. Bladin and M. Saling, 'The "burden of normality": Concepts of adjustment after surgery for seizures', *J. Neurol. Neurosurg. Psychiatry*, 70 (2001), 649–56.

Wilson, S. A. K., 'Some aspects of the problem of the epilepsies', *BMJ*, 2 (1929), 745–9.

Wilson, S. A. K., 'Treatment in general practice: The treatment of epilepsy', *BMJ*, 2 (1935), 959–61.

Wood, R., 'Queer attacks and fits: epilepsy and ecstatic experiences in the novels of J. C. Powys', *Powis Rev.*, 31&32 (n.d.), 21–9.

Woodward, M., 'The role of low intelligence in delinquency', *Br. J. Delinq.*, 5 (1955), 281–303.

Wong, V. S., M. Stevenson and L. Selwa, 'The presentation of seizures and epilepsy in YouTube videos', *Epilepsy Behav* 27 (2013), 247–50.

Worster-Drought, C. C., 'British Medical Association, proceedings of sections at the annual meeting, Bradford, 1924', *BMJ*, 2 (1924), 1043–54.

Wycis, H. T., A. J. Lee and E. A. Spiegel, 'Simultaneous records of thalamic and cortical (scalp) potentials in schizophrenics and epileptics', *Confin. Neurol.*, 9 (1949), 264–72.

Yakovlev, P. I., 'Motility, behavior and the brain: stereodynamic organization and neural coordinates in behavior', *J. Nerv. Mental Dis.*, 107 (1948), 313–35.

Yang, R., W. Wang, D. Snape et al., 'Stigma of people with epilepsy in China: Views of health professionals, teachers, employers, and community leaders', *Epilepsy Behav.*, 21 (2011), 261–6.

Yealland, L. R. and E. D. Adrian, 'The treatment of some common war neuroses', *Lancet*, 189 (1917), 867–72.

Zieliński, J., 'Epilepsy and mortality rate and cause of death', *Epilepsia*, 15 (1974), 191–201.

Zimmerman, F. T. and B. B. Burgemeister, 'A new drug for petit mal epilepsy', *Neurology*, 8 (1958), 769–75.

Zimmerman, H. M., 'The histopathology of convulsive disorders in children', *J. Pediatrics*, 13 (1938), 859–90.

Zottoli, S. J., 'The origins of the Grass Foundation', *Biol. Bull.*, 201 (2001), 218–26.

Zülch, K. J., 'Otfrid Foerster 1873–1941, an appreciation', *J. Neurol. Sci.*, 6 (1968), 384–5.

MISCELLANY

Adolf Meyer Collection of the Alan Mason Chesney Medical Archives of The Johns Hopkins Medical Institutions, Baltimore.

Erven F. Bohn Collection, University of Leiden Library.

ILAE Archive, Wellcome Trust, London. (see also https://www.ilae.org/about-ilae/history-and-archives)

INDEX OF NAMES

Listed here are persons cited in the text with their dates of birth and death and other details.[1] Those who are still alive at the time of writing are not included.

---

[1] The country of birth and where their major work in epilepsy was conducted, are given (but note that their country of birth may not be their nationality).

INDEX

Printed in the United States
by Baker & Taylor Publisher Services